INTRODUCTION TO

Health
Physics

INTRODUCTION TO

Health
Physics

FOURTH EDITION

Herman Cember, PhD
Professor Emeritus
Northwestern University
Evanston, Illinois

Thomas E. Johnson, PhD
Assistant Professor
Department of Environmental and Radiological Health Sciences
Colorado State University
Fort Collins, Colorado

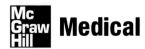

New York   Chicago   San Francisco   Lisbon   London   Madrid   Mexico   City   Milan
New Delhi   San Juan   Seoul   Singapore   Sydney   Toronto

The McGraw·Hill Companies

Introduction to Health Physics, Fourth Edition

1 2 3 4 5 6 7 8 9 0 DOC/DOC 12 11 10 9 8

ISBN 978-0-07-142308-3
MHID 0-07-142308-7

This book was set in New Baskerville by Aptara®, Inc.
The editors were Catherine A. Johnson and Christie Naglieri.
The production supervisor was Philip Galea.
Project management was provided by Satvinder Kaur, Aptara®, Inc.
The cover designer was Libby Pisacreta.
RR Donnelley was printer and binder.

This book is printed on acid-free paper.

Library of Congress Cataloging-in-Publication Data

Cember, Herman.
    Introduction to Health Physics/Herman Cember, Thomas E. Johnson. — 4th ed.
      p. ; cm.
    Includes bibliographical references and index.
    ISBN-13: 978-0-07-142308-3 (hardcover : alk. paper)
    ISBN-10: 0-07-142308-7 (hardcover : alk. paper)
    I. Medical physics.   I. Johnson, Thomas E. (Thomas Edward), 1964-   II. Title.
  3. Radiation Monitoring–methods.   4. Radiation Protection–methods.
    WN 110 C394i 2008]
R895.C454 2008
610.1'53—dc22
                                2007042919

To my wife, Sylvia
and to the memory of
Dr. Elda E. Anderson
and
Dr. Thomas Parran

CONTENTS

PREFACE

The practice of radiation safety is a continually evolving activity. Many of the changes in the practice of ionizing and nonionizing radiation safety, in calculation methodology, and in the methods for demonstrating compliance with the safety standards that have occurred since the publication of the previous edition of *Introduction to Health Physics* are incorporated in the fourth edition.

Since their inception in 1928, the Recommendations of the International Commission on Radiological Protection have formed the scientific basis for ionizing radiation safety standards issued by regulatory authorities throughout the world. Generally, earlier recommendations were successively more restrictive than the previous ones. The 2006 recommendations, however, are essentially the same as the previous recommendations made in 1990. The main difference is that the 2006 recommendations are made on the basis of the increased knowledge acquired since 1990. This is not surprising, since no harmful radiation effects have been observed among the population of radiation workers whose doses had been within the previous standards. The new recommendations continued to stress that all unnecessary exposure be avoided and that all exposures should be kept as low as reasonably achievable, economic and social factors being taken into account. A reasonable question, therefore, that is raised by the ICRP recommendations is "How safe is safe?" This question lies in the field that Dr. Alvin Weinberg, the late director of the Oak Ridge National Laboratory, called *transscience*. Transscientific questions have a scientific basis, but they cannot be answered by science alone. Safety is a subjective concept that can be interpreted only within the context of its application. Policy decisions regarding matters of health and safety should be made in the context of public health. In the practice of public health, we find that numerous diseases and threats to health are always present in every community. The cost of controlling these threats to health is borne by the community. Since the community has limited resources, it must set priorities regarding which of the many real or perceived health threats to control. One of the techniques for quantifying the likelihood of the expression of a potential risk is called *quantitative risk assessment*. In the area of radiation safety, this usually deals with two main risks: (1) failure of a large technological system, such as a nuclear power plant, and (2) the long-term effects of low-level radiation. The results of quantitative risk assessment are often perceived as the determination of a real threat to life or limb, no matter how small the calculated chance of occurrence. However, quantitative risk assessment is a calculation that almost always assumes the most pessimistic, and in many cases entirely unrealistic, values for parameters whose magnitudes include several different uncertainties. In addition to statistical uncertainties, for example, we must choose among several different equally reasonable models to which to apply the statistical data. One of the purposes of this edition is to provide the technical background needed to understand the calculation and use of quantitative risk assessment for radiation hazards in order to help us to allocate our limited resources.

Although it has been a number of years since the ICRP recommended that health physics quantities be expressed in the meter–kilogram–second (MKS) units of the SI system rather than the traditional units based on the centimeter–gram–second (cgs) system, the change to the SI units has not yet been universally implemented. For example, the U.S. Nuclear Regulatory Commission continues to use the traditional system of units in its regulations. For this reason, this edition continues to use both systems, with one or the other equivalent quantity given in parentheses.

I wish to thank the many persons, too numerous to mention by name, for their helpful suggestions. I also owe a debt of gratitude to my former student and now colleague, Thomas Johnson, for his authorship of Chapter 14 and for checking the text of the other chapters, and to his wife, Melissa, for giving up her time with her husband so that he could contribute to this book.

Herman Cember

INTRODUCTION TO

Health Physics

1

INTRODUCTION

Health physics, radiological health, or radiological engineering are synonymous terms for that area of public health and environmental health engineering that deals with the safe use of ionizing and nonionizing radiation in order to prevent harmful effects of the radiation to individuals, to population groups, and to the biosphere. The health physicist is responsible for safety aspects in the design of processes, equipment, and facilities utilizing radiation sources and for the safe disposal of radioactive waste so that radiation exposure to personnel will be minimized and will at all times be within acceptable limits; he or she must keep personnel and the environment under constant surveillance in order to ascertain that these designs are indeed effective. If control measures are found to be ineffective or if they break down, the health physicist must be able to evaluate the degree of hazard and make recommendations regarding remedial action.

Public policy vis-à-vis radiation safety is based on political, economic, moral, and ethical considerations as well as on scientific and engineering principles. This textbook deals only with the scientific and engineering bases for the practice of health physics.

The scientific and engineering aspects of health physics are concerned mainly with (1) the physical measurements of different types of radiation and radioactive materials, (2) the establishment of quantitative relationships between radiation exposure and biological damage, (3) the movement of radioactivity through the environment, and (4) the design of radiologically safe equipment, processes, and environments. Clearly, health physics is a professional field that cuts across the basic physical, life, and earth sciences as well as such applied areas as toxicology, industrial hygiene, medicine, public health, and engineering. The professional health physicist, therefore, in order to perform effectively, must have an appreciation of the complex interrelationships between humans and the physical, chemical, biological, and even social components of the environment. He or she must be competent in the wide spectrum of disciplines that bridge the fields between industrial operations and technology on one hand and health science, including epidemiology, on the other. In addition to these general prerequisites, the health physicist must be technically competent in the subject matter unique to health physics.

The main purpose of this book is to lay the groundwork for attaining technical competency in health physics. Radiation safety standards undergo continuing change as new knowledge is gained and as the public's perception of radiation's benefits and risks evolve. Radiation safety nomenclature too changes in order to accommodate changing standards.

Because of the nature of the subject matter and the topics covered, however, it is hoped that the book will be a useful source of information to workers in environmental health as well as to those who will use radiation as a tool. For the latter group, it is also hoped that this book will impart an appreciation for radiation safety as well as an understanding of the philosophy of environmental health.

2

REVIEW OF PHYSICAL PRINCIPLES

MECHANICS

Units and Dimensions

Health physics is a science and hence is a systematic organization of knowledge about the interaction between radiation and organic and inorganic matter. Quite clearly, the organization must be quantitative as well as qualitative since the control of radiation hazards implies knowledge of the dose–response relationship between radiation exposure and the biological effects of radiation.

Quantitative relationships are based on measurements, which, in reality, are comparisons of the attribute under investigation to a standard. A measurement includes two components: a number and a unit. In measuring the height of a person, for example, the result is given as 70 inches (in.) if the British system of units is used or as 177.8 centimeters (cm) if the metric system is used. The unit *inches* in the first case and *centimeters* in the second tell us what the criterion for comparison is, and the number tells us how many of these units are included in the quantity being measured. Although 70 in. means exactly the same thing as 177.8 cm, it is clear that without an understanding of the units the information contained in the number above would be meaningless. In the United States, the British system of units is used chiefly in engineering, while the metric system is widely used in science.

Three physical quantities are considered basic in the physical sciences: length, mass, and time. In the British system of units, these quantities are measured in feet, slugs (a slug is that quantity of mass that is accelerated at a rate of one foot per second per second by a force of one pound; a mass of 1 slug weighs 32.2 pounds), and seconds, respectively, while the metric system is divided into two subsystems: the mks—in which the three quantities are specified in meters, kilograms, and seconds—and the cgs—in which centimeters, grams, and seconds are used to designate length, mass, and time.

By international agreement, the metric system is being replaced by a third and new system—the Système International, the International System of Units, or simply the SI system. Although many familiar metric units are employed in SI, it should be emphasized that SI is a new system and must not be thought of as a new form of the metric system. All the other units such as force, energy, power, and so on are derived from the three basic units of mass in kilograms (kg), length in meters (m), and time in seconds (s), plus the four additional basic units: electric current in amperes (A), temperature in Kelvin (K) or degrees Celsius (°C), where 1 K = 1°C, amount of a substance in moles (mol), and luminous intensity in candelas (cd). For example, the unit of force, the newton (N), is defined as follows:

> One *newton* is the unbalanced force that will accelerate a mass of one kilogram at a rate of one meter per second per second.

Expressed mathematically:

Force = mass × acceleration,

that is,

$$F = m \times a, \tag{2.1}$$

and the dimensions are

$$F = \text{kg} \times \frac{\text{m/s}}{\text{s}}.$$

Since dimensions may be treated algebraically in the same way as numbers, the dimension for acceleration is written as m/s^2. The dimensions for force in units of newton (N), therefore, are

$$N = \frac{\text{kg} \cdot \text{m}}{\text{s}^2}.$$

In the cgs system, the unit of force is called the *dyne*. The dyne is defined as follows:

> One *dyne* is the unbalanced force that will accelerate a mass of one gram at a rate of one cm per second per second.

For health physics applications, the magnitude of cgs units were closer to the magnitudes being measured than the mks units and, therefore, the cgs system was universally used. However, despite the long history of cgs-based units, the cgs system is being replaced by SI units in order to be consistent with most of the other sciences that have adopted SI units. All the international bodies that deal with radiation safety base their recommendations on SI units. However, the U.S. Nuclear Regulatory Commission continues to use the traditional cgs units in its regulatory activities.

Work and Energy

Energy is defined as the *ability to do work*. Since all work requires the expenditure of energy, the two terms are expressed in the same units and consequently have the same dimensions. Work W is done, or energy expended, when a force f is exerted through some distance r:

$$W = f \times r. \tag{2.2}$$

In the SI system, the *joule* (J) (named after the British scientist who measured the mechanical equivalent of heat energy) is the unit of work and energy and is defined as follows:

One *joule* of work is done when a force of one newton is exerted through a distance of one meter.

Since work is defined as the product of a force and a distance, the dimensions for work and energy are as follows:

$$\text{joule} = \text{newton} \times \text{meter}$$

$$= \frac{\text{kg} \cdot \text{m}}{\text{s}^2} \times \text{m} = \frac{\text{kg} \cdot \text{m}^2}{\text{s}^2}. \tag{2.3}$$

The unit of work or energy in the cgs system is called the *erg* and is defined as follows:

One *erg* of work is done when a force of one dyne is exerted through a distance of one centimeter.

The joule is a much greater amount of energy than an erg.

$$1 \text{ joule} = 10^7 \text{ergs}.$$

Although the erg is very much smaller than a joule, it nevertheless is very much greater than the energies encountered in the submicroscopic world of the atom. When working on the atomic scale, a more practical unit called the *electron volt* (eV) is used. The electron volt is a unit of energy and is defined as follows:

$$1 \text{ eV} = 1.6 \times 10^{-19} \text{J} = 1.6 \times 10^{-13} \text{erg}.$$

When work is done on a body, the energy expended in doing the work is added to the energy of the body. For example, if a mass is lifted from one elevation to another, the energy that was expended during the performance of the work is converted to potential energy. On the other hand, when work is done to accelerate a body, the energy that was expended appears as kinetic energy in the moving body. In the case where work was done in lifting a body, the mass possesses more potential energy at the higher elevation than it did before it was lifted. Work was done, in this case, against the force of gravity and the total increase in potential energy of the mass is equal to its weight, which is the force with which the mass is attracted to the earth, multiplied by the height through which the mass was raised. *Potential energy* is defined as energy that a body possesses by virtue of its position in a force field. *Kinetic energy* is defined as energy possessed by a moving body as result of its motion. For bodies of mass m, moving "slowly" with a velocity v less than about 3×10^7 m/s, the kinetic energy, E_k, is given by

$$E_k = \frac{1}{2} m v^2, \tag{2.3a}$$

and the total energy of the body is equal to the sum of its potential energy and its kinetic energy

$$E_t = E_{pe} + E_k. \tag{2.3b}$$

When the speed of a moving body increases beyond about 3×10^7 m/s, we observe interesting changes in their behavior—changes that were explained by Albert Einstein.

RELATIVISTIC EFFECTS

According to the system of classical mechanics that was developed by Newton and the other great thinkers of the Renaissance period, mass is an immutable property of matter; it can be changed in size, shape, or state but it can neither be created nor be destroyed. Although this law of conservation of mass seems to be true for the world that we can perceive with our senses, it is in fact only a special case for conditions of large masses and slow speeds. In the submicroscopic world of the atom, where masses are measured on the order of 10^{-27} kg, where distances are measured on the order of 10^{-10} m, and where velocities are measured in terms of the velocity of light, classical mechanics is not applicable.

Einstein, in his special theory of relativity, postulated that the velocity of light in a vacuum is constant at 3×10^8 m/s relative to every observer in any reference frame. He also postulated that the speed of light is an upper limit of speed that a material body can asymptotically approach, but never can attain. Furthermore, according to Einstein, the mass of a moving body is not constant, as was previously thought, but rather a function of the velocity with which the body is moving. As the velocity increases, the mass increases, and when the velocity of the body approaches the velocity of light, the mass increases very rapidly. The mass m of a moving object whose velocity is v is related to its rest mass m_0 by the equation

$$m = \frac{m_0}{\sqrt{1 - \dfrac{v^2}{c^2}}},$$
(2.4)

where c is the velocity of light, 3×10^8 m/s.

 EXAMPLE 2.1

Compute the mass of an electron moving at 10% and 90% of the speed of light. The rest mass of an electron is 9.11×10^{-31} kg.

Solution

At $v = 0.1c$,

$$m = \frac{9.11 \times 10^{-31} \text{ kg}}{\sqrt{1 - \dfrac{(0.1\,c)^2}{c^2}}} = 9.16 \times 10^{-31} \text{ kg}$$

and at $v = 0.99\,c$,

$$m = \frac{9.11 \times 10^{-31} \text{ kg}}{\sqrt{1 - \dfrac{(0.99\ c)^2}{c^2}}} = 64.6 \times 10^{-31} \text{ kg}$$

Example 2.1 shows that whereas an electron suffers a mass increase of only 0.5% when it is moving at 10% of the speed of light, its mass increases about sevenfold when the velocity is increased to 99% of the velocity of light.

Kinetic energy of a moving body can be thought of as the income from work put into the body, or energy input, in order to bring the body up to its final velocity. Expressed mathematically, we have

$$W = E_k = f \times r = \frac{1}{2}mv^2. \tag{2.5}$$

However, the expression for kinetic energy in Eqs. (2.3) and (2.5) is a special case since the mass is assumed to remain constant during the time that the body is undergoing acceleration from its initial to its final velocity. If the final velocity is sufficiently high to produce observable relativistic effects (this is usually taken as $v \approx 0.1c = 3 \times 10^7$ m/s, then Eqs. (2.3) and (2.5) are no longer valid.

As the body gains velocity under the influence of an unbalanced force, its mass continuously increases until it attains the value given by Eq. (2.4). This particular value for the mass is thus applicable only to one point during the time that body was undergoing acceleration. The magnitude of the unbalanced force, therefore, must be continuously increased during the accelerating process to compensate for the increasing inertia of the body due to its continuously increasing mass. Equations (2.2) and (2.5) assume the force to be constant and therefore are not applicable to cases where relativistic effects must be considered. One way of overcoming this difficulty is to divide the total distance r into many smaller distances, $\Delta r_1, \Delta r_2, \ldots, \Delta r_n$, as shown in Figure 2-1, multiply each of these small distances by the average force exerted while traversing the small distance, and then sum the products. This process may be written as

$$W = f_1\,\Delta r_1 + f_2\,\Delta r_2 + \cdots + f_n\,\Delta r_n \tag{2.6a}$$

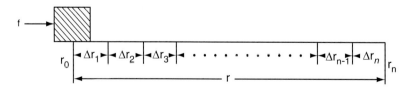

Figure 2-1. Diagram illustrating that the total work done in accelerating a body is $W = \sum\limits_{n=1}^{n} f_n \Delta r_n$.

and symbolized by

$$W = \sum_{n=1}^{n} f_n \Delta r_n \tag{2.6b}$$

As r is successively divided into smaller and smaller lengths, the calculation of the work done, using Eq. (2.6), becomes more accurate. A limiting value for W may be obtained by letting each small distance Δr_n in Eq. (2.6) approach zero, that is, by considering such small increments of distance that the force remains approximately constant during the specified interval. In the notation of the calculus, such an infinitesimally small quantity is called a differential and is specified by prefixing the symbol for the quantity with the letter "d." Thus, if r represents distance, dr represents an infinitesimally small distance and the differential of work done, which is the product of the force and the infinitesimally small distance, is given by

$$dW = f\,dr. \tag{2.7}$$

The total energy expended in going from the point r_0 to point r_n, then, is merely the sum of all the products of the force and the infinitesimally small distances through which it acted. This sum is indicated by the mathematical notation

$$W = \int_{r=0}^{r=n} f\,dr. \tag{2.8}$$

The ratio of two differentials, dW/dr, for example, is called a *derivative*, and the process in which a derivative is obtained is called *differentiation*. Since acceleration is defined as the *rate of change of velocity with respect to time*,

$$a = \frac{v_2 - v_1}{t_2 - t_1} = \frac{\Delta v}{\Delta t}, \tag{2.9}$$

where v_1 and v_2 are the respective velocities at times t_1 and t_2. Then Eq. (2.1) may be written as

$$f = m\frac{\Delta v}{\Delta t}, \tag{2.10}$$

and by letting Δt approach zero we obtain the instantaneous rate of change of velocity or the derivative of velocity with respect to time. Using the differential notation, we have

$$f = m\frac{dv}{dt}. \tag{2.11}$$

This is the expression of Newton's second law of motion for the nonrelativistic case where the mass remains constant. Newton's second law states that the rate of change of momentum of an accelerating body is proportional to the unbalanced force acting on the body. For the general case, where mass is not constant, Newton's second law is written as

$$f = \frac{d\,(mv)}{dt}. \tag{2.12}$$

Substitution of the value of f from Eq. (2.12) into Eq. (2.8) gives

$$W = \int_0^r \frac{d\,(mv)}{dt}\, dr. \tag{2.13}$$

Since $v = dr/dt$, Eq. (2.13) can be written as

$$W = \int_0^t \frac{d\,(mv)}{dt}\, v\,dt = \int_0^{mv} v\,d\,(mv), \tag{2.14}$$

and substituting $m = \dfrac{m_0}{\left(1 - \dfrac{v^2}{c^2}\right)^{1/2}}$, we have

$$W = \int_0^v v\,d \left\{ \frac{m_0 v}{\left(1 - \dfrac{v^2}{c^2}\right)^{1/2}} \right\}. \tag{2.15}$$

Differentiating the term in the parenthesis gives

$$W = m_0 \int_0^v \left\{ \frac{v}{\left(1 - \dfrac{v^2}{c^2}\right)^{1/2}} + \frac{\dfrac{v^3}{c^2}}{\left(1 - \dfrac{v^2}{c^2}\right)^{3/2}} \right\} dv. \tag{2.16}$$

Now, multiply the numerator and denominator of the first term in Eq. (2.16) by $\left[1 - \left(v^2/c^2\right)\right]$ to obtain

$$W = m_0 \int_0^v \left\{ \frac{v - \dfrac{v^3}{c^2}}{\left(1 - \dfrac{v^2}{c^2}\right)^{3/2}} + \frac{\dfrac{v^3}{c^2}}{\left(1 - \dfrac{v^2}{c^2}\right)^{3/2}} \right\} dv \tag{2.17}$$

$$= m_0 \int_0^v \frac{v}{\left(1 - \dfrac{v^2}{c^2}\right)^{3/2}}\, dv = m_0 \int_0^v \frac{1}{v\left(1 - \dfrac{v^2}{c^2}\right)^{3/2}}\, dv. \tag{2.18}$$

The integrand in Eq. (2.18) is almost in the form

$$\int_a^b u^n\, du = \frac{u^{n+1}}{n+1} \bigg|_a^b, \tag{2.19}$$

where

$$u^n = \frac{1}{\left(1 - \dfrac{v^2}{c^2}\right)^{3/2}} \quad \text{and} \quad du = -\frac{2v}{c^2}\, dv.$$

To convert Eq. (2.18) into the form for integration given by Eq. (2.19), it is necessary only to complete du. This is done by multiplying the integrand by $-2/c^2$ and the entire expression by $-c^2/2$ in order to keep the total value of Eq. (2.18) unchanged. The solution of Eq. (2.18), which gives the kinetic energy of a body that was accelerated from zero velocity to a velocity v, is

$$E_k = W = m_0 c^2 \left[\frac{1}{\left(1 - \dfrac{v^2}{c^2}\right)^{1/2}} - 1 \right] = m_0 c^2 \left[\frac{1}{[1 - \beta^2]^{1/2}} - 1 \right], \qquad (2.20)$$

where $\beta = v/c$.

Equation (2.20) is the exact expression for kinetic energy and must be used whenever the moving body experiences observable relativistic effects.

 EXAMPLE 2.2

(a) What is the kinetic energy of the electron in Example 2.1 that travels at 99% of the velocity of light?

Solution

$$E_k = m_0 c^2 \left[\frac{1}{(1 - \beta^2)^{1/2}} - 1 \right]$$

$$= 9.11 \times 10^{-31}\ \text{kg} \left(3 \times 10^8\ \frac{\text{m}}{\text{s}}\right)^2 \left\{ \frac{1}{[1 - (0.99)^2]^{1/2}} - 1 \right\} = 4.99 \times 10^{-13}\ \text{J}$$

(b) How much additional energy is required to increase the velocity of this electron to 99.9% of the velocity of light, an increase in velocity of only 0.91%?

Solution

The kinetic energy of an electron whose velocity is 99.9% of the speed of light is

$$E_k = 9.11 \times 10^{-31}\ \text{kg} \left(3 \times 10^8\ \frac{\text{m}}{\text{s}}\right)^2 \left\{ \frac{1}{[1 - (0.999)^2]^{1/2}} - 1 \right\} = 17.52 \times 10^{-13}\ \text{J}$$

The additional work necessary to increase the kinetic energy of the electron from 99% to 99.9% of the velocity of light is

$$\Delta W = (17.52 - 4.99) \times 10^{-13} \, \text{J}$$

$$= 12.53 \times 10^{-13} \, \text{J}.$$

(c) What is the mass of the electron whose β is 0.999?

Solution

$$m = \frac{m_0}{\left(1 - \beta^2\right)^{1/2}} = \frac{9.11 \times 10^{-31} \, \text{kg}}{\left[1 - (0.999)^2\right]^{1/2}} = 204 \times 10^{-31} \, \text{kg}.$$

The relativistic expression for kinetic energy given by Eq. (2.20) is rigorously true for particles moving at all velocities while the nonrelativistic expression for kinetic energy, Eq. (2.3), is applicable only to cases where the velocity of the moving particle is much less than the velocity of light. It can be shown that the relativistic expression reduces to the nonrelativistic expression for low velocities by expanding the expression $\left(1 - \beta^2\right)^{-1/2}$ in Eq. (2.20) according to the binomial theorem and then dropping higher terms that become insignificant when $v \ll c$. According to the binomial theorem,

$$(a + b)^n = a^n + na^{n-1}b + \frac{n(n-1)\,a^{n-2}b^2}{2!} + \cdots \qquad (2.21)$$

The expansion of $\left(1 - \beta^2\right)^{-1/2}$ according to Eq. (2.21), is accomplished by letting $a = 1$, $b = -\beta^2$, and $n = -1/2$.

$$\left(1 - \beta^2\right)^{-1/2} = 1 + \frac{1}{2}\beta^2 + \frac{3}{8}\beta^4 + \cdots \qquad (2.22)$$

Since $\beta = v/c$, then, if $v \ll c$, terms from β^4 and higher will be insignificantly small and may therefore be dropped. Then, after substituting the first two terms from Eq. (2.22) into Eq. (2.20), we have

$$E_k = m_0 c^2 \left(1 + \frac{1}{2}\frac{v^2}{c^2} - 1\right) = \frac{1}{2}m_0 v^2,$$

which is the nonrelativistic case. Equation (2.3) is applicable when $v \ll c$.

In Example 2.2, it was shown that at a very high velocity ($\beta = 0.99$) a kinetic energy increase of 253% resulted in a velocity increase of the moving body by only 0.91%. In nonrelativistic cases, the increase in velocity is directly proportional to the square root of the work done on the moving body or, in other words, to the kinetic energy of the body. In the relativistic case, the velocity increase due to additional energy is smaller than in the nonrelativistic case because the additional energy serves to increase the mass of the moving body rather than its velocity. This equivalence of mass and energy is one of the most important consequences of Einstein's special theory of relativity. According to Einstein, the relationship between mass and energy is

$$E = mc^2, \tag{2.23}$$

where E is the total energy of a piece of matter whose mass is m and c is the velocity of light in vacuum. The principle of relativity tells us that all matter contains potential energy by virtue of its mass. It is this energy source that is tapped to obtain nuclear energy. The main virtue of this energy source is the vast amount of energy that can be derived from conversion into its energy equivalent of small amounts of nuclear fuel.

 EXAMPLE 2.3

(a) How much energy can be obtained from 1 g of nuclear fuel?

Solution

$$E = mc^2 = 1 \times 10^{-3} \text{ kg} \times \left(3 \times 10^8 \, \frac{\text{m}}{\text{s}}\right)^2 = 9 \times 10^{13} \text{ J}.$$

Since there are 2.78×10^{-7} kilowatt-hours (kW h) per joule, 1 g of nuclear fuel yields

$$E = 9 \times 10^{13} \frac{\text{J}}{\text{g}} \times 2.78 \times 10^{-7} \, \frac{\text{kW} \cdot \text{h}}{\text{J}} = 2.5 \times 10^7 \, \frac{\text{kW} \cdot \text{h}}{\text{g}}$$

(b) How much coal, whose heat content is 13,000 Btu/lb, must be burned to liberate the same amount of energy as 1 g of nuclear fuel?

Solution

$$1 \text{ Btu} = 2.93 \times 10^{-4} \text{ kW h}.$$

Therefore, the amount of coal required is

$$2.5 \times 10^7 \text{ kW} \cdot \text{h} = 1.3 \times 10^4 \frac{\text{Btu}}{\text{lb}} \times 2.93 \times 10^{-4} \frac{\text{kW} \cdot \text{h}}{\text{Btu}}$$

$$\times 2 \times 10^3 \frac{\text{lb}}{\text{ton}} \times C \text{ tons}$$

Therefore,

$$C = 3280 \text{ tons (2981 metric tons)}$$

The loss in mass accompanying ordinary energy transformations is not detectable because of the very large amount of energy released per unit mass and the consequent very small change in mass for ordinary reactions. In the case of coal, for example, the above example shows a loss in mass of 1 g per 3280 tons. The fractional mass loss is

$$f = \frac{\Delta m}{m} = \frac{1 \text{ g}}{3.28 \times 10^3 \text{ tons} \times 2 \times 10^3 \frac{\text{lb}}{\text{ton}} \times 4.54 \times 10^2 \frac{\text{g}}{\text{lb}}} = 3.3 \times 10^{-10}.$$

Such a small fractional loss in mass is not detectable by any of our ordinary weighing techniques.

ELECTRICITY

Electric Charge: The Coulomb

All the elements are electrical in nature and, except for hydrogen, are constructed of multiples of two charged particles and one uncharged particle. Their electrical properties are due to extremely small, charged particles called *protons* and *electrons*. The mass of the proton is 1.6726×10^{-27} kg (1.6726×10^{-24} g) and the mass of the electron is 9.1085×10^{-31} kg (9.1085×10^{-28} g). These two particles have charges of exactly the same magnitude but are qualitatively different. A proton is said to have a positive charge and an electron has a negative charge. Under normal conditions, matter is electrically neutral because the positive and negative charges are homogeneously (on a macroscopic scale) dispersed in equal numbers in a manner that results in no net charge. However, it is possible, by suitable treatment, to induce either net positive or negative charges on bodies. For example, combing the hair with a hard rubber comb transfers electrons to the comb from the hair, leaving a net negative charge on the comb. The uncharged component in every element is called the neutron; it has a mass of 1.67492×10^{-27} kg (1.67492×10^{-24} g). For health physics purposes, these three particles—electron, proton, and neutron—may be considered the basic building blocks of matter (although we now believe that protons and neutrons themselves are made of still smaller particles called quarks). It should be pointed out here that high-energy accelerators produce—in addition to protons, neutrons, and electrons—a number of different extremely short-lived unstable particles. In the context of health physics, the most important of these particles are charged and uncharged *pions (pi-mesons)* and *muons (mu-mesons)* because they give rise to very high-energy electrons and gamma rays when they decay. Muons are also produced by cosmic radiation and contribute to the dose from cosmic radiation.

Charged bodies exert forces on each other by virtue of their electric fields. Bodies with like charges repel each other while those with unlike charges attract each other. In the case of point charges, the magnitude of these electric forces is proportional to the product of the charges and inversely proportional to the square of the distance between the charged bodies. This relationship was described by Coulomb and is known as Coulomb's law. Expressed algebraically, it is

$$f = k\frac{q_1 q_2}{r^2}. \tag{2.24}$$

where k, the constant of proportionality, depends on the nature of the medium that separates the charges. In the SI system, the unit of electric charge, called the *coulomb*

(C), is defined in terms of electric current rather than by Coulomb's law. For this reason, the constant of proportionality has a value not equal to 1 but rather

$$k_0 = 9 \times 10^9 \; \frac{\text{N} \cdot \text{m}^2}{\text{C}^2} \tag{2.25}$$

when the two charges are in a vacuum or in air (air at atmospheric pressure exerts very little influence on the force developed between charges and thus may be considered equivalent to a vacuum). The subscript 0 signifies the value of k in a vacuum. If the charges are separated by materials, other than air, that are poor conductors of electricity (such materials are called *dielectrics*), the value of k is different and depends on the material.

It is convenient to define k_0 in terms of another constant, ε_0, called the *permittivity*:

$$k_0 = \frac{1}{4\pi\,\varepsilon_0} = 9 \times 10^9 \; \frac{\text{N} \cdot \text{m}^2}{\text{C}^2}, \tag{2.26}$$

$$\varepsilon_0 = \frac{1}{4\pi\,k_0} = \frac{1}{4\pi \times 9 \times 10^9 \; \dfrac{\text{N} \cdot \text{m}^2}{\text{C}^2}} = 8.85 \times 10^{-12} \; \frac{\text{C}^2}{\text{N} \cdot \text{m}^2},$$

where ε_0 is the permittivity of a vacuum. The permittivity of any other medium is designated by ε. The relative permittivity, K_e, of a substance is defined by

$$K_e = \frac{\varepsilon}{\varepsilon_0} \tag{2.27}$$

and is called the *dielectric coefficient*.

For all dielectric materials, the dielectric coefficient has a value greater than 1. The permittivity, or the dielectric coefficient, is a measure of the amount of electric energy that can be stored in a medium when the medium is placed into a given electric field. If everything else is held constant, a higher dielectric coefficient leads to a greater amount of stored electric energy.

The smallest natural quantity of electric charge is the charge on the electron or proton, $\pm 1.6 \times 10^{-19}$ C. The reciprocal of the electronic charge, 6.25×10^{18}, is the number of electrons whose aggregate charge is 1 C. In the cgs system, the unit of charge is the *statcoulomb* (sC) and the electronic charge is 4.8×10^{-10} sC. There are 3×10^9 sC in 1 C.

EXAMPLE 2.4

Compare the electrical and gravitational forces of attraction between an electron and a proton separated by 5×10^{-11} m.

Solution

The electrical force is given by Eq. (2.24):

$$f = k_0 \frac{q_1 q_2}{r^2} = 9 \times 10^9 \; \frac{\text{N} \cdot \text{m}^2}{\text{C}^2} \times \frac{1.6 \times 10^{-19} \; \text{C} \; \times \; 1.6 \times 10^{-19} \; \text{C}}{\left(5 \times 10^{-11} \; \text{m}\right)^2}$$

$$= 9.2 \times 10^{-8} \; \text{N}.$$

The gravitational force between two bodies follows the same mathematical formulation as Coulomb's law for electrical forces. In the case of gravitational forces, the force is always attractive. The gravitational force is given by

$$F = \frac{G m_1 m_2}{r^2}. \tag{2.28}$$

G is a universal constant that is equal to 6.67×10^{-11} N $\cdot$ m^2/kg^2 and must be used because the unit of force, the newton, was originally defined using "inertial" mass, according to Newton's second law of motion, given by Eq. (2.1). The mass in Eq. (2.28) is commonly called "gravitational" mass. Despite the two different designations, it should be emphasized that inertial mass and gravitational mass are equivalent. It should also be pointed out that F in Eq. (2.28) gives the weight of an object of mass m_1 when m_2 represents the mass of the earth and r is the distance from the object to the center of the earth. Weight is merely a measure of the gravitational attractive force between an object and the earth and therefore varies from point to point on the surface of the earth, according to the distance of the point from the earth's center. On the surface of another planet, the weight of the same object would be different from that on earth because of the different size and mass of that planet and its consequent different attractive force. In outer space, if the object is not under the gravitational influence of any heavenly body, it must be weightless. Mass, on the other hand, is a measure of the amount of matter and its numerical value is therefore independent of the point in the universe where it is measured.

The gravitational force between the electron and the proton is

$$F = \frac{6.67 \times 10^{-11} \ \dfrac{\text{N} \cdot \text{m}^2}{\text{kg}^2} \times 9.11 \times 10^{-31} \ \text{kg} \times 1.67 \times 10^{-27} \ \text{kg}}{\left(5 \times 10^{-11} \ \text{m}\right)^2}$$

$$= 4.1 \times 10^{-47} \ \text{N}.$$

It is immediately apparent that in the interaction between charged particles, gravitational forces are extremely small in comparison with the electrical forces acting between the particles and may be completely neglected in most instances.

Electrical Potential: The Volt

If one charge is held rigidly and another charge is placed in the electric field of the first charge, it will have a certain amount of potential energy relative to any other point within the electric field. In the case of electric potential energy, the reference point is taken at an infinite distance from the charge that sets up the electric field, that is, at a point far enough from the charge so that its effect is negligible. As a consequence of the great separation, these charges do not interact electrically. Therefore, a value of zero is arbitrarily assigned to the potential energy in the system of charges; the charge at an infinite distance from the one that sets up the electric field has no electric potential energy. If the two charges are of the same sign, bringing them closer together requires work (or the expenditure of energy) in

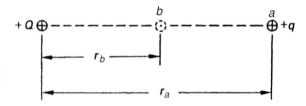

Figure 2-2. Diagram illustrating work done in moving a charge between two points of different potential in an electric field.

order to overcome the repulsive force between the two charges. Since work was done in bringing the two charges together, the potential energy in the system of charges is now greater than it was initially. On the other hand, if the two charges are of opposite signs, then a decrease in distance between them occurs spontaneously because of the attractive forces, and work is done by the system. The potential energy of the system consequently decreases, that is, the potential energy of the freely moving charge with respect to the rigidly held charge, decreases. This is exactly analogous to the case of a freely falling mass whose potential energy decreases as it approaches the surface of the earth. In the case of the mass in the earth's gravitational field, however, the reference point for potential energy of the mass is arbitrarily set on the surface of the earth. This means that the mass has no potential energy when it is lying right on the earth's surface. All numerical values for potential energy of the mass, therefore, are positive numbers. In the case of electric potential energy, however, as a consequence of the arbitrary convention that the point of the zero numerical value is at an infinite distance from the charge that sets up the electric field, the numerical values for the potential energy of a charge, owing to attractive electrical forces, must be negative.

The quantitative aspects of electric potential energy may be investigated with the aid of Figure 2-2, which shows a charge $+Q$ that sets up an electric field extending uniformly in all directions. Another charge, $+q$, is used to explore the electric field set up by Q. When the exploring charge is at point a, at a distance r_a cm from Q, it has an amount of potential energy that depends on the magnitudes of Q, q, and r_a. If the charge q is now to be moved to point b, which is closer to Q, then, because of the repulsive force between the two charges, work is done in moving the charge from point a to point b. The amount of work that is done in moving charge q from point a to point b may be calculated by multiplying the force exerted on the charge q by the distance through which it was moved, in accordance with Eq. (2.2). From Eq. (2.24), however, it is seen that the force is not constant but varies inversely with the square of the distance between the charges. The magnitude of the force, therefore, increases rapidly as the charge q approaches Q, and increasingly greater amounts of work are done when the exploring charge q is moved a unit distance. The movement of the exploring charge may be accomplished by a series of infinitesimally small movements, during each of which an infinitesimally small amount of work is done. The total energy expenditure, or increase in potential energy of the exploring charge, is then merely equal to the sum of all the infinitesimal increments of work. This infinitesimal energy increment is given by Eq. (2.7):

$$\mathrm{d}W = -f\,\mathrm{d}r$$

(the minus sign is used here because an increase in potential energy results from a decrease in distance between the charges) and, if the value for f from Eq. (2.24) is substituted into Eq. (2.7), we have

$$\mathrm{d}W = -k_0 \frac{Qq}{r^2}\mathrm{d}r, \tag{2.29}$$

$$W = -k_0 Qq \int_{r_a}^{r_b} \frac{\mathrm{d}r}{r^2}. \tag{2.30}$$

Integration of Eq. (2.30) gives

$$W = k_0 Qq \left(\frac{1}{r_b} - \frac{1}{r_a}\right). \tag{2.31}$$

If the distances a and b are measured in meters and if the charges are given in coulombs, then the energy W is given in joules.

 # EXAMPLE 2.5

If, in Figure 2-2, Q is $+44.4$ μC, q is $+5$ μC, and r_a and r_b are 2 m and 1 m respectively, then calculate the work done in moving the 5 μC charge from point a to point b.

Solution

The work done is, from Eq. (2.31),

$$W = 9 \times 10^9 \frac{\mathrm{N \cdot m^2}}{\mathrm{C^2}} \times 44.4 \times 10^{-6}\,\mathrm{C} \times 5 \times 10^{-6}\,\mathrm{C} \left(\frac{1}{1\,\mathrm{m}} - \frac{1}{2\,\mathrm{m}}\right)$$

$$= 1\,\mathrm{N \cdot m} = 1\,\mathrm{J}.$$

In this example, 1 J of energy was expended in moving the 5 μC of charge from a to b. The work per unit charge is

$$\frac{W}{q} = \frac{1\,\mathrm{J}}{5 \times 10^{-6}\,\mathrm{C}} = 200,000\,\frac{\mathrm{J}}{\mathrm{C}}$$

We therefore say that the potential difference between points a and b is 200,000 V, since, by definition:

> One *volt* of potential difference exists between any two points in an electric field if one joule of energy is expended in moving a charge of one coulomb between the two points.

Expressed more concisely, the definition of a volt is

$$1\text{ V} = 1\ \frac{\text{J}}{\text{C}}.$$

In Example 2.5, point b is the point of higher potential with respect to point a, because work had to be done on the charge to move it to b from a.

The electrical potential at any point due to an electric field from a point charge Q is defined as the potential energy that a unit positive exploring charge $+q$ would have if it were brought from a point at an infinite distance from Q to the point in question. The electrical potential at point b in Figure 2-2 can be computed from Eq. (2.30) by setting distance r_a equal to infinity. The potential at point b, V_b, which is defined as the potential energy per unit positive charge at b, is, therefore:

$$V_b = \frac{W}{q} = k_0 \frac{Q}{r_b}. \tag{2.32}$$

 EXAMPLE 2.6

(a) What is the potential at a distance of 5×10^{-11} m from a proton?

Solution

$$V = k_0 \frac{Q}{r} = 9 \times 10^9\ \frac{\text{N} \cdot \text{m}^2}{\text{C}^2} \times \frac{1.6 \times 10^{-19}\text{ C}}{5 \times 10^{-11}\text{ m}} = 28.8\ \frac{\text{N} \cdot \text{m}}{\text{C}}$$

$$= 28.8\ \frac{\text{J}}{\text{C}} = 28.8\text{ V}$$

(b) What is the potential energy of another proton at this point?

Solution

According to Eq. (2.32), the potential energy of the proton is equal to the product of its charge and the potential of its location. Therefore,

$$E_\text{p} = qV = 1.6 \times 10^{-19}\text{ C} \times 28.8\text{ V} = 4.6 \times 10^{-18}\text{ J}.$$

Electrical Current: The Ampere

A flow of electrically charged particles constitutes an electric current. The unit for the amount of current is the *ampere (A)*, which is a measure of the time rate of flow of charge. The ampere is defined in the SI system by the interaction between a current flowing through a conductor and a magnetic field. However, a useful working definition is that one ampere represents a flow rate of charge of one coulomb per second. Ordinarily, the charge carrier in an electric current is the electron. Since the charge on an electron is 1.6×10^{-19} C, a current of 1 A represents an electron flow rate of

$$\frac{1 \text{ C/s}}{A} \times \frac{1}{1.6 \times 10^{-19} \dfrac{C}{\text{electron}}} = 6.25 \times 10^{18} \frac{\text{electrons/s}}{A}.$$

A 100-μA electron beam in an X-ray tube represents an electron flow rate of

$$100 \times 10^{-6} \text{ A} \times 6.25 \times 10^{18} \frac{\text{electrons/s}}{A} = 6.25 \times 10^{14} \text{ electrons/s}.$$

Current is determined only by the flow rate of charge. For example, in the case of a beam of alpha particles, whose charge $= 2 \times 1.6 \times 10^{-19}$ C $= 3.2 \times 10^{-19}$ C, 1 A corresponds to 3.125×10^{19} alpha particles.

The direction of current flow was arbitrarily determined, before the discovery of the electron, to be from the positive electrode to the negative electrode of a closed circuit. In fact, the electrons flow in the opposite direction. However, conventional current flow still goes from positive to negative. When we are interested in the actual direction of flow, we use the term "electron current" to indicate current flow from negative to positive.

The Electron Volt: A Unit of Energy

If two electrodes are connected to the terminals of a source of voltage, as shown in Figure 2-3, then a charged particle anywhere in the electric field between the two plates will have an amount of potential energy given by Eq. (2.32),

$$W = qV,$$

where V is the electrical potential at the point occupied by the charged particle. If, for example, the cathode in Figure 2-3 is 1-V negative with respect to the anode and the charged particle is an electron on the surface of the cathode, then the potential

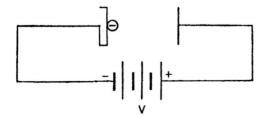

Figure 2-3. Diagram showing the potential energy of an electron in an electric field.

energy of the electron with respect to the anode is

$$W = qV = -1.6 \times 10^{-19} \text{ C} \times (-1 \text{ V})$$
$$= 1.6 \times 10^{-19} \text{ J}$$

This amount of energy, 1.6×10^{-19} J, is called an *electron volt* and is symbolized by eV. Since the magnitude of the electron volt is convenient in dealing with the energetics of atomic and nuclear mechanics, this quantity of energy is taken as a unit and is frequently used in health physics. Multiples of the electron volt are the keV (10^3 eV), the MeV (10^6 eV), and the GeV (10^9 eV).

 EXAMPLE 2.7

How many electron volts of energy correspond to the mass of a resting electron?

Solution

$$E = mc^2$$
$$= 9.11 \times 10^{-31} \text{ kg} \times \left(3 \times 10^8 \, \frac{\text{m}}{\text{s}}\right)^2$$
$$= 81.99 \times 10^{-15} \text{ J}$$

Since there are $1.6 \times 10^{-19} \, \dfrac{\text{J}}{\text{eV}}$,

$$E = \frac{81.99 \times 10^{-15} \text{ J}}{1.6 \times 10^{-19} \, \dfrac{\text{J}}{\text{eV}}} = 0.51 \times 10^6 \text{ eV}.$$

It should be emphasized that, although the numerical value for the electron volt was calculated by computing the potential energy of an electron at a potential of 1 V, the electron volt is not a unit of electrons or volts; it is a unit of energy and may be interchanged (after numerical correction) with any other unit of energy.

 EXAMPLE 2.8

How many electron volts of heat must be added to change 1 L of water whose temperature is 50°C to completely dry steam?

Solution

The specific heat of water is $1 \frac{\text{cal}}{\text{g}}$, and the heat of vaporization of water is 539 $\frac{\text{cal}}{\text{g}}$. Therefore,

$$\text{heat energy added} = 1000 \text{ g} \left[1 \frac{\text{cal}}{\text{g} \cdot \text{deg}} \times (100 - 50) \text{ deg} + 539 \frac{\text{cal}}{\text{g}} \right]$$

$$= 589{,}000 \text{ cal}$$

Since there are $4.186 \frac{\text{J}}{\text{cal}}$ and $1.6 \times 10^{-19} \frac{\text{J}}{\text{eV}}$, we have

$$\text{heat energy added} = \frac{5.89 \times 10^5 \text{ cal} \times 4.186 \frac{\text{J}}{\text{cal}}}{1.6 \times 10^{-19} \frac{\text{J}}{\text{eV}}} = 1.54 \times 10^{25} \text{ eV}$$

The answer to Example 2.8 is an astronomically large number (but not very much energy on the scale of ordinary physical and chemical reactions) and shows why the electron volt is a useful energy unit only for reactions in the atomic world.

 # EXAMPLE 2.9

An alpha particle, whose charge is $+(2 \times 1.6 \times 10^{-19})$ C and whose mass is 6.645×10^{-27} kg, is accelerated across a potential difference of 100,000 V. What is its kinetic energy, in joules and in electron volts, and how fast is it moving?

Solution

The potential energy of the alpha particle at the moment it starts to accelerate is, from Eq. (2.32),

$$W = qV = 2 \times 1.6 \times 10^{-19} \text{ C} \times 10^5 \text{ V}$$

$$= 3.2 \times 10^{-14} \text{ J}$$

In terms of electron volts,

$$W = \frac{3.2 \times 10^{-14} \text{ J}}{1.6 \times 10^{-19} \frac{\text{J}}{\text{eV}}} = 2 \times 10^5 \text{ eV}$$

Since all the alpha particle's potential energy is converted into kinetic energy after it falls through the 100,000 V (100 kV) potential difference, the kinetic energy must then be 200,000 eV (200 keV).

The velocity of the alpha particle may be computed by equating its potential and kinetic energies,

$$q V = \frac{1}{2} m v^2, \tag{2.33}$$

and solving for v:

$$v = \left(\frac{2q V}{m}\right)^{1/2} = \left(\frac{2 \times 10^5 \text{ V} \times 3.2 \times 10^{-19} \text{ C}}{6.645 \times 10^{-27} \text{ kg}}\right)^{1/2}$$

$$= 3.1 \times 10^6 \frac{\text{m}}{\text{s}}.$$

Electric Field

The term *electric field* was used in the preceding sections of this chapter without an explicit definition. Implicit in the use of the term, however, was the connotation by the context that an electric field is any region where electric forces act. "Electric field" is not merely a descriptive term; defining an electric field requires a number in order to specify the magnitude of the electric forces that act in the electric field and a direction in which these forces act, and, thus, it is a vector quantity. The strength of an electric field is called the *electric field intensity* and may be defined in terms of the force (magnitude and direction) that acts on a unit exploring charge that is placed into the electric field. Consider an isolated charge $+Q$ that sets up an electric field and an exploring charge $+q$ that is used to investigate the electric field, as shown in Figure 2-4. The exploring charge will experience a force in the direction shown and of a magnitude given by Eq. (2.24):

$$f = k_0 \frac{Qq}{r^2}.$$

The force per unit charge at the point r meters from charge Q is the electric field intensity at that point and is given by the equation

$$\varepsilon = \frac{f}{q} \frac{\text{N}}{\text{C}} = k_0 \frac{\text{N} \cdot \text{m}^2}{\text{C}^2} \times \frac{Q \text{ C}}{r^2 \text{ m}^2}. \tag{2.34}$$

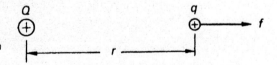

Figure 2-4. The force on an exploring charge $+q$ in the electric field of charge $+Q$.

According to Eq. (2.34), electric field intensity is expressed in units of force per unit charge, that is, in newton per coulomb. It should be emphasized that ε is a vector quantity, that is, it has direction as well as magnitude.

EXAMPLE 2.10

(a) What is the electric field intensity at point P due to the two charges $+6$ C and $+3$ C, shown in Figure 2-5(A)?

Solution

The electric field intensity at point P due to the $+6$ C charge is

$$\varepsilon_1 = k_0 \frac{Q_1}{r_1^2} = 9 \times 10^9 \ \frac{\text{N} \cdot \text{m}^2}{\text{C}^2} \times \frac{6 \ \text{C}}{(2 \ \text{m})^2} = 1.35 \times 10^{10} \ \frac{\text{N}}{\text{C}}$$

and acts in the direction shown in Figure 2-5(A). (The magnitude of the field intensity is shown graphically by a vector whose length is proportional to the field intensity. In Figure 2-5(A), the scale is 1 cm $= 1 \times 10^{10}$ N/C. ε_1 is therefore drawn 1.35-cm long). ε_2, the electric field intensity at P due to the $+3$ C charge, is

$$\varepsilon_2 = k_0 \frac{Q_2}{r_2^2} = 9 \times 10^9 \ \frac{\text{N} \cdot \text{m}^2}{\text{C}^2} \times \frac{3 \ \text{C}}{(1 \ \text{m})^2} = 2.7 \times 10^{10} \ \frac{\text{N}}{\text{C}},$$

and acts along the line $Q_2 P$, as shown in the illustration. The resultant electric intensity at point P is the vector sum of ε_1 and ε_2. If these two vectors are accurately drawn in magnitude and direction, the resultant may be obtained graphically by completing the parallelogram of forces and drawing the diagonal ε_R. The length of

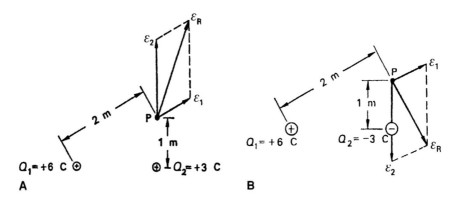

Figure 2-5. Resultant electric field from **(A)** two positive charges and **(B)** two opposite charges.

the diagonal is proportional to the magnitude of the resultant electric field intensity and its direction shows the direction of the electric field at point P. In this case, since 1×10^{10} N/C is represented by 1 cm, the resultant electric field intensity is found to be about 4×10^{10} N/C and it acts in a direction 30° clockwise from the vertical. The value of ε_R may also be determined from the law of cosines

$$a^2 = b^2 + c^2 - 2bc \cos A, \tag{2.35}$$

where b and c are two adjacent sides of a triangle, A is the included angle, and a is the side opposite angle A. In this case, b is 2.7×10^{10}, c is 1.35×10^{10}, angle A is 120°, and a is the resultant ε_R, the electric field intensity whose magnitude is to be calculated. From Eq. (2.35), we find

$$\varepsilon_R^2 = \left(2.7 \times 10^{10}\right)^2 + \left(1.35 \times 10^{10}\right)^2 - 2\left(2.7 \times 10^{10}\right)\left(1.35 \times 10^{10}\right) \cos 120°$$

$$\varepsilon_R = 3.57 \times 10^{10} \frac{N}{C}$$

(b) What is the magnitude and direction of ε_R if the 3 C charge is negative and the 6 C charge is positive?

Solution

In this case, the magnitudes of ε_1 and ε_2 would be exactly the same as in part (a) of this example; the direction of ε_1 would also remain unchanged, but the direction of ε_2 would be toward the −3 C charge, as shown in Figure 2-5(B). From the geometric arrangement, it is seen that the resultant intensity acts in a direction 120° clockwise from the vertical. The magnitude of ε_R, from Eq. (2.35), is

$$\varepsilon_R^2 = \left(2.7 \times 10^{10}\right)^2 + \left(1.35 \times 10^{10}\right)^2 - 2\left(2.7 \times 10^{10}\right)\left(1.35 \times 10^{10}\right) \cos 60°$$

$$\varepsilon_R = 2.34 \times 10^{10} \frac{N}{C}.$$

Point charges result in nonuniform electric fields. A uniform electric field may be produced by applying a potential difference across two large parallel plates made of electrical conductors separated by an insulator, as shown in Figure 2-6.

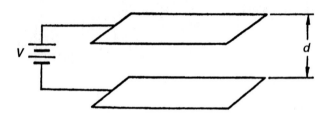

Figure 2-6. Conditions for producing a relatively uniform electric field. The field will be quite uniform throughout the region between the plates, but will be distorted at the edges of the plates.

The electric intensity throughout the region between the two plates is ε newtons per coulomb. The force acting on any charge within this field therefore is

$$f = \varepsilon q \text{ N.} \tag{2.36}$$

If the charge q happens to be positive, then to move it across the distance d, from the negative to the positive plates, against the electric force in the uniform field requires the expenditure of energy given by the equation

$$W = fd = \varepsilon q d. \tag{2.37}$$

However, since potential difference (V) is defined as work per unit charge, Eq. (2.37) may be expressed as

$$V = \frac{W}{q} = \varepsilon d, \tag{2.38}$$

or

$$\varepsilon = \frac{V}{d} \frac{\text{V}}{\text{m}}. \tag{2.39}$$

Equation (2.39) expresses electric field intensity in the units most commonly used for this purpose—volts per meter.

A nonuniform electric field that is of interest to the health physicist (in instrument design) is that due to a potential difference applied across two coaxial conductors, as shown in Figure 2-7. If the radius of the inner conductor is a meters and that of the outer conductor is b meters, then the electric intensity at any point between the two conductors, r meters from the center, is given by

$$\varepsilon = \frac{1}{r} \times \frac{V}{\ln\left(\dfrac{b}{a}\right)} \frac{\text{V}}{\text{m}}, \tag{2.40}$$

where V is the potential difference between the two conductors.

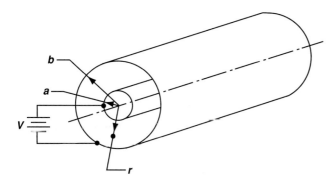

Figure 2-7. Conditions for the nonuniform electric field between two coaxial conductors given by Eq. (2.40).

EXAMPLE 2.11

A Geiger-Müller counter is constructed of a wire anode whose diameter is 0.1 mm and a cathode, coaxial with the anode, whose diameter is 2 cm. If the voltage across the tube is 1000 V, what is the electric field intensity

(a) at a distance of 0.03 mm from the surface of the anode and

(b) at a point midway between the center of the tube and the cathode?

Solution

(a) We know,

$$\varepsilon = \frac{1}{r} \times \frac{V}{\ln\left(\dfrac{b}{a}\right)}.$$

Letting $r = \frac{1}{2}(0.01) + 0.003 = 0.008$ cm $= 8 \times 10^{-5}$ m, we have,

$$\varepsilon = \frac{1}{8 \times 10^{-5}\ \text{m}} \times \frac{1000\ \text{V}}{\ln\left(\dfrac{1}{0.005}\right)} = 2.36 \times 10^6 \frac{\text{V}}{\text{m}}.$$

(b) At $r = 0.005$ m,

$$\varepsilon = \frac{1}{0.005\ \text{m}} \times \frac{1000\ \text{V}}{\ln\left(\dfrac{1}{0.005}\right)} = 3.78 \times 10^4 \frac{\text{V}}{\text{m}}.$$

It should be noted that in the case of coaxial geometry, extremely intense electric fields may be obtained with relatively small potential differences. Such large fields require mainly a small ratio of outer to inner electrode radii.

ENERGY TRANSFER

In a quantitative sense, the biological effects of radiation depend on the amount of energy absorbed by living matter from a radiation field and by the spatial distribution in tissue of the absorbed energy. In order to comprehend the physics of tissue irradiation, some pertinent mechanisms of energy transfer must be understood.

Elastic Collision

An elastic collision is defined as a collision between two bodies in which kinetic energy and momentum are conserved; that is, the sum of the kinetic energy of the two bodies before the collision is equal to their sum after the collision, and the sums of their momenta before and after the collision are the same. In an elastic collision, the total kinetic energy is redistributed between the colliding bodies; one body gains energy at the expense of the other. A simple case is illustrated in the example below.

EXAMPLE 2.12

A block of mass 10 kg, made of a perfectly elastic material, slides on a frictionless surface with a velocity of 2 m/s and strikes a stationary elastic block whose mass is 2 kg (Fig. 2-8). How much energy was transferred from the large block (M) to the small block (m) during the collision?

Solution

If V_1, v_1, and V_2 and v_2 are the respective velocities of the large and small blocks before and after the collision, then, according to the laws of conservation of energy and momentum, we have

$$\frac{1}{2}MV_1^2 + \frac{1}{2}mv_1^2 = \frac{1}{2}MV_2^2 + \frac{1}{2}mv_2^2 \tag{2.41}$$

and

$$MV_1 + mv_1 = MV_2 + mv_2 \tag{2.42}$$

Since $v_1 = 0$, Eqs. (2.41) and (2.42) may be solved simultaneously to give

$$V_2 = 1\frac{1}{3}\,\frac{m}{s} \text{ and } v_2 = 3\frac{1}{3}\,\frac{m}{s}.$$

The kinetic energy transferred during the collision is

$$\frac{1}{2}MV_1^2 - \frac{1}{2}MV_2^2 = \frac{1}{2} \times 10\left(4 - \frac{16}{9}\right) = 11\frac{1}{9}\,\text{J},$$

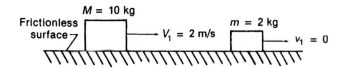

Figure 2-8. Elastic collision between blocks M and m, in which the sum of both kinetic energy and momenta of the two blocks before and after the collision are the same.

and this, of course, is the energy gained by the smaller block:

$$\frac{1}{2}mv^2 = \frac{1}{2} \times 2 \times \frac{100}{9} = 11\frac{1}{9}\,\text{J}.$$

Note that the magnitude of the force exerted by the larger block on the smaller block during the collision was not considered in the solution of Example 2.12. The reason for not explicitly considering the force in the solution can be seen from Eq. (2.10), which may be written as

$$f \times \Delta t = m \times \Delta v.$$

According to Eq. (2.10), the force necessary to change the momentum of a block is dependent on the time during which it acts. The parameter of importance in this case is the product of the force and the time. This parameter is called the impulse; Eq. (2.10) may be written in words as

Impulse = change of momentum.

The length of time during which the force acts depends on the relative velocity of the system of moving masses and on the nature of the mass. Generally, the more the colliding blocks "give in," the greater will be the time of application of the force and the smaller, consequently, will be the magnitude of the force. For this reason, for example, a baseball player who catches a ball moves his hand back at the moment of impact, thereby increasing the time during which the stopping force acts and decreasing the shock to his hand. For this same reason, a jumper flexes his knees as his feet strike the ground, thereby increasing the time that his body comes to rest and decreasing the force on his body. For example, a man who jumps down a distance of 1 m is moving with a velocity of 4.43 m/s at the instant that he strikes the floor. If he weighs 70 kg and if he lands rigidly flat footed and is brought to a complete stop in 0.01 s, then the stopping force, from Eq. (2.10), is 3.1×10^4 N, or 6980 lb. If, however, he lands on his toes and then lowers his heels and flexes his knees as he strikes, thereby increasing his actual stopping time to 0.5 s, the average stopping force is only about 140 lb.

In the case of the two blocks in Example 2.12, if the time of contact is 0.01 s, then the average force of the collision during this time interval is

$$f = \frac{10\ \text{kg} \times 0.0067\ \dfrac{\text{m}}{\text{s}}}{0.01\ \text{s}} = 6.7\ \text{N}$$

The instantaneous forces acting on the two blocks vary from zero at the instant of impact to a maximum value at some time during the collision, then to zero again as the second block leaves the first one. This may be graphically shown in Figure 2-9, a curve of force versus time during the collision. The average force during the collision is the area under the curve divided by the time that the two blocks are in contact.

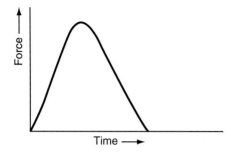

Figure 2-9. The time variation of the force between colliding bodies.

In the case of a collision between two masses, such as that described above, one block exerts a force on the other only while the two blocks are in "contact." During "contact," the two blocks seem to be physically touching each other. Actually, however, the two blocks are merely very close together, too close, in fact, for us to be able to perceive any space between them. Under this condition, the two blocks repel each other by very short-range forces that are thought to be electrical in nature. (These forces will be discussed again in Chapter 3.) This concept of a "collision" without actual contact between the colliding masses may be easily demonstrated with the aid of magnets. If magnets are affixed to the two blocks in Example 2.12, as shown in Figure 2-10, then the magnetic force, which acts over relatively long distances, will repel the two blocks, and the smaller block will move. If the total mass of each block, including the magnet, remains the same as in Example 2.12, then the calculations and results of Example 2.12 are applicable. The only difference between the physical "collision" and the magnetic "collision" is that the magnitude of the force in the former case is greater than in the latter instance, but the time during which the forces are effective is greater in the case of the magnetic "collision." In both instances, the product of average force and time is exactly the same.

Inelastic Collision

If the conditions in Figure 2-8 are modified by fastening the 2-kg block, block *B*, to the floor with a rubber band, then, in order to break the rubber band and cause the block to slide freely, the 10-kg block, block *A*, must transfer at least sufficient energy to break the rubber band. Any additional energy transferred would then appear as kinetic energy of block *B*. If the energy necessary to break the rubber band is called the *binding energy* of block *B*, then the kinetic energy of block *B* after it is struck by block *A* is equal to the difference between the energy lost by *A* and the binding energy of *B*. Algebraically, this may be written as

$$E_B = E_A - \phi, \tag{2.43}$$

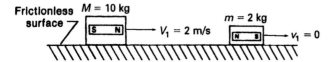

Figure 2-10. "Collision" between two magnetic fields.

where E_A is the energy lost by block A and ϕ is the binding energy of block B. In a collision of this type, where energy is expended to free one of the colliding bodies, kinetic energy is not conserved and the collision is therefore not elastic, that is, it is inelastic.

EXAMPLE 2.13

A stationary block B, whose mass is 2 kg, is held by an elastic cord whose elastic constant is 10 N/m and whose ultimate strength is 5 N. Another block A, whose mass is 10 kg, is moving with a velocity of 2 m/s on a frictionless surface. If block A strikes block B, with what velocity will block B move after the collision?

Solution

From Example 2.12, it is seen that the energy lost by block A in this collision is $11\frac{1}{9}$ J. The energy expended in breaking the rubber band may be calculated from the product of the force needed to break the elastic cord and the distance that the elastic cord stretches before breaking. In the case of a spring, rubber band, or any other substance that is elastically deformed, the deforming force is opposed by a restoring force whose magnitude is proportional to the deformation. That is,

$$f = k \times r, \tag{2.44}$$

where f is the force needed to deform the elastic body by an amount r, and k is the "spring constant" or the force per unit deformation. Since Eq. (2.44) shows that the force is not constant but rather is proportional to the deformation of the rubber band, the work done in stretching the rubber band must be computed by the application of calculus. The infinitesimal work, dW, done in stretching the rubber band through a distance dr is

$$dW = f\,dr,$$

and the total work done in stretching the rubber band from $r = 0$ to r is given by

$$W = \int_0^r f\,dr$$

Substituting Eq. (2.44) for f, we have

$$W = \int_0^r kr\,dr \tag{2.45}$$

and solving Eq. (2.45) shows the work done in stretching the rubber band to be

$$W = \frac{kr^2}{2}. \tag{2.46}$$

Since in this example k is equal to 10 N/m, the ultimate strength of the elastic cord,

5 N, is reached when the rubber band is extended to 0.5 m. With these numerical values, Eq. (2.46) may be solved:

$$W = \frac{10\frac{N}{m} \times (0.5 \text{ m})^2}{2} = 1.25\frac{N}{m} = 1.25 \text{ J}.$$

Therefore, of the $11\frac{1}{9}$ J lost by block A in its collision with block B, 1.25 J are dissipated in breaking the elastic cord (the binding energy) that holds block B. The kinetic energy of block B, using Eq. (2.43), is

$$E_B = 11.11 - 1.25 = 9.86 \text{ J}.$$

$$9.86 \text{ J} = \frac{1}{2} mv^2$$

$$9.86 \text{ J} = \frac{1}{2} (2 \text{ kg}) v^2$$

$$v = 3.14 \frac{m}{s}$$

If block A had less than 1.25 J of kinetic energy, the elastic cord would not have been broken; the restoring force in the elastic cord would have pulled block B back and caused it to oscillate about its equilibrium position. (For this oscillation to actually occur, block A would have to be withdrawn immediately after the collision, otherwise block B, on its rebound, would transfer its energy back to block A and send it back with the same velocity that it had before the first collision. The net effect of the two collisions, then, would have been only the reversal of the direction in which block A traveled.)

Waves

Energy may be transmitted by disturbing a "medium," permitting the disturbance to travel through the medium, and then collecting the energy with a suitable receiver. For example, if work is done in raising a stone and the stone is dropped into water, the potential energy of the stone before being dropped is converted into kinetic energy, which is then transferred to the water when the stone strikes. The energy gained by the water disturbs it and causes it to move up and down. This disturbance spreads out from the point of the initial disturbance at a velocity characteristic of the medium (in this case, the water). The energy can be "received" at a remote distance from the point of the initial disturbance by a bob that floats on the water. The wave, in passing by the bob, will cause the bob to move up and down, thereby imparting energy to it. It should be noted here that the *water* moves only in a vertical direction while the *disturbance* moves in the horizontal direction.

Displacement of water upward from the undisturbed surface produces a crest, while downward displacement results in a trough. The amplitude of a wave is a measure of the vertical displacement, and the distance between corresponding points on adjacent disturbances is called the wavelength (Fig. 2-11). (The wavelength is usually represented by the Greek letter lambda, λ.) The number of disturbances per second

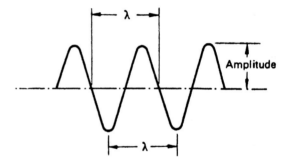

Figure 2-11. Graphical representation of a wave.

at any point in the medium is called the frequency. The velocity with which a wave (disturbance) travels is equal to the product of the wavelength and the frequency,

$$v = f \times \lambda. \tag{2.47}$$

EXAMPLE 2.14

Sound waves, which are disturbances in the air, travel through air at a velocity of 344 m/s. Middle C has a frequency of 264 Hz (cycles per second). Calculate the wavelength of this note.

Solution

$$\lambda = \frac{v}{f} = \frac{344 \dfrac{m}{s}}{264 \dfrac{1}{s}} = 1.3 \text{ m}.$$

If more than one disturbance passes through a medium at the same time, then, where the respective waves meet, the total displacement of the medium is equal to the algebraic sum of the two waves. For example, if two rocks are dropped into a pond, then, if the crests of the two waves should coincide as the waves pass each other, the resulting crest is equal to the height of the two separate crests and the trough is as deep as the sum of the two individual troughs, as shown in Figure 2-12. If, on the other hand, the two waves are exactly out of phase, that is, if the crest of one

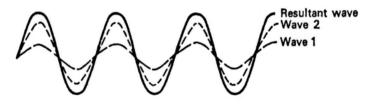

Figure 2-12. The addition of two waves of equal frequency and in phase.

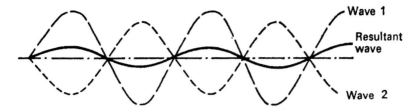

Figure 2-13. The addition of two waves of equal frequency but different amplitude and 180° out of phase.

coincides with the trough of the other, then the positive and negative displacements cancel each other, as shown in Figure 2-13. If, in Figure 2-13, wave 1 and wave 2 are of exactly the same amplitude as well as the same frequency, there would be no net disturbance. For the more general case, in which the component waves are of different frequencies, different amplitudes, and only partly out of phase, complex waveforms may be formed, as seen below in Figure 2-14.

Electromagnetic Waves

In 1820, Christian Oersted, a Danish physicist, observed that a compass needle deflected whenever it was placed in the vicinity of a current-carrying wire. He thus discovered the intimate relationship between electricity and magnetism and found that a magnetic flux coaxial with the wire is always induced in the space around a current-carrying wire. Furthermore, he found that the direction of deflection of the compass needle depended on the direction of the electric current, thus showing that the induced magnetic flux has direction as well as magnitude. The direction of the induced magnetic flux can be determined by the "right-hand rule": If the fingers of the right hand are curled around the wire, as though grasping the wire, with the thumb outstretched and pointing in the direction of conventional current flow, then the curled fingers point in the direction of the induced magnetic flux. If two parallel, current-carrying wires are near each other, they either attract or repel one another, depending on whether the currents flow in the same or in opposite directions. The attractive or repulsive force F per unit length l of wire, as shown in Figure 2-15, is proportional to the product of the currents and inversely proportional to the distance between the wires.

$$\frac{F}{l} \propto \frac{i_1 \times i_2}{r} = k_m \times \frac{i_1 \times i_2}{r}. \tag{2.48}$$

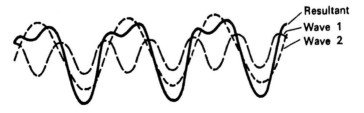

Figure 2-14. Complex wave formed by the algebraic addition of two different pure waves.

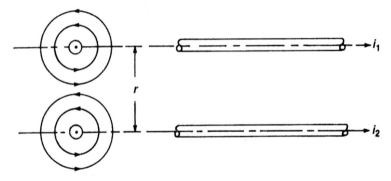

Figure 2-15. Force between two parallel current-carrying wires. The force, attractive in this case, is due to the magnetic fields (shown by the circular lines in the end view) that are generated by the electric current.

If the current-carrying wires are in free space (or in air) and if i_1 and i_2 are 1 A each and if the distance r between the wires is 1 m, then the force per unit length of wire is found to be

$$\frac{F}{l} = 2 \times 10^{-7} \frac{\text{N}}{\text{m}}.$$

The constant of proportionality k_m, therefore, is equal to 2×10^{-7} N/A². It is convenient to define k_m in terms of another constant, μ_0:

$$k_m = \frac{\mu_0}{2\pi} = 2 \times 10^{-7} \frac{\text{N}}{\text{A}^2} \tag{2.49a}$$

$$\mu_0 = 4\pi \times 10^{-7} \frac{\text{N}}{\text{A}^2}. \tag{2.49b}$$

μ_0 is called the *permeability* of free space. Permeability is a property of the medium in which magnetic flux is established. The permeability of any medium other than free space is designated by μ. The *relative permeability* of any medium, K_m is defined by

$$K_m = \frac{\mu}{\mu_0}. \tag{2.50}$$

Iron, cobalt, nickel, and gadolinium have high values of relative permeability, that is, $K_m = 1$; these substances we call *ferromagnetic*. Those substances—such as silver, copper, and bismuth—whose relative permeability is less than 1 are said to be diamagnetic. Most substances, including all biological materials, have relative permeabilities of 1 or slightly greater; these materials are called *paramagnetic*.

The unit of magnetic flux is called the *weber* (Wb):

$$1\,\text{Wb} = 1\frac{\text{J}}{\text{A}} \tag{2.51}$$

and the unit of flux density, which is a measure of magnetic intensity, is called the *tesla* (after the Croatian-born American electrical engineer Nikola Tesla), denoted by symbol T:

$$1\,\text{T} = 1\frac{\text{Wb}}{\text{m}^2}. \tag{2.52}$$

In the cgs system, the unit for magnetic flux is called the *maxwell,* and the unit for flux density is called the *gauss,* where

$$1\,\text{T} = 10{,}000\,\text{gauss}.$$

Since joules $=$ newtons $\times$ meters, the dimensions of μ_0 may be written as

$$\mu_0 = 4\pi \times 10^{-7}\,\frac{\text{J}}{\text{A}^2 \cdot \text{m}}.$$

Furthermore, since webers $\times$ amperes $=$ joules, μ_0 may also be expressed as

$$\mu_0 = 4\pi \times 10^{-7}\,\frac{\text{Wb}}{\text{A} \cdot \text{m}}.$$

The magnetic flux density, symbolized by B, at a distance r from a wire carrying a current i is given by

$$B = \frac{\mu_0}{2\pi} \times \frac{i}{r} = \frac{\text{Wb}}{\text{m}^2}. \tag{2.53}$$

 EXAMPLE 2.15

What is the magnetic flux density at a distance of 0.1 m from a wire that carries a current of 0.25 A?

Solution

Substituting the numerical values into Eq. (2.53) yields

$$B = \frac{4\pi \times 10^{-7}\,\dfrac{\text{Wb}}{\text{A} \cdot \text{m}}}{2\pi} \times \frac{0.25\,\text{A}}{0.1\,\text{m}}$$

$$= 5 \times 10^{-7}\,\frac{\text{Wb}}{\text{m}^2} = 5 \times 10^{-7}\,\text{T}.$$

In comparison, the magnetic flux density at the equator is about 3×10^{-5} T.

Any region in which there is a magnetic flux is called a magnetic field, and the field intensity (or field strength) is directly proportional to the magnetic flux density. Since magnetic flux has direction as well as magnitude, magnetic field strength is a vector quantity. Michael Faraday, a Scottish experimental physicist, found in 1831 that electricity could be generated from a magnetic field and that electricity and magnetism were related.

In 1873, James Clerk Maxwell, a Scottish physicist, published a general theory that related the experimental findings of Oersted and Faraday. He deduced the quantitative relationships among moving charged particles, magnetic fields, and electric fields and formulated an electromagnetic theory that described quantitatively the interaction between moving electric charges and magnetic fields. His theory states that a changing electric field is always associated with a changing magnetic field and a changing magnetic field is always associated with a changing electric field. He showed that an oscillating electric circuit will create an electromagnetic wave as the flowing electrons in the circuit undergo continuous acceleration and deceleration as the current oscillates. When this happens, some of the energy of the charged particle is radiated as electromagnetic radiation. This phenomenon is the basis of radio transmission, in which electrons are accelerated up and down an antenna that is connected to an oscillator. The electromagnetic wave thus generated has a frequency equal to that of the oscillator and a velocity of 3×10^8 m/s in free space. The waves consist of oscillating electric and magnetic fields that are perpendicular to each other and are mutually perpendicular to the direction of propagation of the wave (Fig. 2-16). The energy carried by the waves depends on the strength of the associated electric and magnetic fields.

In dealing with electromagnetic waves, it is more convenient to describe the magnetic component in terms of magnetic field strength H rather than in terms of magnetic flux density B. H can be considered as the magnetizing force that leads to the magnetic field of flux density B. In free space, magnetic field strength H is related to magnetic flux density B by

$$H = \frac{B \dfrac{\text{Wb}}{\text{m}^2}}{\mu_0 \dfrac{\text{Wb}}{\text{A} \cdot \text{m}}} = \frac{B}{\mu_0} \frac{\text{A}}{\text{m}}. \tag{2.54}$$

Since B has dimensions of Wb/m^2 and μ_0 has dimensions of Wb/(A $\cdot$ m), the dimensions of magnetic field strength, H, are A/m. In any medium other than air, the magnetic flux density is equal to the product of the magnetic field strength H and the magnetic permeability of that medium, μ. Safety standards for magnetic field strength are listed in terms of amperes per meter. Thus, in Example 2.15, the magnetic flux density of 5×10^{-7} T corresponds to a magnetic field strength of 0.4 A/m.

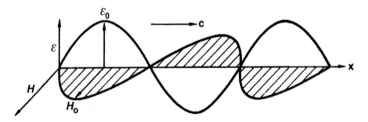

Figure 2-16. Schematic representation of an electromagnetic wave. The electric intensity ε and the magnetic intensity H are at right angles to each other, and the two are mutually perpendicular to the direction of propagation of the wave. The velocity of propagation is c, the electric intensity is $\varepsilon = \varepsilon_0 \sin 2\pi /\lambda \, (x - ct)$, and the magnetic intensity is $H = H_0 \sin 2\pi /\lambda \, (x - ct)$. The plane of polarization is the plane containing the electric field vector.

The relationship between the peak magnetic and electric field intensities H_0 and ε_0 depends on the magnetic permeability μ and the electrical permittivity ϵ of the medium through which the electromagnetic wave is propagating. This relationship is given by

$$H_0\sqrt{\mu} = \varepsilon_0\sqrt{\epsilon}, \qquad (2.55)$$

where ϵ is the permittivity of the medium. Permittivity is a measure of the capacity for storing energy in a medium that is in an electric field. The permittivity of free space is $\epsilon_0 = 8.85 \times 10^{-12}\ \mathrm{C^2/N \cdot m^2}$, and the permittivity of any other medium is the product of the relative permittivity, k_ϵ and the permittivity of free space, ϵ_0: $\epsilon = k_\epsilon \times \epsilon_0$. The greater the value of ϵ, the greater is its interaction with the ε field and the greater is its ability to store energy. Permittivity is frequency dependent and generally decreases with increasing frequency. If the wave is traveling through free space, then

$$H_0\sqrt{\mu_0} = \varepsilon_0\sqrt{\epsilon_0}. \qquad (2.56)$$

Radio waves, microwaves (radar), infrared radiation, visible light, ultraviolet light, and X-rays are all electromagnetic radiations. They are qualitatively alike but differ in wavelength to form a continuous electromagnetic spectrum.

All these radiations are transmitted through the atmosphere (which may be considered, for this purpose, as free space) at a speed very close to 3×10^8 m/s. Since the speed of all electromagnetic waves in free space is a constant, Eq. (2.47), when applied to electromagnetic waves in free space, becomes

$$c = 3 \times 10^8\ \mathrm{m/s} = f \times \lambda. \qquad (2.57)$$

Specifying either the frequency or wavelength of an electromagnetic wave in free space is equivalent to specifying both. Free-space wavelengths may range from 5×10^6 m for 60-Hz electric waves through visible light (green light has a wavelength of about 500 nanometers, or nm, and a frequency of 6×10^{14} Hz) to short-wavelength X- and gamma radiation (whose wavelengths are on the order of 10 nm or less). There is no sharp cutoff in wavelength at either end of the spectrum nor is there a sharp dividing line between the various portions of the electromagnetic spectrum. Each portion blends into the next, and the lines of demarcation, shown in Figure 2-17, are arbitrarily placed to show the approximate wavelength span of the regions of the electromagnetic spectrum.

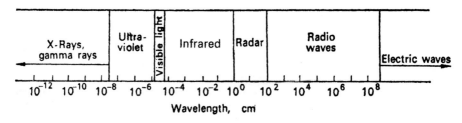

Figure 2-17. The electromagnetic spectrum.

Generally, the speed of an electromagnetic wave in any medium depends on the electrical and magnetic properties of that medium: on the permittivity and the permeability. The speed is given by

$$v = \sqrt{\frac{1}{\epsilon \mu}}. \tag{2.58}$$

In free space,

$$\mu = \mu_0 = 4\pi \times 10^{-7} \frac{N}{A}$$

$$\epsilon = \epsilon_0 = \frac{1}{4\pi \times 9 \times 10^9 \dfrac{N \cdot m^2}{C^2}}.$$

Substituting the values above into Eq. (2.58) gives the speed c of an electromagnetic wave in free space:

$$v = c = \left(\frac{4\pi \times 9 \times 10^9 \dfrac{N \cdot m^2}{C^2}}{4\pi \times 10^{-7} \dfrac{N}{A^2}} \right)^{1/2} = 3 \times 10^8 \frac{m}{s}.$$

An electromagnetic wave travels more slowly through a medium than through free space. The frequency of the electromagnetic wave is independent of the medium through which it travels. The wavelength is decreased, however, so that the relationship (Eq. [2.47]):

$$v = f \times \lambda$$

is maintained. The wavelength in a medium is given by

$$\lambda = \lambda_0 \sqrt{\frac{1}{K_e K_m}}, \tag{2.59}$$

where λ_0 is the free-space wavelength and K_e and K_m are the relative permittivity (dielectric coefficient) and relative permeability of the medium, respectively. Since the relative permeability is ≈ 1 for most biological materials and dielectrics, we can approximate Eq. (2.59) for most biological materials by

$$\lambda = \lambda_0 \sqrt{\frac{1}{K_e}}. \tag{2.60}$$

If the medium is a *lossy dielectric* (a lossy dielectric is one that absorbs energy from an electromagnetic field; all biological media are lossy), the wavelength of our electromagnetic wave within the medium is given by

$$\lambda = \frac{\lambda_0}{\sqrt{K_e}} \left[\frac{1}{2} + \frac{1}{2}\sqrt{1 + \left(\frac{\sigma}{\omega \epsilon}\right)^2} \right]^{-1/2} \tag{2.61}$$

or, in terms of the *loss tangent*,

$$\lambda = \frac{\lambda_0}{\sqrt{K_e}} \left[\frac{1}{2} + \frac{1}{2}\sqrt{1 + \tan^2 \delta} \right]^{-1/2}, \tag{2.62}$$

where

$\lambda_0 = $ free space wavelength,

$K_e = $ dielectric coefficient,

$\sigma = $ conductivity, in reciprocal ohm meters, or siemens per meter,

$\omega = 2\pi \times$ frequency,

$\in = K_e \in_0$, and

$$\tan^2 \delta = \left(\frac{\sigma}{\omega \in} \right)^2 = \text{loss tangent.} \tag{2.63}$$

EXAMPLE 2.16

The dielectric coefficient for brain tissue is $K_e = 82$ and the resistivity is $\rho = 1.88$ ohm-meters at 100 MHz. What is the wavelength of this radiation in the brain?

Solution

$$\lambda_0 = \frac{c}{f} = \frac{3 \times 10^8 \text{ m/s}}{100 \times 10^6 \frac{1}{\text{s}}} = 3 \text{ m}$$

$$\tan^2 \delta = \left(\frac{\sigma}{\omega \in} \right)^2 = \left(\frac{\sigma}{\omega K_e \in_0} \right)^2$$

$$= \left(\frac{\left(\frac{1}{1.88} \right)}{2\pi \times 100 \times 10^6 \times 82 \times \frac{1}{4\pi \times 9 \times 10^9}} \right)^2 = 1.36$$

$$\lambda = \frac{\lambda_0}{\sqrt{K_e}} \left(\frac{1}{2} + \frac{1}{2}\sqrt{1 + \tan^2 \delta} \right)^{-1/2}$$

$$\lambda = \frac{3}{\sqrt{82}} \left(\frac{1}{2} + \frac{1}{2}\sqrt{2.36} \right)^{-1/2} = 0.3 \text{ m.}$$

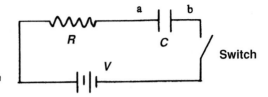

Figure 2-18. A circuit having a capacitance C and a resistance R in series with a voltage source V.

The *loss tangent* is a measure of energy absorption by a medium through which an electromagnetic wave passes; energy absorption by the medium is directly proportional to the loss tangent. The loss tangent is defined as

$$\text{Loss tangent} = \frac{\text{conduction current}}{\text{displacement current}} \qquad (2.64)$$

Conduction current is the ordinary current that consists of a flow of electrons across a potential difference in a circuit. Since no dielectric material is a perfect insulator, some small conduction current will flow through any insulating material under the influence of a potential difference. *Displacement* is a concept proposed by Maxwell to account for the apparent flow of current through an insulator—even a perfect insulator—under the action of a changing voltage.

Consider the circuit shown in Figure 2-18, a capacitor (whose dielectric is a perfect insulator), a resistor, a switch, and a battery are connected in series. While the switch is open, plate a of the capacitor is at the same potential as the positive terminal of the battery to which it is connected through the resistor. When the switch is closed, plate b of the capacitor is connected to the negative pole of the battery, and the capacitor begins to charge under the influence of the potential across the plates. Since the dielectric in this circuit is a perfect insulator, clearly no current can flow through the dielectric. However, connecting the plates of the capacitor to the battery terminals causes electrons to pile up on the negative plate and to be drained off from the positive plate. That is, electrons flow onto the plate connected to the negative terminal and flow from the other plate to the positive terminal until an equilibrium is reached when no more charge flows. Thus, during the time that the capacitor is charging, the circuit behaves *as if* current were flowing through every portion of the circuit, including the dielectric. This apparent current flowing through the dielectric is called the *displacement* current. Since no real dielectric is a perfect insulator, there always is a conduction current through the dielectric in addition to the displacement current. Furthermore, since a conduction current is always accompanied by energy loss through joule heating, there always is some loss of energy when a dielectric is placed in an electric field.

While the capacitor is charging, the displacement current in the circuit is given by

$$i = \frac{V}{R} e^{-t/RC}, \qquad (2.65)$$

and the voltage across the capacitor is given by

$$V_C = V(1 - e^{-t/RC}) \qquad (2.66)$$

where

> t = time after closing the switch (in seconds),
> R = resistance (in ohms),
> C = capacitance (in farads),
> V_C = voltage across capacitor, and
> V = battery voltage.

The product RC is called the *time constant* of the circuit and represents the time (in seconds) after closing the switch, until the current decreases to $1/e$, or 37% of the initial current, and the voltage increases to $V_0(1 - 1/e)$, or 67% of its final voltage. A charged capacitor in a circuit with a series resistor may be considered as the equivalent of a battery whose voltage, V_i, is the voltage across the capacitor. When such a circuit is closed, the capacitor will discharge through the resistor and the capacitor's voltage, V_C, will decrease according to

$$V_c = V_i e^{-t/RC},\tag{2.67}$$

and the charge on each plate of the capacitor is given by

$$Q = C V_C.\tag{2.68}$$

Impedance

While electric current in a circuit is transmitted as electrons flow through conducting wires, electromagnetic waves are transmitted as disturbances in the electromagnetic fields established in various media, including a vacuum (free space). The electric and magnetic components of the field may be considered the analogs of voltage and current in an electrical circuit. The impedance Z of an alternating current is given by Ohm's law:

$$Z = \frac{V}{i},\tag{2.69}$$

where i is the current flow due to the voltage V. By analogy, the impedance of a medium through which an electromagnetic wave is propagated is given by

$$Z = \frac{\varepsilon_0}{H_0},\tag{2.70}$$

where ε_0 and H_0 are the electric and magnetic field strengths respectively. Using the relationship given by Eq. (2.55),

$$H_0 \sqrt{\mu} = \varepsilon_0 \sqrt{\epsilon},$$

we can rewrite Eq. (2.70) as

$$Z = \sqrt{\frac{\mu}{\epsilon}}.\tag{2.71}$$

In free space,

$$\mu = \mu_0 = 4\pi \times 10^{-7} \frac{N}{A^2}$$

$$\epsilon = \epsilon_0 = \frac{1}{4\pi \times 9 \times 10^9 \ \frac{N \cdot m^2}{C^2}}.$$

Using these values in Eq. (2.71), one obtains

$$Z = \left[\frac{4\pi \times 10^{-7} \ \frac{N}{A^2}}{\left(\frac{1}{4\pi \cdot 9 \times 10^9 \ \frac{N \cdot m^2}{C^2}} \right)} \right]^{1/2} = 377 \ \Omega,$$

which is the impedance of free space.

In an electric circuit, the power dissipated in a load whose impedance is Z ohms, across which the voltage drop is V volts and the current is i amperes, is given by

$$P = \frac{V^2}{Z} = i^2 Z. \tag{2.72}$$

The analogous quantities in an electromagnetic field of mean power density $\bar{P} \ \frac{W}{m^2}$ and effective electric field strength, $\bar{\varepsilon} \ \frac{V}{m}$, are related by

$$\bar{P} = \frac{(\bar{\varepsilon})^2}{Z} = \frac{\left(\frac{\varepsilon_0}{\sqrt{2}} \right)^2}{Z} = \left(\frac{H_0}{\sqrt{2}} \right)^2 \times Z, \tag{2.73}$$

where ε_0 is the maximum value of the sinusoidally varying electric field strength and $\varepsilon_0/\sqrt{2}$ is the effective or root-mean-square (rms) value of the electric field strength. In free space, where $Z = 377$ ohms, the effective power density corresponding to $\varepsilon_0 = 1 \frac{V}{m}$ is

$$\bar{P} = \frac{\left(\frac{1}{\sqrt{2}} \right)^2}{377} = 1.33 \times 10^{-3} \frac{W}{m^2} = 1.33 \times 10^{-4} \frac{mW}{cm^2}.$$

Energy in an electromagnetic wave is transported in a direction mutually perpendicular to the electric and magnetic field vectors, as shown in Figure 2-16. The instantaneous rate of energy flow in an electromagnetic wave through a unit area perpendicular to the direction of propagation is given by the vector product

$$\bar{P} = \varepsilon \times H. \tag{2.74}$$

The vector $\bar{\boldsymbol{P}}$, which represents the flow of energy, is called the *Poynting vector*. Since the instantaneous values of $\boldsymbol{\varepsilon}$ and $\boldsymbol{H}$ vary sinusoidally from 0 to their maxima, their effective values are $\varepsilon_0/\sqrt{2}$ and $H_0/\sqrt{2}$. Since the magnetic and electric field vectors are always at $90°$ to each other, Eq. (2.72) may be rewritten as

$$\bar{P} = \frac{\varepsilon_0}{\sqrt{2}} \times \frac{H_0}{\sqrt{2}} = \frac{1}{2}\varepsilon_0 H_0. \tag{2.75}$$

 ## EXAMPLE 2.17

The electric field intensity ε_0 of a plane electromagnetic wave is $1 \frac{V}{m}$. What is the average power density perpendicular to the direction of the propagation of the wave?

Solution

From Eq. (2.73), the average power density is

$$\bar{P} = \frac{1}{2}\varepsilon_0 H_0,$$

and from Eq. (2.56), H_0 is found to be

$$H_0 = \varepsilon_0 \sqrt{\frac{\epsilon_0}{\mu_0}}.$$

If we substitute the expression above for H_0 into Eq. (2.73), and insert the numerical values for ϵ_0 and for μ_0, we have

$$\bar{P} = \frac{1}{2}\left(1\frac{V}{m}\right)\left(1\frac{V}{m^2}\right)\sqrt{\frac{\left(\dfrac{1}{4\pi \cdot 9\times10^9}\dfrac{N \cdot m^2}{C^2}\right)}{4\pi \times 10^{-7}\frac{N}{A^2}}}$$

$$= 1.33 \times 10^{-3} \ \frac{W}{m^2}$$

$$= 1.33 \times 10^{-4} \ \frac{mW}{cm^2}.$$

For health physics purposes, the electromagnetic spectrum may be divided into two major portions: One portion, called *ionizing radiation*, extends from the shortest wavelengths to about several nanometers. Electromagnetic radiation of these wavelengths include X-rays and gamma rays (X-rays and gamma rays are exactly the same type of radiations; they differ only in their manner of origin. Once created, it is impossible to distinguish between these two types.). Electromagnetic radiation whose wavelength exceeds that of ionizing radiation is called *nonionizing radiation*. In this region, the health physicist is interested mainly in laser radiation—which includes ultraviolet, visible, and infrared light—and in the high-frequency bands from about 3 megahertz (MHz) to 300 gigahertz (GHz). Although ultraviolet light is capable of producing ions, it nevertheless is considered as a nonionizing radiation in the context of radiation safety.

QUANTUM THEORY

The representation of light and other electromagnetic radiations as a continuous train of periodic disturbances or a "wave train" in an electromagnetic field is a satisfactory model that can be used to explain many physical phenomena and can serve as a basis for the design of apparatus for transmitting and receiving electromagnetic energy. According to this wave theory, or the classical theory, as it is often called, the amount of energy transmitted by a wave is proportional to the square of the amplitude of the wave. This model, despite its usefulness, fails to predict certain phenomena in the field of modern physics. Accordingly, a new model for electromagnetic radiation was postulated, one that could "explain" certain phenomena which were not amenable to explanation by wave theory. It should be emphasized that hypothesizing a new theory was not synonymous with abandoning the former theory. Models or theories are useful insofar as they describe observed phenomena and permit prediction of the consequences of certain actions. Philosophically, most scientists subscribe to the school of thought known as "logical positivism." According to this philosophy, there is no way to discover or to verify an absolute truth. Science is not concerned with absolute truth or reality—it is concerned with giving the simplest possible unified description of as many experimental findings as possible. It follows, therefore, that several different theories on the nature of electromagnetic radiation (or for the nature of matter, energy, electricity, etc.) are perfectly acceptable provided that each theory is capable of explaining experimentally observed facts that the others cannot explain.

Experimental observations on the nature of electromagnetic radiation, such as the radiation emitted from heated bodies, the photoelectric effect, and Compton scattering could not be explained by classical wave theory. This led to the development of the current theory of electromagnetic radiation, which is called the *quantum theory*. According to this theory, electromagnetic radiation consists of discrete "corpuscles" or "particles" of energy that travel in space at a speed of 3×10^8 m/s. Each particle or "quantum," as it is called, contains a discrete quantity of electromagnetic energy. The energy content of a quantum is proportional to the frequency when it is considered as a wave, and is given by the relationship

$$E = hf. \tag{2.76}$$

The symbol h is called *Planck's constant* and is a fundamental constant of nature whose magnitude in SI units is $h = 6.6 \times 10^{-34}$ J · s. The energy E in Eq. (2.74) therefore is in joules and the frequency is in hertz.

After substituting the value of f from Eq. (2.57) into Eq. (2.74), we have

$$E = h\frac{c}{\lambda}. \tag{2.77}$$

A quantum of electromagnetic energy is also called a *photon*. Equations (2.76) and (2.77) show that a photon is completely described when either its energy, frequency, or wavelength is given.

EXAMPLE 2.18

(a) Radio station KDKA in Pittsburgh, Pennsylvania, broadcasts on a carrier frequency of 1020 kHz.

(1) What is the wavelength of the carrier frequency?

Solution

$$\lambda f = c$$

$$\lambda = \frac{c}{f} = \frac{3 \times 10^8 \frac{m}{s}}{1.02 \times 10^3 \text{ kHz} \times 10^3 \frac{\text{Hz}}{\text{kHz}}} = 294 \text{ m}.$$

(2) What is energy of the KDKA photon in joules and electron volts?

Solution

$$E = hf$$

$$= 6.626 \times 10^{-34} \text{ J} \cdot \text{s} \times 1.02 \times 10^6 \frac{1}{s}$$

$$= 6.8 \times 10^{-28} \text{ J}$$

and

$$E = \frac{6.8 \times 10^{-28} \text{ J}}{1.6 \times 10^{-19} \frac{\text{J}}{\text{eV}}}$$

$$= 4.2 \times 10^{-9} \text{ eV}$$

(b) What is the energy, in electron volts, of an X-ray photon whose wavelength is 1×10^{-10} m?

Solution

$$E = h\frac{c}{\lambda}$$

$$= \frac{6.626 \times 10^{-34} \text{ J} \cdot \text{s} \times 3 \times 10^8 \frac{m}{s}}{10^{-10} \text{ m} \times 1.6 \times 10^{-19} \frac{\text{J}}{\text{eV}}}$$

$$= 1.24 \times 10^4 \text{ eV}$$

The wavelengths of X-rays and gamma rays are very short: on the order of 10^{-10} m or less. Because of this, and in order to avoid writing the factor 10^{-10} repeatedly, another unit of length called the *angstrom unit* is commonly used in X-ray work and in health physics. The angstrom unit, symbolized by Å, is equal to 1×10^{-10} m or 1×10^{-8} cm. Another unit of length that is often used is the nanometer (nm). One nm represents 1×10^{-9} m, which is equal to 10 Å.

It may seem strange that having found the wave theory of electromagnetic radiation inadequate to explain certain observed physical phenomena we should incorporate part of the wave model into the quantum model of electromagnetic radiation. This dualism, however, seems to be inherent in the "explanations" of atomic and nuclear physics. Mass and energy—particle and wave, in the case of electromagnetic energy—and, as will be shown below, wave and particle in the case of subatomic particles, all are part of a dualism in nature; either aspect of this dualism can be demonstrated in the laboratory by appropriate experiments. If the experiment is designed to recognize a particle, a particle will be found. If, on the other hand, an experiment is designed to recognize radiation from the same source as waves, the results show that the same radiation that had been previously identified as being particulate in nature is now a wave!

In the case of the photon, some degree of correspondence with the classical picture of electromagnetic radiation can be demonstrated by a simple thought experiment. It is conceivable that, given a very large number of waves of different frequencies and amplitudes, a wave packet, or quantum, could result from reinforcement of the waves over a very limited region and complete interference ahead and behind of the region of reinforcement. Figure 2-19 is an attempt to graphically portray such a phenomenon.

The model of a photon shown in Figure 2-19 combines wave properties and particle properties. Furthermore, this model suggests that a photon may be considered a moving particle that is guided in its path by the waves that combine to produce the particle. The "mass" of a photon may be found by equating its energy with the relativistic energy of a moving particle.

$$E = hf = mc^2, \tag{2.78a}$$

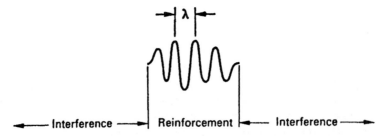

Figure 2-19. Possible combination of electromagnetic waves to produce a wave packet, a quantum of electromagnetic energy called a *photon*. The energy content of the photon is $E = hc/\lambda$.

therefore,

$$m = \frac{hf}{c^2}.$$ (2.78b)

The "momentum" p of the photon is

$$p = mc = \frac{hf}{c}.$$ (2.79)

If the value of f from Eq. (2.57) is substituted into Eq. (2.79), we have

$$p = \frac{h}{\lambda},$$ (2.80)

and the energy of the photon, in terms of its momentum, is

$$E = pc.$$ (2.81)

Matter Waves

In 1924, Louis de Broglie, a French physicist, suggested that all moving particles were associated with wave properties. The length of these waves, according to de Broglie, was inversely proportional to the momentum of the moving particle and the constant of proportionality was Planck's constant h. The length of these matter waves is given by Eq. (2.77b). Since momentum p is equal to mv, Eq. (2.77b) may be rewritten as

$$\lambda = \frac{h}{mv}.$$ (2.82)

Here too, as in the case of the photon, we have in the same equation, properties characteristic of particles and properties characteristic of waves. The mass of the moving particle m in Eq. (2.79) represents a particle, while λ, the wavelength of the "matter wave" associated with the moving particle, is quite clearly a wave concept.

The fact that moving particles possess wave properties is the basis of the electron microscope. In any kind of microscope, whether using beams of light waves or beams of de Broglie matter waves, the resolving power (the ability to separate two points that are close together, or the ability to see the edges of a very small object sharply and distinctly) is an inverse function of the wavelength of the probing beam; a shorter wavelength leads to greater resolution than a longer wavelength. For this reason, optical microscopes are usually illuminated with blue light since blue is near the short-wavelength end of the visible spectrum. Under optimum conditions, the limit of resolution of an optical microscope, using blue light whose wavelength is about 4000 Å, is of the order of 100 nm. Since high-velocity electrons are associated with very much shorter wavelengths than blue light, an electron microscope, which uses a beam of electrons instead of visible light, has a much greater resolving power than the best optical microscope. Since useful magnification is limited by resolving power, the increased resolution of an electron microscope permits much greater useful magnification than could be obtained with an optical microscope.

EXAMPLE 2.19

What is the de Broglie wavelength of an electron that is accelerated across a potential difference of 100,000 V?

Solution

According to Eq. (2.20), the kinetic energy of a moving particle with a velocity $v = \beta c$ is

$$E_k = m_0 c^2 \left(\frac{1}{\sqrt{1 - \beta^2}} - 1 \right),$$

from which it follows that

$$\frac{m_0 c^2}{E_k + m_0 c^2} = \sqrt{1 - \beta^2}. \tag{2.83}$$

In Example 2.7, we found that $m_0 c^2$ for an electron is 5.1×10^5 eV. We therefore have, after substituting the appropriate numerical values into Eq. (2.80),

$$\frac{5.1 \times 10^5 \text{ eV}}{1 \times 10^5 \text{ eV} + 5.1 \times 10^5 \text{ eV}} = \sqrt{1 - \beta^2}$$

$$0.836 = \sqrt{1 - \beta^2}$$

$$(0.836)^2 = 1 - \beta^2$$

$$\beta = 0.55$$

The momentum of the electron is

$$p = mv = \frac{m_0}{\sqrt{1 - \beta^2}} \beta c$$

$$= \frac{9.11 \times 10^{-31} \text{ kg} \times 0.55 \times 3 \times 10^8 \, \frac{\text{m}}{\text{s}}}{0.836}$$

$$= 1.8 \times 10^{-22} \, \frac{\text{kg} \cdot \text{m}}{\text{s}}$$

and the de Broglie wavelength, consequently is

$$\lambda = \frac{h}{p} = \frac{6.626 \times 10^{-34} \text{ J} \cdot \text{s}}{1.8 \times 10^{-22} \text{ kg} \cdot \text{m/s}}$$

$$= 3.7 \times 10^{-12} \text{ m} = 0.037 \, \text{Å}$$

The wave–particle dualism may seem especially abstract when it is extended to include particles of matter whose existence may be confirmed by our experience, our senses, and our intuition. At first it may seem that the wave properties of particles are purely mathematical figments of our imagination whose only purpose is to quantitatively describe experimental phenomena that are not otherwise amenable to theoretical analysis. Even in this regard, the wave–particle dualism serves a useful purpose. It is possible to give a physical interpretation of matter waves. According to the physical theory of waves, the intensity of a wave is proportional to the square of the amplitude of the wave.

In 1926, Max Born applied this concept to the wave properties of matter. In the case of a beam of electrons, the square of the amplitude of the electron waves was postulated to be proportional to the intensity of the electron beam or to the number of electrons per square centimeter per second incident on a plane perpendicular to the direction of the beam. If this beam should strike a crystal, as in the case shown in Figure 2-20, the reflected electron waves would either reinforce or interfere with each other to produce an interference pattern. The waves are reinforced most strongly at certain points and at other points are exactly out of phase, thereby canceling each other out. Where reinforcement occurs, we observe a maximum density of electrons, whereas interference results in a decrease in electron density. The exact distribution of the interference pattern is determined by the crystalline structure of the scatterer and therefore is uniquely representative of the scatterer.

The duality of nature was further verified in 1927 when two experimenters in the Bell Telephone Laboratories, Davisson and Germer, found a beam of electrons to behave like a wave (Fig. 2-20). When they bombarded a nickel crystal with a fine beam of electrons whose kinetic energy was 54 eV, they found the electrons to be reflected only in certain directions, rather than isotropically as expected. Only at angles of 50° and 0° (directly backscattered) were scattered electrons detected. Such a behavior was unexplainable if the bombarding electrons were considered to be particles. By assuming them to be waves, however, the observed distribution of scattered electrons could easily be explained. The explanation was that the electron "waves" underwent destructive interference at all angles except those at which they were observed; there the electron waves reinforced each other. At the same time the British physicist G.P. Thomson (son of the 1906 Nobel laureate in physics, J.J. Thomson), working at the University of Aberdeen, found that a beam of high-energy

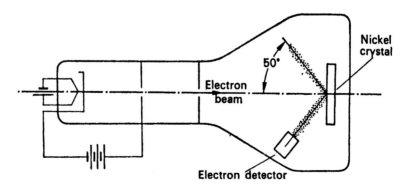

Figure 2-20. Experiment of Davisson and Germer suggesting the wave nature of electrons.

electrons could be diffracted by a thin metal foil, thereby demonstrating the wave properties of electrons. For their work in verifying the wave–particle duality, Davisson, Germer, and Thomson were awarded the Nobel Prize in 1937. Earlier, in 1927, A.H. Compton received the Nobel Prize for demonstrating the particle properties of electromagnetic waves. These experiments led to the development of electron diffraction methods used by physical chemists to identify unknowns.

For a beam of electrons, this relationship between wave and particle properties seems reasonable. In the case of a single electron, however, the electron wave must be interpreted differently. If, instead of bombarding the crystal in Figure 2-20 with a beam of electrons, the electrons were fired at the crystal one at a time and each scattered electron were detected, the single electrons would be found scattered through the same angles as the beam of electrons. The exact coordinates of any particular electron, however, would not be known until it was "seen" by the electron detector. After firing the same number of single electrons as those in the beam and plotting the position of each scattered electron, exactly the same "interference" pattern would be observed as in the case of a beam off electron waves. This experiment shows that, although the behavior of a single electron cannot be precisely predicted, the behavior of a group of electrons can be predicted. From this, it was inferred that the scattering of a single electron was a stochastic event and that the square of the amplitude at any point on the curve of position versus electron intensity gives the probability of a single electron being scattered through that point.

Uncertainty Principle

The implication of Born's probability interpretation of the wave properties of matter were truly revolutionary. According to classical physics, if the position, mass, velocity, and all the external forces on a particle are known, then, in principle, all of its future actions could be precisely predicted. According to the wave-mechanical model, however, precise predictions are not possible—probability replaces certainty. Werner Heisenberg, in 1927, developed these ideas still further and postulated his *uncertainty theory* in which he said that it is impossible, in principle, to know both the exact location and momentum of a moving particle at any point in time. Any one of these two quantities could be determined to any desired degree of accuracy. The accuracy of one quantity, however, decreases as the precision of the other quantity increases. The product of the two uncertainties was shown by Heisenberg to be proportional to Planck's constant h and to be given by the relationship

$$\Delta x \times \Delta p \geq \frac{h}{2\pi}. \tag{2.84}$$

It should be emphasized that the uncertainty expressed by Heisenberg is not due to faulty measuring tools or techniques or due to experimental errors. It is a fundamental limitation of nature, which is due to the fact that any measurement must disturb the object being measured. Precise knowledge about anything can therefore never be attained. In many instances, this inherent uncertainty can be understood intuitively. When students are being tested, for example, it is common knowledge that they may become tense or suffer some other psychological stress that may cast some doubt on the accuracy of the test results. In any case, the tester cannot be absolutely certain that the psychological stress of the examination did not influence the results of the examination. The uncertainty expressed by Eq. (2.84) can be illustrated by an example in which we try to locate a particle by looking at it. To "see" a particle means that light is reflected from the particle into the eye. When a quantum of light strikes the particle and is reflected toward the eye, some energy is transferred from the quantum to the particle, thereby changing both the position and momentum of the particle. The reflected photon tells the observer where the particle *was*, not where it *is*.

SUMMARY

The scientific basis of health physics is the transfer of energy from a radiation field to a biological system or to a nonliving medium. The quantitative aspects of energy transfer are important because radiation bioeffects are dependent on the quantity of energy absorbed by the living system. All measurements include a standard amount (or a unit amount) of the quantity being measured, such as a gram when we are measuring mass, and the number of such units. The *centimeter–gram–second (cgs)* system of units was originally used in health physics. In this system, energy and work are measured in *ergs* and the concentration of absorbed energy is measured in *ergs per gram*. Although the U.S. Nuclear Regulatory Commission continues to use the cgs system in its regulations, the International Commission on Radiological Protection and the International Commission on Radiological Units and Measurements changed from using the cgs system of units to the *International System of Units* commonly called the *SI system*. The SI system is based on *kilogram–meter–second (mks)* units. In this system, the unit of energy is the *joule* (J) and the concentration of energy is expressed in *joules per kilogram*. Power, which is defined as the *rate of energy expenditure,* is expressed in *watts* (W) and is defined as $1W = 1 J/s$.

Energy may be classified either as *potential* or *kinetic* energy or by its physical form such as electrical, mechanical, chemical, heat, electromagnetic, or nuclear. Potential energy is stored and is not doing any work. Potential energy can be converted into kinetic energy, which is defined as the *energy of a moving body*. Kinetic energy is expended in doing work. The total energy in a system is the sum of potential and kinetic energies. According to classical physics, both mass and energy are independent entities and neither one can be created or destroyed. They can only be changed from one form into another. Thus, energy can be changed from chemical to heat to mechanical to electrical, as in the case of generation of electricity in a fossil fuel power plant. Matter can be changed from solid to liquid to gas and from one substance into another, as in the case of chemical reactions. According to modern physics, mass and energy are different manifestations of the same thing. One of Einstein's principles of relativity says that the energy equivalence of mass is directly proportional to the speed of light squared: $E = mc^2$. Since, according to Einstein, nothing can move as fast as the speed of light, energy that is added to a body whose speed is approaching that of light appears as increased mass rather than as increased speed.

The elements may be considered to consist of three elementary particles: one electrically neutral particle called a *neutron* and two electrically charged particles called proton and electron. (Neutrons and protons, in turn, are believed to be made of still more fundamental particles called quarks.). Although the proton and the electron have the same amount of charge, they are qualitatively different; the protons are positively charged and electrons are negatively charged. The unit for measuring the quantity of electric charge is the *coulomb* (C) and the charge on the electron and on the proton is 1.6×10^{-19} C. Charged particles establish electric fields that exert repulsive forces on like charged particles and attractive forces on unlike charged particles. The electric potential at a point in an electric field, which is expressed in units of *volts* (V), is a measure of the potential energy of a charged particle at that point. The potential energy of an electron in a field where the potential is 1 V is

$$1\,V \times\ 1.6 \times 10^{-19}C = 1.6 \times 10^{-19}\,J.$$

Based on this relationship, we define a special unit of energy, the *electron volt* (eV) as

$$1\,eV = 1.6 \times 10^{-19}J.$$

A potential difference of 1 V exists between two points in an electric field if 1 J of energy is expended in moving I C of charge between the two points. Electric current is a flow of charged particles and is measured in *amperes* (A). One ampere represents a flow of 1 C/s. A moving electrically charged particle or an electric current flowing through a conductor generates a magnetic field. Thus, moving charges and electric currents have associated electric and magnetic fields called *electromagnetic fields* or *electromagnetic radiation*. The magnitude of the electromagnetic field is expressed in units of *volts per meter* (V/m) and the magnetic field in units of *amperes per meter* (A/m). The intensities of these fields vary sinusoidally with time. Therefore, an electromagnetic field can be described by a sine wave where the amplitude of the wave at any particular time represents the instantaneous magnitude of the electric or magnetic field at that time. In this representation, the energy content of the electromagnetic wave is proportional to the square of the amplitude of the sine wave. Once generated, the electromagnetic radiations travel through space at a speed c, which is very close to 3×10^8 m/s. The frequency f and wavelength λ of the sine wave representation of an electromagnetic field are related by

$$f \times \lambda = c.$$

Radio waves, microwaves, visible light, ultraviolet radiation, X-rays, and gamma rays are all parts of the continuous electromagnetic spectrum; they differ only in wavelengths and frequencies.

Certain phenomena that had been observed in experiments with light were not amenable to explanation in terms of the wave theory of electromagnetic radiation, experiments in which the energy content of the light was found to depend on the color of the light rather than on the intensity of the light. The *quantum theory* was postulated to explain these observations. This theory says that electromagnetic radiation consists of particles containing discrete quanta of energy and that the energy content of an electromagnetic field is proportional to the density of these quanta and to their energy content. The energy content of a single quantum is directly proportional to its frequency as measured according to the wave model, and is given by

$$E = hf,$$

where h is called Planck's constant, and is equal to 6.6262×10^{-34} J s.

According to quantum theory, high-speed particles have wave properties. The wavelength of a "matter" wave is called the *de Broglie wavelength* after its discoverer. For a particle of mass m moving at a velocity v, the de Broglie wavelength is

$$\lambda = \frac{h}{mv}.$$

These de Broglie waves are the basis for the electron microscope, where the image is formed by matter waves rather than by light waves, as in the optical microscope.

Another consequence of the quantum theory is that we cannot determine simultaneously the exact position and the exact energy of a particle. This is due to the fact that the act of measuring either of these two variables disturbs the particle so that the other variable cannot be precisely measured. The product of the uncertainty in the particle's momentum, Δp, and in its location, Δx, is given by Heisenberg's uncertainty principle as

$$\Delta p \times \Delta x \geq \frac{h}{2\pi}.$$

PROBLEMS

2.1. Two blocks of mass 0.1 kg and 0.2 kg approach each other on a frictionless surface at velocities of 0.4 and 1 m/s respectively. If the blocks collide and remain together, calculate their joint velocity after the collision.

2.2. A bullet whose mass is 50 g travels at a velocity of 500 m/s. It strikes a rigidly fixed wooden block and penetrates a distance of 20 cm before coming to a stop.

(**a**) What is the deceleration rate of the bullet?

(**b**) What is the deceleration force?

(**c**) What was the initial momentum of the bullet?

(**d**) What was the impulse of the collision?

2.3. Compute the mass of the earth, assuming it to be a sphere of 25,000 miles circumference, if at its surface it attracts a mass of 1 g with a force of 980 dynes.

2.4. An automobile weighing 2000 kg and going at a speed of 60 km/h collides with a truck weighing 5 metric tons that was moving perpendicular to the direction of the automobile at a speed of 4 km/h. If the two vehicles become joined in the collision, what is the magnitude and direction of their velocity relative to the automobile's original direction?

2.5. A small electrically charged sphere of mass 0.1 g hangs by a thread 100-cm long between two parallel vertical plates spaced 6-cm apart. If 100 V are across the plates and if the charge on the sphere is 10^{-9} C, what angle does the thread make with the vertical direction?

2.6. A capacitor has a capacitance of 10 μF. How much charge must be removed to cause a decrease of 20 V across the capacitor?

2.7. A small charged particle whose mass is 0.01 g remains stationary in space when it is placed into an upward directed electric field of 10 V/cm. What is the charge on the particle?

2.8. A 1-micron-diameter droplet of oil, whose specific gravity is 0.9, is introduced into an electric field between two large horizontal parallel plates that are 5-mm apart, across which there is a potential difference of V volts. If the oil droplet carries a net charge of 100 electrons, how many volts must be applied across the plates if the droplet is to remain suspended in the space between the plates?

2.9. A diode vacuum tube consists of a cathode and an anode spaced 5-mm apart. If 300 V are applied across the plates:

   (a) What is the velocity of an electron midway between the electrodes and at the instant of striking the plate, if the electrons are emitted from the cathode with zero velocity?

   (b) If the plate current is 20 mA, what is the average force exerted on the anode?

2.10. Calculate the ratios v/c and m/m_0 for a 1-MeV electron and for a 1-MeV proton.

2.11. Assuming an uncertainty in the momentum of an electron equal to one-half its momentum, calculate the uncertainty in position of a 1-MeV electron.

2.12. If light quanta have mass, they should be attracted by the earth's gravity. To test this hypothesis, a parallel beam of light is directed horizontally at a receiver 10 miles away. How far would the photons have fallen during their flight to the receiver if indeed they have mass?

2.13. The maximum wavelength of UV light that can produce the photoelectric effect in tungsten is 2730 Å. What will be the kinetic energy of photoelectrons produced by UV radiation of 1500 Å?

2.14. Calculate the uncertainty in position of an electron that was accelerated across a potential difference of $100,000 \pm 100$ V.

2.15. **(a)** What voltage is required to accelerate a proton from zero velocity to a velocity corresponding to a de Broglie wavelength of 0.01 Å?

   (b) What is the kinetic energy of an electron with this wavelength?

   (c) What is the energy of an X-ray photon whose wavelength is 0.01 Å?

2.16. A current of 25 mA flows through a 25-gauge wire, 0.0179 in. (17.9 mils) in diameter. If there are 5×10^{22} free electrons per cubic centimeter in copper, calculate the average speed with which electrons flow in the wire.

2.17. An electron starts at rest on the negative plate of a parallel plate capacitor and is accelerated by a potential of 1000 volts across a 1-cm gap.

   (a) With what velocity does the electron strike the positive plate?

   (b) How long does it take the electron to travel the 1-cm distance?

2.18. A cylindrical capacitor is made of two coaxial conductors—the outer one's diameter is 20.2 mm and the inner one's diameter is 0.2 mm. The inner conductor is 1000-V positive with respect to the outer conductor. Repeat parts (a) and (b) of Problem 2.17, and compare the results to those of Problem 2.17.

2.19. Two electrons are initially at rest, separated by 0.1 nm. After the electrons are released, they repel each other. What is the kinetic energy of each electron when they are 1.0-nm apart?

2.20. A cyclotron produces a 100-μA beam of 15-MeV deuterons. If the cyclotron were 100% efficient in converting electrical energy into kinetic energy of the deuterons, what is the minimum required power input, (in kilowatts)?

2.21. A 1-μF capacitor is fully charged to 100 V by connecting it across the terminals of a 100-V battery. The charged capacitor is then removed from the battery and connected in parallel to an uncharged 2-μF capacitor as shown below.

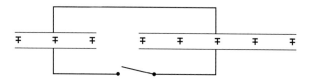

    (a) What is the charge on each capacitor after the switch is closed?

    (b) What is the voltage across the capacitors after the charge is redistributed?

2.22. **(a)** What voltage must be applied across two electrodes separated by 2-cm high vacuum in order to have an electron starting from rest on the negative electrode strike the positive plate in 10^{-8} s?

    (b) With what speed will the electron strike the plate?

2.23. When hydrogen burns, it combines with oxygen according to

$$2H_2 + O_2 \rightarrow 2H_2O.$$

About 2.3×10^5 J of heat energy in the production of 1 mol of water. What is the fractional reduction in the mass of the reactants in this reaction?

2.24. **(a)** A 1000-MW(e) nuclear power plant operates at a thermal efficiency of 33% and at 75% capacity for 1 year. How many kilograms of nuclear fuel are consumed during the year?

    (b) If a coal-fired plant operates at the same efficiency and capacity factor, how many kilograms coal must be burned during the year if the heat content of the coal is 27 MJ/kg (11, 700 Btu/lb)?

2.25. The solar constant is defined as the rate at which solar radiant energy falls on the earth's atmosphere on a surface normal to the incident radiation. The mean value for the solar constant is 1353 W/m^2, and the mean distance of the earth from the sun is 1.5×10^8 km.

    (a) At what rate is energy being emitted from the sun?

    (b) At what rate, in metric tons per second, is the sun's mass being converted into energy?

2.26. What is the energy of a photon whose momentum is equal to that of a 10-MeV electron?

2.27. What is the wavelength of

   (a) an electron whose kinetic energy is 1000 eV?

   (b) a 10^{-8}-kg oil droplet falling at the rate of 0.01 m/s?

   (c) a 1-MeV neutron?

2.28. The specific heat of water in the English system of units is 1 Btu per pound per degree Fahrenheit; in the cgs system, it is 1 calorie per gram per degree Celsius.

   (a) Calculate the number of joules per British thermal unit if there are 4.186 J/cal.

   (b) What is the specific heat of water, in $J/kg \cdot {}^{\circ}C$?

2.29. The maximum amplitude of the electric vector in a plane wave in free space is 275 V/m.

   (a) What is the amplitude of the magnetic field vector?

   (b) What is the rms value of the electric vector?

   (c) What is the power density, in mW/cm^2 in this electromagnetic field?

2.30. An electromagnetic wave has a frequency of 2450 MHz and a maximum electric field intensity of 100 mV/m. What is the

   (a) power density in this field, mW/cm^2?

   (b) maximum magnetic field intensity in this wave?

2.31. A radio station transmits at a power of 50,000 W. Assuming the electromagnetic energy to be isotropically radiated (in the case of a real radio transmitter, emission is not isotropic):

   (a) What is the mean power density (mW/cm^2), at a distance of 50 km?

   (b) What is the maximum electric field strength at that distance?

   (c) What is the maximum magnetic field strength at that distance?

2.32. The mean value for the solar constant is $1.94 \, cal/min \cdot cm^2$. Calculate the electric and magnetic field strengths corresponding to the solar constant.

2.33. How many cubic meters of water must fall over a dam 10-m high in order to generate the electricity needed to keep a 100 W bulb lit for 1 year if the overall efficiency of the hydroelectric generating station is 20%?

2.34. (a) Calculate the speed of a 25-MeV proton.

   (b) What is the percent increase in mass of this proton over its rest mass?

2.35. A neutron passes two points 10.0-m apart in 10 μs. Calculate the neutron's energy in units of

   (a) joules,

   (b) ergs, and

   (c) electron volts.

2.36. A 10-MeV proton is injected into a 2-T magnetic field at an angle of 30° to the field. Calculate the

   (a) velocity of the 10-MeV proton and

   (b) magnitude of the magnetic force acting on the proton.

2.37. **(a)** Calculate the speed of a

   (i) 0.5-MeV electron.

   (ii) 25-MeV electron.

(b) How much greater than the rest mass is the mass of each of the energetic electrons?

SUGGESTED READINGS

Born, M. *Atomic Physics,* 8th ed. Hafner, Darien, CT, 1970.

Einstein, A. *Relativity.* Crown Publishers, New York, 1961.

Feynman, R. P., Leighton, R. B., and Sands, M. *The Feynman Lectures on Physics.* Addison-Wesley, Reading, MA, 1965.

Griffiths, D. *Introduction to Electrodynamics,* 3rd ed. Prentice Hall, Englewood Cliffs, NJ, 1998.

Halliday, D., Resnick, R., and Walker, J. *Fundamentals of Physics,* 7th ed. John Wiley & Sons, New York, 2004.

Hawking, S. *A Brief History of Time.* Bantam Books, New York, 1998.

Heisenberg, W. *Philosophic Problems of Nuclear Science.* Fawcett Publications, Greenwich, CT, 1966.

Hermann, A. *The New Physics.* Heinz Moos Verlag, Munich, 1979.

Holton, G. J. *Thematic Origins of Scientific Thought, Kepler to Einstein.* Harvard University Press, Cambridge, MA, 1973.

Isaacson, W. *Einstein.* Simon and Shuster, New York, 2007.

Lapp, R. E., and Andrews, H. L. *Nuclear Radiation Physics,* 4th ed. Prentice Hall, Englewood Cliffs, NJ, 1972.

Lindley, D. *Uncertainty: Einstein, Heisenberg, Bohr, and the Struggle for the Soul of Science.* Doubleday, New York, 2007.

Magid, L. M. *Electromagnetic Fields, Energy, and Waves.* John Wiley & Sons, New York, 1972.

Peierls, R. E. *The Laws of Nature.* Charles Scribner's Sons, New York, 1956.

Ripley, J. A., Jr. *The Elements and Structure of the Physical Sciences.* John Wiley & Sons, New York, 1964.

Robinson, A. *The Last Man Who Knew Everything: Thomas Young the Anonymous Polymath Who Proved Newton Wrong, Explained How We See, Cured the Sick, and Deciphered the Rosetta Stone, Among Other Feats of Genius.* Pi Press, New York, 2006.

Rogers, E. M. *Physics for the Inquiring Mind.* Princeton University Press, Princeton, NJ, 1960.

Serway, R. A., and Jewett, J. W. *Physics for Scientists and Engineers,* 6th ed., Thomson Brooks Cole, Belmont, CA, 2004.

Serway, R. A., Moses, C. J., and Moyer, C. A. *Modern Physics,* 3rd ed. Brooks Cole, Belmont, CA, 2004.

Taylor, B. N. *The International System of Units (SI).* National Institute of Standards and Technology Special Publication 330, 1991 edition, U.S. Govt. Printing Office, Washington, DC, 1991.

Young, H. D, and Freedman, R. A. *Sears and Zemansky's University Physics with Modern Physics,* 11th ed. Addison Wesley, Reading, MA, 2003.

3

ATOMIC AND NUCLEAR STRUCTURE

ATOMIC STRUCTURE

Matter, as we ordinarily know it, is electrically neutral. Yet the fact that matter can be easily electrified—by walking with rubber-soled shoes on a carpet, by sliding across a plastic auto seat cover when the atmospheric humidity is low, and by numerous other commonplace means—testifies to the electrical nature of matter. The manner in which the positive and negative electrical charges were held together was a matter of concern to the physicists of the early twentieth century.

Rutherford's Nuclear Atom

The British physicist Rutherford had postulated, in 1911, that the positive charge in an atom was concentrated in a central massive point called the *nucleus* and that the negative electrons were situated at some remote points, about one angstrom unit distant from the nucleus. In one of the all-time classic experiments of physics, two of Rutherford's students, Geiger and Marsden, in 1913, tested the validity of this hypothesis by bombarding an extremely thin (6×10^{-5} cm) gold foil with highly energetic, massive, positively charged projectiles called *alpha particles*. These projectiles, whose kinetic energy was 7.68 MeV, were emitted from the radioactive substance polonium. If Rutherford's idea had merit, it was expected that most of the alpha particles would pass straight through the thin gold foil. Some of the alpha particles, however, those that would pass by a gold nucleus closely enough to permit a strong interaction between the electric field of the alpha particle and the positive point charge in the gold nucleus, would be deflected as a result of the repulsive force between the alpha particle and the gold nucleus. An angular scan with an alpha particle detector about the point where the beam of alpha particles traversed the gold foil, as shown in Figure 3-1, permitted Geiger and Marsden to measure the alpha particle intensity at various scattering angles.

The experimental results verified Rutherford's hypothesis. Although most of the alpha particles passed undeflected through the gold foil, a continuous distribution

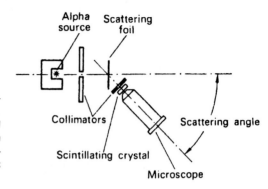

Figure 3-1. Diagram showing the principle of Rutherford's experiment with the scattering of alpha particles. The alpha source, its collimator, and the scattering foil are fixed; the alpha-particle detector—consisting of a collimator, a ZnS scintilling crystal, and a microscope—rotates around the point where the alpha beam strikes the scattering foil.

of scattered alpha particles was observed as the alpha-particle detector traversed a scattering angle from 0° to 150°. Similar results were obtained with other scatterers. The observed angular distributions of the scattered alpha particles agreed with those predicted by Rutherford's theory, thereby providing experimental evidence for the nuclear atom. Matter was found to consist mainly of open space. A lattice of atoms, consisting of positively charged nuclei about 5×10^{-15} m in diameter and separated by distances of about 10^{-10} m, was inferred from the scattering data. Detailed analyses of many experimental data later showed the radius of the nucleus to be as follows:

$$r = 1.2 \times 10^{-15} \times A^{1/3} \text{ m,} \tag{3.1}$$

where A is the atomic mass number. The number of unit charges in the nucleus (1 unit charge is 1.6×10^{-19} C) was found to be approximately equal to the atomic number of the atom and to about one-half the atomic weight.

Later work in Rutherford's laboratory by Moseley and by Chadwick in 1920 showed the number of positive charges in the nucleus to be exactly equal to the atomic number. These data implied that the proton, which carries one unit charge, is a fundamental building block of nature. (Based on data from high-energy particle experiments accumulated over a period of several decades, the American physicist Murray Gell-Mann showed that the proton consisted of three basic particles called quarks and was held together by a nuclear force so strong that the quarks cannot be separated. For this discovery, Gell-Mann was awarded the Nobel Prize in Physics in 1969. Although the proton [as well as the neutron] is an assembly of three smaller particles, for the purpose of health physics, the proton and neutron are considered to be fundamental particles.)

The outer periphery of the atom, at a distance of about 5×10^{-11} m from the nucleus, was thought to be formed by electrons—equal in number to the protons within the nucleus and distributed around the nucleus. However, no satisfactory theory to explain this structure of the atom was postulated by Rutherford. Any acceptable theory must answer two questions: First, how are the electrons held in place outside the nucleus despite the attractive electrostatic forces, and, second, what holds the positive charges in the nucleus together in the face of the repulsive electrostatic forces?

Bohr's Atomic Model

A simple solar system type of model, with the negative electrons revolving about the positively charged nucleus, seemed inviting. According to such a model, the attractive force between the electrons and the nucleus could be balanced by the centrifugal force due to the circular motion of the electrons. Classical electromagnetic theory, however, predicted that such an atom is unstable. The electrons revolving in their orbits undergo continuous radial acceleration. Since classical theory predicts that charged particles radiate electromagnetic energy whenever they experience a change in velocity (either in speed or in direction), it follows that the orbital electrons should eventually spiral into the nucleus as they lose their kinetic energy by radiation. (The radiation produced by the loss of kinetic energy by this mechanism is called *bremsstrahlung* and is very important in health physics. This point will be taken up in more detail in later chapters.) The objection to the solar system type of atomic model, based on the argument of energy loss due to radial acceleration, was overcome in 1913 by the Danish physicist Niels Bohr simply by denying the validity of classical electromagnetic theory in the case of motion of orbital electrons.

Although this was a radical step, it was by no means without precedent. The German physicist Max Planck had already shown that a complete description of blackbody radiation could not be given with classical theory. To do this, he postulated a quantum theory of radiation, in which electromagnetic radiations are assumed to be particles whose energy depends only on the frequency of the radiation. Bohr adopted Planck's quantum theory and used it to develop an atomic model that was consistent with the known atomic phenomena. The main source of experimental data from which Bohr inferred his model was atomic spectra. Each element, when excited by the addition of energy, radiates only certain colors that are unique to it. (This is the basis of neon signs. Neon, sealed in a glass tube, emits red light as a consequence of electrical excitation of the gas. Mercury vapor is used in the same way to produce blue-gray light.) Because of the discrete nature of these colors, atomic spectra are called "sharp-line" spectra to distinguish them from white light or blackbody radiation, which has a continuous spectrum. Hydrogen, for example, emits electromagnetic radiation of several distinct frequencies when it is excited, as shown in Figure 3-2. Some of these radiations are in the ultraviolet region, some are in the visible light region, and some are in the infrared region. The spectrum of hydrogen consists of several well-defined series of lines whose

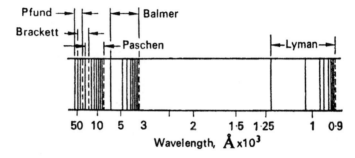

Figure 3-2. Hydrogen spectrum.

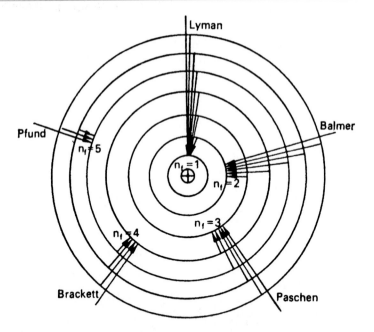

Figure 3-3. Bohr's model of the hydrogen atom showing the origin of the various series of lines seen in the hydrogen spectrum.

wavelengths were described empirically by physicists of the late nineteenth century by the equation

$$\frac{1}{\lambda} = R\left(\frac{1}{n_1^2} - \frac{1}{n_2^2}\right), \tag{3.2}$$

where R is a constant (named after the Swedish scientist Johannes Rydberg) whose numerical value is 1.097×10^{-2} 1/nm, n_1 is any whole number equal to or greater than 1, and n_2 is a whole number equal to or greater than $n_1 + 1$. The Lyman series, which lies in the ultraviolet region, is the series in which $n_1 = 1$ and $n_2 = 2, 3, 4,$ .... The longest wavelength in this series, obtained by setting n_2 equal to 2 in Eq. (3.2), is 121.5 nm. Succeeding lines, when n_2 is 3 and 4, are 102.6 nm and 97.2 nm, respectively. The shortest line, called the series limit, is obtained by solving Eq. (3.2) with n_2 equal to infinity; in this case, the wavelength of the most energetic photon is 91.1 nm.

Bohr's atomic model (Fig. 3-3) is based on two fundamental postulates:

1. The orbital electrons can revolve around the nucleus only in certain fixed radii called *stationary states*. These radii are such that the orbital angular momentum of the revolving electrons must be integral multiples of $h/2\pi$, specifically,

$$mvr = \frac{nh}{2\pi}, \tag{3.3}$$

where m is the mass of the electron, v is its linear velocity, r is the radius of revolution, h is Planck's constant, and n is any positive integer.

2. A photon is emitted only when an electron falls from one orbit to another orbit of lower energy. The energy of the photon is equal to the difference between the energy levels of the electrons in the two orbits.

$$hf = E_2 - E_1 \tag{3.4a}$$

$$f = \frac{E_2}{h} - \frac{E_1}{h}, \tag{3.4b}$$

where f is the frequency of the emitted photon and E_2 and E_1 are the high- and low-energy orbits, respectively.

When the electron revolves around the nucleus, the electrostatic force of attraction between the electron and the nucleus is balanced by the centrifugal force due to the revolution of the electron:

$$k_0 \frac{Ze \times e}{r^2} = \frac{mv^2}{r}, \tag{3.5}$$

where

k_0 is Coulomb's law constant, 9×10^9 $(\text{N} \cdot \text{m}^2)/\text{C}^2$,
Z is the atomic number of the atom, and
e is the electron and proton charge;
Ze, therefore, is the charge on the nucleus.

Substituting the value for v from Eq. (3.3) into Eq. (3.5) and solving for r, we have

$$r = \frac{n^2 h^2}{4\pi^2 m e^2 Z k_0}. \tag{3.6}$$

Equation (3.6) gives the radii of the electronic orbits that will satisfy the condition for the stationary states when whole numbers are substituted for n. The normal condition of the atom, or the ground state, is that state for which n equals 1. When in the ground state, the atom is in its lowest possible energy state and, therefore, in its most stable condition. Transitions from the ground state to higher energy orbits are possible through the absorption of sufficient energy to raise the electron to a larger orbital radius.

The energy in any orbit may be calculated by considering the kinetic energy of the electron due to its motion around the nucleus and the potential energy due to its position in the electric field of the nucleus. Since the kinetic energy of the electron is equal to $1/2 mv^2$ (the electron does not revolve rapidly enough to consider relativistic effects), then, from Eq. (3.5), we have

$$E_k = \frac{1}{2} mv^2 = k_0 \frac{Ze^2}{2r}. \tag{3.7}$$

The potential energy is, from Eq. (2.32),

$$E_p = k_0 \frac{Ze}{r}(-e) = -k_0 \frac{Ze^2}{r}. \tag{3.8}$$

The total energy is the sum of the kinetic and potential energies:

$$E = E_k + E_p$$

$$= \frac{k_0\,Ze^2}{2r} - \frac{k_0\,Ze^2}{r} = -\frac{k_0\,Ze^2}{2r}. \tag{3.9}$$

The total energy given by Eq. (3.9) is negative simply as a result of the convention discussed in Chapter 2. By definition, the point of zero potential energy was set at an infinite distance from the nucleus. Since the force between the nucleus and the electron is attractive, it follows that at any point closer than infinity, the potential energy must be less than that at infinity and therefore must have a negative numerical value.

The total energy in any permissible orbit is found by substituting the value for the radius, from Eq. (3.6), into Eq. (3.9):

$$E = \frac{-2\pi^2 k_0^2\, m\, Z^2 e^4}{h^2} \times \frac{1}{n^2}. \tag{3.10}$$

Equation (3.10) may now be substituted into Eq. (3.4b) to get the frequency of the "light" that is radiated from an atom when an electron falls from an excited state into one of lower energy. Letting n_f and n_i represent respectively the orbit numbers for the lower and higher levels, we have the frequency of the emitted radiation:

$$f = \frac{2\pi^2 k_0^2\, m\, Z^2 e^4}{h^3} \left(\frac{1}{n_f^2} - \frac{1}{n_i^2} \right). \tag{3.11}$$

Since $\lambda = \dfrac{c}{f}$, the reciprocal of the wavelength of this radiation is

$$\frac{1}{\lambda} = \frac{2\pi^2 k_0^2\, m\, Z^2 e^4}{c h^3} \left(\frac{1}{n_f^2} - \frac{1}{n_i^2} \right). \tag{3.12}$$

When numerical values are substituted into the first term of Eq. (3.12), the numerical value for Rydberg's constant is obtained.

Excitation and Ionization

The Bohr equation may be used to illustrate the case of hydrogen by substituting $Z = 1$ into the equations. The radius of the ground state is found to be, from Eq. (3.6), 0.526×10^{-8} cm. The wavelength of the light emitted when the electron falls from the first excited state, $n_i = 2$, to the ground state, $n_f = 1$, may be calculated by substituting these values into Eq. (3.2):

$$\frac{1}{\lambda} = 1.097 \times 10^{-2} \frac{1}{\text{nm}} \left(\frac{1}{1^2} - \frac{1}{2^2} \right)$$

$$\lambda = 121.5 \text{ nm}.$$

The energy of this photon is

$$E = \frac{hc}{\lambda} = \frac{6.6 \times 10^{-34} \, \text{J} \cdot \text{s} \times 3 \times 10^8 \, \text{m/s}}{121.5 \times 10^{-9} \, \text{m} \times 1.6 \times 10^{-19} \, \dfrac{\text{J}}{\text{eV}}} = 10.2 \, \text{eV}.$$

This same amount of energy, 10.2 eV, is necessary to excite hydrogen to the first excited state. Precisely this amount of energy, no more and no less, may be used.

When a sufficient amount of energy is imparted to raise the electron to an infinitely great orbit, that is, to remove it from the electrical field of the nucleus, the atom is said to be *ionized* and the negative electron together with the remaining positively charged atom are called an *ion pair*. This process is called *ionization*. Ionization or excitation may occur when either a photon or a charged particle, such as an electron, a proton, or an alpha particle, collides with an orbital electron and transfers some of its kinetic energy to the orbital electron. Ionization and excitation are of great importance in health physics because this is the avenue through which energy is transferred from radiation to matter. When living matter is irradiated, the primary event in the sequence of events leading to biological damage is either excitation or ionization. The *ionization potential* of an element is the amount of energy necessary to ionize the least tightly bound electron in an atom of that element. To remove a second electron requires considerably more energy than that needed for removing the first electron. For most elements, the first ionization potential is on the order of several electron volts. In the case of hydrogen, the ionization potential, I, may be calculated from Eq. (3.11) by setting n_i equal to infinity:

$$I = hf = \frac{2\pi^2 m Z^2 e^4 k_0^2}{1.6 \times 10^{-19} \, \dfrac{\text{J}}{\text{eV}} \times h^2} \left(\frac{1}{1} - \frac{1}{\infty} \right)$$

$$= \frac{2\pi^2 \times 9.11 \times 10^{-31} \text{kg} \times 1 \times \left(1.6 \times 10^{-19} \, \text{C}\right)^4 \times \left(9 \times 10^9 \, \dfrac{\text{N} \cdot \text{m}^2}{\text{C}^2}\right)^2}{1.6 \times 10^{-19} \, \dfrac{\text{J}}{\text{eV}} \times \left(6.626 \times 10^{-34} \, \text{J} \cdot \text{s}\right)^2}$$

$$= 13.6 \, \text{eV}.$$

A collision in which a rapidly moving particle transfers much more than 13.6 eV to the orbital electron of hydrogen results in the ionization of the hydrogen. The excess energy above 13.6 eV that is transferred in this collision appears as kinetic energy of the electron and of the resulting positive ion, which recoils under the impact of the collision in accordance with the requirements of the conservation of momentum. Such inelastic collisions occur only if the incident particle is sufficiently energetic, about 100 eV or greater, to meet this requirement. In those instances where the energy of the particle is insufficient to meet this requirement, an elastic collision with the atom as a whole occurs.

Einstein, in 1905, in the first of four groundbreaking papers in that year of wonders (*annus mirabilis*), described the interaction between a quantum of light and a bound electron. When a photon, whose energy is great enough to ionize an atom, collides with a tightly bound orbital electron, the photon disappears and the electron is ejected from the atom with a kinetic energy equal to the difference between the energy of the photon and the ionization potential. This mechanism is called the *photoelectric effect* and is described by the equation

$$E_{pe} = hf - \phi, \tag{3.13}$$

where E_{pe} is the kinetic energy of the photoelectron (the ejected electron), hf is the photon energy, and ϕ is the ionization potential (commonly called the *work function*). Einstein won the Nobel Prize in 1921 for his work on the theoretical aspects of the photoelectric effect. His other papers in that annus mirabilis included the theory of Brownian motion, special relativity, and the dependence of inertial mass on energy as well as his doctoral dissertation on Avogadro's number and the size of a molecule.

EXAMPLE 3.1

An ultraviolet photon whose wavelength is 2000 Å strikes the outer orbital electron of sodium; the ionization potential of the atom is 5.41 eV. What is the kinetic energy of the photoelectron?

Solution

The energy of the incident photon is

$$\frac{hf \text{ J}}{1.6 \times 10^{-19} \; \frac{\text{J}}{\text{eV}}} = \frac{hc}{1.6 \times 10^{-19} \times \lambda}$$

$$= \frac{6.626 \times 10^{-34} \text{ J} \cdot \text{s} \times 3 \times 10^{8} \text{ m/s}}{1.6 \times 10^{-19} \; \frac{\text{J}}{\text{eV}} \times 2 \times 10^{-7} \text{m}}$$

$$= 6.21 \text{ eV}.$$

From Eq. (3.13), the kinetic energy of the photoelectron is found to be

$$E_{pe} = 6.21 - 5.41 = 0.80 \text{ eV}.$$

Modifications of the Bohr Atom

The atomic model proposed by Bohr "explains" certain atomic phenomena for hydrogen and for hydrogen-like atoms, such as singly ionized helium (He^{+}) and doubly ionized lithium (Li^{2+}). Calculation of spectra for other atoms according to the Bohr model is complicated by the screening effect of the other electrons, which effectively reduces the electrical field of the nucleus, and by electrical interactions among the electrons. The simple Bohr theory described above is inadequate even for the hydrogen atom. Examination of the spectral lines of hydrogen with spectroscopes of high resolving power shows the lines to have a fine structure. The spectral lines are in reality each made of several lines that are very close together. This observation implies the existence of sublevels of energy within the principal energy levels and that these sublevels are very close together. They can be explained by assuming the orbits to be elliptical instead of circular, with the nucleus at one of the foci, and also assuming that ellipses of different eccentricities have slightly different energy levels. For any given principal energy level, the major axes of these ellipses are the same; eccentricity varies only by changes in the length of the minor axes. The eccentricity of these ellipses is restricted by quantum conditions. The angular momentum of an electron revolving in an elliptical orbit is an integral multiple of $h/2\pi$, as in the case of the circular Bohr orbit. However, the numerical value for this multiple is not the same as that for the circular orbit. In the case of the circular orbit, this multiple, or quantum number, is called the *principal quantum number* and is given the symbol n. For the elliptical orbit, the multiple is called the *azimuthal quantum number*, usually symbolized by the letter l, and may be any integral number between 0 and $n-1$ inclusive.

Elliptical orbits alone were insufficient to account for observed spectral lines because the lines observed with the high-resolution spectroscope were found to exhibit a hyperfine structure of two lines when viewed with a very high resolution spectrometer. To explain the hyperfine structure, it postulated that each orbital electron spins about its own axis in the same manner as the earth spins about its axis as it revolves around the sun. The angular momentum due to this spin also is quantized and can only have a value equal to one-half a unit of angular momentum. It is symbolized by the letter s:

$$s = \pm \frac{1}{2}\left(\frac{h}{2\pi}\right). \tag{3.14}$$

The orbital electron can spin in only one of two directions with respect to the direction of its revolution about the nucleus—either in the same direction or in the opposite direction. This accounts for the plus and minus signs in Eq. (3.14). Since momentum is a vector quantity, the total angular momentum of the electron is therefore equal to the vector sum of the orbital and spin angular momenta.

The magnetic properties of the atom must be considered before the description of the atom is complete. An electron revolving in its orbit around the nucleus may be considered a current flowing through a closed loop. According to electromagnetic theory, this current flow generates a magnetic field. The revolving electron thus may be considered to be a tiny bar magnet. A bar magnet has a magnetic moment given by the product of the pole strength and the distance between the poles. If such a magnet were aligned in a magnetic field, a certain amount of work, depending on the strength of the field, would have to be done in order to rotate the magnet. Magnetic moments therefore are described by joules per tesla in SI units or by ergs per gauss in cgs units. Moments have direction as well as magnitude and therefore are vector quantities.

The spinning of the electron results in an additional magnetic moment, which may be either positive or negative, depending on the direction of spin relative to the direction of the orbital motion. The total magnetic moment is therefore equal to the vector sum of the orbital and spin magnetic moments. If the atoms of any substance are placed in a strong magnetic field, the orbital electrons, because of their magnetic moments, will orient themselves in definite directions relative to the applied magnetic field. These directions are such that the component of the vector representing the orbital angular momentum l, which is parallel to the magnetic field, must have an integral value of angular momentum. This integral number, m, is called the *magnetic quantum* number; it can have numerical values ranging from $l, l - 1, l - 2, \ldots, 0 \ldots$, $-(l - 2), -(l - 1), -l$. The interaction of the magnetic properties of the orbital electrons and an applied magnetic field is the basis for the analytical technique called *electron spin resonance.*

To describe an atom completely, it is necessary to specify four quantum numbers, which have the values given below, for each of the orbital electrons:

SYMBOL	NAME	VALUE
n	Principal quantum number	$1, 2, \ldots$
l	Azimuthal quantum number	0 to $n - 1$
m	Magnetic quantum number	$- l$ to 0 to $+ l$
s	Spin quantum number	$-\frac{1}{2}, +\frac{1}{2}$

By using Bohr's atomic model and assigning all possible numerical values to these four quantum numbers according to certain rules, it is possible to construct the periodic table of the elements.

Periodic Table of the Elements

The periodic table of the elements may be constructed with Bohr's atomic model by applying the *Pauli exclusion principle.* This principle states that no two electrons in any atom may have the same set of four quantum numbers. Hydrogen, the first element, has a nuclear charge of $+1$ and therefore has only one electron. Since the principal quantum number of this electron must be 1, l and m must be 0 and the spin quantum number s may be either plus or minus 1/2. If now we go to the second element, helium, we must have two orbital electrons since helium has a nuclear charge of $+2$. The first electron in the helium atom may have the same set of quantum numbers as the electron in the hydrogen atom. The second electron, however, must differ. This difference can be only in the spin since we may have two different spins for the set of quantum numbers $n = 1, l = 0$, and $m = 0$. This second electron exhausts all the possibilities for $n = 1$. If now a third electron is added when we go to atomic number 3, lithium, it must have the principal quantum number 2. In this principal energy level, the orbit may be either circular or elliptical, that is, the azimuthal quantum number l may be either 0 or 1. In the case of $l = 0$, the magnetic quantum number m can only be equal to 0; when $l = 1$, m may be either -1, 0, or $+1$. Each of these quantum states may contain two electrons, one with spin $+1/2$ and the other with spin $-1/2$. Eight different electrons, each with its own unique set of quantum numbers, are therefore possible in the second principal energy level. These eight different possibilities are utilized by the elements Li, Be, B, C, N, O, F, and Ne (atomic numbers 3–10 inclusive). The additional electron for sodium (atomic number 11) must have the principal quantum number $n = 3$. By assigning all the possible combinations of the four quantum numbers to the electrons in the third principal energy level, it is found that 18 electrons are possible. These energy levels are not filled successively, as were those in the K and L shells. (The principal quantum levels corresponding to $n = 1, 2, 3, 4, 5, 6$, and 7 are called the K, L, M, N, O, P, and Q shells, respectively.) No outermost electron shell contains more than eight electrons. After the M shell contains eight electrons, as in the case of argon, the next element in the periodic table, potassium (atomic number 20), starts another principal energy level with one electron in the N shell. Subsequent elements then may add electrons either in the M or in the N shells, until the M shell contains its full complement of 18 electrons. No electrons appear in the O shell until the N shell has eight electrons. The maximum number of electrons that may exist in any principal energy level is given by the product $2n^2$, where n is the principal quantum number. Thus, the O shell may have a maximum of $2 \times 5^2 = 50$ electrons.

The fact that no outermost electron shell contains more than eight electrons is responsible for the periodicity of the chemical properties of many elements and is the physical basis for the periodic table. Since chemical reactions involve the outer electrons, it is not surprising that atoms with similar outer electronic structures should have similar chemical properties. For example, Li, Na, K, Rb, and Cs behave chemically in a similar manner because each of these elements has only one electron in its outermost orbit. The gases He, Ne, Ar, Kr, Xe, and Rn are chemically inert because their outermost electron shells are filled. Therefore, these elements do not undergo chemical reactions. The elements are thought to have the electronic configurations given in Table 3-1.

Examination of Table 3-1 reveals certain interesting points. The first 20 elements successively add electrons to their outermost shells. The next 8 elements, Sc to Ni, have four shells but add successive electrons to the third shell until it is filled with the maximum number of 18. These elements are called *transition elements*. The same thing happens with elements 39–46 inclusive. Electrons are added to the fourth shell until they number 18, then the fifth shell increases until it contains 8 electrons. In element number 55, Cs, the sixth principal electron orbit, the P shell, starts to fill. Instead of continuing, however, the N level starts to fill. Beginning with Ce, and continuing through Lu, electrons are successively added to the fourth electron shell while the two outermost shells remain about the same. This group of elements is usually called the *rare earths* and sometimes the *lanthanides* because these elements begin immediately after La. The rare earth elements differ from the transition elements in the depth of the electronic orbit that is filling. While the transition elements fill the second outer orbit, the rare earths fill the third electron shell, which is deeper in the atom. Since, in the case of the rare earths, the two outermost electron shells are alike, it is extremely difficult to separate them by chemical means. They are of importance to the health physicist because they include a great number of the fission products. The concern of the health physicist with the rare earths is aggravated by the fact that the analytical chemistry of the rare earths is very difficult and also by the relative dearth of knowledge regarding their metabolic pathways and toxicological properties. Despite their name, the rare earths are not rare; they are found to be widely distributed in nature, albeit in small concentrations. Another group of rare earths is found in the elements starting with Th and continuing to where the O shell fills while the P and Q shells remain about the same. These rare earths are usually called the *actinide* elements. They are of importance to the health physicist because they are all naturally radioactive and include the fuel used in nuclear reactors.

TABLE 3-1. Electronic Structure of the Elements

PERIOD	SYMBOL	ELEMENT	ATOMIC NO.	K SHELL 1	L SHELL 2	M SHELL 3	N SHELL 4	O SHELL 5	P SHELL 6	Q SHELL 7
1	H	Hydrogen	1	1						
	He	Helium	2	2						
2	Li	Lithium	3	2	1					
	Be	Beryllium	4	2	2					
	B	Boron	5	2	3					
	C	Carbon	6	2	4					
	N	Nitrogen	7	2	5					
	O	Oxygen	8	2	6					
	F	Fluorine	9	2	7					
3	Ne	Neon	10	2	8					
	Na	Sodium	11	2	8	1				
	Mg	Magnesium	12	2	8	2				
	Al	Aluminum	13	2	8	3				
	Si	Silicon	14	2	8	4				
	P	Phosphorus	15	2	8	5				
	S	Sulfur	16	2	8	6				
	Cl	Chlorine	17	2	8	7				
4	Ar	Argon	18	2	8	8				
	K	Potassium	19	2	8	8	1			
	Ca	Calcium	20	2	8	8	2			
	Sc	Scandium	21	2	8	9	2			
	Ti	Titanium	22	2	8	10	2			
	V	Vanadium	23	2	8	11	2			
	Cr	Chromium	24	2	8	13	1			
	Mn	Manganese	25	2	8	13	2			
	Fe	Iron	26	2	8	14	2			
	Co	Cobalt	27	2	8	15	2			
	Ni	Nickel	28	2	8	16	2			
	Cu	Copper	29	2	8	18	1			
	Zn	Zinc	30	2	8	18	2			
	Ga	Gallium	31	2	8	18	3			
	Ge	Germanium	32	2	8	18	4			
	As	Arsenic	33	2	8	18	5			
	Se	Selenium	34	2	8	18	6			
	Br	Bromine	35	2	8	18	7			
5	Kr	Krypton	36	2	8	18	8			
	Rb	Rubidium	37	2	8	18	8	1		
	Sr	Strontium	38	2	8	18	8	2		
	Y	Yttrium	39	2	8	18	9	2		
	Zr	Zirconium	40	2	8	18	10	2		
	Nb	Niobium	41	2	8	18	12	1		
	Mo	Molybdenum	42	2	8	18	13	1		
	Tc	Technetium	43	2	8	18	14	1		
	Ru	Ruthenium	44	2	8	18	15	1		
	Rh	Rhodium	45	2	8	18	16	1		
	Pd	Palladium	46	2	8	18	18	0		
	Ag	Silver	47	2	8	18	18	1		
	Cd	Cadmium	48	2	8	18	18	2		
	In	Indium	49	2	8	18	18	3		
	Sn	Tin	50	2	8	18	18	4		
	Sb	Antimony	51	2	8	18	18	5		
	Te	Tellurium	52	2	8	18	18	6		

(continued)

TABLE 3-1. Electronic Structure of the Elements (*Continued*)

PERIOD	SYMBOL	ELEMENT	ATOMIC NO.	K SHELL 1	L SHELL 2	M SHELL 3	N SHELL 4	O SHELL 5	P SHELL 6	Q SHELL 7
	I	Iodine	53	2	8	18	18	7		
6	Xe	Xenon	54	2	8	18	18	8		
	Cs	Cesium	55	2	8	18	18	8	1	
	Ba	Barium	56	2	8	18	18	8	2	
	La	Lanthanum	57	2	8	18	18	9	2	
	Ce	Cerium	58	2	8	18	19	9	2	
	Pr	Praseodymium	59	2	8	18	20	9	2	
	Nd	Neodymium	60	2	8	18	22	8	2	
	Pm	Promethium	61	2	8	18	23	8	2	
	Sm	Samarium	62	2	8	18	24	8	2	
	Eu	Europium	63	2	8	18	25	8	2	
	Gd	Gadolinium	64	2	8	18	25	9	2	
	Tb	Terbium	65	2	8	18	26	9	2	
	Dy	Dysprosium	66	2	8	18	28	8	2	
	Ho	Holmium	67	2	8	18	29	8	2	
	Er	Erbium	68	2	8	18	30	8	2	
	Tm	Thulium	69	2	8	18	31	8	2	
	Yb	Ytterbium	70	2	8	18	32	8	2	
	Lu	Lutetium	71	2	8	18	32	9	2	
	Hf	Hafnium	72	2	8	18	32	10	2	
	Ta	Tantalum	73	2	8	18	32	11	2	
	W	Tungsten	74	2	8	18	32	12	2	
	Re	Rhenium	75	2	8	18	32	13	2	
	Os	Osmium	76	2	8	18	32	14	2	
	Ir	Iridium	77	2	8	18	32	15	2	
	Pt	Platinum	78	2	8	18	32	17	1	
	Au	Gold	79	2	8	18	32	18	1	
	Hg	Mercury	80	2	8	18	32	18	2	
	Tl	Thallium	81	2	8	18	32	18	3	
	Pb	Lead	82	2	8	18	32	18	4	
	Bi	Bismuth	83	2	8	18	32	18	5	
	Po	Polonium	84	2	8	18	32	18	6	
	At	Astatine	85	2	8	18	32	18	7	
7	Rn	Radon	86	2	8	18	32	18	8	
	Fr	Francium	87	2	8	18	32	18	8	1
	Ra	Radium	88	2	8	18	32	18	8	2
	Ac	Actinium	89	2	8	18	32	18	9	2
	Th	Thorium	90	2	8	18	32	19	9	2
	Pa	Protactinium	91	2	8	18	32	20	9	2
	U	Uranium	92	2	8	18	32	21	9	2
	Np	Neptunium	93	2	8	18	32	22	9	2
	Pu	Plutonium	94	2	8	18	32	24	8	2
	Am	Americium	95	2	8	18	32	25	8	2
	Cm	Curium	96	2	8	18	32	25	9	2
	Bk	Berkelium	97	2	8	18	32	27	8	2
	Cf	Californium	98	2	8	18	32	28	8	2
	Es	Einsteinium	99	2	8	18	32	29	8	2
	Fm	Fermium	100	2	8	18	32	30	8	2
	Md	Mendelevium	101	2	8	18	32	31	8	2
	No	Nobelium	102	2	8	18	32	32	8	2
	Lr	Lawrencium	103	2	8	18	32	32	9	2
	Rf	Rutherfordium	104	2	8	18	32	32	10	2

Characteristic X-rays

There are certain virtues of the solar system type of atomic model, in which electrons rotate about the nucleus in certain radii corresponding to unique energy levels. Virtues of the model include the simple explanations that it allows for transfer of energy to matter by excitation and ionization, for the photoelectric effect, and for the origin of certain X-rays called *characteristic X-rays*. It was pointed out that optical and ultraviolet spectra of elements are due to excitation of outer electrons to levels up to several electron volts and that spectral lines represent energy differences between excited states. As more and more electron shells are added, the energy differences between the principal levels increase greatly. In elements with high atomic numbers, these energy levels reach tens of thousands of electron volts. In the case of Pb, for example, the energy difference between the K and L shells is 72,000 eV. If this K electron is struck by a photon whose energy exceeds 87.95 keV (the binding energy of the K electron) the electron is ejected from the atom and leaves an empty slot in the K shell, as shown schematically in Figure 3-4. Instantaneously, one of the outer electrons falls down into the vacant slot left by the photoelectron. When this happens, a photon is emitted whose energy is equal to the difference between the initial and final energy levels, in accordance with Eq. (3.4a). For the Pb atom, when an electron falls from the L to the K levels, the emitted photon has a quantum energy of 72,000 eV. A photon of such high energy is an X-ray. When produced in this manner, the photon is called a *characteristic X-ray* because the energy differences between electron orbits are unique for the different atoms and the X-rays representing these differences are "characteristic" of the elements in which they originate. This process is repeated until all the inner electron orbits are refilled. It is possible, of course, that the first transition is from the M level or even from the outermost electronic orbit. The most likely origin of the first electronic transition, however, is the L shell. When this happens, the resulting X-ray is called a K_α photon; if an electron falls from the M level to the K level, we have a K_β photon. When the vacancy in the L orbit is filled by an electron that falls from the M level, we have an L_α X-ray; if the L vacancy is filled by an electron originally in the N level, then an L_β X-ray results, and so on.

These characteristic X-rays are sometimes called *fluorescent radiation* since they are emitted when matter is irradiated with X-rays. Characteristic radiation is useful as a tool to the analytical chemist for identifying unknown elements. Characteristic radiation is of importance to the health physicist who must consider the fluorescent

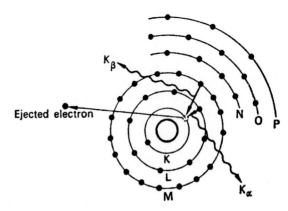

Figure 3-4. Schematic representation of the origin of characteristic X-rays.

radiation that may be produced in radiation absorbers and in certain other cases where inner electrons are ejected from high-atomic-numbered elements.

A characteristic X-ray photon may interact with another electron in the atom where the characteristic photon originated and eject that electron. This second ejected electron is called an *Auger* (pronounced *ozhay*) *electron*. The Auger electron can come from the same orbit as the original photoelectron or it may come from an outer orbit. The kinetic energy of an Auger electron (E_{kA}) is given by

$$E_{kA} = \phi_i - 2\phi_o, \tag{3.15}$$

where

ϕ_i = binding energy of the inner orbit and
ϕ_o = binding energy of the outer orbit.

The Wave Mechanics Atomic Model

The atomic model described above is sufficiently useful to explain most phenomena encountered in health physics. For the study of atomic physics, however, a more abstract concept of the atom was proposed by the Austrian physicist Schrödinger (for which he and the British physicist Dirac shared the Nobel Prize in 1933). Instead of working with particulate electrons as Bohr had done, he treated them as de Broglie waves and developed the branch of physics known as "wave mechanics." Starting with the de Broglie equation for the associated electron wave, Schrödinger derived a general differential equation that must be satisfied by an electron within an atom. The present-day atomic theory consists of solutions of this equation subject to certain conditions. A number of different solutions, corresponding to different energy levels, are possible. However, whereas Bohr pictured an atom with electrons at precisely determined distances from the nucleus, the Schrödinger wave equation gives the probability of finding an electron at any given distance from the nucleus. The two atomic pictures coincide to the extent that the most probable radius for the hydrogen electron is exactly the same as the first Bohr radius. Similarly, the second Bohr radius corresponds to the most probable distance from the nucleus of the electron in the first excited state. Furthermore, the four quantum numbers arbitrarily introduced into the Bohr atom fall naturally out of the solutions of the Schrödinger wave equation. Although the wave model has replaced the Bohr system of atomic mechanics for highly theoretical considerations, the older atomic model is still considered a very useful tool in helping to interpret atomic phenomena.

THE NUCLEUS

The Neutron and Nuclear Force

It has already been pointed out that the positive charges in the atomic nucleus are due to protons and that hydrogen is the simplest nucleus—it consists of only a single proton. If succeeding nuclei merely were multiples of the proton, then the mass numbers of the nuclei, if a mass number of 1 is assigned to the proton, should be equal to the atomic numbers of the nuclei. This was not found to be the case. Except for hydrogen, the nuclear mass numbers were found to be about twice as great as the corresponding atomic numbers and became relatively greater as the atomic numbers increased. Furthermore, it was necessary to account for the stability of the nucleus in the face of the repulsive coulombic forces among the nuclear protons. Example 2.4 shows that the gravitational force of attraction is insufficient to overcome the repulsive electrical forces. Both these problems were solved by the discovery, in 1932, by the British physicist Chadwick, of what was thought to be the third basic building block in nature—the neutron. (Chadwick won the Nobel Prize in 1935 for this discovery.) This particle, whose mass is about the same as that of a proton, 1.67474×10^{-27} kg, is electrically neutral. Its presence in the nucleus accounts for the difference between the atomic number and the atomic mass number; it also supplies the cohesive force that holds the nucleus together. This force is called the *nuclear force*. It is thought to act over an extremely short range—about 2×10^{-15} to 3×10^{-15} m. By analogy to the ordinary case of charged particles, it may be assumed that the neutron and the proton carry certain nuclear charges and that force fields due to these nuclear charges are established around the nucleons (particles within the nucleus). Nuclear forces are all attractive and the interaction between the nuclear force fields supplies the cohesive forces that overcome the repulsive electrical forces. However, since the range of the nuclear force is much shorter than the range of the electrical force, neutrons can interact only with those nucleons to which they are immediately adjacent, whereas protons interact with each other even though they are remotely located within the nucleus. For this reason, the number of neutrons must increase more rapidly than the number of protons.

Quarks

Recent studies in particle physics have shown that protons and neutrons are not the elementary particles that they had been thought to be. They consist of assemblies of three particles, called *quarks,* which are now believed to be elementary particles. Quarks are charged particles and carry charges of either $\pm 2/3$ or $\pm 1/3$ of the charge on a proton. Those that have $\pm 2/3$ of the protonic charge are called *up quarks,* and those that carry $\pm 1/3$ of the protonic charge are called *down quarks*. A proton consists of two positive up quarks and one negative down quark, which results in a single positive charge. A neutron is made of one positive up quark and two negative down quarks, which results in a net charge of zero. The quarks within a particle are held together by an extremely strong force called the *strong force*; it is also known as the *color force* (the area of study of the color force is called *quantum chromodynamics*). This force is so strong that it is not possible at this time to separate a proton or a neutron into its component quarks. In experimental attempts to do this, it was found that the enormous amount of energy needed to separate a proton or a neutron into their component quarks is converted into heavy particles. The mass of these heavy particles accords with Einstein's mass–energy equivalence rather than being expended in separating the quarks.

Isotopes

It has been found that for any particular element the number of neutrons within the nucleus is not constant. Oxygen, for example, consists of three nuclear species: one whose nucleus has 8 neutrons, one of 9 neutrons, and one of 10 neutrons. In each of these three cases, of course, the nucleus contains 8 protons. The atomic mass numbers of these three species are 16, 17, and 18, respectively. These three nuclear species of the same element are called *isotopes* of oxygen. Isotopes of an element are atoms that contain the same number of positive nuclear charges and have the same extranuclear electronic structure but differ in the number of neutrons. Most elements contain several isotopes. The atomic weight of an element is the weighted average of the weights of the different isotopes of which the element is composed. Isotopes cannot be distinguished chemically since they have the same electronic structure and therefore undergo the same chemical reactions. An isotope is identified by writing the chemical symbol with a subscript to the left giving the atomic number and a superscript giving the atomic mass number or the total number of nucleons. Thus, the three isotopes of oxygen may be written as $^{16}_{8}O, ^{17}_{8}O$, and $^{18}_{8}O$. Since the atomic number is synonymous with the chemical symbol, the subscript is usually omitted and the isotope is written as ^{16}O. It should be pointed out that not all isotopes are equally abundant. In the case of oxygen, 99.759% of the naturally occurring atoms are ^{16}O, whereas ^{17}O and ^{18}O include 0.037% and 0.204%, respectively. In other elements, the distribution of isotopes may be quite different. Chlorine, for example, consists of two naturally occurring isotopes, ^{35}Cl and ^{37}Cl, whose respective abundances are 75.77% and 24.23%. Sodium and gold consist of only one naturally occurring isotope, ^{23}Na and ^{197}Au, respectively.

The Atomic Mass Unit

The terms weight and mass are frequently used interchangeably. Weight is the force with which a mass is attracted by gravity. A mass of 1 g weighs 1 g at the earth's surface. One gram of force is equal to 980 dynes. Similarly, a mass of 1 kg weighs 1 kg, and a force of 1 kg is equal to 98 N.

Atomic masses may be given either in grams or in relative numbers called *atomic mass units*. Since one mole of any substance contains 6.02×10^{23} molecules (Avogadro's number) and the weight in grams of one mole is equal numerically to its molecular weight, the weight of a single atom can easily be computed. In the case of ^{12}C, which is a monoatomic molecule, for example, 1 mol weighs 12.0000 g. One atom, therefore, weighs

$$\frac{12.0000 \text{ g/mol}}{6.02 \times 10^{23} \text{ atoms/mol}} = 1.9927 \times 10^{-23} \text{g}.$$

Since the mass of 1 mol of ^{12}C was found to be a whole number, carbon was chosen as the reference standard for the system of relative weights known as atomic weights. (Actually, the atomic weight of an element is the weighted average of all the isotopic weights. The physical scale is based only on the weight of ^{12}C.) Since ^{12}C was assigned an atomic weight of 12.0000, one atomic mass unit, amu (also called a *dalton,* symbolized by D), is

$$1 \text{ amu} = \frac{1.9927 \times 10^{-23} \text{g}}{12} = 1.6605 \times 10^{-24} \text{g}.$$

On this basis, the weight of a neutron m_n is 1.008665 amu, that of a proton m_p is 1.007276 amu, and the weight of an electron is 0.000548 amu. The energy equivalent of one atomic mass unit is (note that the speed of light is rounded in this example)

$$E(1 \text{ amu}) = \frac{mc^2 \text{ J}}{1.6 \times 10^{-13} \dfrac{\text{J}}{\text{MeV}}}$$

$$= \frac{1 \text{ amu} \times 1.6605 \times 10^{-27} \dfrac{\text{kg}}{\text{amu}} \times \left(3 \times 10^8 \dfrac{\text{m}}{\text{s}}\right)^2}{1.6 \times 10^{-13} \dfrac{\text{J}}{\text{MeV}}}$$

$$= 931 \text{ MeV}.$$

Binding Energy

At this point, it is interesting to compare the sum of the weights of the constituent parts of an isotope W with the measured isotopic weight M. For the case of ^{17}O, whose atomic mass is 16.999131 amu, we have

$$W = (Z)m_H + (A - Z)m_n, \tag{3.16}$$

where Z is the atomic number and A is the atomic mass number, which is equal to the number of nucleons within the nucleus, m_H is the mass of a hydrogen atom, and m_n is the mass of a neutron.

$$W = 8(1.00728) + (17 - 8)(1.00867)$$

$$= 17.1363 \text{ amu}.$$

The weight of the sum of the parts is seen to be much greater than the actual weight of the entire atom. This is true not only for ^{17}O but for all nuclei. The difference between the atomic weight and the sum of the weights of the parts is called the *mass defect* and is defined by δ as follows:

$$\delta = W - M. \tag{3.17}$$

The mass defect represents the mass equivalent of the work that must be done in order to separate the nucleus into its individual component nucleons and is therefore called the *binding energy*. In energy units, the binding energy, *BE*, is

$$E_B = (W - M) \text{ amu} \times 931 \frac{\text{MeV}}{\text{amu}}. \tag{3.18}$$

The binding energy is a measure of the cohesiveness of a nucleus. Since the total binding energy of a nucleus depends on the number of nucleons within the nucleus, a more useful measure of the cohesiveness is the average binding energy per nucleon, E_b, as given below:

$$E_b = \frac{931(W - M)}{A} \text{ MeV/nucleon}, \tag{3.19}$$

where A, the atomic mass number, represents the number of nucleons within the nucleus. For the case of ^{17}O, the binding energy is 131.7 MeV and the average binding energy per nucleon is 7.75 MeV.

The binding energy per nucleon is very low for the low-atomic-numbered elements but rises rapidly to a very broad peak at binding energies in excess of 8 MeV/nucleon and then decreases very slowly until a value of 7.58 MeV/nucleon is reached for ^{238}U. Figure 3-5, in which the binding energy per nucleon is plotted against the number of nucleons in the various isotopes, shows that, with very few exceptions, there is a systematic variation of binding energy per nucleon with the number of nucleons within the nucleus.

The most notable departures from the smooth curve are the nuclides ^{4}He, ^{12}C, and ^{16}O. Each of these nuclides lies above the curve, indicating that they are very strongly bound. The ^{12}C and ^{16}O isotopes, as well as ^{20}Ne, which has more binding energy per nucleon than either of the nuclides that flank it, may be thought of as containing three, four, and five subunits of ^{4}He, respectively. The exceptional binding energies in these nuclei, together with the fact that ^{4}He nuclei, as alpha particles, are emitted in certain modes of radioactive transformation, suggest that nucleons tend to form stable subgroups of two protons and two neutrons within the nucleus.

The fact that the binding energy curve (Fig. 3-5) has the shape that it does explains why it is possible to release energy by splitting the very heavy elements and by fusing two very light elements. Since the binding energy per nucleon is greater for nuclei in the center of the curve than for nuclei at both extremes, any change in nuclear

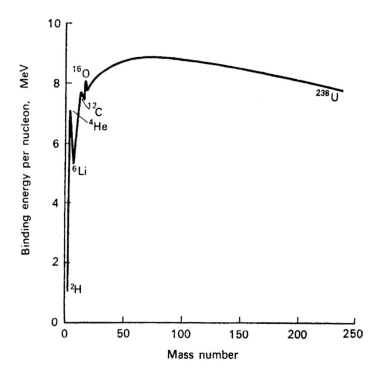

Figure 3-5. Variation of binding energy per nucleon with atomic mass number.

structure that drives the nucleons toward the center of the curve must release the energy difference between the final and the initial states.

Nuclear Models

(a) *Liquid drop model*

Two different nuclear models have been postulated. According to one of these, the nucleus is considered to be a homogenous mixture of nucleons in which all the nucleons interact strongly with each other. As a result, the internal energy of the nucleus is about equally distributed among the constituent nucleons, while surface tension forces tend to keep the nucleus spherical. This is analogous to a drop of liquid and hence is called the *liquid drop model* of the nucleus. This model, which was proposed by Bohr and Wheeler, is particularly successful in explaining nuclear fission and in permitting the calculation of the atomic masses of various nuclides whose atomic masses are very difficult to measure.

From the preceding discussion, we see that the mass of a nucleus of atomic number Z and atomic mass number A is

$$M = (A - Z)\,m_n + Z m_H - \delta. \tag{3.20}$$

Furthermore, the average binding energy per nucleon, and hence the total binding energy, is seen from Figure 3-5 to be a function of Z and A. The liquid drop model permits a semiempirical equation to be formulated that relates the nuclear mass and binding energy to A and Z. According to the liquid drop model, the intranuclear forces and the potential energy resulting from these forces are due to the short-range attractive forces between adjacent nucleons, the long-range repulsive coulomb forces among the protons, and the surface tension effect, in which nucleons on the surface of the nucleus are less tightly bound than those in the nuclear interior. The binding energy due to these forces is modified according to whether the numbers of neutrons and protons are even or odd. On the basis of this reasoning, the following equation was fitted to the experimental data relating nuclear mass, in atomic mass units, with A and Z:

$$M = 0.99389\,A - 0.00081\,Z + 0.014\,A^{2/3}$$

$$+ 0.083\frac{(A/2 - Z)^2}{A} + 0.000627\frac{Z^2}{A^{1/3}} + \Delta, \tag{3.21}$$

where

$$\Delta = 0 \qquad \text{for odd } A,$$
$$\Delta = -0.036/A^{3/4} \qquad \text{for even } A, \text{ even } Z, \text{ and}$$
$$\Delta = +0.036/A^{3/4} \qquad \text{for even } A, \text{ odd } Z.$$

(b) *Shell model*

The alternate nuclear model is called the *shell model*. According to this model of the nucleus, the various nucleons exist in certain energy levels within the nucleus and interact weakly among themselves. Many observations and experimental data lend support to such a nuclear structure. Among the stable nuclides, the "even–even" nuclei—nuclei with even numbers of protons and neutrons—are most numerous, with a total of 162 isotopes. Even–odd nuclei, in which one type of the nucleons—either the protons or the neutrons—is even in number and the other type is odd, are second in abundance with a total of 108 nuclides. Odd–odd nuclei are the fewest in number; only four such stable nuclides are found in nature. Furthermore, "magic numbers" have been found to recur among the stable isotopes. These magic numbers include 2, 8, 20, 50, 82, and 126. Atoms containing these numbers of protons or neutrons or both are most abundant in nature, suggesting unusual stability in their structures. Nuclei containing these magic numbers are relatively inert in a nuclear sense, that is, they do not react easily when bombarded with neutrons. This is analogous to the case of chemically inert elements that have filled electron energy levels.

Nucleons interact with magnetic fields in a manner similar to the orbiting electrons. Protons spin in either one of the two directions, as do the orbiting electrons, and hence behave as tiny magnets and are associated with magnetic moments. The charge on a proton is due to the fact that the proton is an assembly of three electrically charged quarks, two "up" quarks each containing a $+2/3$ charge and one "down" quark whose charge is $-1/3$, resulting in the proton's $+1$ charge. The magnetic moment of a proton is very much smaller than that of an extranuclear electron. In both instances, however, pairs of particles of opposite spin cancel each other's magnetic moments, leaving a net magnetic moment due to an unpaired particle. Neutrons too spin in either one of the two directions. Despite the fact that they are electrically neutral, spinning neutrons nevertheless have a magnetic moment as the neutron consists of three quarks, one positive up quark that contains a $+2/3$ charge and two negative down quarks, each one containing a $-1/3$ charge. Although the net charge is zero, the distribution of charges in the neutron leads to electrical polarization, and hence the ability to generate a magnetic field. The magnetic moment of protons, especially in hydrogen, is the basis for analysis using nuclear magnetic resonance and for magnetic resonance imaging in the practice of medicine.

All these observed facts are compatible with an energy level model of the nucleus similar to the electronic energy level model of the atom. Each nucleon in a nucleus is identified by its own set of four quantum numbers, as in the case of the extranuclear electrons. By application of the Pauli exclusion principle to nucleons, it is possible to construct energy levels that contain successively 2, 8, 20, 28, 50, 82, and 126 nucleons.

As in the case of the extranuclear electrons, nucleons too may be excited by raising them to higher energy levels. When this occurs, the nucleon falls back into its ground state and emits a photon whose energy is equal to the energy difference between the excited and ground states. This is the same type of phenomenon as seen in the case of optical and characteristic X-ray spectra. The photon in this case is called a *gamma ray*. Because nuclear energy levels are usually much further apart than electronic energy levels, gamma rays are usually (though not necessarily) more energetic than X-ray photons. It should be emphasized that from the practical viewpoint of health physics, X-rays and gamma rays are identical. They differ only in their place of origin—X-rays in the extranuclear structure and gamma rays within the nucleus. Once they are produced, it is impossible to distinguish between X-rays and gamma rays.

Nuclear Stability

If a plot is made of the number of protons versus the number of neutrons for the stable isotopes, the curve shown in Figure 3-6 is obtained. The stable isotopes lie within a relatively narrow range, indicating that the neutron-to-proton ratio must lie within certain limits if a nucleus is to be stable. Most radioactive nuclei lie outside this range of stability. The plot also shows that the slope of the curve, which initially has a value of unity, gradually increases as the atomic number increases, thereby showing the continuously increasing ratio of neutrons to protons.

Since all nuclear forces are attractive, it may appear surprising to find unstable nuclei with an excessive number of neutrons. This apparent anomaly may be explained simply in terms of the shell model of the nucleus. According to the Pauli exclusion principle, like nucleons may be grouped in pairs with each pair having all quantum numbers the same except the spin quantum number. Since nuclei with completely filled energy levels are more stable than those with unfilled inner levels, additional neutrons, in the case of nuclei with unfilled proton levels but filled neutron levels, result in unstable nuclei. To achieve stability, the nucleus may undergo an internal rearrangement in which the additional neutron transforms itself into a proton by emitting an electron. The new proton then pairs off with a proton in one

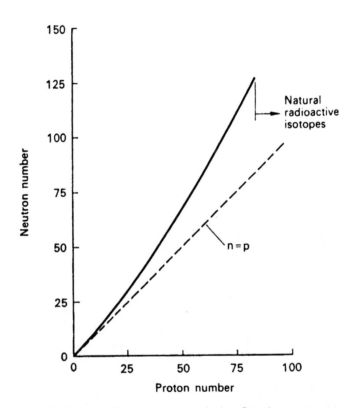

Figure 3-6. Nuclear stability curve. The line represents the best fit to the neutron–proton coordinates of stable isotopes.

of the unfilled proton levels. As an example of this possible mechanism, consider the consequences of the addition of a neutron to $^{31}_{15}$P. This is the stable isotope of phosphorus that occurs naturally. According to the shell model, the 15 protons inside the nucleus may be distributed among seven pairs with one proton remaining unpaired, while the neutrons may be paired off into eight groups. If now an additional neutron is added to the nucleus to make $^{32}_{15}$P, the additional neutron may go into another energy level. This condition, however, is unstable. The additional neutron may therefore become a proton and an electron—with the electron being ejected from the nucleus and the proton pairing off with the single proton, thereby forming stable $^{32}_{16}$S. This internal nuclear transformation is called a *radioactive transformation* or a *radioactive decay*.

SUMMARY

Although the word *atom* is derived from the Greek word *atomos*, which means "indivisible," modern science has found the atom to be a complex structure consisting of a positively charged nucleus surrounded by negatively charged electrons. The nucleus in turn is composed of two different particles—positively charged protons and electrically neutral neutrons. The protons and neutrons consist of an assembly of three smaller particles called quarks. Quarks are considered to be one of the fundamental building blocks in nature. Strong, attractive, short-ranged, nuclear forces act between the nucleons (particles within the nucleus) to overcome the repulsive electric forces that act between the protons. In a neutral atom, the number of extranuclear electrons is equal to the number of intranuclear protons. The overall diameter of the atom is on the order of 10^{-8} cm while the diameter of the nucleus measures about 10^{-13} cm.

The Bohr atomic model resembles a miniature solar system, with the electrons revolving around the nucleus in only certain allowable radii that are described by a set of four quantum numbers. The wave mechanics atomic model pictures the atom as a central nucleus surrounded by a cloud of electrons. The distances of these electrons from the nuclei are not precisely defined, as in the Bohr model, but rather are described by a wavelike probability function. These two atomic models coincide to the extent that the most probable radii of the wave mechanical model correspond to the precisely quantized radii of the Bohr model. Although the wave mechanical model has replaced the Bohr model for highly theoretical considerations, the Bohr model is adequate to explain the phenomena that underlie most health physics measurements and applications.

The atomic number and hence the chemical properties of an element are determined by the number of protons within the nucleus. Different atoms of the same element, however, may have different numbers of neutrons within their nuclei. These different forms of the same element are called *isotopes*. The total number of nucleons within a nucleus is called its *atomic mass number*. An isotope usually is specified by the name of the element and its atomic mass number. In written form, we frequently describe an isotope by its atomic number as a subscript to the left of its chemical symbol and its atomic mass number as a superscript to the left of its symbol. Thus, for uranium 238, whose atomic number is 92, we have $^{238}_{92}$U. The mass of a nucleus is less than the sum of the masses of its constituent parts. This mass difference represents the mass equivalent of the energy that was expended in assembling the nucleus (the binding energy). When a particle is ejected from the nucleus or when an atom undergoes nuclear fission, this potential energy reappears as the kinetic energy of the ejected particle or of the fission fragments and the energy of accompanying radiation. A stable atom requires that the ratio of neutrons to protons within the nucleus be within certain limits. If this ratio is too great or too small then the nucleus is unstable and it spontaneously attempts to become stable by a radioactive transformation.

PROBLEMS

3.1. What is the closest approach that a 5.3-MeV alpha particle can make to a gold nucleus?

3.2. Calculate the number of atoms per cubic centimeter of lead given that the density of lead is 11.3 g/cm^3 and its atomic weight is 207.21.

3.3. A μ^- meson has a charge of -4.8×10^{-10} sC and a mass 207 times that of a resting electron. If a proton should capture a μ^- to form a "mesic" atom, calculate

    (a) the radius of the first Bohr orbit and

    (b) the ionization potential.

3.4. Calculate the ionization potential of a singly ionized ^{4}He atom.

3.5. Calculate the current due to the hydrogen electron in the ground state of hydrogen.

3.6. Calculate the ratio of the velocity of a hydrogen electron in the ground state to the velocity of light.

3.7. Calculate the Rydberg constant for deuterium.

3.8. What is the uncertainty in the momentum of a proton inside a nucleus of ^{27}Al? What is the kinetic energy of this proton?

3.9. A sodium ion is neutralized by capturing a 1-eV electron. What is the wavelength of the emitted radiation if the ionization potential of Na is 5.41 V?

3.10. **(a)** How much energy would be released if 1 g of deuterium were fused to form helium according to the equation ^{2}H $+ ^2$H $\rightarrow ^4$He $+$ Q?

    (b) How much energy is necessary to drive the two deuterium nuclei together?

3.11. The density of beryllium (atomic number 4) is 1.84 g/cm^3, and the density of lead (atomic number 82) is 11.3 g/cm^3. Calculate the density of a ^{9}Be and a ^{208}Pb nucleus.

3.12. Determine the electronic shell configuration for aluminum (atomic number 13).

3.13. What is the difference in mass between the hydrogen atom and the sum of the masses of a proton and an electron? Express the answer in energy equivalent (eV) of the mass difference.

3.14. If the heat of vaporization of water is 540 cal/g at atmospheric pressure, what is the binding energy of a water molecule?

3.15. The ionization potential of He is 24.5 eV. What is the

    (a) minimum velocity with which an electron is moving before it can ionize an unexcited He atom?

    (b) maximum wavelength of a photon in order that it ionizes the He atom?

3.16. In a certain 25-W mercury-vapor ultraviolet lamp, 0.1% of the electric energy input appears as UV radiation of wavelength 2537 Å. What is the UV photon emission rate per second from this lamp?

3.17. The atomic mass of tritium is 3.017005 amu. How much energy in million electron volts is required to dissociate the tritium into its component parts?

3.18. Compute the frequency, wavelength, and energy (in electron volts) for the second and third lines in the Lyman series.

3.19. Using the Bohr atomic model, calculate the velocity of the ground-state electrons in hydrogen and in helium.

3.20. The heat of combustion when H_2 combines with O_2 to form water is 60 kcal/mol water. How much energy (in electron volts) is liberated per molecule of water produced?

3.21. The atomic weights of ^{16}O, ^{17}O, and ^{18}O are 15.994915, 16.999131, and 17.999160 amu, respectively. Calculate the atomic weight of oxygen.

3.22. Calculate the molecular weight of chlorine, Cl_2, using the exact atomic weights of the chlorine isotopes given in appropriate reference sources.

3.23. If 9 g of NaCl were dissolved in 1 L of water, what would be concentration, in atoms per milliliter, of each of the constituent elements in the solution?

3.24. The visual threshold of the normal human eye is about 7.3×10^{-15} W/cm^2 for light whose wavelength is 556 nm. What is the corresponding photon flux, in photons per square centimeter per second?

3.25. What is the binding energy of the last neutron in ^{17}O?

3.26. Calculate the number of hydrogen atoms in 1-g water.

3.27. If all the mass of an electron were converted to electromagnetic energy, what would be the

    (a) energy of the photon, in joules and in million electron volts?

    (b) wavelength of the photon, in angstrom units?

3.28. The thermal energy content of 1 U.S. gal (3.79 L) gasoline is 36.65 kW hours. To what weight of nuclear fuel, grams, does this amount of energy correspond?

3.29. The binding energy of K electrons in copper is 8.980 keV and 0.953 kcV in the L level. What is the wavelength of the K_α characteristic X-ray?

3.30. The first ionization potential of aluminum is 4.2 eV. What is the maximum wavelength of light that can ionize an aluminum atom?

3.31. Two alpha particles are separated by a distance of 4×10^{-15} m. Calculate the

    (a) repulsive electrical force between them.

    (b) attractive gravitational force between them.

3.32. The bonding energy of a C—C bond is about 100 kcal/mol. What is the corresponding energy, expressed as eV/bond?

SUGGESTED READINGS

Born, M. *Atomic Physics*, 8th ed. Hafner, Darien, CT, 1970.

Cohen, B. L. *Concepts of Nuclear Physics*. McGraw-Hill, New York, 1971.

Evans, R. D. *The Atomic Nucleus*. McGraw-Hill, New York, 1955.

Friedlander, G., Kennedy, J. W., Macias, E. S., and Miller, J. M. *Nuclear and Radiochemistry*, 3rd ed. John Wiley & Sons, New York, 1981.

Glasstone, S. *Sourcebook on Atomic Energy,* 3rd ed. D. Van Nostrand, Princeton, NJ, 1967.

Halliday, D., Resnick, R., and Walker, J. *Fundamentals of Physics*, 7th ed. John Wiley & Sons, New York, 2004.

Heisenberg, W. *Philosophic Problems of Nuclear Science*. Fawcett Publications, Greenwich, CT, 1966.

Hunt, S. E. *Nuclear Physics for Engineers and Scientists*. Halstead Press, New York, 1987.

Krane, K. S. *Introductory Nuclear Physics*. John Wiley & Sons, New York, 1987.

Lapp, R. E., and Andrews, H. L. *Nuclear Radiation Physics*, 4th ed. Prentice Hall, Englewood Cliffs, NJ, 1972.

Lilley, J. S. *Nuclear Physics: Principles and Application*. John Wiley & Sons, New York, 2001.

Moore, J. W., Stanitski, C. L., and Jurs, P. C. *Chemistry, the Molecular Science*. Thomson Brooks Cole, Belmont, CA, 2005.

Patel, S. B. *Nuclear Physics: An Introduction*. John Wiley & Sons, New York, 1988.

Peierls, R. E. *The Laws of Nature*. Charles Scribner's Sons, New York, 1956.

Powers, T. *Heisenberg's War*. Little, Brown and Company, Boston, MA, 1993.

Rhodes, R. *The Making of the Atomic Bomb*. Simon and Schuster, New York, 1986.

Rhodes, R. *Dark Sun*. Simon and Schuster, New York, 1996.

Rogers, E. M. *Physics for the Inquiring Mind*. Princeton University Press, Princeton, NJ, 1960.

Rutherford, E. On the scattering of alpha and beta particles by matter and the structure of the atom. *Phil Mag*, **21**:669–688, 1911.

Rutherford, E., Chadwick, J., and Ellis, C. D. *Radiations from Radioactive Substances*. Cambridge University Press, Cambridge, U.K., 1930.

Semat, H., and Albright, J. R. *Introduction to Atomic and Nuclear Physics*, 5th ed. Holt, Rinehart, and Winston, New York, 1972.

Serway, R. A., and Jewett, J. W. *Physics for Scientists and Engineers*, 6th ed. Thomson Brooks Cole, Belmont, CA, 2004.

Smyth, H. D. *Atomic Energy for Military Purposes*. Princeton University Press, Princeton, NJ, 1945.

Wehr, M. R., Richards, J. A., and Adair, T. W. *Physics of the Atom*, 4th ed. Addison Wesley, Reading, MA, 1985.

Young, H. D, and Freedman, R. A. *Sears and Zemansky's University Physics with Modern Physics*, 11th ed. Addison Wesley, Reading, MA, 2003.

RADIATION SOURCES

RADIOACTIVITY

Radioactivity may be defined as spontaneous nuclear transformations in unstable atoms that result in the formation of new elements. These transformations are characterized by one of several different mechanisms, including alpha-particle emission, beta-particle and positron emission, and orbital electron capture. Each of these reactions may or may not be accompanied by gamma radiation. Radioactivity and radioactive properties of nuclides are determined by nuclear considerations only and are independent of the chemical and physical states of the radionuclide. Radioactive properties of atoms, therefore, cannot be changed by any means and are unique to the respective radionuclides. The exact mode of radioactive transformation depends on the energy available for the transition. The available energy, in turn, depends on two factors: on the particular type of nuclear instability—that is, whether the neutron-to-proton ratio is too high or too low for the particular nuclide under consideration—and on the mass–energy relationship among the parent nucleus, daughter nucleus, and emitted particle.

TRANSFORMATION MECHANISMS

All radioactive transformations fall into one of the following categories:

- Alpha emission
- Isobaric transitions (Given the atomic number of the parent nucleus is Z, that of the daughter nucleus is $Z + 1$, if a beta particle is emitted, or $Z - 1$, if a positron is emitted. The atomic mass number of the daughter is same as that of the parent.)
  - Beta (negatron) emission
  - Positron emission
  - Orbital electron capture
- Isomeric transitions (The atomic number and the atomic mass number of the daughter is same as that of the parent.)
  - Gamma ray emission
  - Internal conversion

Alpha Emission

An alpha particle is a highly energetic helium nucleus that is emitted from the nucleus of an unstable atom when the neutron-to-proton ratio is too low. It is a positively charged, massive particle consisting of an assembly of two protons and two neutrons. Since atomic numbers and mass numbers are conserved in alpha transitions, it follows that the result of alpha emission is a daughter whose atomic number is two less than that of the parent and whose atomic mass number is four less than that of the parent. In the case of ^{210}Po, for example, the reaction is

$$^{210}_{84}\text{Po} \rightarrow {}^{4}_{2}\text{He} + {}^{206}_{82}\text{Pb}.$$

In this example, ^{210}Po has a neutron-to-proton ratio of $126:84$, or $1.5:1$. After decaying by alpha-particle emission, a stable daughter nucleus, ^{206}Pb, is formed, whose neutron-to-proton ratio is $1.51:1$. With one exception, $^{147}_{62}$Sm, naturally occurring alpha emitters are found only among elements of atomic number greater than 82. The explanation for this is twofold: First is the fact that the electrostatic repulsive forces in the heavy nuclei increase much more rapidly than the cohesive nuclear forces and the magnitude of the electrostatic forces, consequently, may closely approach or even exceed that of the nuclear force; the second part of the explanation is concerned with the fact that the emitted particle must have sufficient energy to overcome the high potential barrier at the surface of the nucleus resulting from the presence of the positively charged nucleons. This potential barrier may be graphically represented by the curve in Figure 4-1. The inside of the nucleus, because of the negative potential there, may be thought of as a potential well that is surrounded by a wall whose height is about 25 MeV for an alpha particle inside a high-atomic-numbered nucleus. According to quantum mechanical theory, an alpha particle may escape from the potential well by tunneling through the potential barrier. For alpha emission to be observed from the high-atomic-numbered naturally occurring elements, theoretical considerations demand that an alpha particle have a kinetic energy greater than 3.8 MeV. This condition is verified by the experimental finding that the lowest energy alpha particle emitted from the high-atomic-numbered elements is 3.93 MeV. This alpha particle originates in ^{232}Th. (Samarium-147 emits an alpha particle whose energy is only 2.18 MeV. This low energy is consistent, however,

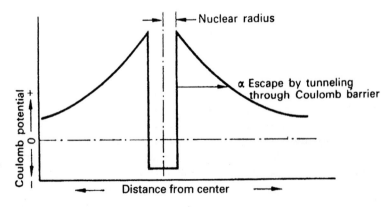

Figure 4-1. Potential inside and in the vicinity of a nucleus.

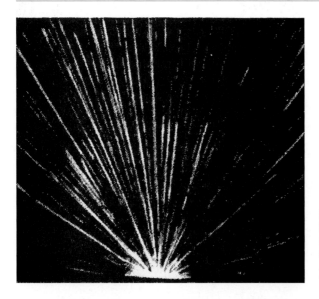

Figure 4-2. Tracks in a Wilson cloud chamber of alpha particles from ThC (^{212}Bi), energy = 8.78 MeV. (Reproduced with permission from Rutherford E, Chadwick J, Ellis CD, *Radiations from Radioactive Substances.* New York, NY: Macmillan; 1930.)

with the theoretical calculations mentioned above if the low atomic number, 62, of samarium is considered.) The question regarding the source of this kinetic energy naturally arises. This energy results from the net decrease in mass following the formation of the alpha particle. Generally, for alpha emission to occur, the following conservation equation must be satisfied:

$$M_p = M_d + M_\alpha + 2M_e + Q, \tag{4.1}$$

where M_p, M_d, M_α, and M_e are respectively equal to the masses of the parent, the daughter, the emitted alpha particle, and the two orbital electrons that are lost during the transition to the lower atomic numbered daughter, while Q is the total energy release associated with the radioactive transformation. In the case of the decay of ^{210}Po, for example, we have, from Eq. (4.1),

$$Q = M_{Po} - M_{Pb} - M_\alpha - 2M_e$$

$$= 210.04850 - 206.03883 - 4.00277 - 2 \times 0.00055$$

$$= 0.0058 \text{ amu (atomic mass units).}$$

In energy units,

$$Q = 0.0058 \text{ amu} \times 931 \text{ MeV/amu} = 5.4 \text{ MeV}$$

This Q value represents the total energy associated with the transformation of ^{210}Po. Since no gamma ray is emitted in this transition, the total released energy appears as kinetic energy and is divided between the alpha particle and the daughter, which recoils after the alpha particle is emitted. The exact energy division between the alpha and recoil nucleus depends on the mass of the daughter and may be calculated by applying the laws of conservation of energy and momentum. If M and m are the masses, respectively, of the recoil nucleus and the alpha particle, and if V and v are their respective velocities, then

$$Q = \frac{1}{2} MV^2 + \frac{1}{2} mv^2. \tag{4.2}$$

We have, according to the law of conservation of momentum,

$$MV = mv \tag{4.3}$$

or

$$V = \frac{mv}{M}.$$

When the value for V from Eq. (4.3) is substituted into Eq. (4.2), we have

$$Q = \frac{1}{2} M \frac{m^2 v^2}{M^2} + \frac{1}{2} mv^2. \tag{4.4}$$

If we let E represent the kinetic energy of the alpha particle, $1/2\ mv^2$, then Eq. (4.4) may be rewritten as

$$Q = E \left(\frac{m}{M} + 1 \right)$$

or

$$E = \frac{Q}{1 + (m/M)}. \tag{4.5}$$

According to Eq. (4.5), the kinetic energy of the alpha particle emitted in the decay of ^{210}Po is

$$E = \frac{5.4 \text{ MeV}}{(1 + 4 \ / \ 206)} = 5.3 \text{ MeV}.$$

The kinetic energy of the recoil nucleus, therefore, is 0.1 MeV.

Alpha particles are essentially monoenergetic. However, alpha-particle spectrograms do show discrete energy groupings, with small energy differences among the different groups. These small differences are attributed to differences in the energy level of the daughter nucleus. That is, a nucleus that emits one of the lower energy alpha particles is left in an excited state, while the nucleus that emits the highest energy alpha particle for any particular nuclide is usually left in the "ground" state. A nucleus left in an excited state usually emits its energy of excitation in the form of a gamma ray. It should be pointed out that this gamma ray is emitted immediately, almost always in $<10^{-12}$ second, after the emission of the charged particle has occurred and, hence, seems to have come from the radioactive parent nucleus, when in fact it was emitted by the daughter nucleus. Because the gamma ray seems to have appeared simultaneously with the charged particle, the parent is said to be a gamma emitter. It should be pointed out that most of the alpha particles are usually emitted with the maximum energy. Very few nuclei, consequently, are left in excited states and gamma radiation, therefore, accompanies only a small fraction

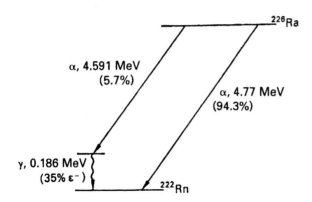

Figure 4-3. Radium-226 transformation (decay) scheme.

of the alpha particles. Radium may be cited as an example of an alpha emitter with a complex spectrum (Fig. 4-3). In the overwhelming majority of transformations of ^{226}Ra (94.3%), alphas are emitted with a kinetic energy of 4.777 MeV. The remaining alpha particles (5.7%) have kinetic energies of only 4.591 MeV. In that instance, where a lower energy alpha is emitted, the daughter nucleus is left in an excited state and rids itself of its energy of excitation by emitting a gamma-ray photon whose energy is equal to the difference between the energies of the two alpha particles: $4.777 - 4.591 = 0.186$ MeV. (About 35% of these gamma-ray photons are internally converted: see the section on "Internal Conversion.") The ^{226}Ra spectrum is among the least intricate of all the complex alpha spectra. Most alpha emitters have several groups of alphas and therefore more gammas. All alpha spectra, however, show the same consistent relationship among the various nuclear energy levels.

Alpha particles are extremely limited in their ability to penetrate matter. The dead outer layer of skin is sufficiently thick to absorb all alpha radiations from radioactive materials. As a consequence, alpha radiation from sources outside the body does not constitute a radiation hazard. In the case of internally deposited alpha-emitting radionuclides, however, the shielding effect of the dead outer layer of skin is absent and the energy of the alpha radiation is dissipated in living tissue. For this reason and others to be discussed in Chapter 7, alpha radiation is a concern when it irradiates the inside of the body from internally deposited radioisotopes.

Isobaric Transitions

Beta Emission

A beta particle is a charged particle that is indistinguishable from an ordinary electron; it is ejected from the nucleus of an unstable radioactive atom whose neutron-to-proton ratio is too high. The particle has a single negative electric charge $(-1.6 \times 10^{-19}$ C), and therefore is also called a negatron, and a very small mass (0.00055 amu). Theoretical considerations preclude the independent existence of an intranuclear electron. It appears as though the beta particle is formed at the instant of emission by the transformation of a neutron into a proton and an electron according to the equation

$$\,_0^1n \rightarrow \,_1^1H + \,_{-1}^0e. \tag{4.6}$$

This transformation shows that beta decay occurs among those nuclides that have a surplus of neutrons. For beta emission to be energetically possible, the exact nuclear mass of the parent must be greater than the sum of the exact masses of the daughter nucleus plus the beta particle.

$$M_p = M_d + M_e + Q. \tag{4.7}$$

This restriction, of course, is analogous to the corresponding restriction on alpha emitters. Because a unit negative charge is lost during beta decay and the mass of the beta particle is $\ll 1$ amu, the daughter nucleus is one atomic number higher than its parent but retains the same atomic mass number as the parent. For example, radioactive phosphorus decays to stable sulfur according to the equation

$$^{32}_{15}P \rightarrow {}^{32}_{16}S + {}_{-1}^{0}e + 1.71 \text{ MeV}.$$

The transformation energy, in this instance 1.71 MeV, is the energy equivalent of the difference in mass between the ^{32}P nucleus and the sum of the masses of the ^{32}S nucleus and the beta particle, and appears as kinetic energy of the beta particle. If neutral atomic masses are used to complete the mass–energy equation, then, of course, the mass of the electron shown in the right-hand side of Eq. (4.7) is not considered since it is implicitly included in the extranuclear electronic structure of the ^{32}S. The mass difference is

$$31.973907 = 31.972070 + Q$$

$$Q = 0.001837 \text{ amu}$$

and the energy equivalent of the mass difference is

$$0.001837 \times 931 \text{ MeV/amu} = 1.71 \text{ MeV}.$$

Examination of Eq. (4.5) shows that in the case of beta emission, an extremely small part of the energy of the reaction is dissipated by the recoil nucleus since m/M (where m is now the mass of the beta particle and M is the mass of the daughter nucleus) is very small. In the example given above,

$$\frac{m}{M} = \frac{0.00055}{32} = 0.000017$$

and Q is only 1.000017 times greater than the kinetic energy of the beta particle.

On the basis of the above analysis, one might expect beta particles to be mo-noenergetic, as in the case of alpha radiation. This expectation is not confirmed by experiment. Instead, beta particles are found to be emitted with a continuous energy distribution ranging from zero to the theoretically expected value based on mass–energy considerations for the particular beta transition. In the case of ^{32}P, for example, although the maximum energy of the beta particle may be 1.71 MeV, most of the betas have considerably smaller kinetic energies, as shown in Figure 4-4. The average energy of a ^{32}P beta particle is 0.7 MeV or about 41% of the maximum energy. Generally, the average energy of the beta radiation from the most beta-active

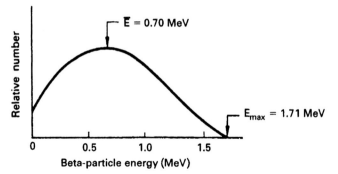

Figure 4-4. Phosphorous-32 beta spectrum.

radioisotopes is about 30–40% of the maximum energy. Unless otherwise specified, whenever the energy of a beta emitter is given, it implies the maximum energy.

The fact that beta radiation is emitted with a continuous energy distribution up to a definite maximum seems to violate the established energy–mass conservation laws. This is explained by the simultaneous emission of a second type of particle, called a *neutrino*,[1] whose energy is equal to the difference between the kinetic energy of the accompanying beta particle and the maximum energy of the spectral distribution. The neutrino, as postulated, has no electrical charge and a vanishingly small mass. Although these two characteristics make detection of the neutrino difficult, neutrinos have been measured and the neutrino hypothesis has been experimentally verified. Equation (4.6) should therefore be modified to

$$\,_{0}^{1}\mathrm{n} \rightarrow \,_{1}^{1}\mathrm{H} + \,_{-1}^{0}\mathrm{e} + \nu, \tag{4.8}$$

where ν represents the neutrino.

Phosphorus-32, like several other beta emitters—including ^{3}H, ^{14}C, ^{90}Sr, and ^{90}Y—emits no gamma rays. These isotopes are known as pure beta emitters. The opposite of a pure beta emitter is a beta–gamma emitter. In this case, the beta particle is followed instantaneously (in most cases) by a gamma ray. For those radionuclides where the gamma-ray emission is delayed, as in the case of ^{99m}Tc and ^{137}Cs, the gamma-ray emission is called an *isomeric transition*. In an isomeric transition, the atomic number and the atomic mass number of the radionuclide is not changed. The explanation for the gamma ray here is the same as that in the case of the alpha. The daughter nucleus, after the emission of a beta, is left in an excited condition and rids itself of the energy of excitation by the emission of a gamma ray. Mercury-203 may be given as an example. It emits a 0.21-MeV beta and a 0.279-MeV gamma, as seen in the transformation scheme shown in Figure 4-5.

Both illustrations given above (^{32}P and ^{203}Hg) are for beta emitters with simple spectra, that is, for emitters with only one group of beta particles. Complex beta emitters are those radionuclides whose beta spectra contain more than one distinct group

---

[1]Technically this is an antineutrino, but in common parlance, unless there is a need to be more specific, this particle is referred to as a neutrino.

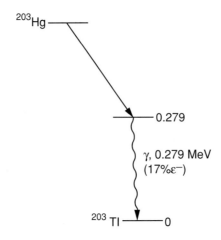

Figure 4-5. Transformation (decay) scheme of ^{203}Hg.

of beta particles. Potassium-42, for example, in about 82% of its transformations, decays to stable ^{42}Ca by emission of a beta particle from a group whose maximum energy is 3.55 MeV and in 18% of its transformations by emitting a 2.04-MeV beta particle (Fig. 4-6). In this case, however, the excited ^{42}Ca immediately emits a gamma-ray whose energy is 1.53 MeV. A commonly used radionuclide that has an even more complex beta–gamma spectrum is ^{131}I. This isotope decays to stable ^{131}Xe by emission of a beta particle. In 90.4% of the transformations, however, the beta particle is a member of a group whose maximum energy is 0.61 MeV, while the remaining beta particles belong to groups whose maximum energies range from 0.81 MeV in 0.6% of the transformations to 0.25 MeV in 1.6% of the transformations. In all instances, each xenon daughter nucleus is left in an excited state and rids itself of its excitation energy by the emission of gamma radiation. The nucleus resulting from the emission of the 0.61-MeV beta particle rids itself of its excitation energy by two competing gamma-ray transitions. About 94% of these nuclei (corresponding to 85.3% of the ^{131}I transformations) emit 0.364-MeV gamma rays, and the remaining excited nuclei emit two gamma rays in cascade—one of 0.284 MeV and one of 0.080 MeV. The transformation scheme for ^{131}I is shown in Figure 4-7.

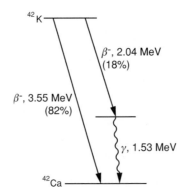

Figure 4-6. Potassium-42 transformation (decay) scheme.

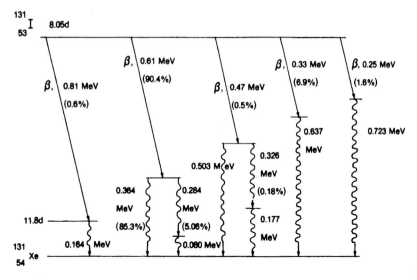

Figure 4-7. Iodine-131 transformation (decay) scheme.

Beta radiation, because of its ability to penetrate tissue to varying depths, depending on the energy of the beta particle, may be an external radiation hazard. The exact degree of hazard, of course, depends on the beta energy and must be evaluated in every case. Generally, however, beta particles whose energies are less than 200 keV have very limited penetrability. Examples of these include ^{3}H, ^{35}S, and ^{14}C. None of these are considered as external radiation hazards. It should be noted, however, that beta particles give rise to highly penetrating X-rays called *bremsstrahlung* when they strike a high-atomic-numbered absorbing material. (This interaction is more fully discussed later, in Chapter 5.) Unless shielding is appropriately designed and proper precautionary measures are adopted, beta radiation may indirectly result in an external radiation hazard through the production of bremsstrahlung radiation. Any beta-emitting radionuclide, of course, is potentially hazardous when it is deposited in the body in amounts exceeding those thought to be safe.

Positron Emission

In those instances where the neutron-to-proton ratio is too low and alpha emission is not energetically possible, the nucleus may, under certain conditions, attain stability by emitting a positron. A positron is a beta particle whose charge is positive (in contrast to a negatively charged beta particle, which is called a *negatron* when there is a need to explicitly distinguish it from a positron). In all other respects, it is the same as the negative beta particle or an ordinary electron. Its mass is 0.000548 amu and its charge is $+1.6 \times 10^{-19}$ C. Because of the fact that the nucleus loses a positive charge when a positron is emitted, the daughter product is one atomic number less than the parent. The mass number of the daughter remains unchanged, as in all nuclear transitions involving electrons. In the case of ^{22}Na, for example, we have

$$^{22}_{11}\text{Na} \rightarrow ^{22}_{10}\text{Ne} + ^{\ 0}_{+1}\text{e} + \nu. \tag{4.9}$$

While negative electrons occur freely in nature, positrons have only a transitory existence. They occur in nature only as the result of the interaction between cosmic rays and the atmosphere and disappear in a matter of microseconds after formation. The manner of disappearance is of interest and great importance to the health physicist. The positron combines with an electron and the two particles are annihilated giving rise to two gamma-rays whose energies are equal to the mass equivalent to the positron and electron. This interaction is discussed in greater detail in Chapter 5. The positron is not thought to exist independently within the nucleus. Rather, it is believed that the positron results from a transformation, within the nucleus, of a proton into a neutron according to the reaction

$$_1^1\text{H} \rightarrow \, _0^1\text{n} + \, _{+1}^{0}\text{e} + \nu. \tag{4.10}$$

For positron emission, the following conservation equation must be satisfied:

$$M_p = M_d + M_{+e} + Q. \tag{4.11}$$

where M_p, M_d, and M_{+e} are the masses of the parent nucleus, daughter nucleus, and positron, respectively and Q is the mass equivalent of the energy of the reaction. Since the daughter is one atomic number less than the parent, it must also lose an orbital electron, M_{-e}, immediately after the nuclear transition. In terms of atomic masses, therefore, the conservation equation is

$$M_p = M_d + M_{-e} + M_{+e} + Q. \tag{4.12}$$

Sodium-22, a useful radioisotope for biomedical research, is transformed into ^{22}Ne by two competing mechanisms, positron emission and K capture (which is discussed in the following section), according to the decay scheme shown in Figure 4-8. Positrons are emitted in 89.8% of the transformations, while the competing decay mode, K capture, occurs in 10.2% of the nuclear transformations. Both modes of decay result in ^{22}Ne, which is in an excited state; the excitation energy instantly appears as a 1.277-MeV gamma ray. The exact atomic mass of the neon may be calculated from the positron transformation data with the aid of Eq. (4.12):

$$M\left(^{22}\text{Ne}\right) = M\left(^{22}\text{Na}\right) - 2M_e - Q_m$$

$$= 22.001404 - 2 \times 0.000548 - \frac{(0.544 + 1.277) \text{ MeV}}{931 \dfrac{\text{MeV}}{\text{amu}}}$$

$$= 21.998353 \text{ amu.}$$

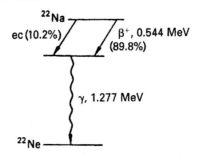

Figure 4-8. Sodium-22 transformation (decay) scheme.

Since positrons are electrons, the radiation hazard from the positrons themselves is very similar to the hazard from beta particles. The gamma radiation resulting from the annihilation of the positron, however, makes all positron-emitting isotopes potential external radiation hazards.

Orbital Electron Capture

Equation (4.12) shows that if a neutron-deficient atom is to attain stability by positron emission, it must exceed the weight of its daughter by at least two electron masses. If this requirement cannot be met, then the neutron deficiency is overcome by the process known as *orbital electron capture* or, alternatively, as *electron capture* or as *K* capture. In this radioactive transformation, one of the extranuclear electrons is captured by the nucleus and unites with an intranuclear proton to form a neutron according to the equation

$$_{-1}^{0}e + {}_{1}^{1}\text{H} \rightarrow {}_{0}^{1}\text{n} + \nu. \tag{4.13}$$

The electrons in the *K* shell are much closer to the nucleus than those in any other shell. The probability that the captured orbital electron will be from the *K* shell is therefore much greater than that for any other shell; hence, the alternate name for this mechanism is *K capture*. In the case of *K* capture, as in positron emission, the atomic number of the daughter is one less than that of the parent while the atomic mass number remains unchanged. The energy conservation requirements for *K* capture are much less rigorous than for positron emission. It is merely required that the following conservation equation be satisfied:

$$M_p + M_e = M_d + \phi + Q, \tag{4.14}$$

where M_p and M_d are the atomic masses (not the atomic mass numbers) of the parent and daughter, M_e is the mass of the captured electron, ϕ is the binding energy of the captured electron, and Q is the energy of the reaction.

Equation (4.14) may be illustrated by the *K*-capture mode of transformation of ^{22}Na. The binding energy ϕ of the sodium *K* electron is 1.08 keV. The energy of decay Q may therefore be calculated as follows:

$$Q = M(^{22}\text{Na}) + M_e - M(^{22}\text{Ne}) - \phi$$

$$= 22.001404 + 0.000548 - 21.998352 - \frac{0.00108 \text{ MeV}}{931 \text{ MeV/amu}}$$

$$= 0.003600 \text{ amu.}$$

In terms of MeV, we have

$$Q = 0.0036 \text{ amu} \times 931 \frac{\text{MeV}}{\text{amu}} = 3.352 \text{ MeV.}$$

Since a 1.277-MeV gamma ray is emitted, we are left with an excess of 3.352–1.277 = 2.075 MeV. The recoil energy associated with the emission of the gamma-ray is insignificantly small. The excess energy, therefore, must be carried away by a neutrino. Although the example given above is for a specific reaction, it is nevertheless typical of all reactions involving *K* capture; a neutrino is always emitted when an orbital electron is captured. It is thus seen that in all types of radioactive decay involving either the capture or emission of an electron, a neutrino must be emitted in order to conserve energy. However, in contrast to positron and negatron (ordinary beta) decay, in which the neutrino carries off the difference between the actual kinetic energy of the particle and the maximum observed kinetic energy and, therefore, has a continuous energy distribution, the neutrino in orbital electron capture is necessarily monoenergetic.

Whenever an atom is transformed by orbital electron capture, an X-ray, characteristic of the daughter element, is emitted as an electron from an outer orbit falls into the energy level that had been occupied by the captured electron. That characteristic X-rays of the daughter should be observed follows from the fact that the X-ray photon is emitted after the nucleus captures the orbital electron and is thereby transformed into the daughter. These low-energy characteristic X-rays must be considered by health physicists when they compute absorbed radiation doses from internally deposited isotopes that decay by orbital electron capture.

Isomeric Transitions

Gamma Rays

Gamma rays are monochromatic electromagnetic radiations that are emitted from the nuclei of excited atoms following radioactive transformations; they provide a mechanism for ridding excited nuclei of their excitation energy without affecting either the atomic number or the atomic mass number of the atom. Since the health physicist is concerned with all radiations that come from radioactive substances and since X-rays are indistinguishable from gamma rays, characteristic X-rays that arise in the extranuclear structure of many nuclides must be considered by the health physicist in evaluating radiation hazards. However, because of the low energy of characteristic X-rays, they are of importance mainly in the case of internally deposited radionuclides. Annihilation radiation—the gamma rays resulting from the mutual annihilation of positrons and negatrons—are usually associated, for health physics purposes, with those radionuclides that emit positrons. In considering the radiation hazard from ^{22}Na, for example, two 0.51-MeV photons (the energy equivalent of the two particles that were annihilated) from the annihilation process, which are not shown on the decay scheme, must be considered together with the 1.277-MeV gamma ray, which is shown on the decay scheme. The general rule in health physics, therefore, is automatically to associate positron emission with gamma radiation in all problems involving shielding, dosimetry, and radiation hazard evaluation.

Internal Conversion

Internal conversion is an alternative isomeric mechanism to radiative transition by which an excited nucleus of a gamma-emitting atom may rid itself of excitation energy. It is an interaction in which a tightly bound electron interacts with its nucleus, absorbs the excitation energy from the nucleus, and is ejected from the atom. Internally converted electrons appear in monoenergetic groups. The kinetic energy of the converted electron is always found to be equal to the difference between the energy of the gamma-ray emitted by the radionuclide and the binding energy of the converted electron of the daughter element. Since electrons in the L energy level of high-atomic-numbered elements are also tightly bound, internal conversion in those elements results in two groups of electrons that differ in energies by the difference between the binding energies of the K and L levels. Internal conversion may be thought of as an internal photoelectric effect, that is, an interaction in which the gamma ray collides with the tightly bound electron and transfers all of its energy to the electron. The energy of the gamma ray is divided between the work done to overcome the binding energy of the electron and the kinetic energy imparted to the electron. This may be expressed by the equation

$$E_\gamma = E_e + \phi, \tag{4.15}$$

where E_γ is the energy of the gamma ray, E_e is the kinetic energy of the conversion electron, and ϕ is the binding energy of the electron. Since conversion electrons are monoenergetic, they appear as line spectra superimposed on the continuous beta-particle spectra of the radionuclide. An interesting example of internal conversion is given by ^{137}Cs. The ^{137}Cs isotope is transformed by beta emission to ^{137m}Ba, which is an excited metastable state of ^{137}Ba. Instead of instantaneously emitting a gamma ray after radioactive decay, a metastable nucleus delays the emission of the gamma ray. In the case of ^{137m}Ba, the nucleus remains in the excited state for an average of 3.75 minutes (half-life = 2.6 minutes) before emitting a 0.661-MeV gamma ray (photon). This photon undergoes internal conversion in 11% of the transitions. The internal conversion coefficient (α), defined as the ratio of the number of conversion electrons per gamma-ray, is given by

$$\alpha = \frac{N_e}{N_\gamma} \tag{4.16}$$

and is equal to 0.11 in this instance. Since the half-life of ^{137m}Ba is 2.6 minutes, it is, for practical purposes, in secular equilibrium with its ^{137}Cs parent. (Secular equilibrium is explained later in this chapter.) The conversion electrons, therefore, seem to come from the ^{137}Cs and are found to be superimposed on the beta spectrum of cesium, as shown in Figure 4-9. After internal conversion, characteristic X-rays are emitted as outer orbital electrons fill the vacancies left in the deeper energy levels by the conversion electrons. These characteristic X-rays may themselves be absorbed by an

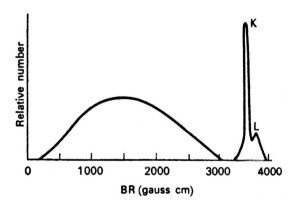

Figure 4-9. Cesium-137 beta spectrum showing conversion electrons from the K and L energy levels.

internal photoelectric effect on the atom from which they were emitted, a process that is of the same nature as internal conversion. The ejected electrons from this process are called *Auger electrons*, and they possess very little kinetic energy.

TRANSFORMATION KINETICS

Half-Life

Different radioactive atoms are transformed at different rates and each radionuclide has its own characteristic transformation rate. For example, when the activity of ^{32}P is measured daily over a period of about 3 months and the percentage of the initial activity is plotted as a function of time, the curve shown in Figure 4-10 is obtained. The data show that one-half of the ^{32}P is gone in 14.3 days, half of the remainder in another 14.3 days, half of what is left during the following 14.3 days, and so on.

If a similar series of measurements were made on ^{131}I, it would be observed that the iodine would disappear at a faster rate. One-half would be gone after 8 days, and three-fourths of the initial activity would be gone after only 16 days, while seven-eighths of the iodine would be gone after 24 days.

The time required for any given radionuclide to decrease to one-half of its original quantity is a measure of the speed with which it undergoes radioactive transformation. This period of time is called the *half-life* and is characteristic of the particular radionuclide. Each radionuclide has its own unique rate of transformation, and no operation, either chemical or physical, is known that will change the transformation rate; the decay rate of a radionuclide is an unalterable property of that nuclide. Half-lives of radionuclides range from microseconds to billions of years.

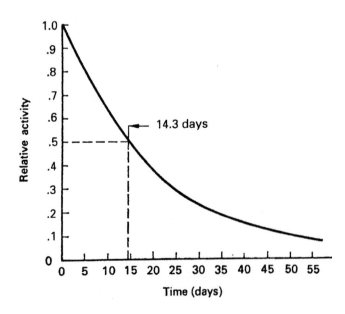

Figure 4-10. Decrease of ^{32}P activity.

From the definition of the half-life, it follows that the fraction of a radionuclide remaining after n half-lives is given by the relationship

$$\frac{A}{A_0} = \frac{1}{2^n},$$ (4.17)

where A_0 is the original quantity of activity and A is the activity left after n half-lives.

EXAMPLE 4.1

Cobalt-60, a gamma-emitting isotope of cobalt whose half-life is 5.3 years, is used as a radiation source for radiographing pipe welds. Because of the decrease in radioactivity with increasing time, the exposure time for a radiograph will be increased annually. Calculate the correction factor to be applied to the exposure time in order to account for the decrease in the strength of the source.

Solution

Equation (4.17) may be rewritten as

$$\frac{A_0}{A} = 2^n.$$

By taking the logarithm of each side of the equation, we have

$$\log \frac{A_0}{A} = n \log 2,$$

where n, the number of ^{60}Co half-lives in 1 year, is $1/(5.3) = 0.189$.

$$\log \frac{A_0}{A} = 0.189 \times 0.301 = 0.0569$$

$$\frac{A_0}{A} = \text{inverse log } 0.0569 = 1.14$$

The ratio of the initial quantity of cobalt to the quantity remaining after 1 year is 1.14. The exposure time after 1 year, therefore, must be increased by 14%. It should be noted that this ratio is independent of the actual amount of activity at the beginning and end of the year. After the second year, the ratio of the cobalt at the beginning of the second year to that at the end will be 1.14. The same correction factor, 1.14, therefore, is applied every year to the exposure time for the previous year.

If the decay data for any radionucide are plotted on semilog paper, with the activity measurements recorded on the logarithmic axis and time on the linear axis,

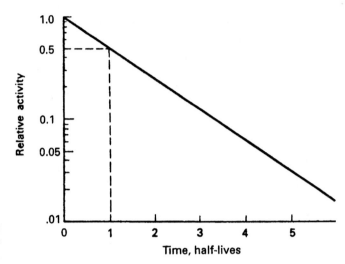

Figure 4-11. Generalized semilog plot of the decrease in activity due to radioactive transformation.

a straight line is obtained. If time is measured in units of half-lives, the straight line shown in Figure 4-11 is obtained.

The illustrative example given above could have been solved graphically with the aid of the curve in Figure 4-11. The ordinate at which the time in units of half-life, 0.189, intersects the curve shows that 87.7% of the original activity is left. The correction factor, therefore, is the reciprocal of 0.877:

$$\text{Correction factor} = \frac{1}{0.877} = 1.14.$$

The fact that the graph of activity versus time, when drawn on semilog paper, is a straight line tells us that the quantity of activity left after any time interval is given by the following equation:

$$A = A_0 \, e^{-\lambda t}, \tag{4.18}$$

where A_0 is the initial quantity of activity, A is the amount left after time t, λ is the transformation rate constant (also called the decay rate constant, or simply the decay constant), and e is the base of the system of natural logarithms.

The transformation rate constant is the fractional decrease in activity per unit time and is defined as

$$\operatorname*{Limit}_{\Delta t \to 0} \frac{\Delta N / N}{\Delta t} = -\lambda, \tag{4.19}$$

where N is a number of radioactive atoms and ΔN is the number of these atoms that are transformed during a time interval Δt. The fraction $\Delta N / N$ is the fractional decrease in the number of radioactive atoms during the time interval Δt. A negative sign is given to λ to indicate that the quantity N is decreasing. For a short-lived radionuclide, λ may be determined from the slope of an experimentally determined transformation curve. For long-lived isotopes, the transformation constant may be determined by measuring N, counting the number of transformations per second, and then calculating the numerical value of λ from Eq. (4.19).

EXAMPLE 4.2

A mass of 1-μg radium is found to emit 3.7×10^4 alpha particles per second. If each of these alphas represents a radioactive transformation of radium, what is the transformation rate constant for radium?

Solution

In this case, ΔN is 3.7×10^4, Δt is 1 s, and N, the number of radium atoms per microgram, may be calculated as follows:

$$N = \frac{6.02 \times 10^{23} \text{ atoms/mol}}{A \text{ g/mol}} \times W \text{ g}, \qquad (4.20)$$

where A is the atomic weight and W is the weight of the radium sample.

$$N = \frac{6.02 \times 10^{23} \text{ atoms/mol}}{2.26 \times 10^2 \text{ g/mol}} \times 10^{-6} \text{ g} = 2.66 \times 10^{15} \text{ atoms}$$

The transformation rate constant, therefore, is

$$\lambda = \frac{\Delta N/N}{\Delta t} = \frac{3.4 \times 10^4 \text{ atoms}/2.66 \times 10^{15} \text{ atoms}}{1 \text{ s}} = 1.27 \times 10^{-11} \frac{1}{\text{s}}$$

On a per-year basis, the transformation rate is

$$\lambda = 1.27 \times 10^{-11} \text{ s}^{-1} \times 8.64 \times 10^4 \frac{\text{s}}{\text{d}} \times 3.65 \times 10^2 \frac{\text{d}}{\text{yr}}$$

$$\lambda = 4.02 \times 10^{-4} \text{ yr}^{-1}$$

This value of λ may be used in Eq. (4.18) to compute the amount of radium left after any given time period.

EXAMPLE 4.3

What percentage of a given amount of radium will decay during a period of 1000 years?

Solution

The fraction remaining after 1000 years is given by

$$\frac{A}{A_0} = e^{-\lambda t} = e^{-4.02 \times 10^{-4} \frac{1}{yr} \times 10^3 \, yr} = e^{-0.402} = 0.67 = 67\%.$$

The percentage that decayed during the 1000-year period, therefore, is

$$100 - 67 = 33\%.$$

The quantitative relationship between half-life T and decay rate constant λ may be found by setting A/A_0 in Eq. (4.18) equal to $1/2$ and solving the equation for t. In this case, of course, the time is the half-life T:

$$\frac{A}{A_0} = \frac{1}{2} = e^{-\lambda T}$$

$$T = \frac{0.693}{\lambda}. \tag{4.21}$$

EXAMPLE 4.4

Given that the transformation rate constant for ^{226}Ra is $4.38 \times 10^{-4} \frac{1}{yr}$, calculate the half-life for radium.

Solution

$$T = \frac{0.693}{\lambda} = \frac{0.693}{4.38 \times 10^{-4} \frac{1}{yr}} = 1.6 \times 10^3 \text{ years.}$$

Average Life

Although the half-life of a particular radionuclide is a unique, reproducible characteristic of that nuclide, it is nevertheless a statistical property and is valid only because of the very large number of atoms involved. (One microgram of radium contains 2.79×10^{15} atoms.) Any particular atom of a radionuclide may be transformed at any time, from zero to infinity. For some applications, as in the case of dosimetry of internally deposited radioactive material (discussed in Chapter 6), it is convenient to use the average life of the radioisotope. The *average life* is defined simply as the *sum of the lifetimes of the individual atoms divided by the total number of atoms originally present.*

The instantaneous transformation rate of a quantity of radioisotope containing N atoms is λN. During the time interval between t and $t + dt$, the total number of transformations is $\lambda N\, dt$. Each of the atoms that decayed during this interval, however, had existed for a total lifetime t since the beginning of observation on them. The sum of the lifetimes, therefore, of all the atoms that were transformed during the time interval between t and $t + dt$, after having survived since time $t = 0$, is $t\lambda N\, dt$. The average life, τ, of the radioactive species is

$$\tau = \frac{1}{N_0} \int_0^\infty t\lambda N\, dt, \tag{4.22}$$

where N_0 is the number of radioactive atoms in existence at time $t = 0$. Since

$$N = N_0 e^{-\lambda t},$$

we have

$$\tau = \frac{1}{N_0} \int_0^\infty t\lambda N_0 e^{-\lambda t}\, dt. \tag{4.23}$$

This expression, when integrated by parts, shows the value for the mean life of a radioisotope to be

$$\tau = \frac{1}{\lambda}. \tag{4.24}$$

If the expression for the transformation constant in terms of the half-life, T, of the radioisotope

$$\lambda = \frac{0.693}{T}$$

is substituted into Eq. (4.22), the relationship between the half-life and the mean life is found to be

$$\tau = \frac{T}{0.693} = 1.44\, T. \tag{4.25}$$

ACTIVITY

The Becquerel

Uranium-238 and its daughter ^{234}Th each contain about the same number of atoms per gram—approximately 2.5×10^{21}. Their half-lives, however, are greatly different; ^{238}U has a half-life of 4.5×10^9 years while ^{234}Th has a half-life of 24.1 days (or 6.63×10^{-2} year). Thorium-234, therefore, is transforming 6.8×10^{10} times faster than ^{238}U.

Another example of greatly different rates of transformation that may be cited is ^{35}S and ^{32}P. These two radionuclides, which have about the same number of atoms per gram, have half-lives of 87 and 14.3 days, respectively. The radiophosphorus, therefore, is decaying about 6 times faster than the ^{35}S. When using radioactive material, the radiations are the center of interest. In this context, therefore, 1/6 g of ^{32}P is about equivalent to 1 g of ^{35}S in radioactivity, while 15 mg of ^{234}Th is about equivalent in activity to 1 g of ^{238}U. These examples show that when interest is centered on radioactivity, the gram is not a very useful unit of quantity. To be meaningful, the unit for quantity of radioactivity must be based on the number of radioactive decays occurring within a prescribed time in the radioactive material. This quantity—the number of decays within a given time—is called the activity. Two units for measuring the activity are used. The SI unit is called the *becquerel*, symbolized by Bq, and is defined as follows:

> The *becquerel* is that quantity of radioactive material in which one atom is transformed per second (tps).

Very often, we use the term disintegration instead of transformation and the becquerel is defined in term of disintegrations per second, dps.

$$1 \text{ Bq} = 1 \text{ tps} = 1 \text{ dps}. \tag{4.26}$$

It must be emphasized that although the becquerel is defined in terms of a number of atoms transformed per second, it is not a measure of the rate of transformation. *The becquerel is a measure only of quantity of radioactive material.* The phrase "one atom transformed per second," as used in the definition of the becquerel, is not synonymous with the number of particles emitted by the radioactive isotope in 1 s. In the case of a pure beta emitter, for example, 1 Bq, or 1 tps, does, in fact, result in one beta particle per second. In the case of a more complex radionuclide, however, such as ^{60}Co (Fig. 4-12), each transformation releases one beta particle and two gamma rays; the total number of radiations, therefore, is 3 s^{-1} Bq^{-1}. In the case of ^{42}K (Fig. 4-6), on the other hand, 18% of the beta transformations are accompanied by a single quantum of gamma radiation. The total number of emissions from 1 Bq of ^{42}K, therefore, is 1.2 s^{-1}. For many purposes, the becquerel is a very small quantity

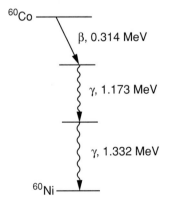

Figure 4-12.   Cobalt-60 decay scheme.

of activity and, therefore, the following multiples of the becquerel are commonly used:

1 kilobecquerel (kBq) = 10^3 Bq
1 megabecquerel (MBq) = 10^6 Bq
1 gigabecquerel (GBq) = 10^9 Bq
1 terabecquerel (TBq) = 10^{12} Bq.

The Curie

The *curie*, symbolized by Ci, is the unit for quantity of radioactivity that was used before the adoption of the SI units and the becquerel. The curie, which originally was defined as the activity of 1 g of ^{226}Ra, is now more explicitly defined as

> The *curie* is the activity of that quantity of radioactive material in which 3.7×10^{10} atoms are transformed in one second.

The curie is related to the becquerel by

$$1 \text{ Ci} = 3.7 \times 10^{10} \text{ Bq}. \tag{4.27}$$

For health physics as well as for many other purposes, the curie is a very large amount of activity. Submultiples of the curie, as listed below, are therefore used:

1 millicurie (mCi) = 10^{-3} Ci
1 microcurie (μCi) = 10^{-6} Ci
1 nanocurie (nCi) = 10^{-9} Ci
1 picocurie (pCi) = 10^{-12} Ci
1 femtocurie (fCi) = 10^{-15} Ci.

Specific Activity

Note that the becquerel (or curie), although used as a unit of quantity, does not imply anything about the mass or volume of the radioactive material in which the specified number of transformations occur. The concentration of radioactivity, or the relationship between the mass of radioactive material and the activity, is called the *specific activity*. Specific activity is the number of becquerels (or curies) per unit mass or volume. The specific activity of a carrier-free (pure) radioisotope—a radioisotope that is not mixed with any other isotope of the same element—may be calculated as follows:

If λ is the transformation constant in units of reciprocal seconds, then the number of transformations per second and, hence, the number of becquerels in an aggregation of N atoms, is simply given by λN.

If the radionuclide under consideration weighs 1 g, then, according to Eq. (4.20), the number of atoms is given by

$$N = \frac{6.02 \times 10^{23} \text{ atoms/mol}}{A \dfrac{\text{g}}{\text{mol}}} \times W \text{ g,}$$

where A is the atomic weight of the nuclide. The activity per unit weight or the specific activity, therefore, is

$$SA = \lambda N = \frac{\lambda \times 6.02 \times 10^{23}}{A} \frac{\text{Bq}}{\text{g}}. \tag{4.28}$$

Equation (4.28) gives the desired relationship between the specific activity and weight of an isotope and can be calculated in terms of the isotope's half-life by substituting Eq. (4.21) for λ in Eq. (4.28):

$$\lambda N = \frac{0.693}{T} \times \frac{6.02 \times 10^{23}}{A}$$

$$SA = \frac{4.18 \times 10^{23}}{A \times T} \frac{\text{Bq}}{\text{g}}. \tag{4.29}$$

Note that Eqs. (4.28) and (4.29) are valid only if λ and T are given in time units of seconds. A more convenient form for calculating specific activity may be derived by making use of the fact that there are 3.7×10^{10} tps in 1 g of ^{226}Ra. The specific activity, therefore, of ^{226}Ra is 3.7×10^{10} Bq/g. The ratio of the specific activity of any radionuclide, SA_i, to that of ^{226}Ra is

$$\frac{SA_i}{3.7 \times 10^{10} \frac{\text{Bq}}{\text{g}}} = \left(\frac{4.18 \times 10^{23}/A_i \times T_i}{4.18 \times 10^{23}/A_{\text{Ra}} \times T_{\text{Ra}}} \right)$$

$$SA_i = 3.7 \times 10^{10} \times \frac{A_{\text{Ra}} \times T_{\text{Ra}}}{A_i \times T_i} \frac{\text{Bq}}{\text{g}}, \tag{4.30}$$

where A_{Ra}, the atomic weight of ^{226}Ra, is 226, A_i is the atomic weight of the radioisotope whose specific activity is being calculated, and T_{Ra} and T_i are the half-lives of the radium and the radionuclide i. The only restriction on Eq. (4.30) is that both half-lives must be in the same units of time. Analogously, the specific activity in units of $\frac{\text{Ci}}{\text{g}}$ is given by

$$SA_i = \frac{A_{\text{Ra}} \times T_{\text{Ra}}}{A_i \times T_i} \frac{\text{Ci}}{\text{g}}. \tag{4.31}$$

EXAMPLE 4.5

Calculate the specific activities of ^{14}C and ^{35}S, given that their half-lives are 5730 years and 87 days, respectively.

Solution

$$SA\left({}^{14}\text{C}\right) = 3.7 \times 10^{10} \times \frac{226 \times 1600 \text{ year}}{14 \times 5700 \text{ year}} \frac{\text{Bq}}{\text{g}}$$

$$= 1.7 \times 10^{11} \frac{\text{Bq}}{\text{g}} \quad \left(4.5 \frac{\text{Ci}}{\text{g}}\right),$$

$$SA\left({}^{35}\text{S}\right) = 3.7 \times 10^{10} \times \frac{226 \times 1600 \text{ year} \times 365 \text{ d/yr}}{35 \times 87 \text{ days}} \frac{\text{Bq}}{\text{g}}$$

$$= 1.6 \times 10^{15} \frac{\text{Bq}}{\text{g}} \quad \left(4.3 \times 10^{4} \frac{\text{Ci}}{\text{g}}\right),$$

The specific activities calculated above are for the carrier-free isotopes of ^{14}C and ^{35}S. Very frequently, especially when radioisotopes are used to label compounds, the radioisotope is not carrier-free but rather constitutes an extremely small fraction, either by weight or number of atoms, of the element that is labeled. In such cases, it is customary to refer to the specific activity either of the element or the compound that is labeled. Generally, the exact meaning of the specific activity is clear from the context.

EXAMPLE 4.6

A solution of $Hg(NO_3)_2$ tagged with ^{203}Hg has a specific activity of 1.5×10^{5} Bq/mL $(4 \frac{\mu\text{Ci}}{\text{mL}})$. If the concentration of mercury in the solution is $5 \frac{\text{mg}}{\text{mL}}$,

(a) what is the specific activity of the mercury?

(b) what fraction of the mercury in the $Hg(NO_3)_2$ is ^{203}Hg?

(c) what is the specific activity of the $Hg(NO_3)_2$?

Solution

(a) The specific activity of the mercury is

$$SA\left(\text{Hg}\right) = \frac{1.5 \times 10^{5} \text{ Bq/mL}}{5 \text{ mg Hg/mL}} = 0.3 \times 10^{5} \frac{\text{Bq}}{\text{mg}} \text{ Hg}.$$

(b) The weight-fraction of mercury that is tagged is given by

$$\frac{SA\left(\text{Hg}\right)}{SA\left({}^{203}\text{Hg}\right)},$$

and the specific activity of ^{203}Hg is calculated from Eq. (4.30):

$$SA\left(^{203}\text{Hg}\right) = 3.7 \times 10^{10} \times \frac{226 \times 1600 \text{ yr} \times 365 \text{ d/yr}}{203 \times 46.5 \text{ days}}$$

$$= 5.2 \times 10^{14} \frac{\text{Bq}}{\text{g}} \quad \left(1.4 \times 10^4 \frac{\text{Ci}}{\text{g}}\right).$$

The weight fraction of ^{203}Hg, therefore, is

$$\frac{0.3 \times 10^8 \text{ Bq/g Hg}}{5.2 \times 10^{14} \text{ Bq/g } ^{203}\text{Hg}} = 5.8 \times 10^{-8} \frac{\text{g } ^{203}\text{Hg}}{\text{g Hg}}.$$

(c) Since an infinitesimally small fraction of the mercury is tagged with ^{203}Hg, it may be assumed that the formula weight of the tagged Hg $(NO_3)_2$ is 324.63 and that the concentration of Hg $(NO_3)_2$ is

$$\frac{324.63 \text{ mg Hg } (NO_3)_2}{200.61 \text{ mg Hg}} \times \frac{5 \text{ mg Hg}}{\text{mL}} = 8.1 \frac{\text{mg Hg } (NO_3)_2}{\text{mL}}.$$

The specific activity, therefore, of the Hg$(NO_3)_2$ is

$$\frac{1.5 \times 10^5 \text{ Bq/mL}}{8.1 \text{ mg Hg } (NO_3)_2} = 1.9 \times 10^4 \frac{\text{Bq}}{\text{mg}} \text{ Hg } (NO_3)_2 \left[0.5 \frac{\mu\text{Ci}}{\text{mg}} \text{ Hg } (NO_3)_2\right].$$

EXAMPLE 4.7

Can commercially available ^{14}C-tagged ethanol, $CH_3-C^*H_2-OH$, whose specific activity is 1 mCi/mol, be used in an experiment that requires a minimum specific activity of 10^7 transformations 1/min.mL? The density of the alcohol is $0.789 \frac{\text{g}}{\text{cm}^3}$.

Solution

The specific activity of ^{14}C, as calculated from Eq. (4.13), is 4.61 $\frac{\text{Ci}}{\text{g}}$. Therefore, 1 mCi of ^{14}C weighs

$$\frac{10^{-3} \text{ Ci}}{4.61 \frac{\text{Ci}}{\text{g}}} = 2.2 \times 10^{-4} \text{ g}$$

and the number of radioactive atoms represented by 0.22-mg ^{14}C is

$$\frac{6.02 \times 10^{23} \text{ atoms/mol}}{14 \frac{\text{g}}{\text{mol}}} \times 2.2 \times 10^{-4} \text{ g} = 9.5 \times 10^{18} \text{ atoms.}$$

Since 1 mol contains Avogadro's number of molecules and each tagged molecule contains only one carbon atom, there are

$$\frac{9.5 \times 10^{18}}{6.02 \times 10^{23}} = 16/\text{million}$$

ethanol molecules that are tagged. For all practical purposes, therefore, the additional mass due to the isotopic carbon may be neglected in calculating the molecular weight of the labeled ethanol and the accepted molecular weight of ethanol, 46.078, may be used to compute the activity per milliliter of the alcohol:

$$1 \frac{\text{mCi}}{\text{mol}} \times \frac{1 \text{ mol}}{46.078 \text{ g}} \times 2.22 \times 10^9 \frac{\text{t/min}}{\text{mCi}} \times 0.789 \frac{\text{g}}{\text{mL}} = 3.8 \times 10^7 \frac{\text{t/min}}{\text{mL}}.$$

The commercially available ethanol may be used.

NATURALLY OCCURRING RADIATION

There are three sources for naturally occurring sources of radiation. The oldest source is cosmic radiation, which is believed to have originated at the birth of the universe, about 13–14 billion years ago. A second source is from primordial radioactive elements that were created when the earth was born about 4.5 billion years ago. Concentrations or quantities of naturally occurring radioactive material of sufficient activity to be of interest to a health physicist are known by the acronym NORM. A third source of naturally occurring radioactivity and radiation is cosmogenic radioactivity. The production of cosmogenic radioactivity is an ongoing process as cosmic radiation interacts with the atmosphere to produce radionuclides. Another transient source of radioactivity was a naturally occurring nuclear reactor in what is now the Republic of Gabon in West Africa, at a site called Oklo, and hence is called the Oklo reactor. The Oklo reactor went critical about 1.7 billion years ago and continued to operate over a period of several hundred thousand years. The operating history of the Oklo reactor is inferred from the fission products that have been found and from the isotopic composition of the uranium at the Oklo site.

Cosmic Radiation

Cosmic radiation was discovered in 1912 by the Austrian physicist Victor Hess, for which he received the Nobel Prize in 1936. Cosmic rays are very high-energy particles from extraterrestrial sources that bombard the earth. One source is the sun, which emits mainly alpha particles and protons. The other radiation, consisting mainly of electrons and protons, originates beyond our solar system and is called *galactic radiation*. These primary particles enter the earth's atmosphere and collide with the atmospheric molecules to produce secondary cosmic rays that bombard the earth's surface and have sufficient energy to penetrate deeply into the ground and the sea. Cosmic ray intensity increases with altitude because of the decreased shielding effect of the atmosphere. For example, the cosmic ray intensity in Denver, CO, which is at an altitude of about 1609 meters (5280 feet), is about twice that in New York, which is at sea level. In a jet aircraft at an altitude of 30,000 feet (9140 meters), the cosmic ray intensity is about six to seven times that at sea level. Cosmic-ray intensity increases with increasing latitude north and south of the equator because the earth's magnetic field deflects the high-velocity charged particles that are cutting across the magnetic force field.

Cosmogenic Radioactivity

Interactions that occur between cosmic radiation and the atmosphere lead to the production of numerous cosmogenic radionuclides. Most of the cosmogenic radionuclides, because of their relative paucity and insignificant contribution to the dose from naturally occurring radioactivity, are of little or no importance in the context of health physics. Two of these, tritium (^{3}H) and radiocarbon (^{14}C), are of interest to health physicists because anthropogenic tritium and radiocarbon are widely used in research and the presence of the naturally occurring isotopes must be considered in interpreting health physics measurements when dealing with these radionuclides. The production of cosmogenic radionuclides is an ongoing process and a steady state has been established whereby the radionuclides are produced at the same rate as they decay. For ^{3}H, the worldwide steady state inventory is estimated to be 34×10^6 Ci (1.26×10^{18} Bq) and the estimated global inventory for ^{14}C is 31×10^7 Ci (1.15×10^{19} Bq).

The long half-life of ^{14}C (5730 years) makes it an excellent tool for "radiocarbon" dating of organic artifacts from the historical past. The production of ^{14}C is still going on due to nuclear transformations induced by the cosmic-ray bombardment of ^{14}N. The environmental burden of ^{14}C before the advent of nuclear bombs was about 1.5×10^{11} MBq (4 MCi) in the atmosphere, 4.8×10^{11} MBq (13 MCi) in plants, and 9×10^{12} MBq (243 MCi) in the oceans. Testing of nuclear weapons has resulted in an increase in the atmospheric level of radiocarbon. It is estimated that about 1.1×10^{11} MBq (3 MCi) ^{14}C were injected into the air by all weapons tests conducted up to 1963, when atmospheric testing was halted. The atmospheric radiocarbon exists as $^{14}CO_2$. It is therefore inhaled by all animals and utilized by plants in the process of photosynthesis. Because only living plants continue to incorporate ^{14}C along with nonradioactive carbon, it is possible to determine the age of organic matter by measuring the specific activity of the carbon present. If, after correcting for the weapons-testing contribution, it is assumed that the rate of production of ^{14}C, as well as its concentration in the air, has remained constant during the past several tens of thousands of years, then a simple correction of specific activity data for half-life permits the estimation of the age of ancient samples of organic matter.

EXAMPLE 4.8

If 2 g of carbon from a piece of wood found in an ancient temple is analyzed and found to have an activity of 10 transformations/minute/gram, what is the age of the wood if the current specific activity of ^{14}C in carbon is assumed to have been constant at 15 transformations/minute/gram?

Solution

The fraction of the original ^{14}C remaining today is, according to Eq. (4.18),

$$\frac{A}{A_0} = \frac{10}{15} = e^{-\lambda t}.$$

Since the half-life for ^{14}C is 5730 years

$$\lambda = \frac{0.693}{5730 \text{ years}} = 1.21 \times 10^{-4} \frac{1}{\text{yr}}$$

$$\frac{10}{15} = e^{-1.21 \times 10^{-4} t}$$

$$t = 3.35 \times 10^3 \text{ years.}$$

Primordial Radioactivity

The naturally occurring radioactive substance that Becquerel discovered in 1896 was a mixture of several radionuclides, which were later found to be related to each other. They were members of a long series of isotopes of various elements, all of which but the last were radioactive (Tables 4-1 to 4-4). Uranium, the most abundant of the radioactive elements in this mixture, consists of three different isotopes: about 99.3% of naturally occurring uranium is ^{238}U, about 0.7% is ^{235}U, and a trace quantity (about 5×10^{-3}%) is ^{234}U. The ^{238}U and ^{234}U belong to one family, the *uranium series*, while the ^{235}U isotope of uranium is the first member of another series called the *actinium series*. Uranium is ubiquitous in the natural environment and is found in the soil at average concentrations of about 3 ppm (parts per million) by weight, which corresponds to ~2 pCi or ~74 mBq/g soil. Uranium forms extremely stable compounds with phosphorous. Phosphate-rich soil, therefore, contains uranium at concentrations much higher than average, from about 7 ppm to about 125 ppm Medium-grade uranium ore contains about 1000–5000 ppm uranium, while the uranium concentration in high-grade ore is about 10,000–40,000 ppm. Uranium concentration in most surface waters in the United States of America are in the range of about 1–10 μg/L, and in most of the groundwater, the concentrations vary from about 1–120 μg/L.

Thorium, another ubiquitous naturally occurring radioactive element, is about 4 times more abundant in nature than uranium. The most abundant thorium isotope, ^{232}Th, is the first member of still another long chain of successive radionuclides.

TABLE 4-1. Thorium Series ($4n$)

NUCLIDE	HALF-LIFE	ALPHA[a]	BETA	GAMMA (PHOTONS/ TRANS.)[b]
			ENERGY (MeV)	
$^{232}_{90}$Th	1.39 10^{10} yrs	3.98		
$^{228}_{88}$Ra (MsTh1)	6.7 yrs		0.01	
$^{228}_{89}$Ac (MsTh2)	6.13 h		Complex decay scheme	1.59 (n.v.) 0.966 (0.2)
			Most intense beta group is 1.11 MeV	0.908 (0.25)
$^{228}_{90}$Th (RdTh)	1.91 yrs	5.421		0.084 (0.016)
$^{224}_{88}$Ra (ThX)	3.64 d	5.681		0.241 (0.038)
$^{220}_{86}$Rn (Tn)	52 s	6.278		0.542 (0.0002)
$^{216}_{82}$Po (ThA)	0.158 s	6.774		
$^{212}_{82}$Pb (ThB)	10.64 h		0.35, 0.59	0.239 (0.40)
$^{212}_{83}$Bi (ThC)	60.5 min	6.086 (33.7%)[c]	2.25 (66.3%)[c]	0.04 (0.034 branch)
$^{212}_{84}$Po (ThC')	3.04×10^{-7} s	8.776		
$^{208}_{81}$Tl (ThC'')	3.1 min		1.80, 1.29, 1.52	2.615 (0.997)
$^{208}_{82}$Pb (ThD)	Stable			

[a]Only the highest-energy alpha is given. Complete information on alpha energies may be obtained from Sullivan's *Trilinear Chart of Nuclides*, Government Printing Office, Washington, DC, 1957.
[b]Only the most prominent gamma rays are listed. For the complete gamma-ray information, consult T. P. Kohman: Natural radioactivity, in H. Blatz (ed.): *Radiation Hygiene Handbook*. McGraw-Hill, New York, 1959, pp. 6–13.
[c]Indicates branching. The percentage enclosed in the parentheses gives the proportional decay by the indicated mode.

All of the isotopes that are members of a radioactive series are found in the upper portion of the periodic table; the lowest atomic number in these groups is 81, while the lowest mass number is 207.

All the radioactive series have several common characteristics. The first member of each series is very long-lived, with a half-life that may be measured in geological time units. That the first member of each must be very long-lived is obvious because, if the time since the creation of the world is considered, relatively short-lived radioactive material would have decayed away during the 4.5 billion years that the earth is believed to have been in existence. This point is well illustrated by considering the artificially produced *neptunium series*. In this case, the first member is the transuranic element ^{241}Pu, which is produced in the laboratory by neutron irradiation of reactor-produced ^{239}Pu. The half-life of ^{241}Pu, however, is only 13 years. Because of this short half-life, even a period of a century is long enough to permit most of the ^{241}Pu to decay away. Even the half-life of the longest-lived member of this series, ^{237}Np, which is 2.2×10^6 years, is sufficiently short for this element to have essentially disappeared if it had been created at the same time as all the other elements of the earth.

A second characteristic common to all three naturally occurring series is that each has a gaseous member and, furthermore, that the radioactive gas in each case is a different isotope of the element radon. In the case of the uranium series, the gas (Rn) is called *radon*; in the thorium series, the gas is called *thoron*; and in the actinium series (Table 4-4), it is called *actinon*. It should be noted that the artificial neptunium series (Table 4-2) has no gaseous member. The existence of the radioactive gases in

TABLE 4-2. Neptunium Series $(4n + 1)^a$

| NUCLIDE | HALF-LIFE | ENERGY (MeV) | | GAMMA (PHOTONS/ TRANS.)^c |
		ALPHA^b	BETA	
$^{241}_{94}$Pu	13.2 yrs		0.02	
$^{241}_{95}$Am	462 yrs	5.496		0.060 (0.4)
$^{237}_{93}$Np	2.2×10^6 yrs	4.77		
$^{233}_{91}$Pa	27.4 d		0.26, 0.15, 0.57	0.31 (very strong)^c
$^{233}_{92}$U	1.62×10^5 yrs	4.823		0.09 (0.02)
				0.056 (0.02)
				0.042 (0.15)
$^{229}_{90}$Th	7.34×10^3 yrs	5.02		
$^{225}_{88}$Ra	14.8 d		0.32	
$^{225}_{89}$Ac	10.0 d	5.80		
$^{221}_{87}$Fr	4.8 min	6.30		0.216 (1)
$^{217}_{85}$At	0.018 s	7.02		
$^{213}_{83}$Bi	47 min	5.86 (2%)^d	1.39 (98%)^d	
$^{213}_{84}$Po	4.2×10^{-6} s	8.336		
$^{209}_{81}$Tl	2.2 min		2.3	0.12 (weak)^e
$^{209}_{82}$Pb	3.32 h		0.635	
$^{209}_{83}$Bi	Stable			

^{a}This series is not found in nature; it is produced artificially.
^{b}Only the highest-energy alpha is given. Complete information on alpha energies may be obtained from Sullivan's *Trilinear Chart of Nuclides*, Government Printing Office, Washington, DC, 1957.
^{c}Only the most prominent gamma rays are listed. For the complete gamma-ray information, consult T. P. Kohman: Natural radioactivity, in H. Blatz (ed.): *Radiation Hygiene Handbook*. McGraw-Hill, New York, 1959, pp. 6–13.
^{d}Indicates branching. The percentage enclosed in the parentheses gives the proportional decay by the indicated mode.
^{e}Exact intensity is not known.

the three chains is one of the chief reasons for the public health concerns about naturally occurring environmental radioactivity. The radon gas diffuses out of the earth into the air and becomes widely dispersed throughout the local atmosphere. The radioactive radon daughters, which are solids under ordinary conditions, attach themselves to atmospheric dust. The health hazard from radon comes not from the radon itself but from inhaled dust particles that had adsorbed radioactive radon progeny on their surfaces. Atmospheric concentrations of radioactivity from this source vary widely around the earth and are dependent on the local concentrations of uranium and thorium in the earth. Although the average atmospheric radon concentration is on the order of 2×10^{-6} Bq/mL ($5 \times 10^{-11} \mu$Ci/mL), concentrations 10 times greater are not uncommon. Since the radioactive radon progeny are found on the surface of atmospheric particles and airborne particles are washed out of the atmosphere by rain, it is reasonable to expect increased background radiation during periods of rain. This phenomenon is, in fact, observed, and it must be considered by health physicists and others in interpreting routine monitoring data. Fallout caused by rain in Upton, NY, is shown in Figure 4-13—a set of curves giving the beta and gamma activity during rainy and dry periods.

TABLE 4-3. Uranium Series $(4n + 2)$

NUCLIDE	HALF-LIFE	ENERGY (MeV)		
		ALPHA[a]	BETA	GAMMA (PHOTONS/ TRANS.)[b]
$^{238}_{92}$U	4.51×10^9 yrs	4.18		
$^{434}_{90}$Th (U X$_1$)	24.10 d		0.193, 0.103	0.092 (0.04)
				0.063 (0.03)
$^{234m}_{91}$Pa (U X$_2$)	1.175 min		2.31	1.0 (0.015)
				0.76 (0.0063), I.T.
$^{234}_{91}$Pa (UZ)	6.66 h		0.5	Many (weak)
$^{234}_{92}$U (UII)	2.48×10^5 yrs	4.763		
$^{230}_{90}$Th (I$_0$)	8.0×10^4 yrs	4.685		0.068 (0.0059)
$^{230}_{90}$Ra	1,622 yrs	4.777		
$^{222}_{86}$Em (Rn)	3.825 d	5.486		0.51 (very weak)
$^{218}_{84}$Po (RaA)	3.05 min	5.998 (99.978%)[c]	Energy not known (0.022%)[c]	0.186 (0.030)
$^{218}_{85}$At (RaA')	2 s	6.63 (99.9%)[c]	Energy not known (0.1%)[c]	
$^{218}_{86}$Em (RaA'')	0.019 s	7.127		
$^{214}_{82}$Pb (RaB)	26.8 min		0.65	0.352 (0.036)
				0.295 (0.020)
				0.242 (0.07)
$^{214}_{83}$Bi (RaC)	19.7 min	5.505 (0.04%)[c]	1.65, 3.7 (99.96%)[c]	0.609 (0.295)
				1.12 (0.131)
$^{214}_{84}$Po (RaC')	1.64×10^{-4} s	7.680		
$^{210}_{81}$Tl (RaC'')	1.32 min		1.96	2.36 (1)
				0.783 (1)
				0.297 (1)
$^{210}_{82}$Pb (RaD)	19.4 yrs		0.017	0.0467 (0.045)
$^{210}_{83}$Bi (RaE)	5.00 d		1.17	
$^{210}_{84}$Po (RaF)	138.40 d	5.298		0.802 (0.000012)
$^{206}_{82}$Pb (RaG)	Stable			

[a]Only the highest-energy alpha is given. Complete information on alpha energies may be obtained from Sullivan's *Trilinear Chart of Nuclides*, Government Printing Office, Washington, DC, 1957.
[b]Only the most prominent gamma rays are listed. For the complete gamma-ray information, consult T. P. Kohman: Natural radioactivity, in H. Blatz (ed.): *Radiation Hygiene Handbook*. McGraw-Hill, New York, 1959, pp. 6–13.
[c]Indicates branching. The percentage enclosed in the parentheses gives the proportional decay by the indicated mode.

When the ground is covered with snow, however, a decrease in airborne radioactivity occurs because of the filtering action of the snow blanket on the effusing radon and its daughters. Increased environmental radioactivity from this source also occurs during temperature inversions, when vertical mixing of the air and consequent dilution of radon and its daughters temporarily ceases. Because of this naturally occurring airborne activity, certain correction factors must be applied in computing the atmospheric concentration of airborne radioactive contaminants from dust samples. These corrections are discussed in more detail in Chapter 13.

TABLE 4-4. Actinium Series $(4n + 3)$

| NUCLIDE | HALF-LIFE | ENERGY (MeV) | | |
		ALPHA[a]	BETA	GAMMA (PHOTONS/TRANS.)[b]
$^{235}_{92}U$	7.13×10^8 yrs	4.39		0.18 (0.7)
$^{231}_{90}Th$ (UY)	25.64 h		0.094, 0.302, 0.216	0.022 (0.7) 0.0085 (0.4) 0.061 (0.16)
$^{231}_{91}Pa$	3.43×10^4 yrs	5.049		0.33 (0.05) 0.027 (0.05) 0.012 (0.01)
$^{227}_{89}Ac$	21.8 yrs	4.94 (1.2%)[a]	0.0455 (98.8%)[c]	
$^{227}_{90}Th$ (RdAc)	18.4 d	6.03		0.24 (0.2) 0.05 (0.15)
$^{223}_{87}Fr$ (AcK)	21 min		1.15	0.05 (0.40) 0.08 (0.24)
$^{223}_{88}Ra$ (AcX)	11.68 d	5.750		0.270 (0.10) 0.155 (0.055)
$^{219}_{86}Em$ (An)	3.92 s	6.824		0.267 (0.086) 0.392 (0.048)
$^{215}_{84}Po$ (AcA)	1.83×10^{-3} s	7.635		
$^{211}_{82}Pb$ (AcB)	36.1 min		1.14, 0.5	Complex spectrum, 0.065–0.829 MeV
$^{211}_{83}Bi$ (AcC)	2.16 min	6.619 (99.68%)[c]	Energy not known (0.32%)[c]	0.35 (0.14)
$^{211}_{84}Po$ (AcC')	0.52 s	7.434		0.88 (0.005) 0.56 (0.005)
$^{207}_{81}Tl$ (AcC'')	4.78 min		1.47	0.87 (0.005)
$^{207}_{82}Pb$	Stable			

[a]Only the highest-energy alpha is given. Complete information on alpha energies may be obtained from Sullivan's *Trilinear Chart of Nuclides*, Government Printing Office, Washington, DC, 1957.

[b]Only the most prominent gamma rays are listed. For the complete gamma-ray information, consult T. P. Kohman: Natural radioactivity, in H. Blatz (ed.): *Radiation Hygiene Handbook*. McGraw-Hill, New York, 1959, pp. 6–13.

[c]Indicates branching. The percentage enclosed in the parentheses gives the proportional decay by the indicated mode.

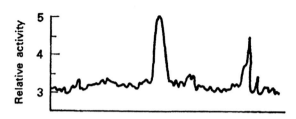

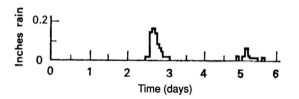

Figure 4-13. Washout of atmospheric radioactivity by rain. (Reproduced with permission from Weiss MM. *Area Survey Manual*. Upton, NY: Brookhaven National Lab; June 15, 1955. BNL 344(T-61).)

A third common characteristic among the three natural radioactive series is that the end product in each case is lead. In the case of the uranium series (Table 4-3), the final member is stable ^{206}Pb; in the actinium series, it is ^{207}Pb; and in the thorium series, it is ^{208}Pb. The artificial neptunium series differs in this characteristic too from the natural series; the terminal member is stable bismuth, ^{209}Bi.

These four radioactive decay series, the three naturally occurring ones and the artificially produced neptunium series, are often designated as the $4n$, $4n + 1$, $4n + 2$, and $4n + 3$ series. These identification numbers refer to the divisibility of the mass numbers of each of the series by 4. The atomic mass number of ^{232}Th, the first member of the thorium series, is exactly divisible by 4. Since all disintegrations in the series are accomplished by the emission of either an alpha particle of 4 atomic mass units or a beta particle of 0 atomic mass units, it follows that the mass numbers of all members of the thorium series are exactly divisible by 4. The uranium series, whose first member is ^{238}U, consists of radionuclides whose mass numbers are divisible by 4 and leave a remainder of 2 ($238 \div 4 = 59 + 2/4$). This series, therefore, is called the $4n + 2$ series. The actinium series, whose first member is ^{235}U (actinouranium), is the $4n + 3$ series. The "missing" series, $4n + 1$, is the artificially produced neptunium series, which begins with ^{241}Pu.

Primordial radionuclides found in nature are not restricted to the thorium, uranium, and actinium series. Several of the elements among the lower-atomic-numbered members of the periodic table also have radioactive isotopes. The most important of these low-atomic-numbered natural emitters are listed in Table 4-5.

Of these naturally radioactive isotopes, ^{40}K—by virtue of the widespread distribution of potassium in the environment (the average concentration of potassium in crustal rocks is about 27 g/kg and in the ocean is about 380 mg/L) and in plants and animals, including humans (the average concentration of potassium in humans is about 1.7 g/kg)—is the most important from the health physics point of view. Estimates of body burden of many radioactive materials, from which the degree of exposure to environmental contaminants may be inferred, are made from radiochemical analysis of urine from persons suspected of overexposure. Potassium, whose concentration in urine is about 1.5 g/L, may interfere with the determination of the suspected contaminant unless special care is taken to remove the potassium from the urine or unless allowance is made for the ^{40}K activity. That this interfering activity must be considered is clearly shown by a comparison of the ^{40}K activity in urine with that of certain isotopic concentrations thought to be indicative of a significant body burden.

TABLE 4-5. Some Low-Atomic-Numbered Naturally Occurring Radioisotopes

NUCLIDE	ISOTOPIC ABUNDANCE (%)	HALF-LIFE (YRS)	PRINCIPAL RADIATIONS	
			PARTICLES (MeV)	GAMMA (MeV)
^{40}K	0.0119	1.3×10^9	1.35	1.46
^{87}Rb	27.85	5×10^{10}	0.275	None
^{138}La	0.089	1.1×10^{11}	1.0	0.80, 1.43
^{147}Sm	15.07	1.3×10^{11}	2.18	None
^{176}Lu	2.6	3×10^{10}	0.43	0.20, 0.31
^{187}Re	62.93	5×10^{10}	0.043	None

TABLE 4-6. *Average Concentrations of Uranium, Thorium, and Potassium in Some Building Materials*

MATERIAL	URANIUM		THORIUM		POTASSIUM	
	ppm	mBq/g (pci/g)	ppm	mBq/g (pci/g)	ppm	mBq/g (pci/g)
Granite	4.7	63 (1.7)	2	8 (0.22)	4	1184 (32)
Sandstone	0.45	6 (0.2)	1.7	7 (0.19)	1.4	414 (11.2)
Cement	3.4	46 (1.2)	5.1	21 (0.57)	0.8	237 (6.4)
Limestone concrete	2.3	31 (0.8)	2.1	8.5 (0.23)	0.3	89 (2.4)
Sandstone concrete	0.8	11 (0.3)	2.1	8.5 (0.23)	1.3	385 (10.4)
Wallboard	1.0	14 (0.4)	3	12 (0.32)	0.3	89 (2.4)
By-product gypsum	13.7	186 (5.0)	16.1	66 (1.78)	0.02	5.9 (0.2)
Natural gypsum	1.1	15 (0.4)	1.8	7.4 (0.2)	0.5	148 (4)
Wood	—	—			11.3	3390 (90)
Clay brick	8.2	111 (3)	10.8	44 (1.2)	2.3	666 (18)

Source: From *Exposure of the Population in the United States and Canada from Natural Background Radiation.* Bethesda, MD: National Council on Radiation Protection and Measurements; 1987. NCRP Report 94.

EXAMPLE 4.9

Calculate the specific activity of urine (in transformations per minute per liter) with respect to ^{40}K.

Solution

The specific activity of urine, in units of transformations per minute per liter, with respect to ^{40}K is

$$SA, \frac{\text{t/min}}{\text{L}} = \frac{3.7 \times 10^{10} \times 1600 \times 226}{1.3 \times 10^9 \times 40} \frac{\text{Bq}}{\text{g} \ ^{40}\text{K}} \times 1.19 \times 10^{-4} \frac{\text{g} \ ^{40}\text{K}}{\text{g K}} \times \frac{1.5 \text{ g K}}{\text{L}}$$

$$\times 60 \frac{\text{t/min}}{\text{Bq}} = 2.8 \times 10^3 \frac{\text{t/min}}{\text{L}}.$$

A gross beta activity in excess of 200 transformations per minute per liter of urine following possible exposure to mixed fission products is considered indicative of internal deposition of the fission products. This activity is less than 10% of that due to the naturally occurring potassium.

SERIAL TRANSFORMATION

In addition to the four chains of radioactive isotopes described above, a number of other groups of sequentially transforming isotopes are important to the health physicist and radiobiologist. Most of these series are associated with nuclear fission, and the first member of each series is a fission fragment. One of the most widely known fission products, for example, ^{90}Sr, is the middle member of a five-member series of beta emitters that starts with ^{90}Kr and finally terminates with stable ^{90}Zr according to the following sequence:

$$^{90}_{36}\text{Kr} \xrightarrow{33\,\text{s}} {}^{90}_{37}\text{Rb} \xrightarrow{2.74\,\text{min}} {}^{90}_{38}\text{Sr} \xrightarrow{28.8\,\text{yr}} {}^{90}_{39}\text{Y} \xrightarrow{64.2\,\text{hr}} {}^{90}_{40}\text{Zr}.$$

Secular Equilibrium

The quantitative relationship among the various members of the series is of great significance and must be considered in dealing with any of the group's members. Intuitively, it can be seen that any amount of ^{90}Kr will, in a time period of 10–15 minutes, have been transformed to such a degree that, for practical purposes, the ^{90}Kr may be assumed to have been completely transformed. Rubidium-90, the ^{90}Kr daughter, because of its 2.74-minute half-life, will suffer the same fate after about an hour. Essentially, all the ^{90}Kr is, as a result, converted into ^{90}Sr within about an hour after its formation. The buildup of ^{90}Sr is therefore very rapid. The half-life of ^{90}Sr is 28.8 years and its transformation, therefore, is very slow. The ^{90}Y daughter of ^{90}Sr, with a half-life of 64.2 hours, transforms rapidly to stable ^{90}Zr. If pure ^{90}Sr is prepared initially, its radioactive transformation will result in an accumulation of ^{90}Y. Because the ^{90}Y transforms very much faster than ^{90}Sr, a point is soon reached at which the instantaneous amount of ^{90}Sr that transforms is equal to that of ^{90}Y. Under these conditions, the ^{90}Y is said to be in *secular equilibrium*. The quantitative relationship between radionuclides in secular equilibrium may be derived in the following manner:

$$A \xrightarrow{\lambda_A} B \xrightarrow{\lambda_B} C$$

where the half-life of isotope A is very much greater than that of isotope B. The decay constant of A, λ_A, is therefore much smaller than λ_B, the decay constant for B. C is stable and is not transformed. Because of the very long half-life of A relative to B, the rate of formation of B may be considered to be constant and equal to K. Under these conditions, the net rate of change of isotope B with respect to time, if N_B is the number of atoms of B in existence at any time t after an initial number, is given by

rate of change = rate of formation − rate of transformation,

that is,

$$\frac{dN_B}{dt} = K - \lambda_B N_B. \tag{4.32}$$

We will integrate Eq. (4.32), and solve for N_B:

$$\int_{N_{B_0}}^{N_B} \frac{dN_B}{K - \lambda_B N_B} = \int_0^t dt. \tag{4.33}$$

The integrand can be changed to the form

$$\int_a^b \frac{dv}{v} = \ln v \big|_a^b \tag{4.34}$$

if it is multiplied by $-\lambda_B$ and the entire integral is multiplied by $-1/\lambda_B$, in order to keep the value of the integral unchanged. Equation (4.33), therefore, may be solved to yield

$$\ln \left(\frac{K - \lambda_B N_B}{K - \lambda_B N_{B_0}} \right) = -\lambda_B t. \tag{4.35}$$

Equation (4.35) may be written in the exponential form as

$$\frac{K - \lambda_B N_B}{K - \lambda_B N_{B_0}} = e^{-\lambda_B t} \tag{4.36}$$

and then may be solved for N_B as

$$N_B = \frac{K}{\lambda_B} (1 - e^{-\lambda_B t}) + N_{B_0} e^{-\lambda_B t}. \tag{4.37}$$

If we start with pure A, that is, if $N_{B_0} = 0$, then Eq. (4.37) reduces to

$$N_B = \frac{K}{\lambda_B} (1 - e^{-\lambda_B t}). \tag{4.38}$$

The rate of formation of B from A is equal to the rate of transformation of A. Therefore, K is simply equal to $\lambda_A N_A$. An alternative way of expressing Eq. (4.38), therefore, is

$$N_B = \frac{\lambda_A N_A}{\lambda_B} (1 - e^{-\lambda_B t}). \tag{4.39}$$

Note that the quantity of both the parent (A) and the daughter (B) is given in the same units, namely, λN, or transforming atoms per unit time. This is a reasonable unit since each parent atom that is transformed changes into a daughter. Any other unit that implicitly states this fact is equally usable in Eq. (4.39). If λN represents transforming atoms per second, then division of both sides of the equation by the proper factor to convert the activity to curies, or multiples thereof, is permissible and converts Eq. (4.39) into a slightly more usable form. For example, if the activity of the parent is given in becquerels or millicuries, then the activity of the daughter must also be in units of becquerels or millicuries, and Eq. (4.39) may be written as

$$Q_B = Q_A (1 - e^{-\lambda_B t}), \tag{4.40}$$

where Q_A and Q_B are the respective activities in becquerels or millicuries of the parent and daughter.

EXAMPLE 4.10

If we have 500-mg radium, how much ^{222}Rn will be collected after 1 day, after 3.8 days, after 10 days, and after 100 days?

Solution

Since the specific activity of radium is 3.7×10^{10} Bq/g (1 Ci/g), 500 mg $= 1.85 \times 10^{10}$ Bq (500 mCi). The half-life of radon is 3.8 days and its decay constant therefore is

$$\lambda_{Rn} = \frac{0.693}{\left(T_{1/2}\right)_{Rn}} = \frac{0.693}{3.8 \text{ days}} = 0.182 \, \frac{1}{d}.$$

From Eq. (4.40), we have

$$Q_{Rn} = Q_{Ra}(1 - e^{-\lambda_{Rn}t}),$$

$$Q_{Rn} = 1.85 \times 10^{10} \text{ Bq } (1 - e^{-0.182 \frac{1}{day} \times t \text{ days}}).$$

Substituting the respective time in days for t in the equation above gives 3.1×10^9 Bq (83 mCi) of Rn after 1 day, 9.25×10^9 Bq (250 mCi) after 3.8 days, 1.55×10^{10} Bq (419 mCi) after 10 days, and 1.85×10^{10} Bq (500 mCi) after 100 days.

Equation (4.40), as well as the illustrative example given above, show a buildup of radon from zero to a maximum activity, which is equal to that of the parent from which it was derived. This buildup of daughter activity may be shown graphically by plotting Eq. (4.40). A generally useful curve showing the buildup of daughter activity under conditions of secular equilibrium may be obtained if t is plotted in units of daughter half-life, as shown in Figure 4-14. As time increases, $e^{-\lambda t}$ decreases and Q_B approaches Q_A. For practical purposes, equilibrium may be considered to be established after about seven half-lives of the daughter. At equilibrium, it should be noted that

$$\lambda_A N_A = \lambda_B N_B. \tag{4.41}$$

Equation (4.41) tells us that under the conditions of secular equilibrium, the activity of the parent is equal to that of the daughter and that the ratio of the decay constants of the parent and daughter are in the inverse ratio of the equilibrium concentrations of the parent and daughter. This relationship enables us to determine the decay rate constant, and hence the half-life, of a very long lived radionuclide.

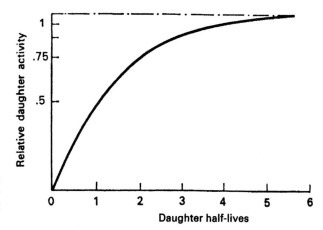

Figure 4-14. Secular equilibrium: Buildup of a very short lived daughter from a very long lived parent. The activity of the parent remains constant.

EXAMPLE 4.11

Deduce the transformation constant and half-life of ^{226}Ra if the radon gas in secular equilibrium with 1 g Ra exerts a partial pressure of 4.8×10^{-4} mm Hg in a 1-L flask and if the half-life of radon is 3.8 days.

Solution

The amount of radon, A, in equilibrium with the radium is computed by

$$\frac{A \text{ mol/L}}{4.8 \times 10^{-4} \text{ mm}} = \frac{1 \text{ mol/22.4 L}}{760 \text{ mm}}$$

$$A = 2.82 \times 10^{-8} \text{ mol.}$$

Since the radon is in equilibrium with 1 g radium and since the number of moles of radium in 1 gram radium is

$$\frac{1 \text{ g}}{226 \text{ g/mol}} = 4.42 \times 10^{-3} \text{ mol radium.}$$

At secular equilibrium, the activities of the parent and daughter are equal. Therefore,

$$\lambda_{Ra} \times N_{Ra} = \lambda_{Rn} \times N_{Rn}$$

$$\lambda_{Ra} \times 4.42 \times 10^{-3} \text{ mol} = \frac{0.693}{3.8 \text{ days}} \times 2.82 \times 10^{-8} \text{ mol}$$

$$\lambda_{Ra} = 1.16 \times 10^{-6} \frac{1}{d} = 4.24 \times 10^{-4} \frac{1}{yr}$$

$$\left(T_{1/2}\right)_{Ra} = \frac{0.693}{4.24 \times 10^{-4} \dfrac{1}{yr}} = 1.63 \times 10^{3} \text{ years}$$

EXAMPLE 4.12

What is the weight of ^{226}Ra, grams, in 1-metric ton (1000 kg) ore containing 1% (W/W) U_3O_8?

Solution

In ore, the Ra is in secular equilibrium with its ^{238}U (U-8) progenitor. The activity of U-8, therefore, is equal to the activity of the Ra (Eq. [4.41]):

$$\lambda_{Ra} \times N_{Ra} = \lambda_{U\text{-}8} \times N_{U\text{-}8}$$

$$N_{Ra} = \frac{\lambda_{U\text{-}8}}{\lambda_{Ra}} \times N_{U\text{-}8}.$$

Since the value of λ varies inversely with the half-life according to Eq. (4.23),

$$\lambda = \frac{0.693}{T},$$

we may substitute Eq. (4.23) into Eq. (4.41) to obtain

$$N_{Ra} = \frac{T_{Ra}}{T_{U\text{-}8}} \times N_{U\text{-}8}. \tag{4.41a}$$

The number of U-8 atoms in 1000 kg (10^6 g) of ore is

$$N_{U\text{-}8} = 10^6 \text{ g ore} \times 0.01 \frac{\text{g } U_3O_8}{\text{g ore}} \times \frac{1 \text{ mol } U_3O_8}{3 \times 238 + 8 \times 16} \frac{\text{g U-8}}{\text{g } U_3O_8}$$

$$\times \frac{3 \text{ mol U}}{1 \text{ mol } U_3O_8} \times \frac{6.02 \times 10^{23} \text{ atoms}}{1 \text{ mol U}} = 2.1 \times 10^{25} \text{ atoms U-8}.$$

Therefore,

$$N_{Ra} = \frac{1620 \text{ yr}}{4.5 \times 10^9 \text{ yr}} \times 2.1 \times 10^{25} \text{ atoms}$$

$$W(Ra) = 7.56 \times 10^{18} \text{ atoms} \times \frac{1 \text{ mol}}{6.02 \times 10^{23} \text{ atoms}} \times 226 \frac{\text{g}}{\text{mol}}$$

$$= 2.8 \times 10^{-3} \text{ g}.$$

Transient Equilibrium

In the case of secular equilibrium discussed above, the quantity of the parent remains substantially constant during the period that it is being observed. Since it is required for secular equilibrium that the half-life of the parent be very much longer than that of the daughter, it follows that secular equilibrium is a special case of a more general situation in which the half-life of the parent may be of any conceivable magnitude, but greater than that of the daughter. For this general case, where the parent activity is not relatively constant,

$$A \xrightarrow{\lambda_A} B \xrightarrow{\lambda_B} C,$$

the time rate of change of the number of atoms of species B is given by the differential equation

$$\frac{dN_B}{dt} = \lambda_A N_A - \lambda_B N_B. \tag{4.42}$$

In this equation, $\lambda_A N_A$ is the rate of transformation of species A and is exactly equal to the rate of formation of species B, the rate of transformation of isotope B is $\lambda_B N_B$, and the difference between these two rates at any time is the instantaneous rate of growth of species B at that time.

According to Eq. (4.18), the value of λ_A in Eq. (4.42) may be written as

$$N_A = N_{A_0} e^{-\lambda t}. \tag{4.43}$$

Equation (4.42) may be rewritten, after substituting the expression above for N_A and transposing $\lambda_B N_B$, as

$$\frac{dN_B}{dt} + \lambda_B N_B = \lambda_A N_{A_0} e^{-\lambda_A t}. \tag{4.44}$$

Equation (4.44) is a first-order linear differential equation of the form

$$\frac{dy}{dx} + P(x) y = Q(x), \tag{4.45}$$

and may be integrable by multiplying both sides of the equation by

$$e^{\int P\, dx} = e^{\int \lambda_B\, dt} = e^{\lambda_B t},$$

and the solution to Eq. (4.45) is

$$y e^{\int P\, dx} = \int e^{\int P\, dx} \cdot Q\, dx. \tag{4.46}$$

Since N_B, λ_B, and $\lambda_A N_{A_0} e^{-\lambda_A t}$ from Eq. (4.44) are represented in Eq. (4.46) by y, P, and Q, respectively, the solution of Eq. (4.44) is

$$N_B e^{\lambda_B t} = \int e^{\lambda_B t} \lambda_A N_{A_0} e^{-\lambda_A t}\, dt + C \tag{4.47}$$

or, if the two exponentials are combined, we have

$$N_B e^{-\lambda_B t} = \int \lambda_A N_{A_0} e^{(\lambda_B - \lambda_A) t}\, dt + C. \tag{4.48}$$

If the integrand in Eq. (4.48) is multiplied by the integrating factor $\lambda_B - \lambda_A$, then Eq. (4.48) is in the form

$$\int e^v dv = e^v + C \tag{4.49}$$

and the solution is

$$N_B e^{\lambda_B t} = \frac{1}{\lambda_B - \lambda_A} \lambda_A N_{A_0} e^{(\lambda_B - \lambda_A)t} + C. \tag{4.50}$$

The constant C may be evaluated by applying the boundary conditions

$$N_B = 0 \text{ when } t = 0$$

$$0 = \frac{1}{\lambda_B - \lambda_A} \lambda_A \times N_{A_0} + C$$

$$C = -\frac{\lambda_A N_{A_0}}{\lambda_B - \lambda_A}. \tag{4.51}$$

If the value for C, from Eq. (4.51), is substituted into Eq. (4.50), the solution for N_B is found to be

$$N_B = \frac{\lambda_A N_{A_0}}{\lambda_B - \lambda_A} (e^{-\lambda_A t - \lambda_B t}). \tag{4.52}$$

For the case in which the half-life of the parent is very much greater than that of the daughter, that is, when $\lambda_A \ll \lambda_B$, Eq. (4.52) approaches the condition of secular equilibrium, which is the limiting case described by Eq. (4.41). Two other general cases should be considered—the case where the parent half-life is slightly greater than that of the daughter ($\lambda_A < \lambda_B$), and the case in which the parent half-life is less than that of the daughter ($\lambda_B < \lambda_A$). In the former case, where the half-life of the daughter is slightly smaller than that of the parent, the daughter activity (if the parent is initially pure and free of any daughter activity) starts from zero, rises to a maximum, and then seems to decay with the same half-life as that of the parent. When this occurs, the daughter is undergoing transformation at the same rate as it is being produced, and the two radionuclides are said to be in a state of *transient equilibrium.*

The quantitative relationships prevailing during transient equilibrium may be inferred from Eq. (4.52). If both sides of the equation are multiplied by λ_B, we have an explicit expression for the activity of the daughter:

$$\lambda_B N_B = \frac{\lambda_B \lambda_A N_{A_0}}{\lambda_B - \lambda_A} (e^{-\lambda_A t} - e^{-\lambda_B t}). \tag{4.53}$$

Since λ_B is greater than λ_A, then, after a sufficiently long period of time, $e^{-\lambda_B t}$ will become much smaller than $e^{-\lambda_A t}$. Under this condition, Eq. (4.53) may be rewritten as

$$\lambda_B N_B = \frac{\lambda_B \lambda_A N_{A_0}}{\lambda_B - \lambda_A} e^{-\lambda_A t}. \tag{4.54}$$

By the use of Eq. (4.43), the mathematical expression for transient equilibrium, Eq. (4.54) may be rewritten as

$$\lambda_B N_B = \frac{\lambda_B \lambda_A N_A}{\lambda_B - \lambda_A}, \tag{4.55}$$

or, in terms of activity units (becquerels, curies, etc.), as

$$Q_B = \frac{\lambda_B}{\lambda_B - \lambda_A} Q_A. \tag{4.56}$$

An example of this equilibrium that is of importance to the health physicist is the ThB to ThC to ThC′ and ThC″ chain, which occurs near the end of the thorium series. In this sequence of transformations, ThB (^{212}Pb), whose half-life is 10.6 hours, decays by beta emission to 60.5-minute ThC (^{212}Bi), which then branches, 35.4% of the transformations going by alpha emission to ThC″ (^{208}Tl) and 64.6% of the transitions being accomplished by beta emission to form ThC′ (^{212}Po). The ThC′ and ThC″ half-lives are very short, 3×10^{-7} seconds and 3.1 minutes, respectively, and both decay to stable ^{208}Pb. Since ThB is a naturally occurring atmospheric isotope, correction for its activity and its daughter's activity must be made before the data on air samples can be accurately interpreted. The growth and decay of ThC are shown in Figure 4-15. These curves graphically emphasize the fact that at transient equilibrium the daughter activity seems to decrease at the same rate as the parent activity.

Figure 4-15 also shows that the daughter activity, which starts from zero, rises to a maximum value and then decreases. It is also seen that the total activity, daughter plus parent, reaches a maximum value that does not coincide in time with that of

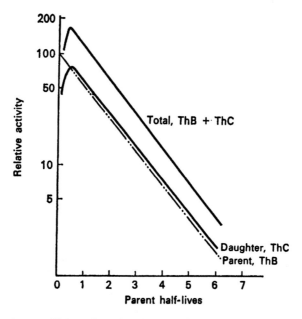

Figure 4-15. Transient equilibrium: Growth and decay of 60.5-minute ThC from 10.6-hour ThB.

the daughter. The time after isolation of the parent that the daughter reaches its maximum activity, t_{md}, may be computed by differentiating Eq. (4.53), the daughter activity, setting the derivative equal to zero, and then solving for the time at which the daughter activity is at its maximum, t_{md}.

$$\lambda_B N_B = \frac{\lambda_B \lambda_A N_{A_0}}{\lambda_B - \lambda_A} (e^{-\lambda_A t} - e^{-\lambda_B t})$$

$$\frac{d(\lambda_B N_B)}{dt} = \frac{\lambda_B \lambda_A N_{A_0}}{\lambda_B - \lambda_A} (-\lambda_A e^{-\lambda_A t} + \lambda_B e^{-\lambda_B t}) = 0,$$

$$\lambda_A e^{-\lambda_A t} = \lambda_B e^{-\lambda_B t}$$

$$\frac{\lambda_B}{\lambda_A} = \frac{e^{-\lambda_A t}}{e^{-\lambda_B t}} = e^{(\lambda_B - \lambda_A)t}$$

$$\ln \frac{\lambda_B}{\lambda_A} = (\lambda_B - \lambda_A) t$$

$$t = t_{md} = \frac{\ln(\lambda_B/\lambda_A)}{\lambda_B - \lambda_A} = \frac{2.3 \log(\lambda_B/\lambda_A)}{\lambda_B - \lambda_A}. \qquad (4.57)$$

For the case illustrated in Figure 4-15,

$$\lambda_A = \frac{0.693}{10.6} = 0.065 \text{ h}^{-1},$$

and

$$\lambda_B = \frac{0.693}{1.01} = 0.686 \text{ h}^{-1}.$$

The time at which the daughter ThC will reach its maximum activity is

$$t_{md} = \frac{\ln (0.686/0.065)}{0.686 - 0.065} = 3.8 \text{ hours.}$$

The time when the total activity is at its peak may be determined in a similar manner. In this case, the total activity $A(t)$ must be maximized. The total activity at any time is given by

$$A(t) = \lambda_A N_A + \lambda_B N_B. \qquad (4.58)$$

Substituting Eqs. (4.43) and (4.52) for N_A and N_B, respectively, in Eq. (4.58), we have

$$A(t) = \lambda_A N_{A_0} e^{-\lambda_A t} + \frac{\lambda_B \lambda_A N_{A_0}}{\lambda_B - \lambda_A} (e^{-\lambda_A t} - e^{-\lambda_B t}). \qquad (4.59)$$

Differentiating Eq. (4.59) yields

$$\frac{dA(t)}{dt} = -\lambda_A^2 N_{A_0} e^{-\lambda_A t} + \frac{\lambda_B \lambda_A N_{A_0}}{\lambda_B - \lambda_A} (-\lambda_A e^{-\lambda_A t} + \lambda_B e^{-\lambda_B t}) = 0. \qquad (4.60)$$

Expanding and collecting terms, we have

$$-\lambda_A^2 N_{A_0} e^{-\lambda_A t}\left(1+\frac{\lambda_B}{\lambda_B-\lambda_A}\right)+\frac{\lambda_A\lambda_B^2}{\lambda_B-\lambda_A}N_{A_0}e^{-\lambda_B t}=0$$

and solving for t_{mt}, the time when the total activity is at its maximum, we get

$$t=t_{mt}=\frac{1}{\lambda_B-\lambda_A}\ln\left(\frac{\lambda_B^2}{2\lambda_A\lambda_B-\lambda_A^2}\right).$$

Referring once more to the example in Figure 4-15, one finds the maximum total activity to occur at

$$t_{mt}=\frac{1}{0.686-0.065}\ln\left[\frac{(0.686)^2}{2\times0.065\times0.686-(0.065)^2}\right]=2.8\text{ hours}$$

after the initial purification of the parent. It should be noted that the maximum total activity occurs earlier than that of the daughter alone.

The time when the parent and daughter isotopes may be considered to be equilibrated depends on their respective half-lives. The shorter the half-life of the daughter relative to the parent, the more rapidly will equilibrium be attained. In the case where the half-life of the daughter exceeds that of the parent, no equilibrium is possible. The daughter activity reaches a maximum at a time that can be calculated from Eq. (4.57) and then reaches a point where it decays at its own characteristic rate. The parent, in the meantime, because of its shorter half-life, decays away. The total activity in this case does not increase to a maximum; it decreases continuously. Equation (4.58), which gives the time after isolation of a parent at which the total activity is maximum, cannot be solved for the case in which the half-life of the daughter exceeds that of the parent or if $\lambda_B<\lambda_A$. These points are all illustrated in Figure 4-16, which shows the course in time of the growth and decay of ^{146}Pr, whose half-life

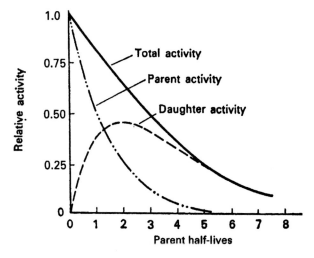

Figure 4-16. No equilibrium growth and decay of 24-minute ^{146}Pm from 14-minute ^{146}Ce.

is 24.4 minutes, from the fission product ^{146}Ce, whose half-life is only 13.9 minutes. Solution of Eq. (4.57) shows the ^{146}Pr activity to reach its peak 26.2 minutes after isolation of ^{146}Ce.

Background Radiation

Background radiation is the sum of the external radiation doses that accrue from the naturally occurring radiation sources (^{238}U, ^{232}Th, ^{226}Ra, ^{40}K, ^{14}C, etc.), cosmic radiation, and anthropogenic sources, such as debris from weapons tests, fallout from accidental releases, and releases from the routine operations of reactors and the nuclear fuel cycle. The exact background dose rate varies from place to place, depending mainly on the mineral content in the ground and the cosmic ray intensity (which in turn depends on the altitude and the latitude). In most places, the external background dose rate varies from about 70 to 150 millirads (700–1500 μGy) per year. (The millirad and the μGy are units of radiation dose that are explained in Chapter 8.) However, there are many places throughout the world where the background is very much higher than the average. These higher background dose rates are due to high concentrations of radioactive minerals (mainly the thorium-bearing mineral monazite) in the ground. In Brazil, there are beaches where the background dose rates reach as high as 43,000 millirads (430,000 μGy) per year.

The soil in the Kerala region of southwest India too is rich in monazite, which results in average external dose rates of 500–600 millirads (5000–6000 μGy) per year. In China, there are large densely populated areas where the external background rate is in the range of 300–400 millirads (3000–4000 μGy) per year. In the United States, the background radiation in Denver, CO, of approximately 200 millirads (2000 μGy) per year is about twice the background dose rate in New York City. It is important to note that no harmful radiation effects have been observed among the populations living in the high-radiation areas.

Background is significant to the health physicist in two ways. First, the background radiation must be accounted for when measuring radiation from a source. Secondly, it substantiates the validity of our radiation safety standards for incremental doses that are within the range of variability of background dose rate levels.

Machine Sources of Radiation

X-ray Tube

Useful radiation can also be generated in several different types of machines. The first of these machine sources was the high-vacuum diode, called a Crooke's tube, which Roentgen was using in a laboratory experiment in the year 1895. In the Crooke's tube, electrons were accelerated across about 25,000 V to a high velocity and then were abruptly stopped when they struck the anode. In accordance with Maxwell's theory of electromagnetic radiation, some of the kinetic energy of the electrons was converted into electromagnetic energy in the form of X-rays due to the abrupt deceleration of the electrons (Fig. 4-17). This method of generating X-rays is the forerunner of the modern X-ray tube used in diagnostic radiology, dentistry, and in industrial radiography. The same type of X-ray generators are used in X-ray spectrometers and diffractometers in analytical chemistry and crystallography, and in inspection and control devices. Most of the X-rays from this type of generator are emitted

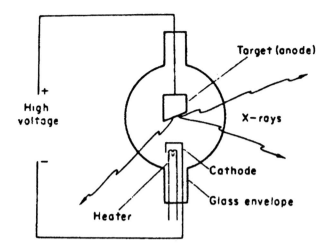

Figure 4-17. A conventional X-ray generator, in which electrons that are emitted by a heated cathode are accelerated by the strong electric field and emit X-rays after being abruptly stopped by striking the target. The useful X-ray beam emerges through an opening in the tube housing (shield).

at right angles to the path of the accelerated electron. In this type of X-ray generator, the full accelerating voltage must be applied across the electrodes of the tube. This limits the maximum kinetic energy of the electrons to several hundred thousand electron volts.

Linear Accelerator

Other methods of accelerating electrons are used to overcome this high voltage limitation in order to generate very high energy X-rays. The most common method is with the linear accelerator (Fig. 4-18). The linear accelerator, in principle, consists of a series of tubular electrodes, called drift tubes, with an electron source at one end and a target at the other end for stopping the high-energy electrons. The electrodes are connected to a source of high-frequency alternating voltage whose frequency is such that the polarity of the electrode changes as the electron exits from one drift tube and thus is attracted to the next drift tube. Each successive drift tube is at a higher voltage than the preceding one. The electron's gain in kinetic energy in eV is thus equal to the voltage difference between successive drift tubes. These gains in kinetic energy are cumulative. Thus, if we had a series of 30 electrode gaps with 100 kV differences between them, and if the electron were injected into the system with a kinetic energy of 100 keV, the electron would emerge at the other end with a kinetic energy of

$$E_k = 100 + (30 \times 100) = 3100 \text{ keV} = 3.1 \text{ MeV}.$$

The energy gradient in linear accelerators typically is 2–4 MeV/ft. At these high energies, the speed of an electron is almost that of the speed of light. A 2-MeV electron has a speed of 2.94×10^8 m/s, while the speed of a 4-MeV electron is 2.98×10^8 m/s, and the speed of a 6-MeV electron is 2.99×10^8 m/s. The increase in kinetic energy goes to increased mass rather than to higher speed, and all the high-energy electrons travel at about the same speed. The drift tubes, therefore, could be made of the same length for high-energy electrons. In practice, the alternating sections of the linear accelerator are coupled to a microwave source, such as a magnetron or

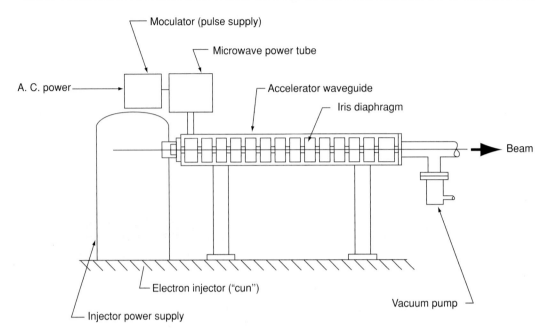

Figure 4-18. Illustration of the operating principle of a linear accelerator. (From Brobeck WM. *Particle Accelerator Safety Manual*, MORP 68-12. Rockville, MD: National Center for Radiological Health; 1968.)

klystron. The high-frequency alternating voltage may be thought of as a voltage wave that is guided down the accelerating tube (called a waveguide) and carries a bunch of electrons with each wave. The microwaves energize the waveguide in pulses of several microseconds each at a pulse repetition rate of about 50 to several thousand pulses per second. In addition to generating X-ray by causing the electron beam to strike an internal target, a linear accelerator can be designed to be an electron irradiator, that is, to bring the electron beam out of the machine and to deliver a radiation dose with the electron beam. Linear accelerators are widely used to treat cancers, as well as in research and industrial applications.

Cyclotron

High-energy charged particles, such as protons and deuterons, can be generated for use in research and for producing radionuclides for medical use. Generally, heavy charged particles are accelerated by driving them in a circular path, with energy gained stepwise as the particle completes a revolution in the accelerator. The earliest machine of this type is the cyclotron, which was invented in 1931 by Ernest Lawrence and Stanley Livingston. In the cyclotron (Fig. 4-19), the heavy charged particle is injected into an evacuated chamber containing two opposing hollow electrodes (called "dees" because of their shape) made of nonmagnetic metal, such as copper. The evacuated chamber is located between the poles of a strong electromagnet, on the order of 1.5 T (15,000 gauss) or more. The magnetic field causes the injected ions to travel in a circular path. The dees, which are separated by a small gap, are connected to a radiofrequency (RF) voltage source whose frequency is the same as the rotational frequency of the circulating ions. The injected positive ion is attracted to and enters

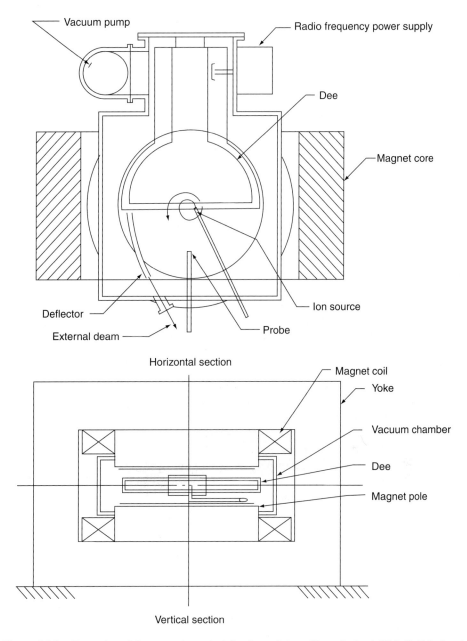

Figure 4-19. Illustration of the operating principle of a cyclotron. (From Brobeck WM. *Particle Accelerator Safety Manual*, MORP 68-12. Rockville, MD: National Center for Radiological Health; 1968.)

into the hollow negatively charged dee. Since there is no electric field inside a hollow conductor, the ion is under the influence only of the magnetic field, and coasts in a circular path at a constant angular velocity until it reaches the other edge of the dee. At the correct, or resonance frequency, the ion arrives at the gap between the dees at the instant that the polarity of the dees reverses. That is, the dee that the ion is leaving becomes positive, thus repelling the exiting ion, while the opposite dee becomes negative, thus attracting the positive ion. The peak oscillating voltage across the dees is on the order of 100 kV. Thus, every time that the ion crosses the gap when the inter-dee voltage is at its peak, its kinetic energy is increased by 100 keV if it is a singly charged ion, such as a proton, and its radius of curvature increases to accommodate the increased energy. In a single complete revolution, the ion crosses the gap twice, and its energy is increased by 200 keV (if the voltage across the dees is 100 kV and if the ion crosses the gap at the peak voltage). If the ion is a singly charged deuteron, it will gain 200 keV per revolution, and a doubly charged helium nucleus will gain 400 keV per revolution. Ions that reach the edge of the dee at other times in the sinusoidal voltage cycle will receive smaller increases in kinetic energy per gap crossing and, thus, will make more revolutions before they reach the outer edge of the dees. As the ion's energy increases, its radius increases, and the ions spiral outward. An electrical deflector at the outermost radius deflects the ions to form a pulse of high-energy protons, deuterons, or whatever other heavier ions were accelerated.

The maximum energy attainable in a cyclotron is limited by the relativistic increase in mass as the particle's energy increases. The operation of the cyclotron as described above, and shown by Eq. (4.61), is based on a constant mass of the accelerated particle and the fact that it takes the same time to travel in a semicircle of large radius as in one of a small radius. If the mass increases, the time to complete a semicircular path will fall out of synchronization with the frequency of the inter-dee voltage. For protons, this upper limit is about 25 MeV. Because of this upper energy limit, cyclotrons are not commonly used in high-energy physics research. Their principal use is as radiation sources, especially for the manufacture of short-lived radionuclides, such as 110-minute ^{18}F, which is widely used in PET (positron emission tomography) scans for medical diagnostic studies.

When the velocity vector of the injected ion is perpendicular to the magnetic field, the ion will follow a circular path at a radius where the magnetic force tending to bend the ion's path into a circle is equal to the centrifugal force acting on the ion:

$$Bqv = \frac{mv^2}{r}, \tag{4.61a}$$

$$r = \frac{mv}{Bq} \tag{4.61b}$$

where

B = magnetic field strength, tesla
q = charge on ion, coulomb
v = velocity of the ion, meters per second
m = mass of the ion, kilogram
r = radius of curvature, meters

The time to travel the semicircular path within the dee is

$$t = \frac{\text{distance}}{\text{velocity}} = \frac{\pi r}{v}. \tag{4.62}$$

Substituting the value of r from Eq. (4.61b) into Eq. (4.62) gives

$$t = \frac{\pi m}{Bq},$$
(4.63)

which shows that the time to travel a circular path within the dee is independent of the radius. For the nonrelativistic case, the kinetic energy of the particle is given, according to Eq. (2.5), by

$$E_k = \frac{mv^2}{2}.$$

Substituting the expression for v^2 from Eq. (4.61a) into Eq. (2.5) gives the kinetic energy of the particle after traversing a radius r:

$$E_k = \frac{\left(B^2 r^2 q^2\right)}{2m}.$$
(4.64)

 EXAMPLE 4.13

Deuterons, mass $= 3.344 \times 10^{-27}$ kg, are accelerated in a cyclotron whose magnetic field is 1.2 T, and the effective dee radius is 21.25 in. (0.54 m). What is the

(a) kinetic energy of the deuterons in the cyclotron's exit beam?

(b) speed of these deuterons?

Solution

Substituting the appropriate values into Eq. (4.64), we have

(a) $E_k = \dfrac{\left(1.2 \text{ T} \times 0.54 \text{ m} \times 1.6 \times 10^{-19} \text{ C}\right)^2}{2 \times 3.344 \times 10^{-27} \text{ kg}} = 1.61 \times 10^{-12}$ J

$E_k = \dfrac{1.61 \times 10^{-12} \text{ J}}{1.6 \times 10^{-13} \dfrac{\text{J}}{\text{MeV}}} = 10 \text{ MeV}.$

(b) $E_k = \dfrac{mv^2}{2}$

$v = \left(\dfrac{2 \times 1.61 \times 10^{-12} \text{ J}}{3.344 \times 10^{-27} \text{ kg}}\right)^{1/2} = 3.1 \times 10^7 \dfrac{\text{m}}{\text{s}}.$

The speed of the 10-MeV deuteron is 10.3% of the speed of light. This speed is considered to be the threshold for relativistic effects to become important.

SUMMARY

Radioactivity is a spontaneously occurring transformation in an unstable nucleus in which radiation is emitted and the nucleus is changed into another element. These transformations are accomplished through the emission of alpha or beta particles, positrons, or by orbital electron capture. Each of these reactions may or may not be accompanied by a gamma ray. Alpha particles are highly energetic ^{4}He nuclei, while beta particles and positrons are highly energetic electrons. Negatrons (negatively charged beta particles) are stable negatively charged electrons, while positrons are unstable positively charged electrons. When a positron loses its kinetic energy and collides with a negatively charged electron, the two electrons are annihilated and two 0.51-MeV photons (0.51 MeV is the energy equivalent of the rest mass of the positron and of the electron) appear in their stead.

All radionuclides are uniquely identified by three characteristics—the type of radiation, the energy of the radiation, and the rate at which the spontaneous transformations occur. The rate is measured in terms of the fraction of the radioisotope that is transformed per unit time. A convenient analog for this measure is the half-life, which is defined as the *time required for one-half the number of radioactive atoms to be transformed*. During the next half-life interval, one-half of the remaining atoms are transformed to leave one-fourth of the initial activity, then another half of this activity is transformed during the next half-life period, and so on. Nothing can be done to a radionuclide to change these radioactive characteristics. The characteristics remain the same regardless of the physical state or the chemical compound in which the radioactive atoms exist.

The quantity of radioactivity is measured by the becquerel (Bq) in the SI system and by the curie (Ci) in the traditional system of radiation units. The *curie* originally was defined as the activity of 1 g of ^{226}Ra, in which 3.7×10^{10} atoms are transformed to ^{222}Rn in 1 second. One *becquerel* is defined as the quantity of radioactivity in which one atom is transformed per second. Thus, 1 Ci is 3.7×10^{10} Bq. The concentration of radioactivity is measured by the specific activity, in terms of Bq or Ci per unit mass or per unit volume. The highest specific activity attainable for any radionuclide is the specific activity of the carrier-free radioisotope, that is, the radioisotope alone, with no other isotope of that element or any other chemical species present.

A number of different radionuclides undergo serial transformations. When this happens in the case of a very long lived parent and a short-lived daughter, an equilibrium condition called *secular equilibrium* develops after about 6–7 daughter half-lives. When secular equilibrium is reached, the activity of the daughter is equal to the activity of the parent. In those cases in which the half-life of the daughter is less than that of the parent, a condition known as *transient equilibrium* develops. In transient equilibrium, the daughter activity exceeds that of the parent by an amount that is determined by the ratio of their half-lives. If the daughter is longer lived than the parent, then no equilibrium condition can be attained.

We find three different series of naturally occurring radioisotopes in the ground: the thorium series, which starts with ^{232}Th; the uranium series, which starts with ^{238}U; and the actinium series, which starts with ^{235}U. All three series begin with a very long lived ancestor; they all end as isotopes of lead and they all have an isotope of the gaseous element radon in the middle of the series. Radon gas that originates in soil near the surface has enough time to diffuse out of the ground into the air before it is transformed into a nongaseous element. Subsequent transformations in the series take place in the air. Thus, radon and its progeny are the principal source of naturally occurring atmospheric radioactivity. In addition to the radionuclides in these series, there are singly occurring natural radionuclides. Chief among the singly occurring radionuclides is ^{40}K, whose half-life is about 1.3×10^9 years and which was created when the world was created. Carbon-14 and tritium, ^3H, are two other radionuclides of interest. Their half-lives are very short in a geological context and they are continuously replenished by the interaction between cosmic radiation and the atmosphere.

X-rays, or bremsstrahlung radiation, are produced whenever high-energy, charged particles are abruptly stopped. This phenomenon is the basis for the conventional X-ray machines that are used in medical diagnosis, in industry, and in science. Because of the energy limitation of conventional X-ray tubes, X-rays whose energy is greater than about 200 keV are generated in linear accelerators. Electrons can be accelerated to hundreds of MeV before they are either caused to strike a target in order to convert some of the electron beam's energy into X-rays, or the electron beam is extracted for electron irradiation. Linear accelerators from about 6 MeV to about 18 MeV are widely used in hospitals to treat deep-seated cancers.

Cyclotrons are used to accelerate heavy ions, such as protons, deuterons, and alpha particles (^4He nuclei), to a velocity that is about 10% of the speed of light. Cyclotrons today are used mainly for the production of short-lived radionuclides for medical uses.

PROBLEMS

4.1. Carbon 14 is a pure beta emitter that decays to ^{14}N. If the exact atomic masses of the parent and daughter are 14.007687 and 14.007520 atomic mass units, respectively, calculate the kinetic energy of the most energetic beta particle.

4.2. If 1.0 MBq (27 mCi) of ^{131}I is needed for a diagnostic test, and if 3 days elapse between shipment of the radioiodine and its use in the test, how many Bq must be shipped? To how many mCi does this correspond?

4.3. The gamma radiation from 1 mL of a solution containing 370-Bq (0.01-μCi) ^{198}Au and 185-Bq (0.005-μCi) ^{131}I is counted daily over a 16-day period. If the detection efficiency of the scintillation counter is 10% for all the quantum energies involved, what will be the relative counting rates of the ^{131}I and ^{198}Au at time $t = 0$, $t = 3$ days, $t = 8$ days, and $t = 16$ days? Plot the daily total counting rates on semilog paper and write the equation of the curve of total count rate versus time.

4.4. The following counting rates were obtained on a sample that was identified as a pure beta emitter:

Day	0	1	2	3	5	10	20
cpm	5500	5240	5000	4750	4320	3400	2050

(a) Plot the data on semilog paper.

(b) Determine the half-life from the graph.

(c) What is the value of the transformation constant (in per day)?

(d) Write the equation for the decay curve.

(e) What is the radionuclide in the sample?

4.5. If we start with 5 mg of ^{210}Pb, what would be the activity of this sample 10-years later?

4.6. The decay constant for ^{235}U is 9.72×10^{-10} yr^{-1}. Compute the number of transformations per second in a 500 mg sample of ^{235}U.

4.7. Two hundred megabecquerels (5.4 mCi) of ^{210}Po are necessary for a certain ionization source. How many grams of ^{210}Po does this represent?

4.8. How long would it take for 99.9% of ^{137}Cs to decay, if its half-life is 30 years?

4.9. How long will it take for each of the following radioisotopes to decrease to 0.0001% of its initial activity?

(a) ^{99}Mo

(b) ^{99m}Tc

(c) ^{131}I

(d) ^{125}I

4.10. For use in carcinogenesis studies, benzo(a)pyrene is tagged with ^{3}H to a specific activity of 4×10^{11} Bq/mmol. If there is only one ^{3}H atom on a tagged molecule, what percentage of the benzo(a)pyrene molecules is tagged with ^{3}H?

4.11. How many alpha particles are emitted per minute by 1 cm^{3} of ^{222}Rn at a temperature of 27°C and a pressure of 100,000 Pa?

4.12. Calculate the number of beta particles emitted per minute by 1 kg of KCl if ^{40}K emits one beta particle per transformation.

4.13. Iodine-125, a widely used isotope in the practice of nuclear medicine, has a half-life of 60 days.

(a) How long will it take for 4 MBq ($\sim$1 μCi) to decrease to 0.1% of its initial activity?

(b) What is the mean life of ^{125}I?

4.14. If uranium ore contains 10% U_3O_8, how many metric tons are necessary to produce 1 g of radium if the extraction process is 90% efficient?

4.15. How much ^{234}U is there in 1 metric ton of the uranium ore containing 10% U_3O_8?

4.16. Compare the activity of the ^{234}U to that of the ^{235}U and the ^{238}U in the ore of problems 4.14 and 4.15.

4.17. Calculate the activity, in becquerels and microcuries, of each of the uranium isotopes in 1 g of natural uranium and then using these results, together with the values for the isotopic abundances, calculate the activity of 1 g of natural uranium.

4.18. What will be the temperature rise after 24 hours in a well-insulated 100-mL aqueous solution containing 1 g of $Na_2(^{35}SO_4)$, if the specific activity of the sulfur is 3.7×10^{12} Bq/g (100 Ci/g)?

4.19. The mean concentration of potassium in crustal rocks is 27 g/kg. If ^{40}K constitutes 0.012% of potassium, what is the ^{40}K activity, in Bq and μCi, in 1 metric ton of rock?

4.20. An aqueous solution of ^{203}Hg is received with the following assay: 1 MBq/mL on March 1, 2005, at 8:00 AM. It is desired to make a solution whose activity will be 0.1 MBq/mL on April 1, 2005, at 8:00 AM. Calculate the dilution factor (mL water:mL Hg stock solution) to give the desired activity. $T_{1/2}$ of $^{203}Hg = 46$ days.

4.21. In a mixture of two radioisotopes, 99% of the activity is due to ^{24}Na and 1% is due to ^{32}P. At what subsequent time will the two activities be equal?

4.22. Low-level waste from a biomedical laboratory consists of a mixture of 100-mCi (3.7-MBq) ^{131}I and 10-mCi (0.37-MBq) ^{125}I. Plot the decay curve for the total activity over a period of 365 days and write the equation for the decay curve.

4.23. ThB is transformed to ThC at a rate of 6.54% per hour, and ThC is transformed at a rate of 1.15% per minute. How long will it take for the two isotopes to reach their equilibrium state?

4.24. How many grams of ^{90}Y are there when ^{90}Y is equilibrated with 10 mg of ^{90}Sr?

4.25. Radiogenic lead constitutes 98.5% of the element as found in lead ore. The isotopic constitution of lead in nature is ^{204}Pb, 1.5%; ^{206}Pb, 23.6%; ^{207}Pb, 22.6%; and ^{208}Pb, 52.3%. How much uranium and thorium decayed completely to produce 985 mg of radiogenic lead?

4.26. How long after 1 kg of ^{241}Pu is isolated will the ^{241}Am activity be at its maximum? What will the activity be at that time?

4.27. How long after 14-minute ^{146}Ce is isolated will the activity of the 24-minute ^{146}Pr daughter be equal to that of the parent?

4.28. 37-MBq (1-mCi) ^{99m}Tc are "milked" from a ^{99}Mo "cow." What will be the activity of the ^{99m}Tc daughter, ^{99}Tc, 1 year after the milking?

4.29. Calculate the specific activity of ^{85}Kr ($T_{1/2} = 10.7$ years) in Bq/m^3 and mCi/cm^3 at 25°C and 760 mm Hg.

4.30. Calculate the specific power of ^{35}S and of ^{14}C in

(a) watts per MBq.

(b) watts per kilogram.

4.31. Calculate the specific power of a ^{90}Sr power source in

(a) watts per MBq.

(b) watts per kilogram.

4.32. How many joules of energy are released in 3 hours by an initial volume of 1-L ^{41}Ar at 0°C and 760 mm Hg?

4.33. (a) Calculate the specific power, in watts per kilogram, of ^{41}Ar.

(b) What is the specific power of ^{41}Ar 4 hours after the ^{41}Ar is isolated in a bottle?

4.34. What volume of radon 222 (at 0°C and 760 torr) is in equilibrium with 0.1 g of radium 226?

4.35. One hundred milligrams of radium as $RaBr_2$ (specific gravity = 5.79) is in a platinum capsule whose inside dimensions are 2 mm (diameter) × 4 cm (length). What will be the gas pressure, at body temperature, inside the capsule 100 years after manufacture if it originally contained air at atmospheric pressure at room temperature (25°C)?

4.36. A volume of 10 cm^3 of tritium gas, $^3H_2$, at NTP dissipates 3.11 J/h.

    (a) What is the activity of the tritium?

    (b) What is the mean beta energy if one beta particle is emitted per transition?

4.37. Barium-140 decays to ^{140}La with a half-life of 12.8 days, and the ^{140}La decays to stable ^{140}Ce with a half-life of 40.5 hours. A radiochemist, after precipitating ^{140}Ba, wishes to wait until he has a maximum amount of ^{140}La before separating the ^{140}La from the ^{140}Ba.

    (a) How long must he wait?

    (b) If he started with 1000 MBq (27 mCi) of ^{140}Ba, how many micrograms of ^{140}La will he collect?

4.38. Strontium-90 is to be used as a heat source for generating electrical energy in a satellite.

    (a) How much of ^{90}Sr activity is required to generate 50 W of electric power if the conversion efficiency from heat to electricity is 30%?

    (b) Weight of the isotopic heat source is an important factor in design of the power source. If weight is to be kept at a minimum and if the source is to generate 50 W after 1 year of operation, would there be an advantage to using ^{210}Po?

4.39. Carbon-14 is produced naturally by the $^{14}N(n, p)^{14}C$ interaction of cosmic radiation with the nitrogen in the atmosphere at a rate of about 1.4×10^{15} Bq/yr. If the half-life of ^{14}C is 5730 years, what is the steady-state global inventory of ^{14}C?

4.40. The global steady-state inventory of naturally produced tritium from the interaction of cosmic rays with the atmosphere is estimated by the United Nations Scientific Committee on the Effects of Atomic Radiation to be 1.26×10^{18} Bq (34 × 10^6 Ci). If the half-life of tritium is 12.3 years, what is the annual production of natural tritium?

4.41. The atomic ratio of ^{235}U to ^{238}U in current uranium is 1:139. What was the ratio of these two isotopes when the Oklo reactor went critical 1.7 billion years ago?

4.42. Highly enriched uranium (HEU) contains 1.5% U-4, 93.5% U-5, and 5.0% U-8 (percentages are by weight). Calculate

    (a) the activity of each uranium isotope in 1-g HEU in Bq and in Ci.

    (b) the total activity of 1 g of this enriched uranium, in Bq and in Ci.

4.43. 100-mCi ^{210}Pb is sealed in a capsule. (^{210}Pb, $T_{1/2} = 22$ years, decays to ^{210}Po, whose $T_{1/2} = 138$ days).

  (a) What will be the activity of the ^{210}Pb (in mCi) after 10 years?

  (b) What will be the activity of the ^{210}Po at that time?

  (c) What is the weight (grams) of the 10-year-old ^{210}Pb?

  (d) What is the weight of the ^{210}Po

   (i) at the time that the ^{210}Pb source was sealed?

   (ii) after 10 years?

4.44. What is the

  (a) half-life

  (b) mean life (in minutes) of a radioisotope whose instantaneous decay rate is 10% per minute?

4.45. Today's terrestrial background radiation is about 50 mrems/yr, mainly due to the uranium and thorium decay chains, and potassium. The approximate current contributions of each of these is ^{232}Th: 11 mrems/yr, ^{238}U: 26 mrems/yr, ^{40}K: 11 mrems/yr.

  The earliest evidence of life on earth consists of unicellular organisms about 3.5 billion years old.

  (a) What is the half-life of each of these three radioisotopes?

  (b) What was the terrestrial background radiation rate when life began 3.5 billion years ago from these three isotopes?

4.46. Potassium constitutes 3.4% by weight of granite. Potassium-40 constitutes 0.012% by weight of natural potassium. The half-life of ^{40}K is 1.3×10^9 years.

  (a) Calculate the specific activity of ^{40}K in

   (i) Ci/g

   (ii) Bq/g

  (b) Calculate the ^{40}K activity of 1-kg granite in

   (i) Ci

   (ii) Bq

4.47. The Environmental Protection Agency's recommended limit for indoor ^{222}Rn in air is 4 pCi/L. Calculate the

  (a) specific activity of ^{222}Rn (in Ci/g).

  (b) weight of 4-pCi ^{222}Rn in 1 L at 25°C and 760 mm Hg.

  (c) quantity (in moles) of the Rn gas in 1 L.

  (d) number of moles of air in 1 L, assuming the air to be a gas whose atomic weight is $0.2 \times 16 + 0.8 \times 14$.

  (e) volumetric percent of 4-pCi ^{222}Rn in 1-L air at 25°C and 760 mm Hg.

4.48. The ratio of ^{206}Pb atoms to ^{238}U atoms in a sample of pre-Cambrian rock is found to be 0.12. Assuming that all the ^{206}Pb atoms are the descendents of ^{238}U, calculate the age of the rock.

4.49. A sealed capsule contains 5550-MBq (150-mCi) ^{222}Rn ($T_{1/2} = 3.8$ days).

    (a) What is the Rn activity 38 days later?

    (b) How many Rn atoms have decayed?

    (c) How many moles of He have been produced from alphas during 38 days?

    (d) What is the volume, at 25°C and 760 mm Hg, of the helium (in mm^3)?

4.50. The Windmill Hill Neolithic village in England was dated by traditional archeological methods to 4300 BCE. If this is correct, how many dpm/g carbon from an artifact there would be expected in a ^{14}C dating? The specific activity of current carbon is 15.3 dpm/g carbon.

4.51. The half-life of ^{35}S is 87 days. How many micrograms of ^{35}S will there be from 1-Ci (3.7×10^{10} Bq) ^{35}S after 1 year?

4.52. The concentration of a ^{99m}Tc radiopharmaceutical is 50 mCi in 20 mL at 7:00 AM. A patient is scheduled to receive 10 mCi (370 MBq) at 10:00 AM. What is the volume of the ^{99m}Tc injectate?

SUGGESTED READINGS

Attix, F. A. *Introduction to Radiological Physics and Radiation Dosimetry*. John Wiley & Sons, New York, 1986.

Born, M. *Atomic Physics*, 8th ed. Hafner, Darien, CT, 1970.

Brobeck, W. M. *Particle Accelerator Safety Manual*, MORP 68-12, National Center For Radiological Health, Rockville, MD, 1968.

Brodsky, A., ed. *Handbook of Radiation Measurement and Protection. Section A, Vol. 1. Physical Science and Engineering Data*. CRC Press, West Palm Beach, FL, 1978.

Cohen, B. L. *Concepts of Nuclear Physics*. McGraw-Hill, New York, 1971.

Etherington, H., ed. *Nuclear Engineering Handbook*. McGraw-Hill, New York, 1958.

Evans, R. D. *The Atomic Nucleus*. McGraw-Hill, New York, 1955.

Faw, R., and Shultis, J. K. *Radiological Assessment*. Prentice Hall, Englewood Cliffs, NJ, 1993.

Friedlander, G., Kennedy, J. W., Macias, E. S., and Miller, J. M. *Nuclear and Radiochemistry*, 3rd ed. John Wiley & Sons, New York, 1981.

Glasstone, S. *Sourcebook on Atomic Energy*, 3rd ed. D. Van Nostrand, Princeton, NJ, 1967.

Haissinsky, M., and Adloff, J. P. *Radiochemical Survey of the Elements*. Elsevier, Amsterdam, 1965.

Hunt, S. E. *Nuclear Physics for Engineers and Scientists*. Halstead Press, New York, 1987.

IAEA. *Radiological Safety Aspects of the Operation of Electron Linear Accelerators*, Technical Report Series No. 188, International Atomic Energy Agency, Vienna, 1979.

Karam, P. A. *The Evolution of Background Beta and Gamma Radiation Fields Through Geologic Time, from Geologic, Cosmic, and Internal Sources*. M.S. Thesis, Ohio State University, Columbus, OH, 1998.

Karzmark, C. J., Nunan, C. S., and Tanabe, E. *Medical Electron Accelerators*, McGraw-Hill, New York, 1993.

Krane, K. S. *Introductory Nuclear Physics*. John Wiley & Sons, New York, 1987.

Lapp, R. E., and Andrews, H. L. *Nuclear Radiation Physics*, 4th ed. Prentice-Hall, Englewood Cliffs, NJ, 1972.

McLaughlin, J. P., Simopoulos, E. S., and Steinhausler, F. *The Natural Radiation Environment VII*. Elsevier, New York, 2005.

National Council on Radiation Protection and Measurements:

    Report No. 77: *Exposures from the Uranium Series with Emphasis on Radon and Its Daughters*, 1984.

    Report No. 79: *Neutron Contamination from Medical Accelerators*, 1984.

    Report No. 93: *Ionizing Radiation Exposure of the Population of the United States*, 1987.

    Report No. 94: *Exposure of the Population in the United States and Canada from Natural Background Radiation*, 1987.

Report No. 103: *Control of Radon in Houses*, 1989.

Report No. 144: *Radiation Protection for Particle Accelerator Facilities*, 2003.

Radiological Health Handbook, Rev. ed. U.S. Dept. of Health, Education and Welfare, Public Health Service, Rockville, MD, 1970.

Patterson, H. W., and Thomas, R. H. *Accelerator Health Physics*. Academic Press, New York, 1973.

Patterson, H. W., and Thomas, R. *A History of Accelerator Radiation Protection*. Ramtrans Publishing, Ashford, Kent, U.K., 1994.

Rutherford, E., Chadwick, J., and Ellis, C. D. *Radiations from Radioactive Substances*. Cambridge University Press, Cambridge, England, 1930.

Semat, H., and Albright, J. R. *Introduction to Atomic and Nuclear Physics*, 5th ed. Holt, Rinehart, and Winston, New York, 1972.

Shleien, B., Slabak, L., and Birkey, B., *Handbook of Health Physics and Radiological Health*. Lippincott Williams & Wilkins, Philadelphia, PA, 1998.

Stannard, J. N. *Radioactivity and Health; A History*. Pacific Northwest Laboratory, Office of Scientific and Technical Information, Publication DOE/RL/01830-T59, National Technical Information Service, Springfield, VA, 1988.

Sullivan, A. H. *A Guide to Radiation and Radioactivity Levels Near High Energy Particle Accelerators,* Ramtrans Publishing, Ashford, Kent, U.K., 1992.

Turner, J. E. *Atoms, Radiation, and Radiation Protection*. John Wiley & Sons, New York, 1995.

Varian. *Linatron High Energy X-Ray Applications*, Varian, Inc., Palo Alto, CA, 1975.

Waltar, A. *Radiation and Modern Life: Marie Curie's Dream Fulfilled*. Prometheus Press, Tonbridge, Kent, U.K., 2004.

INTERACTION OF RADIATION WITH MATTER

In order for health physicists to understand the physical basis for radiation dosimetry and the theory of radiation shielding, they must understand the mechanisms by which the various radiations interact with matter. In most instances, these interactions involve a transfer of energy from the radiation to the matter with which it interacts. Matter consists of atomic nuclei and extranuclear electrons. Radiation may interact with either or both of these constituents of matter. The probability of occurrence of any particular category of interaction, and hence the penetrating power of the several radiations, depends on the type and energy of the radiation as well as on the nature of the absorbing medium. In all instances, excitation and ionization of the absorber atoms result from their interaction with the radiation. Ultimately, the energy that is transferred either to a tissue or to a radiation shield is dissipated as heat.

BETA PARTICLES (BETA RAYS)

Range–Energy Relationship

The attenuation of beta particles (beta rays is used synonymously with beta particles) by any given absorber may be measured by interposing successively thicker absorbers between a beta source and a suitable beta detector, such as a Geiger–Muller counter (Fig. 5-1), and counting the beta particles that penetrate the absorbers. When this is done with a pure beta emitter, it is found that the beta-particle counting rate decreases rapidly at first, and then, as the absorber thickness increases, it decreases slowly. Eventually, a thickness of absorber is reached that stops all the beta particles; the Geiger counter then registers only background counts due to environmental radiation. If semilog paper is used to plot the data and the counting rate is plotted on the logarithmic axis while absorber thickness is plotted on the linear axis, the data approximate a straight line, as shown in Figure 5-2. (Please note that the

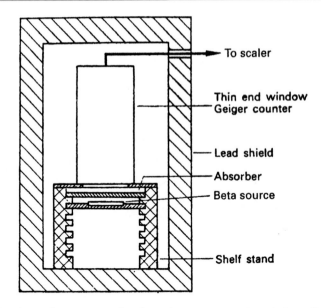

Figure 5-1. Experimental arrangement for absorption measurements on beta particles.

approximation of exponential beta absorption is a fortuitous consequence of the shape of the beta-energy-distribution curve; beta and electron absorption do not follow first-order kinetics and hence are not truly exponential functions.) The end point in the absorption curve, where no further decrease in the counting rate is observed, is called the *range* of the beta in the material of which the absorbers are made. As a rough rule of thumb, a useful relationship is that the absorber half-thickness (that thickness of absorber which stops one-half of the beta particles) is about one-eighth the range of the beta. Since the maximum beta energies for the various isotopes are known, by measuring the beta ranges in different absorbers, the systematic relationship between range and energy shown in Figure 5-3 is established. Inspection of Figure 5-3 shows that the required thickness of absorber for any given beta energy decreases as the density of the absorber increases. Detailed analyses of experimental data show that the ability to absorb energy from beta particles depends mainly on the number of absorbing electrons in the path of the beta—that is, on the areal density (electrons/cm^2) of electrons in the absorber, and, to a much lesser degree, on the atomic number of the absorber. For practical purposes, therefore, in the calculation of shielding thickness against beta particles, the effect of atomic number is neglected. (It should be pointed out that, for reasons to be given later, beta shields are almost always made from low-atomic-numbered materials.) Areal density of electrons is approximately proportional to the product of the density of the absorber material and the linear thickness of the absorber, thus giving rise to the unit of thickness called the *density thickness*. Mathematically, density thickness t_d is defined as

$$t_d \, \text{g/cm}^2 = \rho \, \text{g/cm}^3 \times t_1 \, \text{cm}. \tag{5.1}$$

The units of density and thickness in Eq. (5.1), of course, need not be grams and centimeters; they may be any consistent set of units. Use of the density thickness

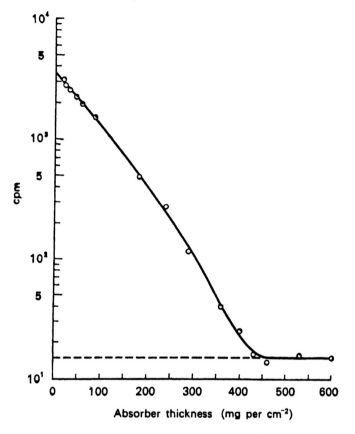

Figure 5-2. Absorption curve (aluminum absorbers) of ^{210}Bi beta particles, 1.17 MeV. The broken line represents the mean background count rate.

unit, such as g/cm^2 or mg/cm^2 for absorber materials, makes it possible to specify such absorbers independently of the absorber material. For example, the density of aluminum is 2.7 g/cm^3. From Eq. (5.1), a 1-cm-thick sheet of aluminum, therefore, has a density thickness of

$$t_d = 2.7 \, \frac{g}{cm^3} \times 1 \, cm = 2.7 \, \frac{g}{cm^2}.$$

If a sheet of Plexiglas whose density is 1.18 g/cm^3 is to have a beta absorbing quality very nearly equal to that of the 1-cm-thick sheet of aluminum—that is, 2.7 g/cm^2—its linear thickness is found, from Eq. (5.1), to be

$$t_l = \frac{t_d}{\rho} = \frac{2.7 \, g/cm^2}{1.8 \, g/cm^3} = 2.39 \, cm.$$

Another practical advantage of using this system of thickness measurement is that it allows the addition of thicknesses of different materials in a radiologically meaningful

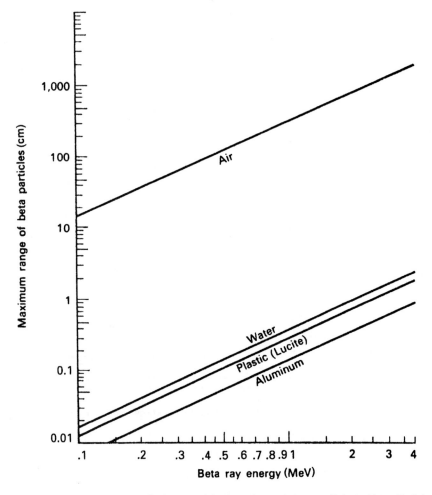

Figure 5-3. Range–energy curves for beta particles in various substances. (Adapted from *Radiological Health Handbook.* Washington, DC: Office of Technical Services; 1960.)

way. The quantitative relationship between beta energy and range is given by the following experimentally determined empirical equations:

$$E = 1.92 R^{0.725} \qquad R \leq 0.3\,\mathrm{g/cm^2} \qquad\qquad (5.2)$$

$$R = 0.407 E^{1.38} \qquad E \leq 0.8\,\mathrm{MeV} \qquad\qquad (5.3)$$

$$E = 1.85 R + 0.245 \qquad R \geq 0.3\,\mathrm{g/cm^2} \qquad\qquad (5.4)$$

$$R = 0.542 E - 0.133 \qquad E \geq 0.8\,\mathrm{MeV} \qquad\qquad (5.5)$$

where

R = range, g/cm^2 and
E = maximum beta energy, MeV.

An experimentally determined curve of beta range (in units of density thickness expressed as mg/cm^2) versus energy is given in Figure 5-4.

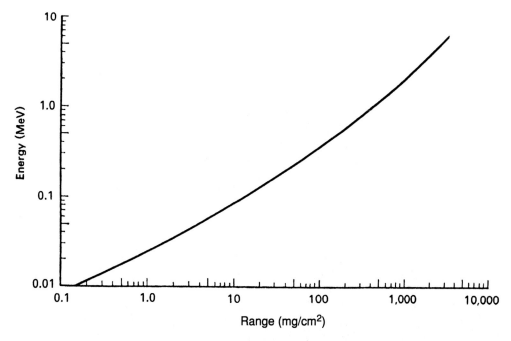

Figure 5-4. Range–energy curve for beta particles and for monoenergetic electrons. (Adapted from *Radiological Health Handbook*. Washington, DC: Office of Technical Services; 1960.)

EXAMPLE 5.1

What must be the minimum thickness of a shield made of (a) Plexiglas and (b) aluminum in order that no beta particles from a ^{90}Sr source pass through?

Solution

Strontium-90 emits a 0.54-MeV beta particle. However, its daughter, ^{90}Y, emits a beta particle whose maximum energy is 2.27 MeV. Since ^{90}Y beta particles always accompany ^{90}Sr beta particles, the shield must be thick enough to stop these more-energetic betas. If we substitute 2.27 MeV for E in Eq. (5.5), we find the range of the betas:

$$R = (0.542 \times 2.27) - 0.133 = 1.1\,\text{g/cm}^2.$$

Alternatively, from Figure 5-4, the range of a 2.27-MeV beta particle is found to be 1.1 g/cm². The density of Plexiglas is 1.18 g/cm³. From Eq. (5.1), the required thickness is found to be

$$t_1 = \frac{t_d}{\rho} = \frac{1.1\,\text{g/cm}^2}{1.18\,\text{g/cm}^3} = 0.932\,\text{cm}.$$

Plexiglas may suffer radiation damage and crack if exposed to very intense radiation for a long period of time. Under these conditions, aluminum is a better choice for a shield. Since the density of aluminum is 2.7 g/cm³, the required thickness of aluminum is found to be 0.41 cm.

The range–energy relationship may be used by the health physicist as an aid in identifying an unknown beta-emitting contaminant. This is done by measuring the range of the beta radiation, calculating the beta particle's energy, and then using published values of beta energies from the various nuclides to find the radionuclide whose beta energy matches the calculated value.

 ## EXAMPLE 5.2

Using the counting setup shown in Figure 5-5, beta radiation from an unidentified radionuclide was stopped by a 0.111-mm-thick aluminum absorber. No measurable decrease of the radioactivity in the sample was observed during a period of 1 month and no other radiation was emitted from the sample.

(a) What was the energy of the beta particle?

(b) What is the isotope?

Solution

The total range of the beta particle is given as:

$$\text{Range} = 1.7 \, \frac{\text{mg}}{\text{cm}^2} \text{ mica} + 1 \text{ cm air} + 0.111 \text{ mm Al}.$$

These different absorbing media may be added together if their thicknesses are expressed as density thickness. The density of air is 1.293 mg/cm³ at standard temperature and pressure (STP). With Eq. (5.1), the density thicknesses of the air

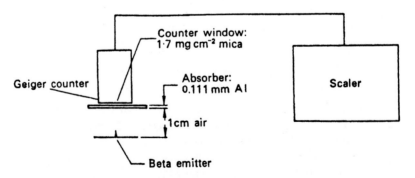

Figure 5-5. Measuring the range of an unknown beta particle to identify the radioisotope.

and aluminum are computed and the range of the unknown beta particle is found to be:

$$\text{Range} = 1.7 \text{ mg/cm}^2 + 1.29 \text{ mg/cm}^2 + 30 \text{ mg/cm}^2 = 32.99 \text{ mg/cm}^2$$

In Figure 5-4, the energy corresponding to this range is seen to be about 0.17 MeV. The unknown radionuclide is therefore likely to be ^{14}C, a pure beta emitter whose maximum beta energy is 0.155 MeV and whose half-life is about 5700 years.

Mechanisms of Energy Loss

Ionization and Excitation

Interaction between the electric fields of a beta particle and the orbital electrons of the absorbing medium leads to electronic excitation and ionization. Such interactions are inelastic collisions, analogous to that described in Example 2.13. The electron is held in the atom by electrical forces, and energy is lost by the beta particle in overcoming these forces. Since electrical forces act over long distances, the "collision" between a beta particle and an electron occurs without the two particles coming into actual contact—as is also the case of the collision between like poles of two magnets. The amount of energy lost by the beta particle depends on its distance of approach to the electron and on its kinetic energy. If ϕ is the ionization potential of the absorbing medium and E_t is the energy lost by the beta particle during the collision, the kinetic energy of the ejected electron E_k is

$$E_k = E_t - \phi. \tag{5.6}$$

In some ionizing collisions, only one ion pair is produced. In other cases, the ejected electron may have sufficient kinetic energy to produce a small cluster of several ionizations; and in a small proportion of the collisions, the ejected electron may receive a considerable amount of energy, enough to cause it to travel a long distance and to leave a trail of ionizations. Such an electron, whose kinetic energy may be on the order of 1000 eV (1 keV), is called a *delta ray*.

Beta particles have the same mass as orbital electrons and hence are easily deflected during collisions. For this reason, beta particles follow tortuous paths as they pass through absorbing media. Figure 5-6 shows the path of a beta particle through a photographic emulsion. The ionizing events expose the film at the points of ionization, thereby making them visible after development of the film.

By using a cloud chamber or film to visualize the ionizing events and by counting the actual number of ionizations due to a single primary ionizing particle of known energy, it was learned that the average energy expended in the production of an ion pair is about two to three times greater than the ionization potential. The difference between the energy expended in ionizing collisions and the total energy lost by the ionizing particle is attributed to electronic excitation. For oxygen and nitrogen, for example, the ionization potentials are 13.6 and 14.5 eV, respectively, while the average energy expenditure per ion pair in air is 34 eV. Table 5-1 shows the ionization potential and mean energy expenditure (w) for several gases of practical importance.

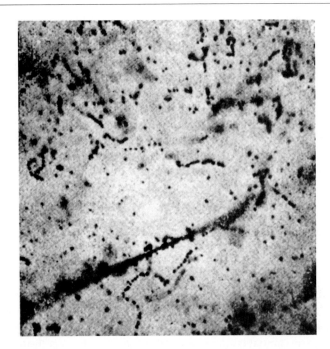

Figure 5-6. Electron tracks in photographic emulsion. The tortuous lines are the electron tracks; the heavy line in the lower half was made by an oxygen nucleus from primary cosmic radiation. (Reproduced with permission from Yagoda H. The tracks of nuclear particles. *Scientific American,* May 1956:40–47.)

Specific Ionization. The linear rate of energy loss of a beta particle due to ionization and excitation, which is an important parameter in health physics instrument design and in the biological effects of radiation, is usually expressed by the *specific ionization.* Specific ionization is the number of ion pairs formed per unit distance traveled by the beta particle. Generally, the specific ionization is relatively high for low-energy betas;

TABLE 5-1. Average Energy Lost by a Beta Particle in the Production of an Ion Pair

GAS	IONIZATION POTENTIAL (eV)	MEAN ENERGY EXPENDITURE PER ION PAIR (eV)
H_2	13.6	36.6
He	24.5	41.5
N_2	14.5	34.6
O_2	13.6	30.8
Ne	21.5	36.2
A	15.7	26.2
Kr	14.0	24.3
Xe	12.1	21.9
Air		33.7
CO_2	14.4	32.9
CH_4	14.5	27.3
C_2H_2	11.6	25.7
C_2H_4	12.2	26.3
C_2H_6	12.8	24.6

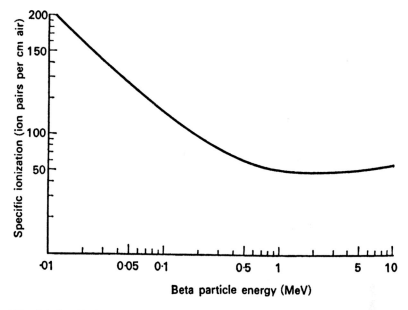

Figure 5-7. Relationship between particle energy and specific ionization of air.

it decreases rapidly as the beta-particle energy increases, until a broad minimum is reached at around 1–3 MeV. Further increase in beta energy results in a slow increase of specific ionization, as shown in Figure 5-7.

The linear rate of energy loss due to excitation and ionization may be calculated from the equation

$$\frac{dE}{dx} = \frac{2\pi q^4 NZ \times (3 \times 10^9)^4}{E_m \beta^2 (1.6 \times 10^{-6})^2} \left\{ \ln\left[\frac{E_m E_k \beta^2}{I^2 (1 - \beta^2)} \right] - \beta^2 \right\} \frac{\text{MeV}}{\text{cm}}, \tag{5.7}$$

where

$q =$ charge on the electron, 1.6×10^{-19} C,
$N =$ number of absorber atoms per cm^3,
$Z =$ atomic number of the absorber,
$NZ =$ number of absorber electrons per $cm^3 = 3.88 \times 10^{20}$ for air at 0° and 76 cm Hg,
$E_m =$ energy equivalent of electron mass, 0.51 MeV,
$E_k =$ kinetic energy of the beta particle (MeV),
$\beta =$ speed of the ionizing particle/speed of light $= v/c$,
$I =$ mean ionization and excitation potential of absorbing atoms (MeV), and
$I = 8.6 \times 10^{-5}$ for air; for other substances, $I = 1.35 \times 10^{-5} Z$.

If the mean energy, w, expended in the creation of an ion pair (ip) is known, then the specific ionization may be calculated from the equation below:

$$SI, \frac{\text{ip}}{\text{cm}} = \frac{\frac{dE}{dx} \text{ eV/cm}}{w \text{ eV/ip}}. \tag{5.8}$$

EXAMPLE 5.3

What is the specific ionization resulting from the passage of a 0.1-MeV beta particle through standard air?

Solution

β^2 is found from Eq. (2.20):

$$E_k = m_0 c^2 \left[\frac{1}{\sqrt{(1 - \beta^2)}} - 1 \right]$$

$$0.1 = 0.51 \left[\frac{1}{\sqrt{(1 - \beta^2)}} - 1 \right]$$

$$\beta^2 = 0.3010.$$

Substituting the respective values into Eq. (5.7), we have

$$\frac{dE}{dx} = \frac{2\pi \, (1.6 \times 10^{-19})^4 \times 3.88 \times 10^{20} \times (3 \times 10^9)^4}{0.51 \times 0.3010 \times (1.6 \times 10^{-6})^2}$$

$$\times \left\{ \ln \left[\frac{0.51 \times 0.1 \times 0.3010}{(8.6 \times 10^{-5})^2 \, (1 - 0.3010)} \right] - 0.3010 \right\} \frac{\text{MeV}}{\text{cm}}$$

$$\frac{dE}{dx} = 4.75 \times 10^{-3} \frac{\text{MeV}}{\text{cm}}.$$

For air, $w = 34$ eV/ip. The average specific ionization, therefore, from Eq. (5.8), is

$$\text{S.I.} = \frac{4750 \text{ eV/cm}}{34 \text{ eV/cm}} = 140 \text{ ip/cm}.$$

It is very important to note that Eq. (5.7) shows that the rate of energy loss due to excitation and ionization increases rapidly with decreasing velocity and with increasing charge.

Very often, the unit of length used in expressing rate of energy loss is density thickness, that is, in units of $\frac{\text{MeV}}{\text{g/cm}^2}$. This is called the *mass stopping power*, it is defined as the ratio of the linear stopping power to the density of the stopping medium:

$$S = \frac{dE/dx}{\rho}. \tag{5.9}$$

Since the density of standard air is 1.293×10^{-3} g/cm³, the mass rate of energy loss, or the mass stopping power, in Example 5.3 is given as

$$S = \frac{4.75 \times 10^{-3} \text{ MeV/cm}}{1.293 \times 10^{-3} \text{ g/cm}^3} = 3.67 \frac{\text{MeV}}{\text{g/cm}^2}.$$

Linear Energy Transfer. The term *specific ionization* is used when attention is focused on the energy lost by the radiation. When attention is focused on the absorbing medium, as is the case in radiobiology and radiation effects, we are interested in the linear rate of energy absorption by the absorbing medium as the ionizing particle traverses the medium. As a measure of the rate of energy absorption, we use the *linear energy transfer* (LET), which is defined by the equation:

$$LET = \frac{dE_L}{dl}, \tag{5.10}$$

where dE_L is the average energy locally transferred to the absorbing medium by a charged particle of specified energy in traversing a distance of dl. In health physics and radiobiology, LET is usually expressed in units of kilo electron volts per micron (keV/μm). As used in the definition above, the term "locally transferred" may refer either to a maximum distance from the track of the ionizing particle or to a maximum value of discrete energy loss by the particle beyond which losses are no longer considered local. In either case, LET refers to energy transferred to a limited volume of absorber.

Relative Mass Stopping Power. The relative mass stopping power is used to compare quantitatively the energy absorptive power of different media. It will be shown later that the mass stopping power of different absorbers relative to that of air is important in the practice of health physics. Relative mass stopping power, ρ_m is defined by

$$\rho_m = \frac{S_{medium}}{S_{air}}. \tag{5.11}$$

EXAMPLE 5.4

What is the relative (to air) mass stopping power of graphite, density = 2.25 g/cm³, for a 0.1-MeV beta particle?

Solution

The mass rate of energy loss in graphite is found by first finding the mean rate of linear energy loss with Eq. (5.7), and then using Eq. (5.9) to calculate the energy loss per unit mass. The values for NZ and for I (the mean ionization and excitation potential of the absorbing atoms) are calculated, as well as the appropriate values for the other factors, and substituted into Eqs. (5.7) and (5.9):

$$NZ = \frac{6.02 \times 10^{23} \frac{\text{atoms}}{\text{mol}} \times 2.25 \frac{\text{g}}{\text{cm}^3} \times 6 \frac{\text{electrons}}{\text{atom}}}{12 \frac{\text{g}}{\text{mol}}}$$

$$= 6.77 \times 10^{23} \text{ electrons/cm}^3,$$

$$I = 1.35 \times 10^{-5} \times 6 = 8.1 \times 10^{-5} \text{ MeV}.$$

Substituting these values, together with the other appropriate values into Eq. (5.7), we have

$$\frac{dE}{dx} = \frac{2\pi (1.6 \times 10^{-19})^4 \times 6.77 \times 10^{23} \times (3 \times 10^9)^4}{0.51 \times 0.3010 \times (1.6 \times 10^{-6})^2}$$

$$\times \left\{ \ln \left[\frac{0.51 \times 0.1 \times 0.3010}{(8.1 \times 10^{-5})^2 (1 - 0.3010)} \right] - 0.3010 \right\} \frac{\text{MeV}}{\text{cm}}$$

$$\frac{dE}{dx} = 8.33 \frac{\text{MeV}}{\text{cm}}.$$

The mass stopping power of graphite for a 0.1-MeV beta particle (or a 0.1-MeV electron) is calculated with Eq. (5.9):

$$S\,(\text{graphite}) = \frac{\frac{dE}{dx}}{\rho} = \frac{8.33 \text{ MeV/cm}}{2.25 \text{ g/cm}^3} = 3.70 \frac{\text{MeV}}{\text{g/cm}^2}.$$

For air, the mass stopping power for 0.1-MeV beta particles is 3.67 MeV/g/cm². From Eq. (5.10), the relative mass stopping power of graphite for a 0.1-MeV electron is

$$\rho_m = \frac{S_{\text{medium}}}{S_{\text{air}}} = \frac{3.70 \frac{\text{MeV}}{\text{g/cm}^2}}{3.67 \frac{\text{MeV}}{\text{g/cm}^2}} = 1.01.$$

Bremsstrahlung

Bremsstrahlung, which is the German word meaning *braking radiation,* consists of X-rays that are produced when high-velocity charged particles undergo a rapid change in velocity, that is, when they are very rapidly accelerated. Since velocity is a vector quantity that includes both speed and direction, a change in direction, even if the speed should remain unchanged, is a change in velocity. When a beta particle or an electron passes close to a nucleus, the strong attractive coulomb force causes the beta particle to deviate sharply from its original path. This change in

TABLE 5-2. Bremsstrahlung Spectrum from Beta Radiation

X-RAY ENERGY INTERVALS IN FRACTIONS OF $E_m(\beta)$	% TOTAL PHOTON INTENSITY IN ENERGY INTERVAL
0.0–0.1	43.5
0.1–0.2	25.8
0.2–0.3	15.2
0.3–0.4	8.3
0.4–0.5	4.3
0.5–0.6	2.0
0.6–0.7	0.7
0.7–0.8	0.2
0.8–0.9	0.03
0.9–1.0	<0.01

direction is a radial acceleration and the beta particle, in accordance with Maxwell's classical theory, loses energy by electromagnetic radiation at a rate proportional to the square of the acceleration. (Radiation emitted by electrons that are undergoing radial acceleration when caused to travel in a circular path by a magnetic field in an accelerator is called *synchrotron* radiation.) Electrons or betas are decelerated at various rates in their interaction with matter. Bremsstrahlung photons (x-rays), therefore, have a continuous energy distribution that ranges downward from a theoretical maximum equal to the kinetic energy of the most energetic beta particle. The energy distribution of the bremsstrahlung photons from a beta source is very heavily skewed toward the low energy relative to the maximum energy of the betas, as shown in Table 5-2. This occurs for two reasons: First, the proportion of betas near the maximum energy is very small, that is, most of the betas are found in the lower half of the beta spectrum (Fig. 4-4), and second, most of the betas are decelerated by a series of collisions in which small amounts of energy are lost, rather than in one or two large energy-loss collisions before being stopped.

It is important for users of radionuclides to know that bremsstrahlung X-rays are not a property of beta-emitting isotopes and hence are not shown in decay schemes. The X-rays are a result of the interaction of the betas with surrounding matter, such as its container or a shield. For example, the bremsstrahlung dose rate at a distance of 10 cm from an aqueous solution of 4000 MBq (~100 mCi) ^{32}P in a 25-mL volumetric flask is about 0.03 mGy/h (3 mrad/h); for 4×10^9 Bq (~100 mCi) ^{90}Sr in a brass container, the bremsstrahlung dose rate is about 1 mGy/h (~100 mrad/h) at a distance of 10 cm. (The mGy and the mrad will be formally introduced in the next chapter. At this point it is sufficient to know that they are units for measuring radiation absorbed dose.) The likelihood of bremsstrahlung production increases with increasing beta energy and with increasing atomic number of the absorber (Eq. [5.12]). Beta shields are therefore made with materials of the minimum practicable atomic number. In practice, beta shields of atomic number higher than 13 (aluminum) are seldom used. For purposes of *estimating* the bremsstrahlung hazard from beta radiation, the following empirically determined relationship may be used:

$$f_\beta = 3.5 \times 10^{-4}\, ZE_m, \tag{5.12}$$

where

f_β = the fraction of the incident beta energy converted into photons,
Z = atomic number of the absorber, and
E_m = maximum energy of the beta particle (MeV).

 # EXAMPLE 5.5

A very small source (physically) of 3.7×10^{10} Bq (1 Ci) of ^{32}P is inside a lead shield just thick enough to prevent any beta particles from emerging. What is the bremsstrahlung energy flux at a distance of 10 cm from the source (neglect attenuation of the bremsstrahlung by the beta shield)?

Solution

Since Z for lead is 82 and the maximum energy of the ^{32}P beta particle is 1.71 MeV, we have, from Eq. (5.12), the fraction of the beta energy converted into photons (x-rays),

$$f = 3.5 \times 10^{-4} \times 82 \times 1.71 = 0.049.$$

Since the average beta-particle energy is about one-third of the maximum energy, the energy E_β carried by the beta particles from the 1-Ci source that is incident on the shield is

$$E_\beta \text{ (MeV/s)} = \frac{1}{3} \frac{E_{max} \text{MeV}}{\beta} \times 3.7 \times 10^{10} \frac{\beta}{s}.$$

For health physics purposes, it is assumed that all the bremsstrahlung photons are of the beta particle's maximum energy, E_{max}. The photon flux ϕ of bremsstrahlung photons at a distance r cm from a point source of beta particles whose activity is 3.7×10^{10} Bq (1 Ci) is therefore given as

$$\phi = \frac{f E_\beta}{4\pi r^2 E_{max}}$$

$$= \frac{0.049 \times \frac{1}{3} \times 1.71 \frac{\text{MeV}}{\beta} \times 3.7 \times 10^{10} \frac{\beta}{s}}{4\pi \times (10 \text{ cm})^2 \times 1.71 \text{ MeV/photon}} = 4.8 \times 10^5 \frac{\text{photons/s}}{\text{cm}^2}. \qquad \textbf{(5.13)}$$

X-ray Production

When a beam of monoenergetic electrons that had been accelerated across a high potential difference is abruptly decelerated by stopping the electron beam (as in the case of an X-ray tube, a cathode ray tube, or a klystron microwave generator), a small fraction of the energy in the electron beam (Eq. [5.14]) is converted into X-rays.

$$f_e = 1 \times 10^{-3} \times ZE, \tag{5.14}$$

where

f_e = fraction of the energy in the electron beam that is converted into X-rays,

Z = atomic number of the target in the X-ray tube or whatever the electron beam strikes in any other device, and

E = voltage across the X-ray tube or other device (mega volts, MV). The numerical value of the voltage E is equal to the kinetic energy of the electron, expressed in eV, as it strikes the target. Thus, an electron that has been accelerated across a voltage of 0.1 MV has acquired a kinetic energy of 0.1 MeV (or 100 keV).

This is the operating principle of traditional diagnostic, industrial, and analytical X-ray tube (Fig. 5-8). The American physicist William D. Coolidge invented this type of X-ray tube in 1913. In 1937, Dr. Coolidge was awarded an honorary MD degree by the University of Zurich in recognition of his many contributions of physics to medical science. It is interesting to note that Coolidge lived to the age of 101 years, despite his extensive experience with X-rays.

An electron beam, usually on the order of milliamperes, is generated by heating the cathode. A voltage difference on the order of tens to hundreds of kilo volts across the tube accelerates the electrons to form a monoenergetic beam in which the kinetic energy of the electrons in electron volts is numerically equal to the voltage across the tube. The high-speed electrons are stopped by a high-atomic-numbered metal target

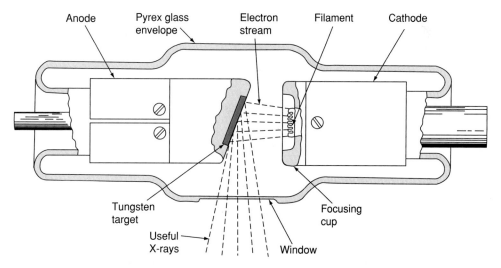

Figure 5-8. Coolidge type stationary target X-ray tube. A beam of useful X-rays is formed by the bremsstrahlung that passes through an open port in the shielding that encloses the X-ray tube. (Figure 3 2A, p. 34 from RADIATION BIOPHYSICS, 2nd ed, by Howard Lucius Andrews. Copytight © 1974 by Prentice-Hall, Inc. Reprinted by permission of Pearson Education, Inc.)

that is embedded in the anode. Some of the kinetic energy in the electron beam is converted into X-rays (bremsstrahlung) when the electrons are suddenly stopped. In X-ray generators where the voltage is less than several hundred thousand volts, the X-rays (photons) are emitted mainly at angles around 90° to the direction of the electron beam. A hole in the protective shielding that houses the X-ray tube allows a useful X-ray beam to emerge from the shielded tube.

The X-rays that are produced in this manner have a continuous energy distribution that approaches a maximum energy equal to the kinetic energy of the electron that was stopped instantaneously and thus all of its kinetic energy was converted into an X-ray photon. If an electron were to be instantaneously stopped by the target, all of its kinetic energy would be converted into an X-ray photon. This would represent the maximum-energy (or shortest-wavelength) photon possible with the given voltage across the tube. However, this maximum limit can only be approached, since no electron can be stopped instantaneously. The fact that the electrons are slowed down at different rates due to different ionization and excitation collisions leads to a continuous energy distribution up to the theoretical maximum energy that is determined only by the high voltage across the X-ray tube (Fig. 5-9). If we have a full-wave rectified, but unfiltered AC voltage across the X-ray tube, then the voltage varies cyclically from zero to the maximum voltage. This condition skews the X-ray

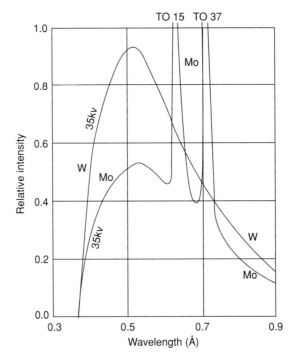

Figure 5-9. X-ray spectrum from a tungsten target (W) and from a molybdenum target (Mo) bombarded by electrons accelerated through 35 kV. The limiting wavelength for both targets, representing the 35-keV maximum-energy photon, is 0.3543 Å. The two peaks on the Mo curve represent the K_β (to 15) and K_α (to 37). (Figure 3-4B, p. 37 from RADIATION BIOPHYSICS, 2nd ed, by Howard Lucius Andrews. Copyright © 1974 by Prentice-Hall, Inc. Reprinted by permission of Pearson Education, Inc.)

energy distribution toward the lower energies since most of the electrons are accelerated across a varying voltage that is less than its peak. A highly filtered, high-voltage power supply produces a constant high voltage across the tube, and consequently a "harder," that is, a higher effective energy beam than an unfiltered high-voltage power supply. To distinguish between X-rays produced by these two power supplies, we call the first kV$_P$ (kV peak) and X-rays from the filtered generator are labelled kV$_{cp}$ (kV constant potential).

The theoretical maximum photon energy ($hc/\lambda_{\text{minimum}}$) is equal to the electron's kinetic energy when it strikes the target, which in turn is equal to potential energy of the electron before it is accelerated, qV. Thus, the relationship between applied voltage and the minimum wavelength, which is known as the *Duane-Hunt law*, is

$$qV = \frac{hc}{\lambda_m} \tag{5.15}$$

$$\lambda_m = \frac{6.6 \times 10^{-34}\,\text{J} \cdot \text{s} \times 3 \times 10^8\,\text{m/s}}{1.6 \times 10^{-19}\,\text{C} \times E\,\text{eV}} \times 10^{10}\,\text{Å/m}$$

$$\lambda_m = \frac{12,400}{E}\,\text{Å}. \tag{5.16}$$

 # EXAMPLE 5.6

Calculate the lower wavelength limit of the X-ray spectrum from a tube with 100 kV across it.

Solution

The lower wavelength limit of the X-ray spectrum from a tube with 100 kV across it is calculated with Eq. (5.16):

$$\lambda_m = \frac{12,400}{E} = \frac{12,400}{100,000\ \text{volts}} = 0.124\ \text{Å}.$$

The power, P watts, in the electron beam of an X-ray machine is given by the product of the high voltage across the tube, V volts, and the beam current i amperes.

$$P\,(\text{beam}) = V \times i. \tag{5.17}$$

Since the fraction of the beam power that is converted to X-rays is proportional to ZV, the intensity of the X-ray beam, I, is proportional to the product of ZV and Vi:

$$I(\text{X-rays}) \propto (ZV \times Vi) \propto ZV^2 i. \tag{5.18}$$

Equation (5.17) shows that the X-rays from an X-ray generator varies directly with the beam current and with the square of the high voltage across the tube.

The kinetic energy of an electron that has been accelerated across V volts is eV (electron volts); Eq. (5.16) may be adapted to relate the wavelength to the energy, in electron volts, of any photon:

$$\lambda = \frac{12,400}{eV}. \tag{5.19}$$

EXAMPLE 5.7

Calculate the wavelength of the 0.364-MeV photon from ^{131}I.

Solution

The wavelength of the 0.364-MeV photon from ^{131}I is calculated as follows:

$$\lambda = \frac{12,400}{E} = \frac{12,400}{0.364 \times 10^6} = 0.0341 \text{ Å}.$$

ALPHA PARTICLES (ALPHA RAYS)

Range–Energy Relationship

Alpha particles (The terms alpha rays and alpha particles are synonymous, and are used interchangibly) are the least penetrating of the radiations. In air, even the most energetic alphas from radioactive substances travel only several centimeters, while in tissue, the range of alpha radiation is measured in microns (1 $\mu = 10^{-4}$ cm). The term *range*, in the case of alpha particles, may have two different definitions—mean range and extrapolated range. The difference between these two ranges can be seen in the alpha-particle absorption curve (Fig. 5-10).

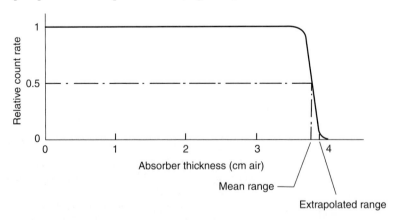

Figure 5-10. Alpha-particle absorption curve.

An alpha-particle absorption curve is flat because alpha radiation is essentially monoenergetic. Increasing thickness of absorbers serves merely to reduce the energy of the alphas that pass through the absorbers; the number of alphas is not reduced until the approximate range is reached. At this point, there is a sharp decrease in the number of alphas that pass through the absorber. Near the very end of the curve, absorption rate decreases due to straggling, or the combined effects of the statistical distribution of the "average" energy loss per ion and the scattering by the absorber nuclei. The mean range is the range most accurately determined and corresponds to the range of the "average" alpha particle. The extrapolated range is obtained by extrapolating the absorption curve to zero alpha particles transmitted.

Air is the most commonly used absorbing medium for specifying range–energy relationships of alpha particles. The range (in cm) of air, R_a, at $0°C$ and 760 mm Hg pressure of alphas whose energy E is between 2 MeV and 8 MeV is closely approximated (within 10%) by the following empirically determined equation:

$$R_a = 0.322E^{3/2}. \tag{5.20}$$

The range of alpha particles in any other medium whose atomic mass number is A and whose density is ρ may be computed from the following relationship:

$$R_a \times \rho_a \times (A_m)^{0.5} = R_m \times \rho_a \times (A_a)^{0.5}, \tag{5.21}$$

where

R_a and R_m = range in air and tissue (cm),
A_a and A_m = atomic mass number of air and the medium, and
ρ_a and ρ_m = density of air and the medium (g/cm^3).

 EXAMPLE 5.8

What thickness of aluminum foil, density 2.7 g/cm^3, is required to stop the alpha particles from ^{210}Po?

Solution

The energy of the ^{210}Po alpha particle is 5.3 MeV. From Eq. (5.20), the range of the alpha particle in air is

$$R = 0.322 \times (5.3)^{3/2} = 3.93 \text{ cm}.$$

Substituting

$R_a = 3.93$ cm,
$A_m = 27$,
$A_a = (0.2 \times 16 + 0.8 \times 14)$,

$\rho_m = 2.7\ \text{g/cm}^3$, and
$\rho_a = 1.293 \times 10^{-3}\ \text{g/cm}^3$ into Eq. (5.21), we have

$$R_m = \frac{R_a \times \rho_a \times (A_m)^{0.5}}{\rho_m \times (A_a)^{0.5}} = \frac{3.93\ \text{cm} \times 1.293 \times 10^{-3}\ \text{g/cm}^3 \times (27)^{0.5}}{2.7\ \text{g/cm}^3 \times (0.2 \times 16 + 0.8 \times 14)^{0.5}}$$

$$= 2.58 \times 10^{-3}\ \text{cm}.$$

The range of the 5.3 MeV-alpha, in units of density thickness, from Eq. (5.1), is

$$t_d = t_d \times \rho = 2.58 \times 10^{-3}\ \text{cm} \times 2.7\ \frac{\text{g}}{\text{cm}^3} = 7 \times 10^{-3}\ \frac{\text{g}}{\text{cm}^2}.$$

Because the effective atomic composition of tissue is not very much different from that of air, the following relationship may be used to calculate the range of alpha particles in tissue:

$$R_a \times \rho_a = R_t \times \rho_t, \tag{5.22}$$

where

R_a and R_t = range in air and tissue and
ρ_a and ρ_t = density of air and tissue.

EXAMPLE 5.9

What is the range in tissue of a ^{210}Po alpha particle?

Solution

The range in air of this alpha particle was found in Example 5.8 to be 3.93 cm. Assuming tissue to have unit density, the range in tissue is, from Eq. (5.22):

$$R_t = \frac{R_t \times \rho_a}{\rho_t} = \frac{3.93\ \text{cm} \times 1.293 \times 10^{-3}\ \text{g/cm}^3}{1\ \frac{\text{g}}{\text{cm}^3}} = 5.1 \times 10^{-3}\ \text{cm}.$$

Energy Transfer

The major energy-loss mechanisms for alpha particles that are considered to be significant in health physics are collisions with the electrons in the absorbing medium. These interactions result in electronic excitation and ionization of the absorber atoms.

In a collision between a heavy ionizing particle and an orbital electron in an absorbing medium, the energy transferred from the ionizing particle to the orbital electron is given by:

$$\Delta E = \frac{2\,(9 \times 10^9 \times Q \times q)^2}{ma^2v^2},\qquad\qquad (5.23)$$

where

Q = charge on the ionizing particle,
q = charge on the electron,
m = mass of the electron, and
a = closest distance of approach of the ionizing particle to the electron (called the *impact parameter*).

 # EXAMPLE 5.10

The first ionization potential, ϕ, of the O_2 molecule $= 12.06$ eV. A 5.3-MeV alpha particle from ^{210}Po passes the molecule at a distance of 0.2 Å from an outer electron.

(a) How much energy does the alpha particle transfer to the electron?

(b) If this amount of energy exceeds the ionization potential, what is the kinetic energy of the ejected electron?

Solution

(a) Equation (5.23) will be used to calculate the transferred energy. First, we will calculate v^2 for substitution into Eq. (5.23). Relativity effects are trivial at an alpha particle energy of 5.3 MeV. We, therefore, may use the Newtonian expression for kinetic energy, (Eq. [2.5]):

$$E_k = \frac{1}{2}mv^2.$$

Solving for v^2, we have:

$$v^2 = \frac{2E_k}{m} = \frac{2 \times 5.3 \text{ MeV} \times 1.6 \times 10^{-13} \text{ J/MeV}}{6.64424 \times 10^{-27} \text{ kg}} = 2.55 \times 10^{14} \left(\frac{\text{m}}{\text{s}}\right)^2.$$

For an alpha particle, $Q = 2q$, therefore,

$$\Delta E_\alpha = \frac{2(9 \times 10^9 \times 2q^2)^2}{ma^2v^2} = \frac{2(81 \times 10^{18} \times 4q^4)}{ma^2v^2} = \frac{648 \times 10^{18} \times q^4}{ma^2v^2}.\qquad (5.24)$$

Substituting the appropriate values for m, a, and v^2 into Eq. (5.24) yields:

$$\Delta E_{5.3\,\text{MeV}}\,\alpha = \frac{648 \times 10^{18} \times \left(1.6 \times 10^{-19}\ \text{C}\right)^4}{9.11 \times 10^{-31}\ \text{kg} \times \left(2 \times 10^{-11}\ \text{m}\right)^2 \times 2.55 \times 10^{14}\ \left(\frac{\text{m}^2}{\text{s}^2}\right)}$$

$$= 4.57 \times 10^{-18}\ \text{J}.$$

Converting 4.57×10^{-18} J into electron volts, we have

$$\Delta E_{5.3\,\text{MeV}}\,\alpha = \frac{4.57 \times 10^{-18}\ \text{J}}{1.6 \times 10^{-19}\ \dfrac{\text{J}}{\text{eV}}} = 28.6\ \text{eV}.$$

(b) $E_{\text{k,electron}} = \Delta E - \varphi = 28.6\ \text{eV} - 12.1\ \text{eV} = 16.5\ \text{eV}.$

In passing through air or soft tissue, an alpha particle loses, on average, 35.5 eV per ion pair that it creates. The specific ionization of an alpha particle is very high, on the order of tens of thousands of ion pairs per centimeter in air. This is due to its high electrical charge and relatively slow speed because of its great mass. The slow speed allows a long interaction time between the electric fields of the alpha particle and an orbital electron of an atom in the medium through which the alpha particle passes, thus allowing sufficient energy transfer to ionize the atom with which it collides. As the alpha particle undergoes successive collisions and slows down, its specific ionization increases because the electric fields of the alpha particle and the electron have longer times to interact, and thus more energy can be transferred per collision. This increasing ionization density leads to a maximum specific ionization near the end of the alpha particle's range, as shown in Figure 5-11. This maximum is called the *Bragg peak*, after the British physicist Sir William Henry Bragg, who studied radioactivity during the early years of the 1900s.

An alpha particle loses energy at an increasing rate as it slows down until the Bragg peak is reached near the end of its range. Because of its inertia due to its heavy mass,

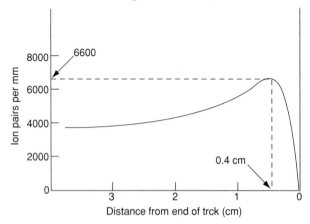

Figure 5-11. Specific ionization of a ^{210}Po alpha particle as a function of its remaining distance to the end of its range in standard air. (Lamarsh, John R.; Baratta, Anthony J., *Introduction to Nuclear Engineering*. 3rd Edition. © 2001, Pgs. 103–104. Reprinted by permission of Pearson Education, Inc., Upper Saddle River, NJ.)

an alpha particle undergoes very little deviation in a collision and therefore travels essentially in a straight line. Its average rate of energy loss may therefore be calculated as follows:

$$\frac{d\bar{E}}{dR} = \frac{\text{Kinetic energy}}{\text{Range}}. \tag{5.25}$$

The mass stopping power of air for a ^{210}Po alpha particle is, according to Eq. (5.9), is given by

$$S\,(\text{air}) = \frac{d\bar{E}/dR}{\rho\,(\text{air})} = \frac{1.35\ \text{MeV/cm}}{1.293 \times 10^{-3}\ \text{g/cm}^3} = 1.04 \times 10^3\ \frac{\text{MeV}}{\text{g/cm}^2}.$$

The relative mass stopping power for alpha particles is defined in the same way as for electrons and betas (Eq. [5.11]). In Example 5.9, it was shown that the range in tissue of a 5.3-MeV alpha particle is 5.1×10^{-3} cm. Its mean rate of energy loss in tissue, therefore, is

$$\frac{d\bar{E}}{dR}\,(\text{tissue}) = \frac{5.3\ \text{MeV}}{5.1 \times 10^{-3}\ \text{cm}} = 1.04 \times 10^3\ \frac{\text{MeV}}{\text{cm}},$$

and its mass stopping power, S, is

$$S\,(\text{tissue}) = \frac{d\bar{E}/dR}{\rho} = \frac{1.04 \times 10^3\ \text{MeV/cm}}{1\ \text{g/cm}^3} = 1.04 \times 10^3\ \frac{\text{MeV}}{\text{g/cm}^2}.$$

Using Eq. (5.11), we calculate the relative stopping power of tissue, ρ_t, for 5.3-MeV alpha particles:

$$\rho_t = \frac{S_{\text{tissue}}}{S_{\text{air}}} = \frac{1.04 \times 10^3\ \dfrac{\text{MeV}}{\text{g/cm}^2}}{1.04 \times 10^3\ \dfrac{\text{MeV}}{\text{g/cm}^2}} = 1.$$

GAMMA RAYS

Exponential Absorption

The attenuation of gamma radiation (photons) by an absorber is qualitatively different from that of either alpha or beta radiation. Whereas both these corpuscular radiations have definite ranges in matter and therefore can be completely stopped, gamma radiation can only be reduced in intensity by increasingly thicker absorbers; it cannot be completely absorbed. If gamma-ray attenuation measurements are made under conditions of *good geometry*, that is, with a well-collimated, narrow beam of radiation, as shown in Figure 5-12, and if the data are plotted on semilog paper, a straight line results, as shown in Figure 5-13, if the gamma rays are monoenergetic. If the

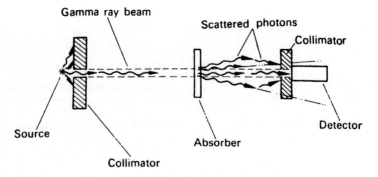

Figure 5-12. Measuring attenuation of gamma rays under conditions of good geometry. Ideally, the beam should be well collimated and the source should be as far away as possible from the detector; the absorber should be midway between the source and the detector and should be thin enough so that the likelihood of a second scattering of a photon already scattered by the absorber is negligible; and there should be no scattering material in the vicinity of the detector.

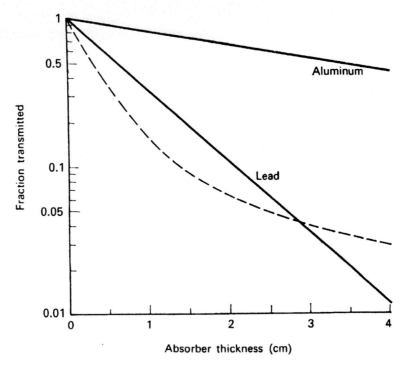

Figure 5-13. Attenuation of gamma rays under conditions of good geometry. The solid lines are the attenuation curves for 0.662-MeV (monoenergetic) gamma rays. The dotted line is the attenuation curve for a heterochromatic beam.

gamma-ray beam is heterochromatic, a curve results, as shown by the dotted line in Figure 5-13. The equation of the straight line in Figure 5-13 is

$$\ln I = -\mu t + \ln I_0 \tag{5.26a}$$

or

$$\ln \frac{I}{I_0} = -\mu t. \tag{5.26b}$$

Taking the inverse logs of both sides of Eq. (5.26b), we have,

$$\frac{I}{I_0} = e^{-\mu t}, \tag{5.27}$$

where

I_0 = gamma-ray intensity at zero absorber thickness,
t = absorber thickness,
I = gamma-ray intensity transmitted through an absorber of thickness t,
e = base of the natural logarithm system, and
μ = slope of the absorption curve = the attenuation coefficient.

Since the exponent in an exponential equation must be dimensionless, μ and t must be in reciprocal dimensions, that is, if the absorber thickness is measured in centimeters, then the attenuation coefficient is called the *linear attenuation coefficient*, μ_l, and it must have dimensions of "per cm." If t is in g/cm^2, then the absorption coefficient is called the *mass attenuation coefficient*, μ_m, and it must have dimensions of per g/cm^2 or cm^2/g. The numerical relationship between μ_l and μ_m, for a material whose density is ρ g/cm^3, is given by the equation

$$\mu_l \, \text{cm}^{-1} = \mu_m \, \frac{\text{cm}^2}{\text{g}} \times \rho \, \frac{\text{g}}{\text{cm}^3}. \tag{5.28}$$

The *attenuation coefficient* is defined as the fractional decrease, or attenuation of the gamma-ray beam intensity per unit thickness of absorber, as defined by the equation below:

$$\lim_{\Delta t \to 0} \frac{\Delta I / I}{\Delta t} = -\mu, \tag{5.29}$$

where $\Delta I / I$ is the fraction of the gamma-ray beam attenuated by an absorber of thickness Δt. The attenuation coefficient thus defined is sometimes called the *total attenuation coefficient*. Values of the attenuation coefficients for several materials are given in Table 5-3.

For some purposes, it is useful to use the *atomic attenuation coefficient*, μ_a. The atomic attenuation coefficient is the fraction of an incident gamma-ray beam that is attenuated by a single atom. Another way of saying the same thing is that the atomic attenuation coefficient is the probability that an absorber atom will interact with one of the photons in the beam. The atomic attenuation coefficient may be defined by the equation

$$\mu_a \, \text{cm}^2 = \frac{\mu_l \, \dfrac{1}{\text{cm}}}{N \, \dfrac{\text{atoms}}{\text{cm}^3}}, \tag{5.30}$$

TABLE 5-3. Linear Attenuation Coefficients, cm^{-1}

	ρ, (g/cm^3)	QUANTUM ENERGY (MeV)												
		0.1	0.15	0.2	0.3	0.5	0.8	1.0	1.5	2	3	5	8	10
C	2.25	0.335	0.301	0.274	0.238	0.196	0.159	0.143	0.117	0.100	0.080	0.061	0.048	0.044
Al	2.7	0.435	0.362	0.324	0.278	0.227	0.185	0.166	0.135	0.117	0.096	0.076	0.065	0.062
Fe	7.9	2.72	1.445	1.090	0.838	0.655	0.525	0.470	0.383	0.335	0.285	0.247	0.233	0.232
Cu	8.9	3.80	1.830	1.309	0.960	0.730	0.581	0.520	0.424	0.372	0.318	0.281	0.270	0.271
Pb	11.3	59.7	20.8	10.15	4.02	1.64	0.945	0.771	0.579	0.516	0.476	0.482	0.518	0.552
Air	1.29×10^{-3}	1.95×10^{-4}	1.73×10^{-4}	1.59×10^{-4}	1.37×10^{-4}	1.12×10^{-4}	9.12×10^{-5}	8.45×10^{-5}	6.67×10^{-5}	5.75×10^{-5}	4.6×10^{-5}	3.54×10^{-5}	2.84×10^{-5}	2.61×10^{-5}
H$_2$O	1	0.167	0.149	0.136	0.118	0.097	0.079	0.071	0.056	0.049	0.040	0.030	0.024	0.022
Concrete[a]	2.35	0.397	0.326	0.291	0.251	0.204	0.166	0.149	0.122	0.105	0.085	0.067	0.057	0.054

[a]Ordinary concrete of the following composition: 0.56%H, 49.56% O, 31.35%Si, 4.56%Al, 8.26%Ca, 1.22%Fe, 0.24%Mg, 1.71%Na, 1.92%K, 0.12%S.

Source: From White G. *X-ray Attenuation Coefficients.* Washington, DC: US Government Printing Office; 1952. NBS Report 1003.

where N is the number of absorber atoms per cm^3. Note that the dimensions of μ_a are cm^2, the units of area. For this reason, the atomic attenuation coefficient is almost always referred to as the *cross section* of the absorber. The unit in which the cross section is specified is the *barn*, b.

$$1\,b = 10^{-24}\,cm^2.$$

The atomic attenuation coefficient is also called the *microscopic cross section* and is symbolized by σ, while the linear attenuation coefficient is often called the *macroscopic cross section* and is given by the symbol Σ. This nomenclature is almost always used in dealing with neutrons. Equation (5.30) can thus be written as

$$\Sigma\,cm^{-1} = \sigma\,\frac{cm^2}{atom} \times N\frac{atoms}{cm^3}. \tag{5.31}$$

Using the relationship given in Eq. (5.31), Eq. (5.27) may be rewritten as

$$\frac{I}{I_0} = e^{-\mu_a t} = e^{-\sigma N t}. \tag{5.32}$$

The linear attenuation coefficient for a mixture of materials or an alloy is given by

$$\mu_l = \mu_{a1} \times N_1 + \mu_{a2} \times N_2 + \cdots = \sum_{n=1}^{n} \mu_{an} \times N_n, \tag{5.33}$$

where

μ_n = atomic coefficient of the nth element and
N_n = number of atoms per cm^3 of the nth element.

The numerical values for μ_a have been published for many elements and for a wide range of quantum energies.[*] With the aid of atomic cross sections and Eq. (5.33), we can compute the attenuation coefficients of compounds or alloys containing several different elements.

 EXAMPLE 5.11

Aluminum bronze, an alloy containing 90% Cu (atomic weight = 63.57) and 10% Al (atomic weight = 26.98) by weight, has a density of $7.6\,g/cm^3$. What are the linear and mass attenuation coefficients for 0.4-MeV gamma rays if the cross sections for Cu and Al for this quantum energy are 9.91 and 4.45 b?

Solution

From Eq. (5.33), the linear attenuation coefficient of aluminum bronze is

$$\mu_l = (\mu_a)_{Cu} \times N_{Cu} + (\mu_a)_{Al} \times N_{Al}.$$

---

[*]Gladys White Groodstein: *X-Ray Attenuation Coefficients from 10 KeV to 100 MeV*. NBS Circular 583, U.S. Government Printing Office, Washington, DC, 1957.

The number of Cu atoms per cm^3 in the alloy is

$$N_{Cu} = \frac{6.02 \times 10^{23} \text{ atoms/mol}}{63.57 \text{ g/mol}} \times (7.6 \times 0.9) \frac{\text{g}}{\text{cm}^3} = 6.5 \times 10^{22} \frac{\text{atoms}}{\text{cm}^3}$$

and for Al, it is given by

$$N_{Al} = \frac{6.02 \times 10^{23} \text{ atoms/mol}}{27 \frac{\text{g}}{\text{mol}}} \times (7.6 \times 0.1) \frac{\text{g}}{\text{cm}^3} = 1.7 \times 10^{22} \frac{\text{atoms}}{\text{cm}^3}.$$

The linear attenuation coefficient therefore is

$$\mu_l = 9.91 \times 10^{-24} \frac{\text{cm}^2}{\text{atom}} \times 6.5 \times 10^{22} \frac{\text{atoms}}{\text{cm}^3}$$

$$+ 4.45 \times 10^{-24} \frac{\text{cm}^2}{\text{atom}} \times 1.7 \times 10^{22} \frac{\text{atoms}}{\text{cm}^3} = 0.72 \text{ cm}^{-1}.$$

The mass attenuation coefficient is, from Eq. (5.28),

$$\mu_m = \frac{\mu_l}{\rho} = \frac{0.72 \text{ cm}^{-1}}{7.6 \text{ g/cm}^3} = 0.095 \frac{\text{cm}^2}{\text{g}}.$$

The attenuating properties of matter vary systematically with the atomic number of the absorber and with the energy of the gamma radiation, as shown in Figure 5-13. It should be noted, however, that in the region where the Compton effect (this effect is more fully discussed below) predominates, the mass attenuation coefficient is almost independent of the atomic number of the absorber (Fig. 5-14).

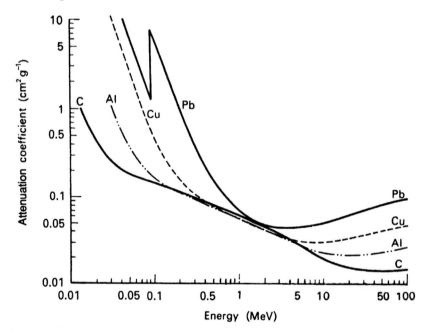

Figure 5-14. Curves illustrating the systematic variation of attenuation coefficient with atomic number of absorber and with quantum energy.

EXAMPLE 5.12

(a) Compute the thickness of Al and Pb to transmit 10% of a narrow beam of 0.1-MeV gamma radiation.

Solution

From Table 5-2, μ_1 for Al is 0.435 cm^{-1}, and for Pb it is 59.7 cm^{-1}. From Eq. (5.27) we have for Al:

$$\frac{I}{I_0} = e^{-\mu t} = \frac{1}{10} = e^{-(0.435\,\text{cm}^{-1})(t\,\text{cm})}$$

$$\ln 10 = 0.435\,t$$

$$t = \frac{\ln 10}{0.435} = \frac{2.3}{0.435} = 5.3\,\text{cm Al.}$$

In a similar manner, we have for Pb:

$$\frac{1}{10} = e^{-(59.7\,\text{cm}^{-1})(t\,\text{cm})}$$

$$t = \frac{2.3}{59.7\,\text{cm}^{-1}} = 0.04\,\text{cm Pb.}$$

(b) Repeat part (a) for a 1.0-MeV gamma ray; given

μ_1 for Al = 0.166 cm^{-1} and

μ_1 for Pb = 0.771 cm^{-1}.

Solution

For Al, we have

$$\frac{1}{10} = e^{-(0.166\,\text{cm}^{-1})(t\,\text{cm})}$$

$$t = 13.9\,\text{cm Al}$$

and for Pb,

$$\frac{1}{10} = e^{-(0.771\,\text{cm}^{-1})(t\,\text{cm})}$$

$$t = 3\,\text{cm Pb.}$$

(c) Compare the density thickness of the Al and Pb in each part of the illustrative example above.

Solution

The density thicknesses for the Al and Pb in the case of the 0.1-MeV photon are, from Eq. (5.1),

t_d (Al) $= 2.7\,\mathrm{g/cm}^3 \times 5.3\,\mathrm{cm} = 14.3\,\mathrm{g/cm}^2$ and
t_d (Pb) $= 11.34\,\mathrm{g/cm}^3 \times 0.04\,\mathrm{cm} = 0.45\,\mathrm{g/cm}^2$.

For the 1.0-MeV photons, the density thicknesses for the Al and Pb are given as follows:

t_d (Al) $= 2.7\,\mathrm{g/cm}^3 \times 13.9\,\mathrm{cm} = 37.5\,\mathrm{g/cm}^2$ and
t_d (Pb) $= 11.34\,\mathrm{g/cm}^3 \times 3\,\mathrm{cm} = 34\,\mathrm{g/cm}^2$.

Example 5.12 shows that for high-energy gamma rays, Pb is only a slightly better absorber, on a mass basis, than Al. For low-energy photons, on the other hand, Pb is a very much better absorber than Al. Generally, for energies between about 0.75 and 5 MeV, almost all materials have, on a mass basis, about the same gamma-ray attenuating properties. To a first approximation in this energy range, therefore, shielding properties are approximately proportional to the density of the shielding material. For lower and higher quantum energies, absorbers of high atomic number are more effective than those of low atomic number. To understand this behavior, we must examine the microscopic mechanisms of the interaction between gamma rays and matter.

Half Value Layer and Tenth Value Layer

The half value layer (HVL) is defined as the thickness of a shield or an absorber that reduces the radiation level by a factor of 2, that is to half the initial level. (The HVL is also called a *half value thickness*.) The relationship of the HVL of a shielding material to the attenuation coefficient for that material is analogous to that between the half-life and the decay rate constant for a radioisotope. The shield thickness necessary to reduce the intensity of a beam, under conditions of good geometry, to 1/2 is calculated from Eq. (5.27) in the following manner:

$$\frac{I}{I_0} = \frac{1}{2} = e^{-\mu t}$$

$$\ln\frac{1}{2} = -0.693 = -\mu t_{1/2}$$

$$t_{1/2} = \frac{0.693}{\mu} = \mathrm{HVL}. \tag{5.34}$$

When calculating shielding thickness, it may be convenient to determine the number of HVLs required to reduce the radiation to the desired level. For example, to reduce the radiation level to 1/10 its original level would require between 3 HVLs (which would reduce the level to $1/2^3 = 1/8$) and 4 HVLs (which would reduce the beam to $1/2^4 = 1/16$). Generally, the number of HVLs (n) required to reduce the beam level from I_0 to I is given by

$$\frac{I}{I_0} = \frac{1}{2^n}. \tag{5.35}$$

To calculate the number of HVLs to reduce the gamma ray beam level to 10%, as in Example 5.12 using Eq. (5.35):

$$\frac{I}{I_0} = \frac{1}{10} = \frac{1}{2^n}$$

$$n = 3.3 \text{ HVLs.}$$

For the case of 1-MeV gammas, whose $\mu_1 = 0.166 \text{ cm}^{-1}$,

$$HVL = \frac{0.693}{\mu_1} = \frac{0.693}{0.166 \text{ cm}^{-1}} = 4.17 \text{ cm Al.}$$

Therefore,

$$\text{Shield thickness} = 3.3 \text{ HVL} \times 4.17 \frac{\text{cm Al}}{\text{HVL}} = 13.8 \text{ cm Al.}$$

A shield that will attenuate a radiation beam to 10% of its radiation level, as in the case of the illustration above, is called a *tenth value layer*, which is symbolized by TVL. The concepts of HVLs and TVLs are widely used in shielding design. Table 10.7 lists the TVLs of ordinary concrete, steel, and lead for X-rays of several energies.

Interaction Mechanisms

For radiation protection purposes, four major mechanisms for the interaction of gamma-ray energy are considered significant. Two of these mechanisms, photoelectric absorption and Compton scattering, which involve interactions only with the orbital electrons of the absorber, predominate in the case where the quantum energy of the photons does not greatly exceed 1.02 MeV, the energy equivalent of the rest mass of two electrons. In the case of higher-energy photons, pair production, which is a direct conversion of electromagnetic energy into mass, occurs. These three gamma-ray interaction mechanisms result in the emission of electrons from the absorber. Very high-energy photons, $E \gg 2m_0 c^2$, may also be absorbed into the nuclei of the absorber atoms; they then initiate photonuclear reactions that result in the emission of other radiations from the excited nuclei.

Pair Production

A photon whose energy exceeds 1.02 MeV may, as it passes near a nucleus, spontaneously disappear, and its energy reappears as a positron and an electron, as pictured in Figure 5-15. Each of these two particles has a mass of $m_0 c^2$, or 0.51 MeV, and the total kinetic energy of the two particles is very nearly equal to E (gamma) $- 2m_0 c^2$. This transformation of energy into mass must take place near a particle, such as a nucleus, for the momentum to be conserved. The kinetic energy of the recoiling nucleus is very small. For practical purposes, therefore, all the photon energy in excess of that needed to supply the mass of the pair appears as kinetic energy of the pair. This same phenomenon may also occur in the vicinity of an electron, but the probability of occurrence near a nucleus is very much greater. Furthermore, the threshold energy for pair production near an electron is $4m_0 c^2$. This higher threshold

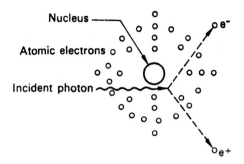

Figure 5-15. *Schematic representation of pair production. The positron–electron pair is generally projected in the forward direction (relative to the direction of the photon). The degree of forward projection increases with increasing photon energy.*

energy is necessary because the recoil electron, which conserves momentum, must be projected back with a very high velocity, since its mass is the same as that of each of the newly created particles. The cross section, or the probability of the production of a positron–electron pair, is approximately proportional to $Z^2 + Z$ and is therefore increasingly important as the atomic number of the absorber increases. The cross section increases slowly with increasing energy between the threshold of 1.02 MeV and about 5 MeV. For higher energies, the cross section is proportional to the logarithm of the quantum energy. This increasing cross section with increasing quantum energy above the 1.02-MeV threshold accounts for the increasing attenuation coefficient, shown in Figure 5-14, for high-energy photons. Note that the curves for each of the coefficients have a minimum value; for lead, the minimum attenuation is for 3-MeV photons (gamma rays).

After production of a pair, the positron and electron are projected in a forward direction (relative to the direction of the photon) and each loses its kinetic energy by excitation, ionization, and bremsstrahlung, as with any other high-energy electron. When the positron has expended all of its kinetic energy, it combines with an electron and the masses of the two particles are converted to energy in the form of two quanta of 0.51 MeV each of *annihilation* radiation. Thus, a 10-MeV photon may, in passing through a lead absorber, be converted into a positron–electron pair in which each particle has about 4 MeV of kinetic energy. This kinetic energy is then dissipated in the same manner as beta particles. The positron is then annihilated by combining with an electron in the absorber, and two photons of 0.51 MeV each may emerge from the absorber (or they may undergo Compton scattering or photoelectric absorption). The net result of the pair production interaction in this case was the conversion of a single 10-MeV photon into two photons of 0.51 MeV each and the dissipation of 8.98 MeV of energy.

Compton Scattering

Compton scattering is an elastic collision between a photon and a "free" electron (an electron whose binding energy to an atom is very much less than the energy of the photon), as shown diagrammatically in Figure 5-16.

In a collision between a photon and a free electron, it is impossible for all the photon's energy to be transferred to the electron if momentum and energy are to

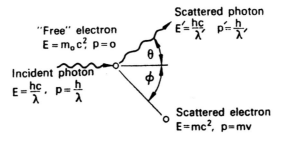

Figure 5-16. *Compton scattering: An elastic collision between a photon and an electron.*

be conserved. This can be shown by assuming that such a reaction is possible. If this were true, then, according to the conservation of energy, all the energy of the photon is imparted to the electron, and we have, from Eq. (2.23),

$$E = mc^2.$$

According to the law of conservation of momentum, all the momentum p of the photon must be transferred to the electron if the photon is to disappear:

$$p = \frac{E}{c} = mv. \tag{5.36}$$

Eliminating m from these two equations and solving for v, we find $v = c$, an impossible condition. The original assumption, that the photon transferred all of its energy to the electron, must therefore be false.

Since all the photon's energy cannot be transferred, the photon must be scattered, and the scattered photon must have lesser energy—or a longer wavelength—than the incident photon. Only the energy difference between the incident and scattered photons is transferred to the free electron. The amount of energy transferred in any collision can be calculated by applying the laws of conservation of energy and momentum to the situation pictured in Figure 5-16. To conserve energy, we must have

$$\frac{hc}{\lambda} + m_0 c^2 = \frac{hc}{\lambda'} + mc^2 \tag{5.37}$$

and to conserve momentum in the horizontal and vertical directions respectively, we have

$$\frac{h}{\lambda} = \frac{h}{\lambda'}\cos\theta + mv\cos\phi \tag{5.38}$$

and

$$0 = \frac{h}{\lambda'}\sin\theta - mv\sin\phi. \tag{5.39}$$

The solution of these equations shows the change in wavelength of the photon to be

$$\Delta\lambda = \lambda' - \lambda = \frac{h}{m_0 c}(1 - \cos\theta) \text{ cm} \tag{5.40}$$

and the relation between the scattering angles of the photon and the electron to be

$$\cot\frac{\theta}{2} = \left\{1 + \frac{h}{\lambda m_0 c}\right\} \tan\phi. \tag{5.41}$$

When the numerical values are substituted for the constants and centimeters are converted into angstrom units, Eq. (5.40) reduces to

$$\Delta\lambda = 0.0242(1 - \cos\theta)\ \text{Å}. \tag{5.42}$$

Equation (5.42) shows that the change in wavelength following a scattering event depends only on the scattering angle; it neither depends on the energy of the incident photon nor on the nature of the scatterer. As a consequence, a low-energy, long-wavelength photon will lose a smaller percentage of its energy than a high-energy, short-wavelength photon for the same scattering angle.

Equation (5.41) shows that the electron cannot be scattered through an angle greater than 90°. This scattered electron is of great importance in radiation dosimetry because it is the vehicle by means of which energy from the incident photon is transferred to an absorbing medium. The Compton electron dissipates its kinetic energy in the same manner as a beta particle and is one of the primary ionizing particles produced by gamma radiation (photons). Compton scattering is also important in health physics engineering because a high-energy photon loses a greater fraction of its energy when it is scattered than a low-energy photon does. By taking advantage of this fact, the required shielding thickness can be reduced and economic savings thereby effected.

 EXAMPLE 5.13

What percentage of their energies do 1-MeV and 0.1-MeV photons lose if they are scattered through an angle of 90°?

Solution

We will solve this problem by first calculating the wavelength of the photons before and after the scattering event, then converting the scattered wavelengths into the corresponding energies, and then calculating the percent energy loss of each photon.

- Using Eq. (5.19), we calculate the wavelength of each photon:

$$\lambda(0.1\,\text{MeV}) = \frac{12{,}400}{\text{eV}} = \frac{1.24 \times 10^4}{1 \times 10^5} = 0.124\ \text{Å}$$

$$\lambda(1.0\,\text{MeV}) = \frac{12{,}400}{\text{eV}} = \frac{1.24 \times 10^4}{1 \times 10^6} = 0.0124\ \text{Å}$$

- The wavelength change due to the scatter depends only on the scattering angle, as shown by Eq. (5.42). $\Delta\lambda$ is therefore the same for both photons.

$$\Delta\lambda = 0.0242(1 - \cos\theta) = 0.0242\ (1 - \cos 90°) = 0.0242\ \text{Å}.$$

- The wavelength of each photon after scattering is

$$\lambda'(0.1\ \text{MeV}) = \lambda + \Delta\lambda = 0.124 + 0.0242 = 0.1482\ \text{Å}$$

$$\lambda'(1.0\ \text{MeV}) = \lambda + \Delta\lambda = 0.0124 + 0.0242 = 0.0366\ \text{Å}.$$

- The energy of each scattered photon, E' is

$$E'(0.1482\ \text{Å}) = \frac{12,400}{0.1482\ \text{Å}} = 83,670\ \text{eV} = 0.08367\ \text{MeV}$$

$$E'(0.0366\ \text{Å}) = \frac{12,400}{0.0366\ \text{Å}} = 338,500\ \text{eV} = 0.3385\ \text{MeV}.$$

- The percentage decrease in the energy each of the photons is

$$\Delta E(1.0\ \text{MeV}) = E - E' = \frac{1.0000\ \text{MeV} - 0.3385\ \text{MeV}}{1.0000\ \text{MeV}} \times 100 = 66.2\%$$

$$\Delta E\ (0.1\ \text{MeV}) = E - E' = \frac{0.10000\ \text{MeV} - 0.08367\ \text{MeV}}{0.10000\ \text{MeV}} \times 100 = 16.3\%.$$

The energy of the scattered photon can be calculated more directly than in the above method by substituting $\lambda = hc/E$ and $\lambda' = hc/E'$ into Eq. (5.40) and solving for E':

$$E' = \frac{E}{1 + (E/m_0 c^2)(1 - \cos\theta)}, \tag{5.43}$$

and the fraction of the incident photon energy that is carried by the scattered photon would be

$$\frac{E'}{E} = \frac{1}{1 + (E/m_0 c^2)(1 - \cos\theta)}, \tag{5.44}$$

where $m_0 c^2$ is the energy equivalent of the rest mass of the electron, 0.51 MeV.

The probability of a Compton interaction with an electron decreases with increasing quantum energy and is independent of the atomic number of the interacting material. In Compton scattering, every electron acts as a scattering center and the bulk scattering properties of matter depends mainly on the electron density per unit mass. Probabilities for Compton scattering are therefore given on a per-electron basis. The theoretical cross sections for Compton scattering were derived by Klein and

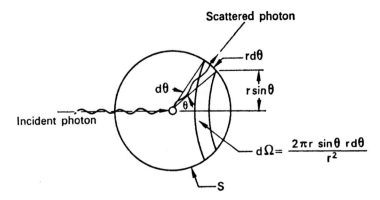

Figure 5-17. *Compton scattering diagram to illustrate differential scattering cross section. S is a sphere of unit radius whose center is the scattering electron.*

Nishina. For scattering into a differential solid angle $d\Omega$ at an angle θ to the direction of the incident photon (Fig. 5-17) they give the differential total scattering coefficient as

$$\frac{d\sigma_t}{d\Omega} = \frac{e^4}{2m_0^2 c^4}\left[\frac{1}{1 + a\,(1 - \cos\,\theta)}\right]^2\left[\frac{1 + \cos^2\theta + a^2(1 - \cos\theta)^2}{1 + a\,(1 - \cos\,\theta)}\right],\qquad(5.45)$$

where e, m_0, and c have the usual meaning and $a = hf/m_0 c^2$. Equation (5.45) and Figure 5-18 give the probability of scattering a photon into a solid angle $d\Omega$ through an angle θ. The total probability of scattering, Ω, can be obtained by substituting $d\Omega = 2\pi\,\sin\,\theta\,d\theta$ and integrating the differential scattering coefficient over the entire sphere. The result of this calculation, for quantum energies up to 10 MeV, is presented graphically in Figure 5-19.

Photoelectric Absorption

The photoelectric effect, in which the photon disappears, is an interaction between a photon and a tightly bound electron whose binding energy is equal to or less than the energy of the photon, as discussed in Chapter 3. The primary ionizing particle resulting from this interaction is the photoelectron, whose energy is given by Eq. (3.13), as

$$E_{pe} = hf - \phi.$$

The photoelectron dissipates its energy in the absorbing medium mainly by excitation and ionization. The binding energy ϕ is transferred to the absorber by means of the fluorescent radiation that follows the initial interaction. These low-energy photons are absorbed by outer electrons or in other photoelectric interactions not far from their points of origin. The photoelectric effect is favored by low-energy photons and high-atomic-numbered absorbers. The cross section for this reaction varies approximately as $Z^4\lambda^3$ (Z^4/E^3). It is this very strong dependence of photoelectric absorption on the atomic number Z that makes lead such a good material for shielding against X-rays. For very low-atomic-numbered absorbers, the photoelectric effect is relatively unimportant.

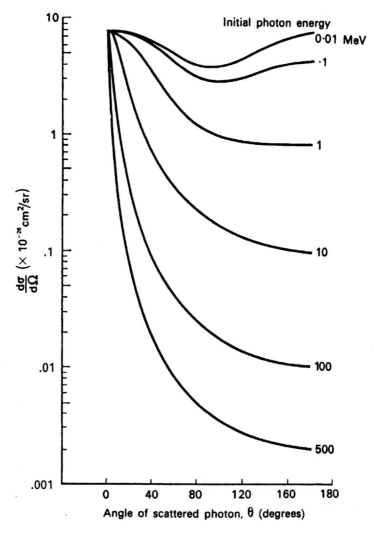

Figure 5-18. Differential scattering coefficient showing the probable angular distribution of Compton-scattered photons.

Photonuclear Reactions (Photodisintegration)

Photodisintegration is a photonuclear reaction in which the absorber nucleus captures a high-energy photon and, in most instances, emits a neutron. This is a threshold reaction in which the quantum energy must exceed a certain minimum value that depends on the absorbing nucleus. This is a high-energy reaction and, with few exceptions, is not an absorption mechanism for gamma rays (photons) from radionuclides. An important exception is the case of ^{9}Be, in which the threshold energy is only 1.666 MeV. The reaction ^{9}Be$(\gamma, n)^8$Be is useful as a laboratory source of monoenergetic neutrons. Photodisintegration is an important reaction in the case of very high energy photons from high-energy electron accelerators such as linear accelerators and electron synchrotrons. Here, too, interest is centered on the fact that

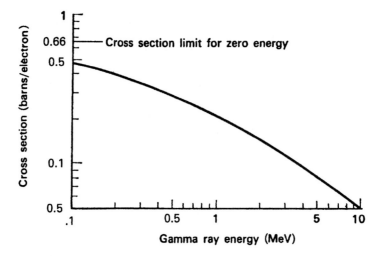

Figure 5-19.   Total Compton cross section for a free electron.

photodisintegration results in neutron production and neutrons can be absorbed by many materials and can make them radioactive. Generally, the cross sections for photodisintegration are very much smaller than the total cross section given in Eq. (5.46). In many shielding calculations, therefore, the photodisintegration cross sections are usually considered insignificant and are neglected. High-energy accelerators, however, produce copious amounts of high-energy (>10 MeV) photons. Photonuclear reactions, therefore, become important in shielding design.

Photodisintegration is a threshold reaction because the energy added to the absorber nucleus must be at least equal to the binding energy of a nucleon. Furthermore, a neutron is preferentially emitted rather than a proton because it has no coulombic potential barrier to overcome in order to escape from the nucleus and hence has a lower threshold. The range of energy thresholds for photodisintegration by neutron emission varies from 1.67 MeV for beryllium to about 8 MeV. For light nuclei, the thresholds fluctuate unsystematically; in the range of atomic mass numbers 20–130, the thresholds increase slowly to about 8.5 MeV and then decreases slowly to about 6 MeV as the atomic mass numbers increase. Quantum energies greater than the threshold appear as kinetic energy of the emitted neutrons or, if great enough, may cause the emission of charged particles from the absorber nucleus.

Combined Effects

The attenuation coefficients or cross sections give the probabilities of removal of a photon from a beam under conditions of good geometry, where it is assumed that any of the possible interactions remove the photon from the beam. The total attenuation coefficient, therefore, is the sum of the coefficients for each of the three reactions discussed above:

$$\mu_t = \mu_{pe} + \mu_{Cs} + \mu_{pp}, \tag{5.46}$$

where the three right-hand terms are the attenuation coefficients for the photoelectric effect, for Compton scattering, and for pair production, respectively. In computing attenuation of radiation for purposes of shielding design, the total attenuation coefficient as defined in Eq. (5.46) is used.

Equation (5.46) gives the fraction of the energy in a beam that is removed, per unit absorber thickness. The fraction of the beam's energy that is deposited in the absorber considers only the energy transferred to the absorber by the photoelectron, by the Compton electron, and by the electron pair. Energy carried away by the scattered photon in a Compton interaction and the energy carried off by the annihilation radiation after pair production is not included. The *energy absorption coefficient*, which is also called the *true absorption coefficient*, is given by

$$\mu_e = \mu_{pe} + \mu_{Ce} + \mu_{pp}\left(\frac{hf - 1.02}{hf}\right) \tag{5.47}$$

and is used in the calculation of radiation dose. The total attenuation and true absorption coefficients for air are shown in Figure 5-20, and the energy absorption coefficients for water, air, compact bone, and muscle are listed in Table 5-4.

NEUTRONS

Production

The most prolific source of neutrons is the nuclear reactor. The splitting of a uranium or a plutonium nucleus in a nuclear reactor is accompanied by the emission of several

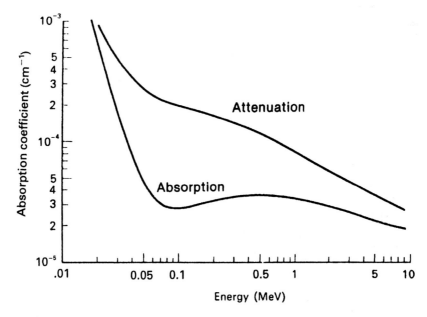

Figure 5-20. Linear attenuation coefficients and absorption coefficients of air for gamma rays as a function of energy.

TABLE 5-4. Values of the Mass Energy–Absorption Coefficients

PHOTON ENERGY (MeV)	MASS-ENERGY-ABSORPTION COEFFICIENT $(\mu_{en}/\rho)cm^2/g$			
	Water	Air	Compact Bone	Muscle
0.010	4.89	4.66	19.0	4.96
0.015	1.32	1.29	5.89	1.36
0.020	0.523	0.516	2.51	0.544
0.030	0.147	0.147	0.743	0.154
0.040	0.0647	0.0640	0.0305	0.0677
0.050	0.0394	0.0384	0.158	0.0409
0.060	0.0304	0.0292	0.0979	0.0312
0.080	0.0253	0.0236	0.0520	0.0255
0.10	0.0252	0.0231	0.0386	0.0252
0.15	0.0278	0.0251	0.0304	0.0276
0.20	0.0300	0.0268	0.0302	0.0297
0.30	0.0320	0.0288	0.0311	0.0317
0.40	0.0329	0.0296	0.0316	0.0325
0.50	0.0330	0.0297	0.0316	0.0327
0.60	0.0329	0.0296	0.0315	0.0326
0.80	0.0321	0.0289	0.0306	0.0318
1.0	0.0311	0.0280	0.0297	0.0308
1.5	0.0283	0.0255	0.0270	0.0281
2.0	0.0260	0.0234	0.0248	0.0257
3.0	0.0227	0.0205	0.0219	0.0225
4.0	0.0205	0.0186	0.0199	0.0203
5.0	0.0190	0.0173	0.0186	0.0188
6.0	0.0180	0.0163	0.0178	0.0178
8.0	0.0165	0.0150	0.0165	0.0163
10.0	0.0155	0.0144	0.0159	0.0154

Source: From *Physical Aspects of Irradiation.* Washington, DC: US Government Printing Office; March 1964. NBS Handbook 85.

neutrons. These fission neutrons have a wide range of energies, as shown in Figure 5-21. The distribution peaks at 0.7 MeV and has a mean value of 2 MeV.

Except for several fission fragments of very short half-life, there are no radionuclides that decay by emitting neutrons. Californium-252, however, an alpha emitter, undergoes spontaneous nuclear fission at an average rate of 10 fissions for every 313 alpha transformations. Since the half-life of ^{252}Cf due to alpha emission is 2.73 years, its effective half-life, including spontaneous nuclear fission, is 2.65 years. Californium-252 thus simulates a neutron-emitting radionuclide. The neutron emission rate has been found to be 2.31×10^6 neutrons per second per μg ^{252}Cf. The emitted neutrons span a wide range of energies. The most probable energy is about 1 MeV, while the average value of the energy distribution is about 2.3 MeV.

All other neutron sources depend on nuclear reactions for the emission of neutrons. Copious neutron beams may be produced in accelerators by many different reactions. For example, bombardment of beryllium by high-energy deuterons in a cyclotron produces neutrons according to the reaction

$$\begin{smallmatrix}9\\4\end{smallmatrix}\text{Be} + \begin{smallmatrix}2\\1\end{smallmatrix}\text{D} \rightarrow \left(\begin{smallmatrix}11\\5\end{smallmatrix}\text{B}\right)^* \rightarrow \begin{smallmatrix}10\\5\end{smallmatrix}\text{B} + \begin{smallmatrix}1\\0\end{smallmatrix}\text{n}. \tag{5.48}$$

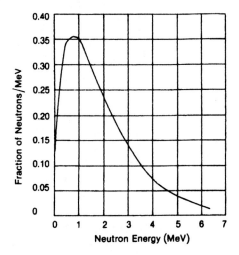

Figure 5-21. *Energy distribution of fission neutrons. The most probable energy is 0.7 MeV and the average energy is 2 MeV.*

The term in the parentheses is called a *compound nucleus,* and the asterisk shows that it is in an excited state. The compound nucleus rids itself of its excitation energy instantaneously ($<10^{-8}$ s) by proceeding to the next step in the reaction. For small laboratory sources of neutrons, the photodisintegration of beryllium may be used. Another commonly used neutron source depends on the bombardment of beryllium with alpha particles. The reaction, in this case, is

$$^{9}_{4}\text{Be} + {}^{4}_{2}\text{He} \rightarrow \left({}^{13}_{6}\text{C}\right)^{*} \rightarrow {}^{12}_{6}\text{C} + {}^{1}_{0}\text{n}. \tag{5.49}$$

For the source of the alpha particles, radium, polonium, or plutonium is used. The alpha emitter, as a powder, is thoroughly mixed with finely powdered beryllium, and the mixture is sealed in a capsule, as shown in Figure 5-22. The neutrons that are produced are all high-energy neutrons. In all cases of neutrons based on this reaction, the neutron energy is spread over a broad spectrum, as shown in

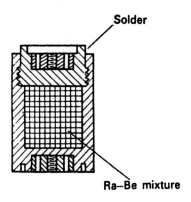

Figure 5-22. *Typical construction of an α, n neutron source in a sealed container. Here Ra serves as the α source.*

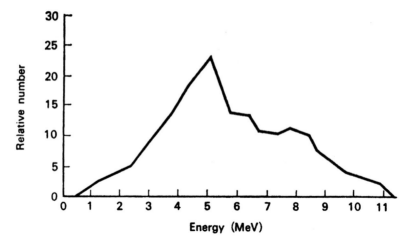

Figure 5-23. Energy distribution of Po–Be neutrons. (Reproduced with permission from *Technical Bulletin NS-2*. Ottawa, Ontario, Canada: Atomic Energy of Canada, Ltd; 1966.)

Figure 5-23. This spread of energies from a $^9Be(\alpha, n)^{12}C$ source is in sharp contrast to the monoenergetic neutrons from a photodisintegration source using monoenergetic photons. In the α, n reaction, the energy equivalent of the difference in mass between the reactants and the products plus the kinetic energy of the bombarding particle is divided between the neutron and the recoil nucleus. In practical α, n sources, some of the alpha-particle energy is dissipated by self-absorption within the source. As a consequence, the alphas that initiate the reaction have a wide range of energies, thereby contributing to the spectral spread of the neutrons. The neutron yield for an α, n source increases with increasing alpha energy because of the greater ease with which higher-energy alphas penetrate the coulomb barrier at the nucleus. Tables 5-5 and 5-6 list some γ, n and α, n neutron sources, respectively.

TABLE 5-5. γ, n Photoneutron Sources

SOURCE	HALF-LIFE	AVERAGE NEUTRON ENERGY (MeV)	YIELD $\frac{n}{s}$/Ci	$\frac{n}{s}$/MBq
$^{24}Na + Be$	15 h	0.83	1.3×10^5	3.5
$^{24}Na + D_2O$	15 h	0.22	2.7×10^5	7.3
$^{56}Mn + Be$	2.58 h	0.1(90%), 0.3(10%)	2.9×10^4	0.8
$^{56}Mn + D_2O$	2.58 h	0.22	3.1×10^3	0.08
$^{72}Ga + Be$	14.2 h	0.78	5×10^4	1.4
$^{72}Ga + D_2O$	14.2 h	0.13	6×10^4	1.6
$^{88}Y + Be$	88 d	0.16	1×10^5	2.7
$^{88}Y + D$	88 d	0.31	3×10^3	0.08
$^{116}In + Be$	54 min	0.30	8.2×10^3	0.2
$^{124}Sb + Be$	60 d	0.024	1.9×10^5	5.1
$^{140}La + Be$	40 h	0.62	3×10^3	0.08
$^{140}La + D_2O$	40 h	0.15	8×10^3	0.2
$Ra + D_2O$	1600 yrs	0.12	1×10^3	0.03

TABLE 5-6. α, n Neutron Sources

SOURCE	HALF-LIFE	AVERAGE NEUTRON ENERGY (MeV)	YIELD $\frac{n}{s}$/Ci	YIELD $\frac{n}{s}$/MBq
Ra + Be	1600 yrs	5	1.7×10^7	459
Ra + B	1600 yrs	3	6.8×10^6	184
^{222}Rn + Be	3.8 d	5	1.5×10^7	405
^{210}Po + Be	138 d	4	3×10^6	81.1
^{210}Po + B	138 d	2.5	9×10^5	24.3
^{210}Po + F	138 d	1.4	4×10^5	10.8
^{210}Po + Li	138 d	0.42	9×10^4	2.4
^{239}Pu + Be	24,000 yrs	4	10^6	27

Classification

Neutrons are classified according to their energy because the type of reaction that a neutron undergoes depends very strongly on its energy. High-energy neutrons, those whose energies exceed about 0.1 MeV, are called *fast neutrons*. *Thermal neutrons,* on the other hand, have the same kinetic energy distribution as gas molecules in their environment. In this respect, thermal neutrons are indistinguishable from gas molecules at the same temperature. The kinetic energies of gas molecules are related to temperature by the Maxwell–Boltzmann distribution (Fig. 5-24):

$$f(E) = \frac{2\pi}{(\pi kT)^{3/2}} e^{-E/kT} E^{1/2}, \tag{5.50}$$

where $f(E)$ is the fraction of the gas molecules (or neutrons) of energy E per unit energy interval; k is the Boltzmann constant, 1.38×10^{-23} J/K (Kelvin) or 8.6×10^{-5} eV/K; and T is the absolute temperature of the gas, K.

The most probable energy, represented by the peak of the curve in Figure 5-24, is given by

$$E_{\text{mp}} = kT, \tag{5.51}$$

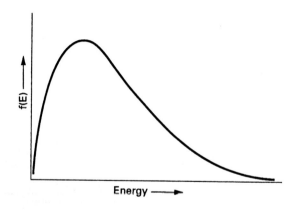

Figure 5-24.   Maxwell–Boltzmann distribution of energy among gas molecules.

and the average energy of gas molecules at any given temperature is

$$\bar{E} = \frac{3}{2}kT. \tag{5.52}$$

For neutrons at a temperature of 293 K, the most probable energy is 0.025 eV. This is the energy often implied by the term "thermal" neutrons. The velocity corresponding to this energy, is calculated as

$$\frac{1}{2}mv^2 = kT = 0.025 \text{ eV} \times 1.6 \times 10^{-19} \frac{\text{J}}{\text{eV}}$$

$$v = \left(\frac{2 \times 0.025 \text{ eV} \times 1.6 \times 10^{-19} \text{ J/eV}}{1.67 \times 10^{-27} \text{kg}}\right)^{1/2} = 2.2 \times 10^3 \frac{\text{m}}{\text{s}}.$$

The average velocity of a neutron in a thermal neutron beam, if the most probable velocity is v_0, is given by

$$\bar{v} = \frac{2}{\sqrt{\pi}}v_0 = 1.13 \ v_0. \tag{5.53}$$

In the region of energy between thermal and fast, neutrons are called by various names including *intermediate neutrons, resonance neutrons,* and *slow neutrons.* All these descriptive adjectives are used loosely, and their exact meaning must be inferred from the context in which they are used.

Interaction

All neutrons at the time of their birth are fast. Generally, fast neutrons lose energy by colliding elastically with atoms in their environment, and then, generally after being slowed down to thermal or near thermal energies, they are captured by nuclei of the absorbing material. Although a number of possible neutron reaction types exist, the chief reactions for the health physicist are elastic scattering and capture followed by the emission of a photon or another particle from the absorber nucleus.

When absorbers are placed in a collimated beam of neutrons and the transmitted neutron intensity is measured, as was done for gamma rays in Figure 5-12, it is found that neutrons too are removed exponentially from the beam. Instead of using linear or mass absorption coefficients to describe the ability of a given absorber material to remove neutrons from the beam, it is customary to designate only the microscopic cross section σ for the absorbing material. The product σN, where N is the number of absorber atoms per cm^3, is the macroscopic cross section Σ. The removal of neutrons from the beam is thus given by

$$I = I_0 e^{-\sigma Nt}. \tag{5.54}$$

Neutron cross sections are strongly energy dependent. If removal of a neutron from the beam may be effected by more than one mechanism, the total cross section is the sum of the cross sections for the various possible reactions.

EXAMPLE 5.14

In an experiment designed to measure the total cross section of lead for 10-MeV neutrons, it was found that a 1-cm-thick lead absorber attenuated the neutron flux to 84.5% of its initial value. The atomic weight of lead is 207.21 and its specific gravity is 11.3. Calculate the total cross section from these data.

Solution

The atomic density of lead is

$$\rho_{atomic} = \frac{6.02 \times 10^{23} \text{ atoms/mol}}{207.21 \frac{\text{g}}{\text{mol}}} \times 11.3 \frac{\text{g}}{\text{cm}^3} = 3.3 \times 10^{22} \frac{\text{atoms}}{\text{cm}^3}$$

$$\frac{I}{I_0} = e^{-\sigma N t}$$

$$0.845 = e^{-\sigma \times 3.3 \times 10^{22} \times 1}$$

$$\ln \frac{1}{0.845} = 3.3 \times 10^{22} \sigma$$

$$\sigma = \frac{0.168}{3.3 \times 10^{22} \frac{\text{atoms}}{\text{cm}^3} \times 1 \text{ cm}} = 5.1 \times 10^{-24} \frac{\text{cm}^2}{\text{atom}}.$$

$\sigma = 5.1$ b and the macroscopic cross section is

$$\sum = \sigma N = 5.1 \times 10^{-24} \text{ cm}^2/\text{atom} \times 3.3 \times 10^{22} \text{ atoms/cm}^3 = 0.168 \text{ cm}^{-1}.$$

Scattering

Neutrons may collide with nuclei and undergo either inelastic or elastic scattering. In the former case, some of the kinetic energy that is transferred to the target nucleus excites the nucleus and the excitation energy is emitted as a gamma-ray (photon). This interaction is best described by the compound nucleus model in which the neutron is captured and then reemitted by that target nucleus together with the gamma ray (photon). This is a threshold phenomenon; the neutron energy threshold varies from infinity for hydrogen (inelastic scattering cannot occur) to about 6 MeV for oxygen to less than 1 MeV for uranium. Generally, the cross section for inelastic scattering is small (on the order of 1 b or less) for low-energy fast neutrons, but it increases with increasing energy and approaches a value corresponding to the geometric cross section of the target nucleus.

Elastic scattering is the most likely interaction between fast neutrons and low-atomic-numbered absorbers. This interaction is a "billiard-ball" type collision, in which kinetic energy and momentum are conserved. By applying these conservation laws, it can be shown that the energy E of the scattered neutron after a head-on collision is

$$E = E_0 \left\{ \frac{M - m}{M + m} \right\}^2 \tag{5.55}$$

where

E_0 = energy of the incident neutron,
m = mass of the incident neutron, and
M = mass of the scattering nucleus.

The energy transferred to the target nucleus is $E_0 - E$. From Eq. (5.55), we have

$$E_0 - E = E_0 \left[1 - \left(\frac{M - m}{M + m} \right)^2 \right]. \tag{5.56}$$

According to Eqs. (5.55) and (5.56), it is possible, in a head-on collision with a hydrogen nucleus, for a neutron to transfer all its energy to the hydrogen nucleus. With heavier nuclei, all the kinetic energy of the neutron cannot be transferred in a single collision. In the case of oxygen, for example, Eq. (5.56) shows that the maximum fraction, $(E_0 - E) = E_0$, of the neutron's kinetic energy that can be transferred during a single collision is only 22.2%. This shows that nuclei with small mass numbers are more effective, on a "per collision" basis, than nuclei with high mass numbers for slowing down neutrons.

Equations (5.55) and (5.56) are valid only for head-on collisions. Most collisions are not head-on, and the energy transferred to the target nuclei are consequently less than the maximum given by the two equations above.

In the course of the successive collisions suffered by a fast neutron as it passes through a slowing-down medium, the average decrease, per collision, in the logarithm of the neutron energy (which is called the *average logarithmic energy decrement*) remains constant. It is independent of the neutron energy and is a function only of the mass of scattering nuclei. The average logarithmic energy decrement is defined as

$$\xi = \overline{\Delta \ln E} = \overline{\ln E_0 - \ln E} = \overline{\ln \frac{E_0}{E}} = \overline{-\ln \frac{E}{E_0}} \tag{5.57}$$

and can be shown to be given by

$$\xi = 1 + \frac{\alpha \ln \alpha}{1 - \alpha} \tag{5.58}$$

where $\alpha = [(M - m)/(M + m)]^2$, as used in Eq. (5.55). If the slowing-down medium contains n kinds of nuclides, each of microscopic scattering cross section σ_s and average logarithmic energy decrement ξ, then the mean value of ξ for the n species is

$$\xi = \frac{\sum_{i=1}^{n} \sigma_{si} N_i \xi_i}{\sum_{i=1}^{n} \sigma_{si} N_i} \tag{5.59}$$

since

$$\overline{\ln\frac{E}{E_0}} = -\xi,$$

$$\frac{E}{E_0} = e^{-\xi},$$

and the median fraction of the incident neutron's energy that is transferred to the target nucleus during a collision is

$$f = 1 - \frac{E}{E_0} = 1 - e^{-\xi}. \tag{5.60}$$

Thus, for hydrogen ($\xi = 1$), the median energy transfer during a collision with a fast neutron is 63% of the neutron's kinetic energy. In the case of carbon, $\xi = 0.159$, and an average of only 14.7% of the neutron's kinetic energy is transferred to the struck nucleus during an elastic collision. The struck nucleus, as a result of the kinetic energy imparted to it by the neutron, becomes an ionizing particle and dissipates its kinetic energy in the absorbing medium by excitation and ionization.

The distance traveled by a fast neutron between its introduction into a slowing-down medium and its thermalization depends on the number of collisions made by the neutron and the distance between collisions. Although the actual path of the neutron is tortuous because of deflections due to collisions, the average straight-line distance covered by the neutron can be determined; it is called the *fast-diffusion length*, or the *slowing-down length*. (The square of the fast-diffusion length is called the *Fermi age* of the neutron.) The distance traveled by the thermalized neutron until it is absorbed is measured by the *thermal diffusion length*. The thermal diffusion length is defined as the thickness of a slowing-down medium that attenuates a beam of thermal neutrons by a factor of e. Thus, attenuation of a beam of thermal neutrons by a substance of thickness t cm whose thermal diffusion length is L cm is given by

$$n = n_0 e^{-t/L}. \tag{5.61}$$

(The terms *fast diffusion length* and *thermal diffusion length* are applicable only to materials in which the absorption cross section is very small. When this condition is not met, as in the case of boron or cadmium, the attenuation of a beam of thermal neutrons is given by Eq. [5.54].) Although fast and thermal diffusion lengths may be calculated, the assumptions inherent in the calculations make it preferable to use measured values for these parameters. Values for fast and thermal diffusion lengths for fission neutrons in certain slowing-down media are given in Table 5-7.

TABLE 5-7. Fast and Thermal Diffusion Lengths of Selected Materials

SUBSTANCE	FAST DIFFUSION LENGTH (cm)	THERMAL DIFFUSION LENGTH (cm)	DIFFUSION COEFFICIENT (cm)
H_2O	5.75	2.88	0.16
D_2O	11	171	0.87
Be	9.9	24	0.50
C (graphite)	17.3	50	0.84

For the case of a point source of S thermal neutrons per second in a spherically shaped nonmultiplying medium (a medium which contains no fissile material) of radius R, thermal diffusion length L, and diffusion coefficient D, the flux of neutrons escaping from the surface is

$$\phi = \frac{S}{4\pi\, RD} \times e^{-R/L}. \tag{5.62}$$

 # EXAMPLE 5.15

A Pu–Be neutron source that emits 10^6 neutrons/s is in the center of a spherical water shield whose diameter is 50 cm. How many thermal neutrons are escaping per square centimeter per second from the surface of the shield?

Solution

Since the radius of the water shield is much greater than the fast diffusion length given in Table 5-7, we may assume (for the purpose of this calculation) that essentially all the fast neutrons are thermalized and that the thermal neutrons are diffusing outward from the center. Substituting the appropriate numbers into Eq. (5.62), we have

$$\phi = \frac{10^6 \text{ neutrons/s}}{4\pi \times 25 \text{ cm} \times 0.16 \text{ cm}} e^{-25 \text{ cm}/2.88 \text{ cm}} = 3.4 \; \frac{\text{neutrons/s}}{\text{cm}^2}.$$

Absorption

The discussion above shows that fast neutrons are rapidly degraded in energy by elastic collisions if they interact with low-atomic-numbered substances. As neutrons reach thermal or near thermal energies, their likelihood of capture by an absorber nucleus increases. The absorption cross section of many nuclei, as the neutron energy becomes very small, has been found to be inversely proportional to the square root of its kinetic energy and thus to vary inversely with its velocity:

$$\sigma \; \propto \; \frac{1}{\sqrt{E}} \propto \frac{1}{v}. \tag{5.63}$$

Equation (5.63) is called the *one-over-v law* for slow neutron absorption. For ^{10}B, this relationship is valid for the span of energies from 0.02 to 1000 eV, as shown in Figure 5-25. Thermal neutron cross sections are usually given for neutrons whose most probable energy is 0.025 eV. If the cross section at energy E_0 is σ_0, then the

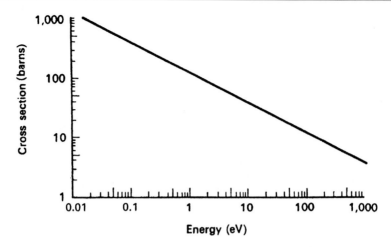

Figure 5-25. Neutron absorption cross sections for boron, showing the validity of the 1/v law for neutrons from 0.02 to 1000 eV in energy. The equation for the curve is $\sigma = 116 \, (\text{eV})^{1/2}$.

cross section for any other energy within the range of validity of the $1/v$ law is given by

$$\frac{\sigma}{\sigma_0} = \frac{v_0}{v} = \sqrt{\frac{E_0}{E}}.$$
(5.64a)

Since neutron energy varies directly with the temperature, Eq. (5.67a) can be written as

$$\frac{\sigma}{\sigma_0} = \frac{v_0}{v} = \sqrt{\frac{T_0}{T}},$$
(5.64b)

where $T_0 = 293$ K.

EXAMPLE 5.16

The cross section of boron for the $^{10}\text{B}(n, \alpha)\,^{7}\text{Li}$ reaction is 753 b for 0.025 eV neutrons. What is the boron cross section for 50-eV neutrons?

Solution

Substituting into Eq. (5.64a) gives

$$\sigma \,(50 \text{ eV}) = 753 \text{ b} \sqrt{\frac{0.025 \text{ eV}}{50 \text{ eV}}} = 16.8 \text{ b}.$$

Some capture reactions of practical importance in health physics include the following:

$$^1H(n, \gamma)^2H \qquad\qquad \sigma = 0.33\,b \tag{5.65}$$

$$^{14}N(n, p)^{14}C \qquad\qquad \sigma = 1.70\,b \tag{5.66}$$

$$^{10}B(n, \alpha)^7Li \qquad\qquad \sigma = 4.01 \times 10^3\,b \tag{5.67}$$

$$^{113}Cd(n, \gamma)^{114}Cd \qquad\qquad \sigma = 2.1 \times 10^4\,b \tag{5.68}$$

Equations (5.65) and (5.66) are important in neutron dosimetry, since H and N are major constituents of tissue. Equation (5.67) is important in the design of instruments for measuring neutrons as well as neutron shielding, while the last equation is important mainly in shielding. It should be noted that the neutron reactions with hydrogen and with cadmium result in the emission of high-energy gamma rays, while the capture of a thermal neutron by ^{10}B releases a low-energy (0.48 MeV) gamma ray in 93% of the reactions. When a thermal neutron is captured by ^{14}N, a 0.6-MeV proton is emitted.

Neutron Activation

Neutron activation is the production of a radionuclide by absorption of a neutron, such as the n, p reaction of Eq. (5.66). In that instance, ^{14}C is produced. Activation by neutrons is important to the health physicist for several reasons. First, it means that any substance that was irradiated by neutrons may be radioactive; a radiation hazard may therefore persist after the irradiation by neutrons is terminated. Secondly, it provides a convenient tool for measuring neutron flux. This is done simply by irradiating a known quantity of the material to be activated, measuring the induced activity, and then, with a knowledge of the activation cross section, computing the neutron flux. In case of a criticality accident (an accidental attainment of an uncontrolled chain reaction), the measurement of induced radioactivity due to neutron irradiation permits calculation of the neutron dose. The same principle is applied by the chemist in neutron-activation analysis. This method, which for many elements is more sensitive than other physical or chemical procedures, involves irradiation of the unknown sample in a neutron field of known intensity and radiospectrometric examination of the induced radiation to identify the isotope, which, in turn, helps to identify the unknown isotope from which it came and the amount of the unknown in the sample.

If a radionuclide is being made by neutron irradiation and is decaying at the same time, the net number of radioactive atoms present in the sample at any time is the difference between the rate of production and the rate of decay. This may be expressed mathematically by the following activity–balance equation:

net rate of increase of radioactive atoms = production rate − decay rate,

that is,

$$\frac{dN}{dt} = \phi\sigma n - \lambda N, \tag{5.69}$$

where

ϕ = flux, neutrons/cm^2/s,

σ = activation cross section, cm^2,

λ = transformation constant of the induced activity,

N = number of radioactive atoms, and

n = number of target atoms (assumed to remain constant during the irradiation).

Equation (5.72) is a linear differential equation of exactly the same form as Eq. (4.32), and may be integrated in a similar manner to yield

$$\lambda N = \phi \sigma n \left(1 - e^{-\lambda t}\right). \tag{5.70}$$

In Eq. (5.70), $\phi \sigma n$ is sometimes called the *saturation activity*. For an infinitely long irradiation time, it represents the maximum obtainable activity with any given neutron flux.

EXAMPLE 5.17

A sample containing an unknown quantity of chromium is irradiated for 1 week in a thermal neutron flux of 10^{11} neutrons/cm^2/s. The resulting ^{51}Cr gamma rays give a counting rate of 600 counts/min in a scintillation counter whose overall efficiency is 10%. How many grams of chromium were there in the original sample?

Solution

The reaction in this case is

$$^{50}\text{Cr} + {}_0^1\text{n} \rightarrow {}^{51}\text{Cr} + \gamma.$$

The thermal neutron activation cross section for ^{50}Cr is 13.5 b, and ^{50}Cr forms 4.31% by number of the naturally occurring chromium atoms. Chromium-51 decays by orbital electron capture with a half-life of 27.8 days and emits a 0.323-MeV gamma-ray in 9.8% of the decays. The atomic weight of Cr is 52.01 D.

The activity is given by λN in Eq. (5.70). This equation may therefore be solved for n, the number of target atoms. Substituting the numerical values into Eq. (5.73), we have

$$10\frac{\text{counts}}{\text{s}} \times 10\frac{\text{decays}}{\text{count}} = 10^{11}\frac{\text{neutrons}}{\text{cm}^2 \cdot \text{s}} \times 1.35$$

$$\times 10^{-23}\frac{\text{cm}^2}{\text{atom}} \times 0.098 \times n \text{ atoms } {}^{50}\text{Cr} \times \left(1 - e^{-\frac{0.693}{27.8 \text{ d}} \times 7 \text{ d}}\right)$$

$$n = 4.7 \times 10^{15} \text{ atoms } {}^{50}\text{Cr}.$$

Since the abundance of ^{50}Cr atoms is 4.31%, the total number of Cr atoms in the sample is

$$\text{No. Cr atoms} = \frac{n}{0.0431} = \frac{4.7 \times 10^{15}}{0.0431} = 1.1 \times 10^{17} \text{Cr atoms}$$

Since there are 52.01 g Cr/mol, the weight of chromium in the sample is

$$\frac{1.1 \times 10^{17} \text{ atoms}}{6.02 \times 10^{23} \text{ atoms/mol}} \times 52.01 \ \frac{\text{g}}{\text{mol}} = 9.5 \times 10^{-6} \text{ g}.$$

SUMMARY

Energy transfer from a radiation field to the absorbing medium is the basis for all types of radiation effects. Charged particles, including betas, positrons, protons, and alphas excite or ionize the atoms in the absorbing media by colliding with their extranuclear electrons. These primary ionizing particles lose a finite amount of energy in each collision. The average loss per ionization in air or in soft tissue is 34 eV for betas and 35.5 eV for alphas. The linear density of the ions thus produced is called the *specific ionization* and is a measure of the rate of energy loss by the primary ionizing particle. Beta particles have a relatively low specific ionization on the order of 100 ip/cm in air. Alphas, because of their double charge and their relatively slow speed, have a high specific ionization, producing on the order of tens of thousands ion pairs per centimeter air. Successive collisions ultimately lead to the expenditure of the entire kinetic energy of the primary ionizing particle. The distance traveled in the absorber until this point is reached is called the *range of the ionizing particle*, and it is determined by the energy of the primary ionizing particle and by the nature of the absorber. If we measure the distance in terms of the density thickness, we find that the range is approximately independent of the nature of the absorber.

Primary ionizing particles can also interact with the nuclei of the absorbing media. This interaction is especially important in the case of high-energy betas and electrons. When this happens, some of the electron's kinetic energy is converted into electromagnetic energy that is radiated as X-ray photons called *bremsstrahlung*. The production of bremsstrahlung is enhanced by high-atomic-numbered absorbing media.

The interaction of X-rays and gamma radiation with matter differs qualitatively from that of alpha and beta particles. Although gamma rays are called *ionizing radiations*, they are indirectly ionizing. The photons of electromagnetic radiation interact with the extranuclear electrons in absorbing media by knocking out electrons by one of two different mechanisms. In one, called *Compton scattering*, an outer electron is ejected and the photon, now reduced in energy by the energy imparted to the electron, is scattered. The ejected electron is called a *Compton electron*. In the other mechanism, called *photoelectric absorption*, the photon knocks out a tightly bound electron, all the photon's energy is transferred to the absorbing atom, and the photon disappears. Some of the photon's energy is used in freeing the tightly bound electron from the atom and the rest of the photon's energy is converted into kinetic energy of the ejected photoelectron. If the energy of the photon exceeds 1.02 MeV, another interaction mechanism, called *pair production*, can occur. In pair production, the photon interacts with the nucleus of the absorbing atom and all of its energy is converted into mass through the production of a positron and a negative electron. The 1.02-MeV threshold energy required for pair production represents the energy equivalent of the mass of the two newly created particles. Any energy that the photon may have in excess of 1.02 MeV is transferred to the pair of particles as kinetic energy. The Compton electrons and photoelectrons as well as the electron and positron pair become primary ionizing particles and proceed to lose their energy by ionization and excitation in the media in which they were produced. They are the agents through which energy is transferred from the X-ray or gamma field to the absorbing medium. When the positron loses all its kinetic energy, it combines with a negative electron. The two particles are annihilated and two photons, called *annihilation radiation,* of 0.51 MeV are created.

The interactions of alpha and beta radiation are governed by deterministic processes and therefore alphas and betas have a finite range and can be completely stopped. Gamma (photon) interactions, on the other hand, are stochastic events. Since the interactions are governed by laws of probability, a gamma-ray (photon) beam does not have a finite range; it can only be reduced in intensity by increasingly thicker absorbers. The fractional reduction in intensity per unit thickness of absorber is called the *attenuation coefficient,* while the fractional absorption of energy from the beam per unit thickness of absorber is called the *absorption coefficient of the absorbing material.* Both these coefficients are functions of the photon energy and the absorber material.

In the context of interaction with matter, neutrons are classified according to their kinetic energy as *thermal* and *fast.* Neutrons are produced through nuclear reactions and by nuclear fission. All neutrons have kinetic energy when they are produced and hence may be considered to be fast. These fast neutrons lose energy by colliding elastically with atoms in their path, and then, after being slowed to thermal energy, they are captured by nuclei in the absorbing medium. Many nonradioactive isotopes become radioactive after capturing a neutron. When a hydrogen nucleus is struck by a fast neutron, the nucleus is knocked out of the atom and becomes a proton, which is a positively charged, high specific ionization primary ionizing particle. It loses its kinetic energy by ionization and excitation interactions with the absorber atoms.

PROBLEMS

5.1. The density of Hg is 13.6 g/cm^3 and its atomic weight is 200.6. Calculate the number of Hg atoms/cm^3.

5.2. The density of quartz (SiO$_2$) crystals is 2.65 g/cm^3. What is the atomic density (atoms/cm^3) of silicon and oxygen in quartz?

5.3. Compare the electronic densities of a 5-mm-thick piece of aluminum and a piece of iron of the same density thickness.

5.4. In surveying a laboratory, a health physicist wipes a contaminated surface and runs an absorption curve using a thin end window counter and aluminum absorbers. The range of the beta particles (no gammas were found) was 800 mg/cm² Al. What could the contaminant be? What further studies could be done on the smear sample to help verify the identification of the contaminant?

5.5. A health physicist finds an unknown contaminant that proves to be a pure beta emitter. To help identify the contaminant, he runs an absorption curve to determine the maximum energy of the beta particles. He uses an end window G.M. counter whose mica window (density = 2.7 g/cm³) is 0.1-mm thick, and he finds that 1.74-mm Al stops all the beta particles. The distance between the sample and the G.M. counter was 2 cm. What was the energy of the beta particle? What is the contaminant?

5.6. A 5-MeV photon produces a positron–electron pair in a lead shield. If both particles are of equal energy, how far will they travel in the shield?

5.7. A Compton electron that was scattered straight forward ($\phi = 0°$) was completely stopped by an aluminum absorber 460 mg/cm² thick. What was the

(a) kinetic energy of the Compton electron?

(b) energy of the incident photon?

5.8. Monochromatic 0.1-MeV gamma rays are scattered through an angle of 120° by a carbon block. What is the

(a) energy of the scattered photon?

(b) kinetic energy of the Compton electron?

5.9. A 1.46-MeV gamma from naturally occurring ^{40}K is scattered twice: first through an angle of 30° and then through an angle of 150°. What is the

(a) energy of the photon after the second scattering?

(b) energy of the scattered photon if the angular sequence is reversed?

5.10. What is the energy of the Compton edge for the 0.661-MeV gamma from ^{137}Cs?

5.11. The energy of a scattered photon is 0.2 MeV after it was scattered through an angle of 135°. What was the photon's energy before the scattering collision?

5.12. What is the energy of the Compton edge for the following gammas:

(a) 0.136 MeV from ^{57}Co,

(b) 0.811 MeV from ^{58}Co, and

(c) 1.33 MeV from ^{60}Co.

5.13. The following gamma-ray absorption data were taken with lead absorbers:

thickness (mm)	0	2	4	6	8	10	15	20	25
counts/min	1000	880	770	680	600	530	390	285	210

(a) Determine the linear, mass, and atomic attenuation coefficients.

(b) What was the energy of the gamma ray?

5.14. The following absorption data were taken with aluminum absorbers:

thickness (mm)	0	0.2	0.4	0.6	0.8	1	1.2	1.4	1.6	2	4	8	15	20	28
counts/min	1000	576	348	230	168	134	120	107	96	95	90	82	68	60	50

(a) Plot the data. What types of radiation does the curve suggest?

(b) If a beta particle is present, what is its energy?

(c) If a gamma ray is present, what is its energy?

(d) What isotope is compatible with the absorption data?

(e) Write the equation that fits the absorption data.

5.15. A collimated gamma ray beam consists of equal numbers of 0.1-MeV and 1.0-MeV photons. If the beam enters a 15-cm-thick concrete shield, what is the relative portion of 1-MeV photons to 0.1-MeV photons in the emergent beam?

5.16. Three collimated gamma-ray beams of equal flux, whose photon energies are 2, 5, and 10 MeV, respectively, pass through 5-cm thick lead. What is the ratio of the emergent fluxes?

5.17. A collimated beam of 0.2-MeV gamma radiation delivers an incident energy flux of $2 \text{ J/m}^2/\text{s}$ to a lead shield 1 g/cm^2 thick. What is the

(a) incident photon flux, $\text{photons/cm}^2/\text{s}$?

(b) rate of energy absorption in the shield, erg/g/s and J/kg/s?

5.18. Calculate the thickness of Al and Cu required to attenuate narrow, collimated, monochromatic beams of 0.1-MeV and 0.8-MeV gamma rays to

(a) one-half the incident intensity (HVL),

(b) one-tenth the incident intensity (TVL). Express the answers in cm and in g/cm^2.

(c) What is the relationship between an HVL and a TVL?

5.19. The mass attenuation coefficient of muscle tissue for 1-MeV gamma radiation is $0.070 \text{ cm}^2/\text{g}$. What is the mean free path of a 1-MeV photon in muscle?

5.20. A laminated shield consists of two layers each of alternating thickness of aluminum and lead, each layer having a density thickness of 1.35 g/cm^2. The shield is irradiated with a narrow collimated beam of 0.2-MeV photons.

(a) What is the overall thickness of the laminated shield, in cm?

(b) Calculate the shield attenuation factor when

(i) the aluminum layer is first.

(ii) the lead layer is first.

5.21. Calculate the probability that a 2-MeV photon in a narrow, collimated beam will be removed from the beam by each of the following shields:

(a) Lead, 1-cm thick

(b) Iron, 1-cm thick

(c) Lead, 1 g/cm^2 thick

(d) Iron, 1 g/cm^2 thick

5.22. Calculate the gamma-ray threshold energy for the reaction $^{11}C(n, \gamma)^{12}C$, if the prompt capture gamma ray is 21.5 MeV.

5.23. X-rays are generated as bremsstrahlung by causing high-speed electrons to be stopped by a high-atomic-numbered target, as shown in the figure below. If the electrons are accelerated by a constant high voltage of 250 kV and if the electron beam current is 10 mA, calculate the X-ray energy flux at a distance of 1 m from the tungsten target. Neglect absorption by the glass tube and assume that the bremsstrahlung is emitted isotropically.

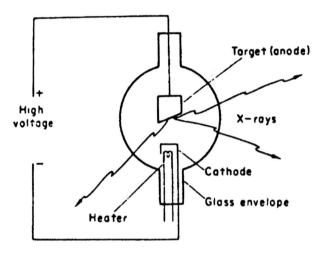

5.24. If the most energetic photon results from the instantaneous stopping of an electron in a single collision, what voltage must be applied across an X-ray tube in order to generate X-rays whose shortest wavelength approaches 0.124 Å?

5.25. A beta particle whose kinetic energy is 0.159 MeV passes through a 4 mg/cm^2 window into a helium-filled Geiger tube. How many ion pairs will the beta particle produce inside the tube?

5.26. If the neutron emission rate from ^{252}Cf is 2.31×10^6 neutrons/s/μg, and the transformation rate constant for alpha emission is 0.25 yr^{-1}, what is the neutron emission rate per MBq and per μCi?

5.27. Calculate the speed of a "slow" neutron whose kinetic energy is 0.1 eV. To what temperature does this energy correspond?

5.28. When ^9Be is irradiated with deuterons, neutrons are produced according to the reaction $^9Be(d, n)^{10}B$. The cross section for this reaction for 15-MeV deuterons is 0.12 b. What is the neutron flux at a distance of 25 cm from a 1-g Be target that is irradiated with a 100-μA beam of deuterons, 1.13-cm diameter, assuming an isotropic distribution of neutrons?

5.29. What is the thickness of Cd that will absorb 50% of an incident beam of thermal neutrons? The capture cross section for the element Cd is 2550 b for thermal neutrons; the specific gravity of Cd is 8.65 and its atomic weight is 112.4 D.

5.30. A small ^{124}Sb gamma-ray source, whose activity is 3.7×10^{10} Bq (1 Ci), is completely surrounded by a 25-g sphere of Be. Calculate the number of neutrons/s from the $^9Be(\gamma, n)^8Be$ reaction if the cross section is 1 mb, and if the diameter of the spherical cavity enclosing the gamma ray source is 1 cm.

5.31. Cadmium is used as a thermal neutron shield in an average flux of 10^{12} neutrons/cm^2/s. How long will it take to use up 10% of the ^{113}Cd atoms?

5.32. The cross section for the ^{32}S$(n, p)^{32}$P reaction is 300 mb for neutron energies greater than 2.5 MeV. How many microcuries of ^{32}P activity can we expect if 100-mg ^{32}S is irradiated in a fast flux of 10^2 neutrons/cm^2/s for 1 week?

5.33. If the absorption coefficient of the high-energy component of cosmic radiation is 2.5×10^{-3} m^{-1} of water, calculate the reduction in intensity of these cosmic rays at the bottom of the ocean, at the depth of 10,000 m.

5.34. If deuterium is irradiated with 2.62-MeV gamma rays from ^{208}Tl (ThC″), the nucleus disintegrates into its component parts of 1 proton and 1 neutron. If the neutron and proton each has 0.225 MeV of kinetic energy, and if the proton has a mass of 1.007593 amu, calculate the mass of the neutron.

5.35. A beam of fast neutrons includes two energy groups. One group, of 1-MeV neutrons, includes 99% of the total neutron flux. The remaining 1% of the neutrons have an energy of 10 MeV.

(a) What will be the relative proportions of the two groups after passing through 25 cm of water?

(b) What would be the relative proportion of the two groups after passing through a slab of lead of the same density thickness? The removal cross sections are as follows:

	CROSS SECTION (BARNS)	
	1-MeV Neutrons	**10-MeV Neutrons**
H	4.2	0.95
O	8	1.5
Pb	5.5	5.1

5.36. Boral is an aluminum boron carbide alloy used as a shield against thermal neutrons. If the boron content is 35% by weight and if the density of boral is 2.7 g/cm^3, calculate the half-thickness of boral for thermal neutrons at room temperature. The capture cross sections are: boron = 755 b, aluminum = 230 mb, carbon = 3.2 mb.

5.37. The scattering cross sections for N and O for thermal neutrons are 10 and 4.2 b, respectively.

(a) Calculate the macroscopic cross section for air at STP. Air consists of 79 volume percent nitrogen and 21 volume percent oxygen.

(b) What is the scattering mean free path of thermal neutrons in air?

5.38. How many scattering collisions in graphite are required to reduce the energy of 2.5-MeV neutrons to

(a) 0.1% of the initial energy?

(b) 0.025 eV?

5.39. A cobalt foil, 1 cm (diameter) × 0.1 mm (thickness), is irradiated in a mean thermal flux of 1×10^{11} neutrons/cm^2/s for a period of 7 days. If the activation cross section is 36 b and if the density of cobalt is 8.9 g/cm^3, what is the activity, in becquerels and in microcuries, at the end of the irradiation period? Note that natural cobalt is 100% ^{59}Co.

5.40. Type 304 stainless steel consists of 71% (weight percent) Fe, 19% Cr, and 10% Ni. The isotopic abundance, percentage, and the respective 2200 m/s capture cross sections (barns) of each of the elements are given below:

Fe			Cr			Ni		
A	Abun. (%)	σ_C (b)	A	Abun. (%)	σ_C (b)	A	Abun. (%)	σ_C (b)
54	5.84	2.9	50	4.31	17	58	67.76	4.4
56	91.68	2.7	52	83.76	0.8	60	21.16	2.6
57	2.17	2.5	53	9.55	18	61	1.25	2
58	0.31	1.1	54	2.38	0.38	62	3.66	15
						64	1.16	1.5

(a) Calculate the macroscopic capture cross section.

(b) If a 1-cm-diameter collimated beam of 2200 m/s neutrons is incident on a 2-mm-thick sheet of type 304 stainless steel, how many neutrons per second will be captured if the flux is 5×10^{11} neutrons/cm^2/s?

5.41. A 1-M solution of boric acid, H_3BO_3, is irradiated for 7 days in a thermal neutron flux of 10^{11} neutrons/cm^2/s at a temperature of 40°C. What is the concentration of Li, moles per liter, after the irradiation?

5.42. How far in standard air will the 5.5-MeV alpha particle from ^{241}Am travel?

5.43. What is the range in soft tissue of betas from

(a) ^{14}C ($E_m = 0.156$ MeV)

(b) ^{32}P ($E_m = 1.71$ MeV)

(c) ^{90}Y ($E_m = 2.273$ MeV)

5.44. Each of the following photons undergoes a Compton scattering in which the maximum energy is transferred to the electron. Calculate the energy of the scattered electron and the percent energy loss suffered by each photon.

(a) 2 MeV

(b) 0.2 MeV

(c) 0.02 MeV

5.45. What is the shortest wavelength of X-rays from a 250-kV machine?

5.46. An X-ray machine with a tungsten target is operated at 250-kV constant potential and a beam current of 25 mA. At what rate must heat be removed from the target in order to have an insignificant temperature rise? Express the answer in Joules per second and in calories per second.

5.47. The hydrogen capture cross section for thermal neutrons is 0.33 b, and for oxygen the capture cross section is 2×10^{-4} b. What is the macroscopic capture cross section for water, cm^{-1}?

5.48. Trace amounts of La (lanthanum), A = 139, will be investigated by irradiating a 10-g soil sample in a thermal neutron flux of 10^{12} neutrons/cm^2/s for 14 days, and determining the induced ^{140}La. If the ^{140}La activity was found to be 10 Bq 1 hour after the end of the irradiation time, calculate the La concentration in the soil in units of μg or g and ppm (pats per million by weight). Given:

^{139}La abundance $= 100\%$

σ (activation) $= 9$ b

$T_{1/2}$ (^{140}La) $= 1.7$ days

5.49. A 1.33-MeV ^{60}Co photon is backscattered 180°. Calculate

    (a) the energy of the backscattered photon and

    (b) the Compton edge.

5.50. A 0.321-MeV ^{51}Cr photon is backscattered 180°. Calculate

    (a) the energy of the backscattered photon and

    (b) the Compton edge.

SUGGESTED READINGS

Andrews, H. L. *Radiation Biophysics.* Prentice-Hall, Englewood Cliffs, NJ, 1974.

Attix, F. H. *Introduction to Radiological Physics and Radiation Dosimetry.* John Wiley & Sons, New York, 1986.

Attix, F. H., and Roesch, W. C., eds. *Radiation Dosimetry,* 2nd ed. *Vol. 1: Fundamentals.* Academic Press, New York, 1968.

Blatz, H., ed. *Radiation Hygiene Handbook.* McGraw-Hill, New York, 1959.

Born, M. *Atomic Physics,* 8th ed. Hafner, Darien, CT, 1970.

Brodsky, A., ed. *Handbook of Radiation Measurement and Protection. Vol. 1: Physical Science and Engineering Data.* CRC Press, West Palm Beach, FL, 1978.

Bureau of Radiological Health. *Radiological Health Handbook,* Rev. ed. U.S. Dept. of Health, Education, and Welfare, Public Health Services, Rockville, MD, 1970.

Cohen, B. L. *Concepts of Nuclear Physics.* McGraw-Hill, New York, 1971.

Compton, A. H., and Allison, S. K. *X-rays in Theory and Experiment.* D. Van Nostrand, Princeton, NJ, 1935.

Etherington, H., ed. *Nuclear Engineering Handbook.* McGraw-Hill, New York, 1958.

Evans, R. D. *The Atomic Nucleus.* McGraw-Hill, New York, 1955.

Faw, R., and Shultis, J. *Radiological Assessment.* Prentice-Hall, Englewood Cliffs, NJ, 1993.

Glasstone, S. *Sourcebook on Atomic Energy,* 3rd ed. D. Van Nostrand, Princeton, NJ, 1967.

Hunt, S. E. *Nuclear Physics for Engineers and Scientists.* Halsted Press, New York, 1987.

International Commission on Radiation Units and Measurements, Washington, DC:

    Report Number 10b: *Physical Aspects of Radiation,* 1964.

    Report Number 16: *Linear Energy Transfer,* 1970.

    Report Number 28: *Basic Aspects of High Energy Particle Interactions and Radiation Dosimetry,* 1978.

    Report Number 37: *Stopping Powers for Electrons and Positrons,* 1984.

    Report Number 49: *Stopping Powers and Ranges for Protons and Alpha Particles,* 1993.

    Report Number 60: *Fundamental Quantities and Units for Ionizing Radiation,* 1998.

Johns, H. E., and Cunningham, J. R. *The Physics of Radiology,* 4th ed. Charles C Thomas, Springfield, IL, 1983.

Kleinknecht, K. *Detectors for Particle Radiation.* Cambridge University Press, Cambridge, England, 1986.

Knoll, G.F. *Radiation Detection and Measurement,* 3rd ed., John Wiley and Sons, New York, 1999.

Krane, K. S. *Introductory Nuclear Physics.* John Wiley & Sons, New York, 1987.

Lapp, R. E., and Andrews, H. L. *Nuclear Radiation Physics,* 4th ed. Prentice-Hall, Englewood Cliffs, NJ, 1972.

National Nuclear Data Center. *Neutron Cross Sections, Report BNL-325 and Supplements.* Brookhaven National Laboratory, Upton, New York, 1965.

Rutherford, E. On the Scattering of alpha and beta particles by matter and the structure of the atom. *Phil Mag,* **21:**669–688, 1911.

Rutherford, E., Chadwick, J., and Ellis, C.D. *Radiations from Radioactive Substances,* Cambridge University Press, Cambridge, U.K., 1930.

Shleien, B., Slabak, L., and Birkey, B., *Handbook of Health Physics and Radiological Health.* Lippincott Williams & Wilkins, Philadelphia, PA, 1998.

Semat, H., and, Albright, J. R. *Introduction to Atomic and Nuclear Physics,* 5th ed. Holt, Rinehart, and Winston, New York, 1972.

Serway, R.A. and Jewett, J.W. *Physics for Scientists and Engineers,* 6th ed. Thomson Brooks Cole, Belmont, CA, 2004.

Turner, J. E. *Atoms, Radiation, and Radiation Protection.* John Wiley & Sons, New York, 1995.

Turner, J.E. Interaction of ionizing radiation with matter. *Health Phys,* **88:**520–544, 2005.

RADIATION DOSIMETRY

UNITS

During the early days of radiological experience, there was no precise unit of radiation dose that was suitable either for radiation protection or for radiation therapy. For purposes of radiation protection, a common "dosimeter" used was a piece of dental film with a paper clip attached. A daily exposure great enough just to produce a detectable shadow, called a "paper-clip" unit, was considered a maximum permissible dose. For greater doses and for therapy purposes, the dose unit was frequently the "skin erythema unit." Because of the great energy dependence of these dose units as well as other inherent shortcomings, neither of these two units could be biologically meaningful or useful either in the quantitative study of the biological effects of radiation or for radiation safety purposes. Furthermore, since the fraction of the energy in a radiation field that is absorbed by the body is energy dependent, it is necessary to distinguish between radiation *exposure* and radiation *absorbed dose*.

Absorbed Dose

Gray

Radiation damage depends on the absorption of energy from the radiation and is approximately proportional to the mean concentration of absorbed energy in irradiated tissue. For this reason, the basic unit of radiation dose is expressed in terms of absorbed energy per unit mass of tissue, that is,

$$\text{radiation absorbed dose} = \frac{\Delta E}{\Delta m}. \tag{6.1}$$

The unit for radiation absorbed dose in the SI system is called the *gray* (Gy) and is defined as follows:

One *gray* is an absorbed radiation dose of one joule per kilogram.

$$1\,\text{Gy} = 1\,\frac{\text{J}}{\text{kg}}. \tag{6.2}$$

The gray is universally applicable to all types of ionizing radiation dosimetry—irradiation due to external fields of gamma rays, neutrons, or charged particles as well as that due to internally deposited radionuclides.

rad (Radiation Absorbed Dose)

Before the introduction of the SI units, radiation dose was measured by a unit called the *rad*.

One *rad* is defined as an absorbed radiation dose of $100 \frac{\text{ergs}}{\text{g}}$.

$$1 \text{ rad} = 100 \frac{\text{ergs}}{\text{g}}. \tag{6.3a}$$

Since $1 \text{ J} = 10^7$ ergs, and since $1 \text{ kg} = 1000$ g,

$$1 \text{ Gy} = 100 \text{ rads}. \tag{6.3b}$$

$$1 \text{ rad} = 0.01 \text{ Gy} = 1 \text{ centigray (cGy)}. \tag{6.3c}$$

Although the gray is the newer unit and will eventually replace the rad, the rad and its derivatives nevertheless continue to be useful units and are used in the official radiation safety regulations in the United States.

It is important to understand that radiation absorbed dose concept, the gray and the rad, is a macroscopic construct and is not intended for microdosimetry on the cellular or subcellular levels. Radiation absorbed dose has been found to be correlated with biomedical effects on the tissue, organ, and organism levels and thus is appropriate for radiation safety measurements and for medical diagnostic and therapeutic uses of radiation. The radiation absorbed dose concept implies that the absorbed energy is uniformly distributed throughout the entire mass of the tissue of interest. On the cellular and subcellular levels that are of interest to molecular biologists, the biological effects are proportional to the number and types of intramolecular bonds that are broken rather than to the concentration of absorbed energy within the cell. On the tissue level, the number of such intramolecular breaks in the tissue is proportional to the radiation absorbed dose. The distinction between microdosimetry and radiation absorbed dose may be illustrated with the following thought experiment.

 EXAMPLE 6.1

Consider a single cell, with dimensions $10 \ \mu\text{m} \times 10 \ \mu\text{m} \times 10 \ \mu\text{m}$ and mass $= 10^{-12}$ kg, in a tissue of weight 0.1 g, in which a low LET particle, 1 keV/μm, transfers 1 keV to the cell as it passes through the cell. Calculate the radiation absorbed dose to the tissue.

Solution

The radiation absorbed dose to the tissue is calculated as

$$\text{radiation absorbed dose (tissue)} = \frac{10 \,\text{keV} \times 1.6 \times 10^{-16} \,\dfrac{\text{J}}{\text{keV}} \times 1\dfrac{\text{Gy}}{\text{J/kg}}}{1 \times 10^{-4} \,\text{kg}}$$

$$= 1.6 \times 10^{-11} \,\text{Gy},$$

which is an infinitesimally small dose. However, if the absorbed dose were to be (erroneously) applied to the single cell, the calculated dose would be

$$\text{radiation absorbed dose (cell)} = \frac{10 \,\text{keV} \times 1.6 \times 10^{-16} \,\dfrac{\text{J}}{\text{keV}} \times 1 \,\text{Gy} \cdot \text{kg/J}}{1 \times 10^{-12} \,\text{kg}}$$

$$= 1.6 \times 10^{-3} \,\text{Gy}.$$

EXTERNAL EXPOSURE

X- and Gamma Radiation

Exposure Unit

For external radiation of any given energy flux, the absorbed dose to any region within an organism depends on the type and energy of the radiation, the depth within the organism at the point at which the absorbed dose is required, and elementary constitution of the absorbing medium at this point. For example, bone, consisting of higher-atomic-numbered elements (Ca and P) than soft tissue (C, O, H, and N), absorbs more energy from an X-ray beam per unit mass of absorber than soft tissue. For this reason, the X-ray fields to which an organism may be exposed are frequently specified in *exposure units*. The exposure unit is a *radiometric* unit rather than a dosimetric unit. That is, it is a measure of the photon fluence and is related to the amount of energy transferred from the X-ray field to a unit mass of *air*. If the amount of exposure, measured in exposure units, is known, then knowing the energy of the X-rays and the composition of the irradiated medium, we can calculate the absorbed dose to any part of the irradiated medium.

One exposure unit is defined as that quantity of X- or gamma radiation that produces, in air, ions carrying one coulomb of charge (of either sign) per kilogram of air. It does not have a special name, and is being called an "X unit" in this textbook for convenience.

$$1 \,\text{X unit} = 1 \,\text{C/kg air.} \tag{6.4}$$

The exposure unit is based on ionization of air because of the relative ease with which radiation-induced ionization can be measured. At quantum energies less than several kilo electron volts and more than several mega electron volts, it becomes difficult to fulfill the requirements for measuring the exposure unit. Accordingly, the use of the exposure unit is limited to X- or gamma rays whose quantum energies do not exceed 3 MeV. For higher energy photons, exposure is expressed in units of watt-seconds per square meter and exposure rate is expressed in units of watts per square meter. The operational definition of the exposure unit may be converted into the more fundamental units of energy absorption per unit mass of air by using the fact that the charge on a single ion is 1.6×10^{-19} C and that the average energy dissipated in the production of a single ion pair in air is 34 eV. Therefore,

$$1 \text{ X unit} = 1\frac{C}{kg}\text{air} \times \frac{1 \text{ ion}}{1.6 \times 10^{-19} \text{ C}} \times 34\frac{eV}{ion} \times 1.6 \times 10^{-19}\frac{J}{eV}$$

$$\times 1\frac{Gy}{J/kg} = 34 \text{ Gy (in air)}. \tag{6.5}$$

It should be noted that the exposure unit is an integrated measure of exposure and is independent of the time over which the exposure occurs. The strength of an X-ray or gamma-ray field is usually expressed as an exposure rate, such as coulombs per kilogram per hour. The total exposure, of course, is the product of exposure rate and time.

Roentgen

Formerly, before the SI system was introduced, the unit of X-ray exposure was called the *roentgen* and was symbolized by R. The roentgen was defined as that quantity of X-or gamma radiation that produces ions carrying one statcoulomb (sC) ($1 \text{ sC} = 3 \times 10^9$ C) of charge of either sign per cubic centimeter of dry air at $0°$C and 760 mm Hg:

$$1 \text{ R} = 1 \text{ sC/cm}^3. \tag{6.6}$$

Since 1 ion carries a charge of 4.8×10^{-10} sC and the mass of 1 cm^3 of standard air is 0.001293 g, we can calculate the dose to the air from an exposure of 1 R:

$$1 \text{ R} = 1 \text{ sC/cm}^3 \text{ air} \times \frac{1 \text{ cm}^3 \text{ air}}{1.29 \times 10^{-3} \text{ g/cm}^3 \text{ air}} \times \frac{1 \text{ ion}}{4.8 \times 10^{-10} \text{ sC}} \times 34\frac{eV}{ion}$$

$$\times 1.6 \times 10^{-12}\frac{erg}{eV} \times \frac{1 \text{ rad}}{100\frac{erg}{g}}$$

$$1 \text{ R} = 0.877 \text{ rad (to air)}.$$

When exposure is measured in roentgens, X-ray or gamma-ray field strength is measured in units such as roentgens per minute or milliroentgens per hour. (A milliroentgen, which is symbolized by "mR," is equal to 0.001 R.)

The relationship between the coulomb per kilogram exposure unit and the roentgen may be calculated as follows:

$$\frac{34 \frac{J/kg}{C/kg} \times 10^7 \frac{ergs}{J} \times \frac{1 \text{ kg}}{1000 \text{ g}}}{87.7 \frac{ergs/g}{R}} = 3881 \frac{R}{C/kg}$$

or

$$1 \text{ X unit} = 3881 \text{ R.} \tag{6.7a}$$

$$1 \text{ R} = (1/3881) \text{X unit} = 2.58 \times 10^{-4} \text{ X unit.} \tag{6.7b}$$

EXAMPLE 6.2

Health physics measurements of X-ray and gamma ray fields are usually made in units of milliroentgen per hour. If a health physicist finds a gamma ray field of 1 mR/h, what is the corresponding exposure expressed in SI units?

Solution

According to Eq. (6.7b),

$$1 \frac{mR}{h} \times 10^{-3} \frac{R}{mR} = 2.58 \times 10^{-4} \times 10^{-3} \frac{C}{kg}$$

$$1 \text{ mR/h} = 2.58 \times 10^{-7} \frac{C}{kg} = 0.258 \frac{\mu C}{h}.$$

Exposure Measurement: The Free Air Chamber

The operational definition of the exposure unit can be satisfied by the instrument shown in Figure 6-1. The X-ray beam enters through the portal and interacts with the cylindrical column of air defined by the entry port diaphragm. All the ions resulting from interactions between the X-rays and the volume of air (A–B–C–D), which is determined by the intersection of the X-ray beam with the electric lines of force from the edges of the collector plate C, is collected by the plates, causing current to flow in the external circuit. Most of these collected ions are those produced as the primary ionizing particles lose their energy by ionizing interactions as they pass through the air. (The primary ionizing particles are the Compton electrons and the photoelectrons resulting from the interaction of the x-rays (photons) with the air.) The guard ring G and the guard wires W help to keep these electric field lines straight and perpendicular to the plates. The electric field intensity between the plates is on the order of 100 V/cm—high enough to collect the ions before they recombine but not great enough to accelerate the secondary electrons produced by the primary ionizing particles to ionizing energy. The guard wires are connected to a voltage-dividing

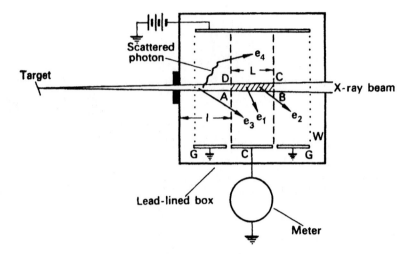

Figure 6-1. Schematic diagram of a parallel-plate ionization chamber. (From *Design of Free Air Ionization Chamber.* Washington, DC: National Bureau of Standards; 1957. NBS Handbook 64.)

network to ensure a uniform potential drop across the plates. The number of ions collected because of X-ray interactions in the collecting volume is calculated from the current flow and the exposure rate, in roentgens per unit time, is then computed. For the exposure unit to be measured in this way, all the energy of the primary electrons must be dissipated in the air within the meter. This condition can be satisfied by making the air chamber larger than the maximum range of the primary electrons. (For 300-keV X-rays, the spacing between the collector plates is about 30 cm and the overall box is a cube of about 50-cm edge.) The fact that many of the ions produced as a consequence of X-ray interactions within the sensitive volume are not collected is of no significance if as many electrons from interactions elsewhere in the X-ray beam enter the sensitive volume as leave it. This condition is known as *electronic equilibrium.* When electronic equilibrium is attained, an electron of equal energy enters into the sensitive volume for every electron that leaves. A sufficient thickness of air, dimension *l* in Figure 6-1, must be allowed between the beam entrance port and the sensitive volume in order to attain electronic equilibrium. For highly filtered 250-kV X-rays, 9 cm of air is required; for 500-kV X-rays, the air thickness required for electronic equilibrium in the sensitive volume increases to 40 cm.

Under conditions of electronic equilibrium and assuming negligible attenuation of the X-ray beam by the air in length *l*, the ions collected from the sensitive volume result from primary photon interactions at the beam entrance port; the measured exposure, consequently, is at that point and not in the sensitive volume. Free air chambers are in use that measure the quantity of X-rays whose quantum energies reach as high as 500 keV. Higher energy radiation necessitates free air chambers of much greater size. The technical problems arising from the use of such large chambers make it impractical to use the free air ionization chamber as a primary measuring device for quantum energies in excess of 500 keV. These problems include recombination of ions in the large chamber before they can be collected and secondary ionization due to acceleration of the initial ions by the great potential difference required for large chambers.

The use of the free air ionization chamber to measure X-ray exposure rate in coulombs per kilogram per second may be illustrated by the following example:

EXAMPLE 6.3

The opening of the diaphragm in the entrance port of a free air ionization chamber is 1 cm in diameter, and the length AB of the sensitive volume is 5 cm. A 200-kV X-ray beam projected into the chamber produces a steady current in the external circuit of 0.01 μA. The temperature at the time of the measurement was 20°C and the pressure was 750 mm Hg. What is the exposure rate in this beam of X-rays?

Solution

A current of 0.01 μA corresponds to a flow of electrical charge of 10^{-8} C/s. The sensitive volume in this case, $\pi \times (0.5 \text{ cm})^2 \times 5 \text{ cm} = 3.927 \text{ cm}^3$. When the pressure and temperature are corrected to standard conditions, we have

$$\dot{X} = \frac{10^{-8} \text{ C/s}}{3.927 \text{ cm}^3 \times 1.293 \times 10^{-6} \dfrac{\text{kg}}{\text{cm}^3}} \times \frac{293}{273} \times \frac{760}{750}$$

$$= 2.14 \times 10^{-3} \frac{\text{C/kg}}{\text{s}}.$$

In the traditional system of units, this exposure rate corresponds to

$$2.14 \times 10^{-3} \frac{\text{C/kg}}{\text{s}} \times 3.881 \times 10^3 \frac{\text{R}}{\text{C/kg}} = 8.31 \frac{\text{R}}{\text{s}}.$$

Exposure Measurement: The Air Wall Chamber

The free air ionization chamber described above is practical only as a primary laboratory standard. For field use, a more portable instrument is required. Such an instrument could be made by compressing the air around the measuring cavity. If this were done, then the conditions for defining the exposure unit would continue to be met. In practice, of course, it would be quite difficult to construct an instrument whose walls were made of compressed air. However, it is possible to make an instrument with walls of "air-equivalent" material—that is, a wall material whose X-ray absorption properties are very similar to those of air. Such a chamber can be built in the form of an electrical capacitor; its principle of operation can be explained with the aid of Figure 6-2.

The instrument consists of an outer cylindrical wall, about 4.75-mm thick, made of electrically conducting plastic. Coaxial with the outer wall, but separated from it by a very high-quality insulator, is a center wire. This center wire, or central anode, is positively charged with respect to the wall. When the chamber is exposed to

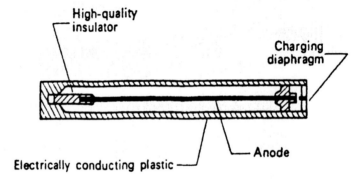

Figure 6-2. Non-self-reading condenser-type pocket ionization chamber.

X-radiation or to gamma radiation, the ionization, which is produced in the measuring cavity as a result of interactions between photons and the wall, discharges the condenser, thereby decreasing the potential of the anode. This decrease in the anode voltage is directly proportional to the ionization produced in the cavity, which in turn is directly proportional to the radiation exposure. For example, consider the following instance:

 EXAMPLE 6.4

Given

> chamber volume = 2 cm^3,
> chamber is filled with air at STP,
> capacitance = 5 pF,
> voltage across chamber before exposure to radiation = 180 V,
> voltage across chamber after exposure to radiation = 160 V, and
> exposure time = 0.5 h.

Calculate the radiation exposure and the exposure rate.

Solution

The exposure is calculated as follows:

$$C \times \Delta V = \Delta Q \tag{6.8}$$

where

> C = capacitance, farads
> V = potential, volts
> Q = charge, coulombs

$$5 \times 10^{-12} \, \text{F} \times (180 - 160) \, \text{V} = 1 \times 10^{-10} \, \text{C}.$$

Since one exposure unit is equal to 1 C/kg, the exposure measured by this chamber is

$$\frac{1 \times 10^{-10} \text{ C}}{2 \text{ cm}^3 \times 1.293 \times 10^{-6} \frac{\text{kg}}{\text{cm}^3}} = 3.867 \times 10^{-5} \frac{\text{C}}{\text{kg}},$$

which corresponds to

$$3.867 \times 10^{-5} \frac{\text{C}}{\text{kg}} \times 3881 \frac{\text{R}}{\text{C/kg}} = 0.150 \text{ R} = 150 \text{ mR},$$

and the exposure rate was

$$\frac{3.867 \times 10^{-5} \text{ C/kg}}{0.5 \text{ h}} = 77.3 \times 10^{-6} \frac{\text{C/kg}}{\text{h}} = 77.3 \frac{\mu\text{C/kg}}{\text{h}}$$

or $300 \frac{\text{mR}}{\text{h}}$.

A chamber built according to this principle is called an "air wall" chamber. When such a chamber is used, care must be taken that the walls are of the proper thickness for the energy of the radiation being measured. If the walls are too thin, an insufficient number of photons will interact to produce primary electrons; if they are too thick, the primary radiation will be absorbed to a significant degree by the wall and an attenuated primary-electron fluence will result.

The determination of the optimum thickness may be illustrated by an experiment in which the ionization produced in the cavity of an ionization chamber is measured as the wall thickness is increased from a very thin wall until it becomes relatively thick. When this is done and the cavity ionization is plotted against the wall thickness, the curve shown in Figure 6-3 results.

Since the cavity ionization is caused mainly by primary electrons resulting from photon (gamma-ray) interactions with the wall, increasing the wall thickness allows more photons to interact, thereby producing more primary electrons, which ionize the gas in the chamber as they traverse the cavity. However, when the wall thickness reaches a point where a primary electron produced at the outer surface of the wall is not sufficiently energetic to pass through the wall into the cavity, the ionization in the cavity begins to decrease. The wall thickness at which this just begins is the *equilibrium wall thickness.*

As the wall material departs from air equivalence, the response of the ionization chamber becomes energy dependent. By proper choice of wall material and thickness, the maximum in the curve of Figure 6-3 can be made quite broad, and the ionization chamber, as a consequence, can be made relatively energy independent over a wide range of quantum energies. In practice, this approximately flat response spans the energy range from about 200 keV to about 2 MeV. In this range of energies, the Compton effect is the predominant mechanism of energy transfer. For lower energies, the probability of a Compton interaction increases approximately in direct proportion to the wavelength, while the probability of a photoelectric interaction is approximately proportional to the cube of the photon's wavelength.

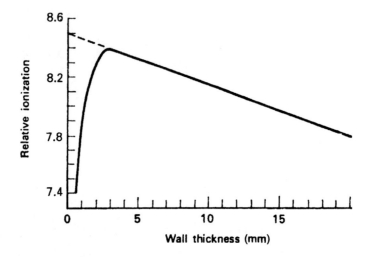

Figure 6-3. Ion pairs per unit volume as a function of wall thickness. The ionization chamber in this case was made of pure carbon and was a 20-mm long cylinder with an inside diameter of 20 mm. (Reproduced with permission from Mayneord WV, Roberts JE. An attempt at precision measurements of gamma rays. *Br J Radiol.* 1937;10(113):365–386.)

The total number of primary electrons increases and therefore the sensitivity of the chamber also increases; the increased sensitivity, however, reaches a peak as the quantum energy decreases and then, because of the severe attenuation of the incident radiation by the chamber wall, the sensitivity rapidly decreases. These effects are shown in Figure 6-4, a curve showing the energy correction factor for a pocket dosimeter.

For quantum energies greater than 3 MeV, neither coulombs per kilogram nor roentgen is used as the unit of measurement of exposure. This is due to the fact that the high energy, and consequently the long range of the primary electrons produced in the wall, makes it impossible to build an instrument that meets the criteria for measuring the exposure. Because of the long range of the primary electrons,

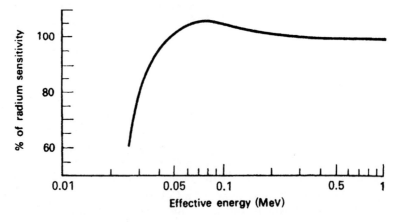

Figure 6-4. Energy dependence characteristics of the pocket dosimeter shown in Figure 9-18.

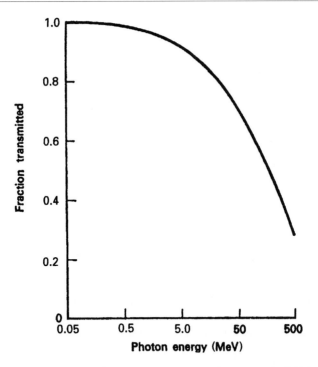

Figure 6-5. Fractional number of photons transmitted through an air wall of thickness equal to the maximum range of the secondary electrons. (From *Protection Against Betatron–Synchrotron Radiations up to 100 Million Electron Volts*. Washington, DC: US Government Printing Office; 1955. NBS Handbook 55.)

very thick walls are necessary. However, when the walls are sufficiently thick, on the basis of the range of the primary electrons, they attenuate the photons (gamma radiation) to a significant degree, as shown in Figure 6-5. Under these conditions, it is not possible to attain electronic equilibrium since the radiation intensity within the wall is not constant and the primary electrons, consequently, are not produced uniformly throughout the entire volume of wall from which they may reach the cavity.

Exposure–Dose Relationship

The air-wall chamber, as the name implies, measures the energy absorption in air. In most instances, we are interested in the energy absorbed in tissue. Since energy absorption is approximately proportional to the electronic density of the absorber in the energy region where exposure units are valid, it can be shown that the tissue dose is not necessarily equal to the air dose for any given radiation field. For example, if we consider muscle tissue to have a specific gravity of 1 and to have an elementary composition of 5.98×10^{22} hydrogen atoms per gram, 2.75×10^{22} oxygen atoms per gram, 0.172×10^{22} nitrogen atoms per gram, and 6.02×10^{21} carbon atoms per gram, then the electronic density is 3.28×10^{23} electrons per gram. For air, whose density is 1.293×10^{-3} g/cm^3, the electronic density is 3.01×10^{23} electrons/gram. The energy absorption, in joules per kilogram of tissue, corresponding to an exposure of 1 C/kg air is, therefore,

$$\frac{3.28}{3.01} \times 34 \frac{J}{kg} \text{ air} = 37 \frac{J}{kg} \text{ tissue.}$$

This value agrees very well with calorimetric measurements of energy absorption by soft tissue from an exposure of 1 C/kg air. By analogy, an exposure of 1 R, which corresponds to 87.7 ergs/g of air, leads to an absorption of 95 ergs/g muscle tissue. This tissue dose from a 1-R exposure is very close to the tissue dose of 100 ergs/g, which corresponds to 1 rad. For this reason, an exposure of 1 R is frequently considered approximately equivalent to an absorbed dose of 1 rad, and the unit "roentgen" is loosely (but incorrectly) used to mean "rad." Because of this simple approximate one-to-one relationship of the roentgen to the rad, the roentgen continues to be used. To be up to date vis-à-vis measurement units, an exposure of 1 R is often called a dose of 1 centigray (cGy).

The exposure unit bears a simple quantitative relationship to the dosimetric unit (the gray or the rad) that permits the calculation of absorbed dose in any medium whose exposure (in coulombs per kilogram or statcoulombs per cubic centimeter air) is known. This relationship may be illustrated by the following example.

EXAMPLE 6.5

Consider a gamma-ray beam of quantum energy 0.3 MeV. If the photon flux is 1000 quanta/cm^2/s and the air temperature is 20°C, what is the exposure rate at a point in this beam and what is the absorbed dose rate for soft tissue at this point?

Solution

From Figure 5-20, the linear energy absorption coefficient for air, μ_a, at STP, for 300-keV photons is found to be 3.46×10^{-5} cm^{-1}. The exposure rate, $\dot{X}$, in C/kg/s in a photon flux ϕ is given by

$$\dot{X} = \frac{\phi \frac{\text{photons}}{\text{cm}^2/\text{s}} \times E \frac{\text{MeV}}{\text{photon}} \times 1.6 \times 10^{-13} \frac{J}{\text{MeV}} \times \mu_{air}/\text{ cm}}{\rho_{air} \frac{kg}{\text{cm}^3} \times 34 \frac{J/kg}{C/kg}},$$

(6.9)

where

μ_a is the linear energy absorption coefficient for air for the photon energy and
ρ_a is the density of air.

The radiation absorbed dose rate from this exposure is given by

$$\dot{D} = \frac{\phi \dfrac{\text{photons}}{\text{cm}^2 \cdot \text{s}} \times E \dfrac{\text{MeV}}{\text{photon}} \times 1.6 \times 10^{-13} \dfrac{\text{J}}{\text{MeV}} \times \mu_{\text{m}} \text{ cm}^{-1}}{\rho_{\text{m}} \dfrac{\text{kg}}{\text{cm}^3} \times 1 \dfrac{\text{J/kg}}{\text{Gy}}},$$

where

μ_{m} is the linear energy absorption coefficient of the medium and
ρ_{m} is the density of the medium.

Substituting the appropriate numerical values into Eq. (6.9), we have

$$\dot{X} = \frac{10^3 \times 0.3 \times 1.6 \times 10^{-13} \times 3.46 \times 10^{-5}}{(1.293 \times 10^{-6} \times \frac{273}{293}) \times 34}$$

$$\dot{X} = 4 \times 10^{-11} \frac{\text{C/kg}}{\text{s}}.$$

Since health physics measurements are usually given in units of per hour, this exposure rate corresponds to

$$4 \times 10^{-11} \frac{\text{C/kg}}{\text{s}} \times 3.6 \times 10^3 \frac{\text{s}}{\text{h}} = 1.5 \times 10^{-7} \frac{\text{C/kg}}{\text{h}}$$

$$= 0.15 \frac{\mu\text{C/kg}}{\text{h}}.$$

Since $0.258 \dfrac{\mu\text{C}}{\text{kg}} = 1$ mR, the exposure rate expressed in traditional units is

$$\dot{R} = 0.15 \frac{\mu\text{C/kg}}{\text{h}} \times \frac{1 \text{ mR}}{0.258 \dfrac{\mu\text{C}}{\text{kg}}} = 0.58 \frac{\text{mR}}{\text{h}}$$

The absorbed dose rate, in grays per second, is given by Eq. (6.10) as

$$\dot{D} = \frac{\phi \dfrac{\text{photons}}{\text{cm}^2 \cdot \text{s}} \times E \dfrac{\text{MeV}}{\text{photon}} \times 1.6 \times 10^{-13} \dfrac{\text{J}}{\text{MeV}} \times \mu_{\text{m}} \text{ cm}^{-1}}{\rho_{\text{m}} \dfrac{\text{kg}}{\text{cm}^3} \times 1 \dfrac{\text{J/kg}}{\text{Gy}}}.$$

The ratio of absorbed dose rate to the exposure dose rate is given by the ratio of Eq. (6.10) to Eq. (6.9):

$$\frac{\dot{D}}{\dot{X}} = \frac{\left(\phi \times E \times 1.6 \times 10^{-13} \times \mu_{\text{med}} \right) / \rho_{\text{med}}}{\left[\dfrac{\left(\phi \times E \times 1.6 \times 10^{-13} \times \mu_{\text{air}} \right)}{\left(\rho_{\text{air}} \times 34 \dfrac{\text{J/kg}}{\text{C/kg}} \right)} \right]}.$$

The absorbed dose rate, in Gy per unit time, resulting from an exposure of $\dot{X}$ C/kg per unit time, therefore is

$$\dot{D}, \frac{Gy}{time} = 34\frac{Gy}{\dfrac{C}{kg}} \times \frac{\left(\dfrac{\mu_{med}\ cm^{-1}}{\rho_{med}\ \dfrac{g}{cm^3}}\right)}{\left(\dfrac{\mu_{air}\ cm^{-1}}{\rho_{air}\ \dfrac{g}{cm^3}}\right)} \times \dot{X}\frac{C/kg}{time}. \tag{6.10}$$

Since the mass absorption coefficient is given by Eq. (5.28) as

$$\mu_{mass} = \frac{\mu_{linear}}{\rho},$$

Eq. (6.10) may be written as

$$\dot{D}, Gy = 34\frac{Gy}{C/kg} \times \left(\frac{\mu_{medium}}{\mu_{air}}\right)_{mass} \times \dot{X}\ \frac{C/kg}{time}. \tag{6.12a}$$

Equation (6.12a) is also applicable to the calculation of the absorbed dose if the exposure dose is used instead of the exposure dose rate.

To obtain a dose in rads to any medium when the exposure is given in roentgens, we use the analogous expression

$$rads = \frac{87.7}{100} \times \left(\frac{\mu_{medium}}{\mu_{air}}\right)_{mass} \times roentgens. \tag{6.12b}$$

EXAMPLE 6.6

What is the radiation absorbed dose corresponding to an exposure dose of 25.8 μC/kg (100 mR) from 300-keV photons?

Solution

When the value for the energy absorption coefficient for muscle tissue for 0.3-MeV photons, $\mu_{medium} = 0.0317$ cm^2/g and $\mu_{air} = 0.0288$ cm^2/g, from Table 5-4, are substituted into Eq. (6.12a), we have

$$Dose = 34\frac{Gy}{C/kg} \times \frac{0.0317\ cm^2/g}{0.0288\ cm^2/g} \times 25.8 \times 10^{-6}\ \frac{C}{kg} = 9.7 \times 10^{-4}\ Gy$$

$$= 0.97\ mGy = 97\ mrads.$$

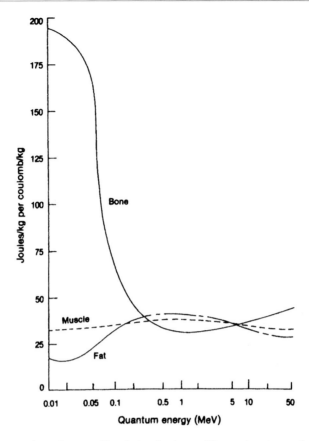

Figure 6-6. Energy absorption per X unit (coulomb per kilogram) exposure for several tissues. (Adapted with permission from Glasser O. *Medical Physics.* Vol 2. Chicago, IL: Year Book Medical Publishers, Inc; 1950.)

Equations (6.12a) and (6.12b) show that the radiation dose absorbed from any given exposure is determined by the ratio of the mass absorption coefficient of the medium to that of air. In the case of tissue, the ratio of dose to exposure remains approximately constant over the quantum energy range of about 0.1–10 MeV because the chief means of interaction between the tissue and the radiation is Compton scattering, and the cross section for Compton scattering depends mainly on electronic density of the absorbing medium. In the case of lower energies, photoelectric absorption becomes important, and the cross section for this mode of interaction increases with atomic number of the absorber. As a consequence of this dependence on atomic number, bone, which contains approximately 10% by weight of calcium, absorbs much more energy than soft tissue from a given air dose of low-energy X-rays. This point is illustrated in Figure 6-6, which shows the number of joules per kilogram absorbed per coulomb per kilogram of exposure for fat, muscle, and bone as a function of quantum energy.

Absorbed Dose Measurement: Bragg–Gray Principle

If a cavity ionization chamber is built with a wall material whose radiation absorption properties are similar to those of tissue, then, by taking advantage of the *Bragg–Gray principle*, an instrument can be built to measure tissue dose directly. According to the Bragg–Gray principle, the amount of ionization produced in a small gas-filled cavity surrounded by a solid absorbing medium is proportional to the energy absorbed by the solid. Implicit in the practical application of this principle is that the gas cavity be small enough relative to the mass of the solid absorber to leave the angular and velocity distributions of the primary electrons unchanged. This requirement is fulfilled if the primary electrons lose only a very small fraction of their energy in traversing the gas-filled cavity. If the cavity is surrounded by a solid medium of proper thickness to establish electronic equilibrium, then the energy absorbed per unit mass of wall, dE_m/dM_m, is related to the energy absorbed per unit mass of gas in the cavity, dE_g/dM_g, by

$$\frac{dE_m}{dM_m} = \frac{S_m}{S_g} \times \frac{dE_g}{dM_g},$$

(6.13)

where

S_m is the mass stopping power of the wall material and
S_g is the mass stopping power of the gas.

Since the ionization per unit mass of gas is a direct measure of dE_g/dM_g, Eq. (6.13) can be rewritten as

$$\frac{dE_m}{dM_m} = \rho_m \times w \times J$$

(6.14)

where

$\rho_m = S_m/S_g$,
w = the mean energy dissipated in the production of an ion pair in the gas, and
J = the number of ion pairs per unit mass of gas.

Using the appropriate equations for stopping power given in Chapter 5, we can compute ρ_m for electrons of any given energy. For those cases where the gas in the cavity is the same substance as the chamber wall, such as methane and paraffin, ρ_m is equal to unity. Table 6-1 shows the stopping power ratios, relative to air, of several substances for monoenergetic electrons. For gamma radiation, however, the problem of evaluating ρ_m is more difficult. The relative fraction of the gamma rays that will interact by each of the competing mechanisms, as well as the spectral distribution of the primary electrons (Compton, photoelectric, and pair-produced electrons) must be considered, and a mean value for relative stopping power must be determined. For the equilibrium electron spectra generated by gamma rays from ^{198}Au, ^{137}Cs, and ^{60}Co, the values for the mean mass relative stopping powers are given in Table 6-2. For air, w, the mean energy loss for the production of an ion pair in air, has a value of 34 eV. To determine the radiation absorbed dose, it is necessary only to measure the ionization J per unit mass of gas.

TABLE 6-1. Mean Mass Stopping Power Ratios, Relative to Air, for Electronic Equilibrium Spectra Generated by Intially Monoenergetic Electrons

Initial Energy (MeV)	ELEMENT AND STATE OF MOLECULAR BINDING								
	Hydrogen, Saturated	Hydrogen, Unsaturated	Carbon, Saturated	Carbon, Unsaturated	Carbon, highly Chlorinated	Nitrogen, amines, Nitrates	Nitrogen Ring	Oxygen, —O—	Oxygen, O=
0.1	2.52	2.59	1.016	1.021	1.047	0.976	1.018	0.978	0.994
0.2	2.52	2.59	1.015	1.019	1.043	0.978	1.016	0.979	0.995
0.3	2.48	2.55	1.014	1.018	1.040	0.979	1.016	0.981	0.995
0.327	2.48	2.54	1.014	1.018	1.040	0.979	1.015	0.981	0.995
0.4	2.46	2.53	1.014	1.018	1.038	0.980	1.015	0.981	0.996
0.5	2.44	2.51	1.013	1.017	1.037	0.980	1.015	0.982	0.996
0.6	2.44	2.50	1.012	1.016	1.035	0.980	1.013	0.981	0.995
0.654	2.43	2.49	1.011	1.014	1.034	0.979	1.012	0.981	0.994
0.7	2.42	2.48	1.010	1.013	1.033	0.978	1.011	0.980	0.993
0.8	2.40	2.46	1.009	1.012	1.031	0.978	1.010	0.979	0.992
1.0	2.39	2.44	1.004	1.008	1.026	0.975	1.005	0.977	0.988
1.2	2.37	2.42	1.001	1.004	1.022	0.973	1.002	0.974	0.985
1.308	2.36	2.42	0.999	1.002	1.019	0.971	1.000	0.972	0.983
1.5	2.35	2.39	0.995	0.998	1.015	0.967	0.996	0.969	0.980

Source: From *Physical Aspects of Irradiation*. Washington, DC: National Bureau of Standards, US Government Printing Office; 1964. NBS Handbook 85.

TABLE 6-2. Mean Mass Stopping Power Ratios, S^m/S_{air} for Equilibrium Electron Spectra Generated by ^{198}Au, ^{137}Cs, and ^{60}Co, on the Assumption That the Electrons Slow Down in a Continuous Manner

ENERGY (MeV)	MEDIUM		
	Graphite	Water	Tissue
0.411 (^{198}Au)	1.032		
0.670 (^{137}Cs)	1.027	1.162	1.145
1.25 (^{60}Co)	1.017	1.155	1.137

Source: From *Report of the International Commission on Radiological Units and Measurements.* Washington, DC: National Bureau of Standards, US Government Printing Office; 1959. NBS Handbook 78.

EXAMPLE 6.7

Calculate the absorbed dose rate from the following data on a tissue-equivalent chamber with walls of equilibrium thickness embedded within a phantom and exposed to ^{60}Co gamma rays for 10 minutes. The volume of the air cavity in the chamber is 1 cm^3, the capacitance is 5 μF, and the gamma-ray exposure results in a decrease of 72 V across the chamber.

Solution

The charge collected by the chamber is

$$Q = C \times \Delta V$$
$$= 5 \times 10^{-12} \text{ F} \times 72 \text{ V}$$
$$= 3.6 \times 10^{-10} \text{ C}.$$

The number of electrons collected, which corresponds to the number of ion pairs formed in the air cavity, is

$$\frac{3.6 \times 10^{-10} \text{ C}}{1.6 \times 10^{-19} \dfrac{\text{C}}{\text{electron}}} = 2.25 \times 10^9 \text{ electrons}.$$

Since 34 eV are expended per ion pair formed in air and since the stopping power of tissue relative to air is 1.137 (Table 6-2), we have from the Bragg–Gray relationship of Eq. (6.14):

$$\frac{\mathrm{d}E_m}{\mathrm{d}M_m} = \rho_m \times w \times J$$

$$= \frac{1.137 \times 34 \dfrac{\text{eV}}{\text{ip}} \times 2.25 \times 10^9 \dfrac{\text{ip}}{\text{cm}^3} \times 1.6 \times 10^{-19} \dfrac{\text{J}}{\text{eV}}}{1.293 \times 10^{-6} \dfrac{\text{kg}}{\text{cm}^3} \times 1 \dfrac{\text{J/kg}}{\text{Gy}}}$$

$$= 0.0108 \text{ Gy} = 10.8 \text{ mGy } (1.08 \text{ rad} = 1080 \text{ mrad}).$$

The exposure time was 10 minutes and the dose rate therefore is 1.08 mGy/min (108 mrad/min).

Kerma

In the case of indirectly ionizing radiation, such as X-rays, gamma rays, and fast neutrons, we are sometimes interested in the initial kinetic energy of the primary ionizing particles (the photoelectrons, Compton electrons, or positron–negatron pairs in the case of photon radiation and the scattered nuclei in the case of fast neutrons) that result from the interaction of the incident radiation with a unit mass of interacting medium. This quantity of transferred energy is called the *kerma, K,* and is measured in SI units in joules per kilogram, or grays. In the traditional system of units, it is measured in ergs per gram or in rads. Although kerma and dose are both measured in the same units, they are different quantities. The kerma is a measure of all the energy transferred from the uncharged particle (photon or neutron) to primary ionizing particles per unit mass, whereas absorbed dose is a measure of the energy absorbed per unit mass.

Not all the energy transferred to the primary ionizing particles in a given volume of material may be absorbed in that volume. Some of this energy may leave that volume and be absorbed elsewhere. This could result from bremsstrahlung or annihilation radiation which is generated by the primary ionizing particles, but which leave the volume element without further interactions within that volume. It may also be the result of failure to attain electronic equilibrium within the volume element under consideration. In a large medium, where electronic equilibrium exists and where we have insignificant energy loss by bremsstrahlung, kerma is equal to absorbed dose. The difference between kerma and dose is illustrated by Example 6.8.

EXAMPLE 6.8

A 10-MeV photon penetrates into a 100-g mass and undergoes a single interaction, a pair-production interaction that leads to a positron and an electron of 4.5 MeV each. Both charged particles dissipate all their kinetic energy within the mass through ionization and bremsstrahlung production. Three bremsstrahlung photons of 1.6, 1.4, and 2 MeV each that are produced escape from the mass before they interact. The positron, after expending all its kinetic energy, interacts with an ambient electron within the mass and they mutually annihilate one another to produce two photons of 0.51 MeV each, and both these photons escape before they can interact within the mass. Calculate

(a) the kerma and

(b) the absorbed dose.

Solution

(a) Kerma is defined as the *sum of the initial kinetic energies per unit mass of all charged particles produced by the radiation.* In this case, a positron–negatron pair of

4.5 MeV each (2 × 4.5 MeV) represents all the initial kinetic energy. The kerma, K, in this case is

$$K = \frac{\text{kinetic energy released}}{\text{mass}} = \frac{2 \times 4.5 \text{ MeV} \times 1.6 \times 10^{-13} \frac{\text{J}}{\text{MeV}}}{0.1 \text{ kg} \times 1 \frac{\text{J/kg}}{\text{Gy}}}$$

$$= 1.44 \times 10^{-11} \text{Gy}.$$

(b) Dose is defined as the *energy absorbed per unit mass*. Here we have the 9 MeV of initial kinetic energy, of which $(1.6 + 1.4 + 2)$ MeV was converted into bremsstrahlung and into 2 photons of 0.51-MeV annihilation radiation. All these photons escaped from the 100-g mass. The absorbed dose, therefore, is

$$D = \frac{\text{absorbed energy}}{\text{mass}}$$

$$= \frac{[10 \text{ MeV} - (1.6 + 1.4 + 2 + 2 \times 0.51) \text{ MeV}] \times 1.6 \times 10^{-13} \frac{\text{J}}{\text{MeV}}}{0.1 \text{ kg} \times 1 \frac{\text{J/kg}}{\text{Gy}}}$$

$$= 6.4 \times 10^{-12} \text{ Gy}.$$

The National Council on Radiation Protection and Measurements (NCRP) specifies X-ray machine output and X-ray levels in units of *air kerma*. Since electronic equilibrium generally is attained in an X-ray field in air, air kerma is, for practical purposes, a measure of exposure. The numerical relationship between air kerma and exposure in C/kg and in R is demonstrated as follows:

1 C/kg = 34 Gy (in air)

$$1 \text{ Gy (air kerma)} = \frac{1}{34} \frac{\text{C}}{\text{kg}} = 0.02941 \frac{\text{C}}{\text{kg}}$$

$$1 \text{ mGy (air kerma)} = 0.02941 \times 10^{-3} \frac{\text{C}}{\text{kg}} = 2.94 \times 10^{-5} \frac{\text{C}}{\text{kg}} = 29.4 \frac{\mu\text{C}}{\text{kg}}.$$

In traditional units, exposure measured in R that corresponds to 1 Gy air kerma is

$$1 \text{ Gy (air kerma)} = 0.02941 \frac{\text{C}}{\text{kg}} \times 3881 \frac{\text{R}}{\text{C/kg}} = 114 \text{ R}$$

$$1 \text{ mGy (air kerma)} = 114 \text{ mR}.$$

Thus, to convert a measurement in the traditional units of roentgens, we divide the roentgen measurement by 114 to obtain the equivalent exposure in air kerma. Because of the differences between the energy absorption of air and soft tissue, an exposure of 1 mGy air kerma leads to a soft tissue absorbed dose of 1 mGy, or 100 mrads.

EXAMPLE 6.9

The NCRP recommends 0.1 mGy air kerma in 1 week as the shielding design criterion for limiting occupational exposure to medical X-rays. What is the corresponding weekly exposure limit in units of

   (a) mR?

   (b) $\dfrac{\mu C}{kg}$?

Solution

   (a) $0.1 \text{ mGy air kerma} \times 114 \dfrac{mR}{mGy} = 11.4 \text{ mR in 1 week.}$

   (b) $0.1 \text{ mGy air kerma} \times 29.4 \dfrac{\mu C/kg}{mGy} \text{ air kerma} = 2.94 \dfrac{\mu C}{kg}$ in 1 week.

   Kerma decreases continuously with increasing depth in an absorbing medium because of the continuous decrease in the flux of the indirectly ionizing radiation. The absorbed dose, however, is initially less at the surface of an absorbing medium than below the surface. It increases as electronic equilibrium is approached and the ionization density increases due to the increasing number of secondary ions produced by the primary ionizing particles (the positron–electron pairs, Compton electrons, and photoelectrons in the case of photon beams and scattered nuclei in the case of fast neutrons). This increase in absorbed dose continues until a maximum is reached, after which the absorbed dose decreases with continuing increase in depth. The maximum absorbed dose occurs at a depth approximately equal to the maximum range of the primary ionizing particles. The relation between kerma and dose for photon radiation and for fast neutrons is shown in Figure 6-7.

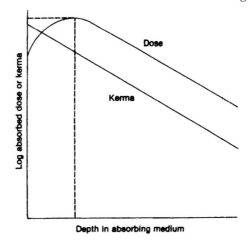

Figure 6-7.   Relation between kerma and absorbed dose for photon radiation and for fast neutrons.

For reasons discussed in Chapter 7, for health physics purposes, the air kerma is called a *sievert* (Sv) in SI units and a *rem* in traditional units (1 Sv = 100 rems).

Source Strength: Specific Gamma-Ray Emission

The radiation intensity from any given gamma-ray source is used as a measure of the strength of the source. The gamma-radiation exposure rate from a point source of unit activity at unit distance is called the *specific gamma-ray constant* and is given in units of sieverts per hour at 1 m from a 1-MBq point source (or, in the traditional system, roentgen per hour at 1 m from a 1-Ci point source). The source strength may be calculated if the decay scheme of the isotope is known. In the case of ^{131}I, for example, whose gamma rays are shown in Figure 4-7 and whose corresponding true absorption coefficients are found in Figure 5-20, we have the following:

MeV/PHOTON	PHOTONS/TRANSFORMATION	μ (ENERGY ABSORPTION), m^{-1}
0.723	0.016	3.8×10^{-3}
0.673	0.069	3.9×10^{-3}
0.503	0.003	3.8×10^{-3}
0.326	0.002	3.8×10^{-3}
0.177	0.002	3.4×10^{-3}
0.365	0.853	3.8×10^{-3}
0.284	0.051	3.7×10^{-3}
0.080	0.051	3.2×10^{-3}
0.164	0.006	3.3×10^{-3}

The gamma-radiation exposure level, in Sv/h (Gy/h air kerma), is calculated by considering the energy absorbed per unit mass of air at the specified distance from the 1-MBq point source due to the photon flux at that distance, as shown in Eq. (6.15). For a distance of 1 m from the point source, we have

$$\dot{X} = \frac{f \, \dfrac{\text{photons}}{t} \times E \, \dfrac{\text{MeV}}{\text{photon}} \times 1.6 \times 10^{-13} \dfrac{\text{J}}{\text{MeV}} \times 1 \times 10^{6} \dfrac{\text{tps}}{\text{MBq}} \times 3.6 \times 10^{3} \dfrac{\text{s}}{\text{h}} \times \dfrac{\mu}{\text{m}}}{4\pi \, (1 \text{ m})^{2} \times \rho \, \dfrac{\text{kg}}{\text{m}^{3}} \times 34 \dfrac{\text{J/kg}}{\text{C/kg}}}$$

$$(6.15)$$

where

$\dot{X} =$ exposure rate, Sv/h (air kerma),
$f =$ fraction of transformations that result in a photon of energy E,
$E =$ photon energy, MeV,
$\mu =$ linear energy absorption coefficient, m^{-1},
$\rho =$ density of air, kg/m^{3}, and
$d =$ distance from the source, m.

This calculation is made for each different quantum energy and the results are summed to obtain the source strength. For the 0.080-MeV gamma ray, at a distance of 1 m, we have

$$\dot{X} = \frac{5.1 \times 10^{-2} \times 8 \times 10^{-2} \times 1.6 \times 10^{-13} \times 1 \times 10^{6} \times 3.6 \times 10^{3} \times 3.2 \times 10^{-3}}{4\pi \, (1)^{2} \times 1.293 \times 1 \times 1}$$

$$= 4.628 \times 10^{-10} \frac{\text{Sv}}{\text{h}} \text{ (air kerma).}$$

The exposure rate for each of the other quanta emitted by ^{131}I is calculated in a similar manner, except that the corresponding frequency and absorption coefficient is used for each of the quanta of different energy. The results of this calculation are tabulated below:

PHOTON ENERGY (MeV)	Sv/h at 1m
0.723	1.558×10^{-9}
0.637	6.048×10^{-9}
0.503	0.203×10^{-9}
0.326	0.088×10^{-9}
0.177	0.043×10^{-9}
0.365	41.960×10^{-9}
0.284	18.930×10^{-9}
0.080	46.280×10^{-9}
0.164	0.116×10^{-9}
	$\sum = 1.152 \times 10^{-7} \dfrac{\text{Sv - m}^2}{\text{MBq - h}}$

Equation (6.15) contains several constants: 1×10^{6} tps/MBq, 3.6×10^{3} s/h, 1.6×10^{-13} J/MeV, 4π (1 m)^{2}, and 1.293 kg/m^{3}. If all these constants are combined, the source strength Γ, in Sv air kerma per MBq per hour at 1 m, is given by

$$\Gamma = 3.54 \times 10^{-5} \sum_{i} f_i \times E_i \times \mu_i \, \frac{\text{Sv-m}^2}{\text{MBq-h}}. \tag{6.16a}$$

where

f_i = fraction of the transformations that yield a photon of the ith energy,
E_i = energy of the ith photon, MeV, and
μ_i = linear energy absorption coefficient in air of the ith photon.

For many practical purposes, Eq. (6.16a) may be simplified. For quantum energies from about 60 keV to about 2 MeV, Figure 5-20 shows that the linear energy absorption coefficient varies little with energy; over this range, μ is about 3.5×10^{-3} m^{-1}. With this value, Eq. (6.16) may be approximated as

$$\Gamma = 1.24 \times 10^{-7} \sum f_i \times E_i \, \frac{\text{Sv-m}^2}{\text{MBq-h}}. \tag{6.16b}$$

If we divide Eq. (6.16b) by 34 Sv per C/kg, we obtain the specific gamma ray emission in exposure units:

$$\Gamma = \frac{1.24 \times 10^{-7}}{34 \dfrac{\text{Sv air kerma}}{\text{C/kg}}} \sum_i f_i \times E_i \; \frac{(\text{ Sv air kerma}) \text{-} \text{m}^2}{\text{MBq - h}}$$

$$\hspace{2cm} \text{(6.17)}$$

$$= 3.65 \times 10^{-9} \sum_i f_i \times E_i \; \frac{(\text{C/kg}) - \text{m}^2}{\text{MBq-h}}.$$

When exposure is measured in roentgens and activity in curies, the specific gamma-ray emission is closely approximated by

$$\Gamma = 0.5 \sum_i f_i \times E_i \; \frac{\text{R - m}^2}{\text{Ci - h}} \hspace{2cm} \text{(6.18)}$$

Table 6-3 lists the specific gamma ray emission of some isotopes that are frequently encountered by health physicists.

Beta Radiation

Examination of a beta-particle absorption curve, such as the one in Figure 5-2, shows it to be approximately linear when plotted on semilog paper. This means that the decrease in beta intensity with increasing depth into an absorbing medium, for depths less than the beta range, can be approximated by

$$\varphi = \varphi_0 e^{-\mu_\beta t}, \hspace{2cm} \text{(6.19)}$$

TABLE 6-3. Specific Gamma-Ray Emission Constant of Some Radioisotopes

ISOTOPE	Γ $\dfrac{\text{R-m}^2}{\text{Ci-h}}$	Air kerma $\left(\dfrac{\text{Sv-m}^2}{\text{MBq-h}}\right)$
Antimony-122	0.24	5.68E−08
Cesium-137	0.33	7.82E−08
Chromium-51	0.016	3.77E−09
Cobalt-60	1.32	3.13E−07
Gold-198	0.23	5.44E−08
Iodine-125	0.07	1.66E−08
Iodine-131	0.22	5.20E−08
Indium-192	0.48	1.14E−07
Iron-59	0.64	1.52E−07
Mercury-203	0.13	3.08E−08
Potassium-42	0.14	4.73E−08
Radium-226	0.825	1.96E−07
Sodium-22	1.20	2.84E−07
Sodium-24	1.84	4.35E−07
Zinc-65	0.27	6.39E−08

From *Radiological Health Handbook*. Rev ed. Rockville, MD: US Public Health Service, Bureau of Radiological Health; 1970.

where

φ = intensity at depth t,
φ_0 = initial intensity, and
μ_β = beta absorption coefficient.

If the maximum beta energy E_m is given in MeV, then the beta absorption coefficients for air and for tissue are

$$\mu_{\beta_a} \,(\text{air}) = 16 \,(E_m - 0.036)^{-1.4} \,\frac{\text{cm}^2}{\text{g}} \tag{6.20}$$

and

$$\mu_{\beta,t} \,(\text{tissue}) = 18.6 \,(E_m - 0.036)^{-1.37} \,\frac{\text{cm}^2}{\text{g}}. \tag{6.21}$$

Skin Contamination

When we refer to "skin dose", or to "shallow dose", we mean the dose to the viable, actively growing basal cells in the basement membrane of the skin. These cells are covered by a tissue layer of nonliving cells whose nominal thickness is 0.007 g/cm^2.

If the skin is contaminated with a radionuclide, we can calculate the dose rate to the contaminated tissue by assuming that 50% of the radiation goes down into the skin and 50% goes up and leaves the skin. If the skin is contaminated at a level of 1 Bq/cm^2 and the mean beta energy is $\bar{E}$ MeV, then the energy fluence rate, φ_b, to the basal cells at a depth of 0.007 g/cm^2 in the skin is

$$\varphi_b, \text{J/cm}^2/\text{h} = 1 \text{ Bq/cm}^2 \times 1 \text{ tps/Bq} \times 0.5 \times \bar{E} \text{ MeV/t} \times 1.6 \times 10^{-13} \text{ J/MeV}$$
$$\times 3.6 \times 10^3 \,\frac{\text{s}}{\text{h}} \times e^{-(\mu_{\beta,t} \text{ cm}^2/\text{g} \times 0.007 \text{ g/cm}^2)}. \tag{6.22}$$

The dose rate to the basal cells, $\dot{D}_b$, is

$$\dot{D}_b = \frac{\varphi_b \,\dfrac{\text{J}}{\text{cm}^2/\text{h}} \times \mu_{\beta,t} \,\dfrac{\text{cm}^2}{\text{g}}}{10^{-6} \,\dfrac{\text{J/g}}{\text{mGy}}} \,\frac{\text{mGy}}{\text{h}}. \tag{6.23}$$

After substituting Eq. (6.22) into Eq. (6.23) and simplifying, we have

$$\dot{D}_b = 2.9 \times 10^{-4} \bar{E} \times \mu_{\beta,t} \times e^{-(\mu_{\beta,t} \times 0.007)} \,\frac{\text{mGy}}{\text{h}}. \tag{6.24}$$

EXAMPLE 6.10

A worker accidentally spills 3700 Bq (10 μCi) of a ^{32}P solution over an area of 10 cm^2 on her skin. What is the dose rate to the contaminated skin?

For ^{32}P:
$E_m = 1.71$ MeV and
$\bar{E} = 0.7$ MeV.

Solution

For ^{32}P, the absorption coefficient for tissue is calculated from Eq. (6.21):

$$\mu_{\beta,t} \text{ (tissue)} = 18.6\,(E_m - 0.036)^{-1.37} = 18.6(1.71 - 0.036)^{-1.37} = 9.18\frac{cm^2}{g}.$$

Substituting the values for $\bar{E}$ and for $\mu_{\beta,t}$ into Eq. (6.24), which gives the dose rate from 1 Bq/cm^2, yields the dose conversion factor (DCF) for skin contamination with ^{32}P:

$$\text{DCF } (^{32}\text{P, skin}) = 1.74 \times 10^{-3}\frac{mGy/h}{Bq/cm^2}.$$

The dose rate to the contaminated skin, therefore, is

$$\dot{D},\ \frac{mGy}{h} = \text{DCF}\ \frac{mGy/h}{Bq/cm^2} \times C_a\ \frac{Bq}{cm^2}. \tag{6.25}$$

$$\dot{D} = 1.74 \times 10^{-3}\frac{mGy/h}{Bq/cm^2} \times \frac{3.7 \times 10^3\ Bq}{10\ cm^2} = 0.64\ \frac{mGy}{h}\ \left(64\ \frac{mrads}{h}\right).$$

Dose from Surface Contamination

If we have a plane beta-emitting surface, such as a contaminated area, then the surface dose rate may be easily calculated. If the surface concentration is C_a Bq per cm^2, then we may assume that 50% of the betas go up from the surface and 50% go down into the surface. Furthermore, some of the downward directed betas are backscattered. Under these conditions, the energy fluence rate at the contaminated surface, $\varphi_0(E)$, is

$$\varphi_0\ \frac{J/cm^2}{h} = C_a\ \frac{Bq}{cm^2} \times 1\ \frac{tps}{Bq} \times 0.5 \times f_b \times \bar{E}\ \frac{MeV}{t}$$

$$\times 1.6 \times 10^{-13}\ \frac{J}{MeV} \times 3.6 \times 10^3\ \frac{s}{h}. \tag{6.26}$$

Assuming that 25% of the beta energy is backscattered, then $f_b = 1.25$ and Eq. (6.26) simplifies to

$$\varphi_0 = 3.6 \times 10^{-10} \times C_a \times \bar{E} \; \frac{\text{J/cm}^2}{\text{h}}. \tag{6.27}$$

At a height d above the center of the contaminated surface, the beta energy flux will be reduced by the thickness of air d and will be closely approximated by

$$\varphi_d = \varphi_0 \times e^{-(\mu_{\beta,a} \times d)} \; \frac{\text{J/cm}^2}{\text{h}} \qquad \text{for } d < \text{range of the betas} \tag{6.28}$$

$$= 3.6 \times 10^{-10} \times C_a \times \bar{E} \times e^{-(\mu_{\beta,a} \times d)} \; \frac{\text{J/cm}^2}{\text{h}}. \tag{6.29}$$

The energy fluence rate to the basal cells will be further reduced by the shielding effect of 0.007 g/cm^2 of nonviable surface skin. Therefore, the energy flux φ_b to the basal cells is

$$\varphi_b = \varphi_d \times e^{-(\mu_{\beta,t} \text{ cm}^2/\text{g} \times 0.007 \text{ g/cm}^2)} \; \frac{\text{J/cm}^2}{\text{h}}. \tag{6.30}$$

Substituting Eq. (6.29) for φ_d into Eq. (6.30), we have

$$\varphi_b = 3.6 \times 10^{-10} \times C_a \times \bar{E} \times \exp -(\mu_{\beta,a} \times d) \times e^{-(\mu_{\beta,t} \times 0.007)} \; \frac{\text{J/cm}^2}{\text{h}}. \tag{6.31}$$

The dose rate to the basal cells in mGy/h, at a height $d \text{ g/cm}^2$ above a contaminated area, is

$$\dot{D}_b, \text{ mGy/h} = \frac{\varphi_b \dfrac{\text{J/cm}^2}{\text{h}} \times \mu_{\beta,t} \dfrac{\text{cm}^2}{\text{g}}}{10^{-6} \dfrac{\text{J/g}}{\text{mGy}}}, \tag{6.32}$$

which yields, after we substitute Eq. (6.31) for φ_b in Eq. (6.32),

$$\dot{D}_b = \frac{3.6 \times 10^{-10} \times C_a \times \bar{E} \times e^{-(\mu_{\beta,a} \times d)} \times e^{-(\mu_{\beta,t} \times 0.007)} \times \mu_{\beta,t}}{10^{-6} \dfrac{\text{J/g}}{\text{mGy}}}. \tag{6.33a}$$

After dividing by $10^{-6} \dfrac{\text{J/g}}{\text{mGy}}$, we have

$$\dot{D}_b = 3.6 \times 10^{-4} \times C_a \times \bar{E} \times e^{-(\mu_{\beta,a} \times d)} \times e^{-(\mu_{\beta,t} \times 0.007)} \times \mu_{\beta,t} \; \frac{\text{mGy}}{\text{h}}. \tag{6.33b}$$

EXAMPLE 6.11

A solution of ^{32}P is spilled and it contaminates a large surface to an areal concentration of 37 $\dfrac{\text{Bq}}{\text{cm}^2}$. What is the estimated beta dose rate to the skin at a height of 1 m above the contaminated area? Temperature in the laboratory is 27°C. (Neglect shielding by clothing.)

For ^{32}P:

$$\text{Range} = (0.542 \times 1.71) - 0.133 = 0.8\,\frac{\text{g}}{\text{cm}^2},$$

$$E_m = 1.71 \text{ MeV},$$

$$\bar{E} = 0.7 \text{MeV},$$

$$\text{Air density at } 27°\text{C} = 1.293 \times 10^{-3} \times (273 \div 300) = 1.2 \times 10^{-3} \text{ g/cm}^3, \text{ and}$$

$$d = 100 \text{ cm} \times 1.2 \times 10^{-3} \text{ g/cm}^3 = 0.12 \text{ g/cm}^2.$$

The beta absorption coefficient in tissue was calculated in example 6.10 and was found to be 9.18 cm^2/g. For air, the beta absorption coefficient is calculated by substituting 1.71 for the value of E_m in Eq. (6.20):

$$\mu_{\beta,a} = 16(1.71 - 0.036)^{-1.4}\,\frac{\text{cm}^2}{\text{g}} = 7.78\,\frac{\text{cm}^2}{\text{g}}.$$

The dose rate to the skin at 1 m above the contaminated area is calculated with Eq. (6.33b):

$$\dot{D}_b = 3.6 \times 10^{-4} \times C_a \times \bar{E} \times e^{-\mu_{\beta,a} \times d} \times e^{-\mu_{\beta,t} \times 0.007} \times \mu_{\beta,t} \frac{\text{mGy}}{\text{h}}$$

$$= 3.6 \times 10^{-4} \times 37 \times 0.7 \times e^{-7.78 \times 0.12} \times e^{-9.18 \times 0.007} \times 9.18$$

$$= 3.2 \times 10^{-2}\,\frac{\text{mGy}}{\text{h}}\,(3.2\,\frac{\text{mrads}}{\text{h}}).$$

In the traditional system of units, if the contamination concentration is given as $\mu\text{Ci/cm}^2$ and dose rate is measured in $\dfrac{\text{mrads}}{\text{h}}$ at a height $d\,\dfrac{\text{g}}{\text{cm}^2}$ above a large contaminated area, Eq. (6.33b) becomes

$$\dot{D}_b = 1.3 \times 10^3 \times C_a \times \bar{E} \times e^{-\mu_{\beta,a} \times d} \times e^{-\mu_{\beta,t} \times 0.007} \times \mu_{\beta,t} \frac{\text{mrads}}{\text{h}}. \tag{6.34}$$

Submersion Dose

Inside an infinite cloud of a radionuclide

rate of energy emission = rate of energy absorption.

In an infinite cloud containing C Bq/m^3 of a beta emitter whose mean beta energy is $\bar{E}$ MeV, the dose rate is

$\dot{D}_\infty(\text{air}), \text{mGy/h}$

$$= \frac{C\dfrac{\text{Bq}}{\text{m}^3} \times 1\dfrac{\text{tps}}{\text{Bq}} \times \bar{E}\dfrac{\text{MeV}}{\text{t}} \times 1.6 \times 10^{-13}\dfrac{\text{J}}{\text{MeV}} \times 3.6 \times 10^3\dfrac{\text{s}}{\text{h}}}{1.293\dfrac{\text{kg}}{\text{m}^3} \times 1\dfrac{\text{J/kg}}{\text{Gy}} \times \dfrac{1\,\text{Gy}}{10^3\,\text{mGy}}}. \tag{6.35}$$

When we combine the constants in Eq. (6.35), we have

$$\dot{D}_\infty(\text{air}) = 4.45 \times 10^{-7} \times C_a \times \bar{E} \text{ mGy/h}. \tag{6.36}$$

Since the skin of a person in an infinite medium is irradiated from one side only, and since soft tissue absorbs about 10% more energy per kilogram than air does, the dose rate to the basal cells of the skin in a semi-infinite medium is

$$\dot{D}_b = 0.5 \times 1.1 \times \dot{D}_\infty(\text{air}) \times e^{-(\mu_{\beta,t} \times 0.007)}. \tag{6.37}$$

If we combine Eqs. (6.36) and (6.37), we have the beta dose to the skin of a person immersed in a large cloud of concentration C Bq/m^3:

$$\dot{D}_b = 2.45 \times 10^{-7} \times C \times \bar{E} \times e^{-(\mu_{\beta,t} \times 0.007)} \text{ mGy/h}. \tag{6.38}$$

Generally, if there are f_i betas of average energy $\bar{E}_i$ MeV whose absorption coefficient is $\mu_{\beta_i,t}$ each, then the beta dose rate is

$$\dot{D}_b = 2.45 \times 10^{-7} \times C \sum_i f_i \bar{E}_i \times e^{-(\mu_{\beta_i,t} \times 0.007)} \frac{\text{mGy}}{\text{h}}, \tag{6.39}$$

and if we divide by the concentration C, we obtain DCF:

$$\text{DCF (submersion)} = 2.45 \times 10^{-7} \times \sum_i f_i \bar{E}_i \times e^{-(\mu_{\beta_i,t} \times 0.007)} \frac{\text{mGy/h}}{\text{Bq/m}^3}. \tag{6.40}$$

EXAMPLE 6.12

Calculate the dose rate to the skin of a person immersed in a large cloud of ^{85}Kr at a concentration of 37 kBq/m^3 (10^{-6} μCi/mL).

Solution

Krypton-85 is a pure beta emitter that is transformed to ^{85}Rb by the emission of a beta particle whose maximum energy is 0.672 MeV and whose average energy is 0.246 MeV. The tissue absorption coefficient is calculated with Eq. (6.21):

$$\mu_{\beta,t} = 18.6(0.672 - 0.036)^{-1.37} = 34.6 \text{ cm}^2/\text{g},$$

and the skin dose is calculated with Eq. (6.38):

$$\dot{D}_b = 2.45 \times 10^{-7} \times C \times \bar{E} \times e^{-(\mu_{\beta,t} \times 0.007)} \text{ mGy/h}$$

$$\dot{D}_b = 2.45 \times 10^{-7} \times 3.7 \times 10^4 \times 0.246 \times e^{-(34.6 \times 0.007)}$$

$$\dot{D}_b = 1.8 \times 10^{-3} \text{ mGy/h} \ (0.18 \text{ mrads/h}).$$

In the traditional system of units, if the concentration is given in μCi/mL, Eqs. (6.39) and (6.40) become

$$\dot{D}_b = 9 \times 10^5 \times C \sum_i f_i \bar{E}_i \times e^{-(\mu_{\beta_i, t} \times 0.007)} \text{ mrads/h} \qquad (6.39a)$$

and

$$\text{DCF (submersion)} = 9 \times 10^5 \times \sum_i f_i \bar{E}_i \times e^{-(\mu_{\beta_i, t} \times 0.007)} \frac{\text{mrads/h}}{\mu\text{Ci/mL}}. \qquad (6.40a)$$

Volume Source

In an infinitely thick (thickness $\geq$ beta range) volume source, the rate of energy emission is equal to the rate of energy absorption. If C_v Bq/kg is the concentration of a beta emitter whose mean energy is $\bar{E}$ MeV/beta, then the dose rate inside the infinite volume is given by

$\dot{D}_{\infty v}$, mGy/h

$$= \frac{C_v \dfrac{\text{Bq}}{\text{kg}} \times 1 \dfrac{\text{tps}}{\text{Bq}} \times \bar{E} \dfrac{\text{MeV}}{t} \times 1.6 \times 10^{-13} \dfrac{\text{J}}{\text{MeV}} \times 3.6 \times 10^3 \dfrac{\text{s}}{\text{h}}}{10^{-3} \dfrac{\text{J/kg}}{\text{mGy}}} \qquad (6.41)$$

$$\dot{D}_{\infty v} = 5.76 \times 10^{-7} \times C_v \times \bar{E} \text{ mGy/h}. \qquad (6.42)$$

Since the surface of an "infinitely thick" volume source is irradiated from one side only, the dose rate at the surface is

$$\dot{D}_{\text{surf.}\infty v} = \frac{1}{2} \times \dot{D}_{\infty v} = 2.88 \times 10^{-7} \times C_v \times \bar{E} \text{ mGy/h}. \qquad (6.43)$$

If there are f_i betas per transformation of $\bar{E}_i$ MeV each, then

$$\dot{D}_{\text{surf.}\infty v} = 2.88 \times 10^{-7} \times C_v \times \sum f_i \bar{E}_i \frac{\text{mGy}}{\text{h}}. \qquad (6.44)$$

In traditional units, if C_v is in μCi/g, then Eq. (6.44) is transformed to

$$\dot{D}_{\text{surf.}\infty v} = 1.1 \times 10^3 \times C_v \times \sum f_i \bar{E}_i \frac{\text{mrads}}{\text{h}}. \qquad (6.44a)$$

EXAMPLE 6.13

A 5-L polypropylene (specific gravity $= 0.95$) bottle, 3-mm wall thickness, contains 5 mCi (185 MBq) ^{32}P aqueous waste. Calculate the beta dose rate at the outside surface of the bottle.

Solution

Phosphorus-32 is transformed to ^{32}S by the emission of a beta particle whose maximum energy is 1.7 MeV and whose average energy is 0.7 MeV. Since the solution is infinitely thick relative to the range of the beta particles, the dose rate at the liquid-wall interface is calculated with Eq. (6.44a):

$$\dot{D}_{\text{surf.}\infty v} = 1.1 \times 10^3 \times C_v \times \sum f_i \bar{E}_i \ \frac{\text{mrads}}{\text{h}}$$

$$\dot{D}_{\text{surf.},\infty v} = 1.1 \times 10^3 \times \frac{5 \times 10^3 \mu\text{Ci}}{5 \times 10^3 \text{g}} \times 0.7 \,\text{MeV}$$

$$= 770 \ \frac{\text{mrads}}{\text{h}} \left(7.7 \ \frac{\text{mGy}}{\text{h}}\right).$$

The wall will attenuate the beta dose rate according to Eq. (6.19):

$$\varphi = \varphi_0 e^{-\mu_\beta t}.$$

In this case, the wall thickness is 0.285 g/cm^2, and $\mu_\beta = 9.18$ cm^2/g (from Example 6.10), and we have

$$\dot{D}_\beta = 770 \times e^{-9.18 \times 0.285} = 56 \text{ mrads/h } (0.56 \,\text{mGy/h}).$$

INTERNALLY DEPOSITED RADIONUCLIDES

Corpuscular Radiation

Radiation dose from internal emitters cannot be measured directly; it can only be calculated. The calculated dose is based on both physical and biological factors. The physical factors include the type and energy of the radiation and the radiological half-life. The biological factors include the distribution of the radioisotope within the body and the kinetic behavior, such as absorption rates, turnover rates, and retention times in the various organs and tissues. The biological factors for internal dosimetry are derived from pharmacologically based biokinetic models of the in vivo behavior of the radioisotopes.

The calculation of the absorbed dose from internally deposited radioisotopes follows directly from the definition of the gray. For an infinitely large medium containing a uniformly distributed radionuclide, the concentration of absorbed energy must be equal to the concentration of energy emitted. The energy absorbed per unit tissue mass per transformation is called the *specific effective energy* (*SEE*). For practical health physics purposes, "infinitely large" may be approximated by a tissue mass whose dimensions exceed the range of the radiation from the distributed isotope. For the case of alpha and most beta radiations, this condition is easily met in practice, and the *SEE* is simply the average energy of the radiation divided by the mass of the tissue in which it is distributed:

$$SEE(\alpha \text{ or } \beta) = \frac{\bar{E}}{m}\frac{\text{MeV/t}}{\text{kg}}. \tag{6.45}$$

The computation of the radiation-absorbed dose from a uniformly distributed beta emitter within a tissue may be illustrated with the following example:

EXAMPLE 6.14

Calculate the daily dose rate to a testis that weighs 18 g and has 6660 Bq of ^{35}S uniformly distributed throughout the organ.

Solution

Sulfur is a pure beta emitter whose maximum-energy beta particle is 0.1674 MeV and whose average energy is 0.0488 MeV. The beta dose rate from q Bq uniformly dispersed in m kg of tissue, if the specific effective energy is *SEE* MeV per transformation per kg, is

$$\dot{D}_\beta, \frac{\text{Gy}}{\text{d}}$$

$$= \frac{q\text{Bq} \times 1\,\frac{\text{tps}}{\text{Bq}} \times SEE\,\frac{\text{MeV/t}}{\text{kg}} \times 1.6 \times 10^{-13}\,\frac{\text{J}}{\text{MeV}} \times 8.64 \times 10^4\,\frac{\text{s}}{\text{d}}}{1\,\frac{\text{J/kg}}{\text{Gy}}}. \tag{6.46}$$

Substituting Eq. (6.45) into Eq. (6.46) yields

$$\dot{D}_\beta = \frac{q\text{Bq} \times 1\,\frac{\text{tps}}{\text{Bq}} \times \bar{E}\,\frac{\text{MeV}}{\text{t}} \times 1.6 \times 10^{-13}\,\frac{\text{J}}{\text{MeV}} \times 8.64 \times 10^4\,\frac{\text{s}}{\text{d}}}{m\,\text{kg} \times 1\,\text{J/kg/Gy}}$$

$$= \frac{6.66 \times 10^3 \times 1 \times 4.88 \times 10^{-2} \times 1.6 \times 10^{-13} \times 8.64 \times 10^4}{0.018 \times 1}$$

$$= 2.5 \times 10^{-4}\,\frac{\text{Gy}}{\text{d}}\left(0.025\,\frac{\text{rad}}{\text{d}}\right). \tag{6.47}$$

Effective Half-Life

The total dose absorbed during any given time interval after the deposition of the sulfur in the testis (in Example 6.14) may be calculated by integrating the dose rate over the required time interval. In making this calculation, two factors must be considered, namely:

(1.) in situ radioactive decay of the radionuclide and
(2.) biological elimination rate of the radionuclide.

In most instances, biological elimination follows first-order kinetics. In this case, the equation for the quantity of radioactive material within an organ at any time t after deposition of a quantity Q_0 is given by

$$Q = \left(Q_0 e^{-\lambda_R t}\right)\left(e^{-\lambda_B t}\right), \tag{6.48}$$

where λ_R is the radioactive decay constant and λ_B is the biological elimination constant. The two exponentials in Eq. (6.48) may be combined

$$Q = Q_0 e^{-(\lambda_R + \lambda_B)t}, \tag{6.49}$$

and, if

$$\lambda_E = \lambda_R + \lambda_B, \tag{6.50}$$

we have

$$Q = Q_0 e^{-\lambda_E t} \tag{6.51}$$

where λ_E is called the *effective* elimination constant. The effective half-life is then

$$T_E = \frac{0.693}{\lambda_E}. \tag{6.52}$$

From the relationship among λ_E, λ_R, and λ_B, we have

$$\frac{1}{T_E} = \frac{1}{T_R} + \frac{1}{T_B}, \tag{6.53}$$

or

$$T_E = \frac{T_R \times T_B}{T_R + T_B}. \tag{6.54}$$

In Example 6.14, for ^{35}S, $T_R = 87.1$ days. T_B, the biological half-life in the testis, is reported to be 623 days. The effective half-life in the testis, therefore, is

$$T_E = \frac{87.1 \times 623}{87.1 + 623} = 76.4 \text{ days},$$

and the effective elimination rate constant is

$$\lambda_E = \frac{0.693}{76.4 \text{ days}} = 0.009 \text{ d}^{-1}.$$

It should be noted that the effective half-life of ^{35}S in the testis is less than either the radiological or the biological half-lives. This must be so because the quantity of a radionuclide in the body is continually decreasing due to radioactive decay and biological elimination. For this reason, the effective half-life can never be greater than the shorter of either the biological or radiological half-life.

Total Dose: Dose Commitment

The dose dD during an infinitesimally small period of time dt at a time interval t after an initial dose rate $\dot{D}_0$ is

$$dD = \text{instantaneous dose rate} \times dt.$$

$$= \dot{D}_0 \times e^{-\lambda_E t} dt. \tag{6.55}$$

The total dose during a time interval t after deposition of the radionuclide is

$$D = \dot{D}_0 \int_0^t e^{-\lambda_E t} dt, \tag{6.56}$$

which, when integrated, yields

$$D = \frac{\dot{D}_0}{\lambda_E} \left(1 - e^{-\lambda_E t}\right). \tag{6.57}$$

For an infinitely long time—that is, when the radionuclide is completely gone—Eq. (6.57) reduces to

$$D = \frac{\dot{D}_0}{\lambda_E}. \tag{6.58}$$

For practical purposes, an "infinitely long time" corresponds to about six effective half-lives. It should be noted that the dose due to total decay is merely equal to the product of the initial dose rate $\dot{D}_0$ and the average life of the radionuclide within the organ $1/\lambda_E$. For the case in Example 6.14, the total absorbed dose during the first 5 days after deposition of the radiosulfur in the testis is, according to Eq. (6.57),

$$D = \frac{2.5 \times 10^{-4} \text{ Gy/d}}{0.009 \text{ d}^{-1}} \left(1 - e^{-0.009 \, \text{d}^{-1} \times 5 \, \text{d}}\right)$$

$$= 1.2 \times 10^{-3} \text{Gy} \qquad (0.12 \text{ rad}),$$

and the dose from complete decay is, from Eq. (6.58),

$$D = \frac{2.5 \times 10^{-4} \text{ Gy/d}}{0.009 \text{ d}^{-1}} = 0.028 \text{ Gy} \qquad (2.8 \text{ rads}).$$

The 0.028-Gy total dose absorbed from the deposition of the radiosulfur is called the *dose commitment* to the testes from this incident. This is defined as the absorbed dose from a given practice or from a given exposure. Although the dose commitment in this example was due to an internally deposited radionuclide, the dose commitment concept is applicable to external radiation as well as to radiation from internally deposited radionuclides.

In the example cited above, the testis behaved as if the radionuclide were stored in a single compartment. In many cases, an organ or tissue behaves as if the radioisotope were stored in more than one compartment. Each compartment follows first-order kinetics and is emptied at its own clearance rate. Thus, for example, cesium is found to be uniformly distributed throughout the body, although the body behaves as if the cesium were stored in two compartments. One compartment contains 10% of the total body burden and has a retention half-time of 2 days, while the second compartment contains the other 90% of the body's cesium content and has a clearance half-time of 110 days. The retention curve for cesium, therefore, is given by the equation

$$q(\text{t}) = 0.1 \, q_0 \, e^{-(0.693 \, t/2 \, \text{days})} + 0.9 \, q_0 \, e^{-(0.693 \, t/110 \, \text{days})}, \tag{6.59}$$

where $q(t)$ is the body burden at time t after deposition of q_0 amount of cesium in the body. Ten percent of the total is deposited in compartment 1 and 90% is deposited in compartment 2. Generally, if there is more than one compartment, the body burden at any time t after deposition of q_0 units of a radionuclide is given by

$$q(t) = f_1 q_0 \, e^{-\lambda_1 t} + f_2 q_0 \, e^{-\lambda_2 t} + \cdots + f_n q_0 \, e^{-\lambda_n t}, \tag{6.60}$$

where $f_1, f_2, \ldots, f_n$ = fraction of the total activity deposited in compartments $1, 2, \ldots, n$, and $\lambda_1, \lambda_2, \ldots, \lambda_n$ = effective clearance rates for compartments $1, 2, \ldots, n$.

Since the activity in each compartment contributes to the dose to that organ or tissue, Eq. (6.57) becomes, for the multicompartment case,

$$D = \frac{\dot{D}_{10}}{\lambda_{1E}} \left(1 - e^{-\lambda_{1E} t}\right) + \frac{\dot{D}_{20}}{\lambda_{2E}} \left(1 - e^{-\lambda_{2E} t}\right) + \cdots + \frac{\dot{D}_{n0}}{\lambda_{nE}} \left(1 - e^{-\lambda_{nE} t}\right), \tag{6.61}$$

and when the radionuclide has completely been eliminated, Eq. (6.61) reduces to

$$D(t) = \frac{\dot{D}_{10}}{\lambda_{1E}} + \frac{\dot{D}_{20}}{\lambda_{2E}} + \cdots + \frac{\dot{D}_{n0}}{\lambda_{nE}}. \tag{6.62}$$

Gamma Emitters

For gamma-emitting isotopes, we cannot simply calculate the absorbed dose by assuming the organ to be infinitely large because gammas, being penetrating radiations, may travel great distances within the tissue and leave the tissue without interacting. Thus, only a fraction of the energy carried by photons originating in the radioisotope-containing tissue is absorbed within that tissue. Before the advent of computers that made complex computational methods possible, gamma ray doses from internal radionuclides were calculated by assuming the body to be made of spheres and cylinders and then using simple calculation techniques to determine internal dose. For example, in the case of a uniformly distributed gamma-emitting nuclide, the dose rate at any point p due to the radioactivity in the infinitesimal volume dV at any other point at a distance r from point p, as shown in Figure 6-8, is

$$d\dot{D} = C\Gamma \frac{e^{-\mu r}}{r^2} dV, \tag{6.63}$$

where C is the concentration of the isotope, Γ is the specific gamma-ray emission, and μ is the linear energy absorption coefficient. The dose rate at point p due to all

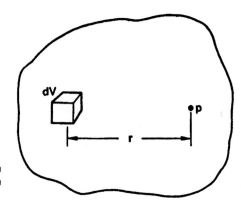

Figure 6-8. Diagram for calculating dose at a point p from the gamma rays emitted from the volume element dV in a tissue mass containing a uniformly distributed radioisotope.

the isotope in the tissue is computed by the contributions from all the infinitesimal volume elements:

$$\dot{D} = C\Gamma \int_{0}^{V} \frac{e^{-\mu r}}{r^2} dV. \tag{6.64}$$

For the case of a sphere, the dose rate at the center (Fig. 6-9) is

$$\dot{D} = 4C\Gamma \int_{r=0}^{r=R} \int_{\theta=0}^{\theta=\pi/2} \int_{\varphi=0}^{\varphi=\pi} \frac{e^{-\mu r}}{r^2} \cdot r\, d\theta \cdot r\cos\theta\, d\varphi \cdot dr. \tag{6.65}$$

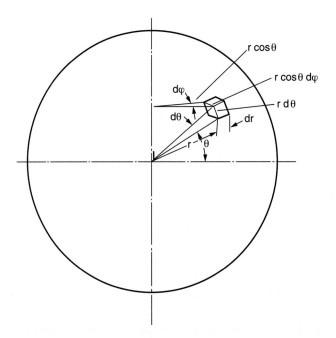

Figure 6-9. Geometry for evaluating Eq. (6.65) for the center of a sphere.

Integrating with respect to each of the variables, we have, for the dose rate at the center of the sphere,

$$\dot{D} = C\Gamma \cdot \frac{4\pi}{\mu} \left(1 - e^{-\mu R}\right). \tag{6.66}$$

From an examination of Eqs. (6.63), (6.64), (6.65), and (6.66) it is seen that the factor that multiplies $C\Gamma$ depends only on the geometry of the tissue mass and hence is called the *geometry factor*.[1] The geometry factor g is defined by

$$g = \int\limits_0^V \frac{e^{-\mu r}}{r^2} dV. \tag{6.67}$$

Equation (6.64) may therefore be rewritten as

$$D = C \times \Gamma \times g. \tag{6.68}$$

The definition of g in Eq. (6.67) applies to a given point within a volume of tissue. In many health physics instances, we are interested in the average dose rate rather than the dose rate at a specific point. For this purpose, we may define an average geometry factor as follows:

$$\bar{g} = \frac{1}{V} \int g \, dV. \tag{6.69}$$

For a sphere,

$$\bar{g} = \frac{3}{4} (g)_{\text{center}}. \tag{6.70}$$

At any other point in the sphere at a distance d from the center, the geometry factor is given by

$$g_{\text{p}} = (g)_{\text{center}} \left[0.5 + \frac{1 - (d/R)^2}{4(d/R)} \ln \frac{1 + d/R}{|1 - d/R|} \right]. \tag{6.71}$$

For a cylinder, the average geometry factor depends on the radius and height. Table 6-4 gives the numerical values of average geometry factors for cylinders of various heights and radii.

---

[1] This material is mainly of historical importance in the evolution of internal dosimetry; it has been replaced by the MIRD system, which is discussed later in this chapter.

TABLE 6-4. Average Geometry Factors for Cylinders Containing a Uniformly Distributed Gamma Emitter

CYLINDER HEIGHT (cm)	RADIUS OF CYLINDER (cm)							
	3	5	10	15	20	25	30	35
2	17.5	22.1	30.3	34.0	36.2	37.5	38.6	39.3
5	22.3	31.8	47.7	56.4	61.6	65.2	67.9	70.5
10	25.1	38.1	61.3	76.1	86.5	93.4	98.4	103
20	25.7	40.5	68.9	89.8	105	117	126	133
30	25.9	41.0	71.3	94.6	112	126	137	146
40	25.9	41.3	72.4	96.5	116	131	143	153
60	26.0	41.6	73.0	97.8	118	134	148	159
80	26.0	41.6	73.3	98.4	119	135	150	161
100	26.0	41.6	73.3	98.5	119	136	150	162

Reproduced with permission from Hine GJ, Brownell GL. *Radiation Dosimetry.* New York, NY: Academic Press, Inc; 1956.

EXAMPLE 6.15

A spherical tank, capacity 1 m^3 and radius 0.62 m, is filled with aqueous ^{137}Cs waste containing a total activity of 37,000 MBq (1 Ci). What is the dose rate at the tank surface if we neglect absorption by the tank wall?

Solution

From Table 6-3 we find $\Gamma = 7.82 \times 10^{-8}$ Sv-m^2/MBq-h. The absorption coefficient of water for the 0.661-MeV gammas from ^{137}Cs is listed (by interpolation between 0.6 and 0.8 MeV) in Table 5.4 as 0.0327 cm^2/g. Since the density of water is 1 g/cm^3, the linear absorption coefficient is 0.0327 cm^{-1}, or 3.27 m^{-1}. The dose rate at the center of the sphere is found by substituting the respective values into Eq. (6.66):

$$\dot{D}_0 = 37 \times 10^3 \, \frac{\text{MBq}}{\text{m}^3} \times 7.82 \times 10^{-8} \, \frac{\text{Sv} \cdot \text{m}^2}{\text{MBq} \cdot \text{h}} \times \frac{4\pi}{3.27 \, \text{m}^{-1}} \left(1 - e^{-3.27 \times 0.62}\right)$$

$$= 9.66 \times 10^{-3} \, \frac{\text{Sv}}{\text{h}} \quad \left(0.966 \, \frac{\text{rem}}{\text{h}}\right).$$

From Eq. (6.71), we see that the surface dose rate is $0.5 \times \dot{D}_0$. Therefore,

$$\dot{D}_{\text{surface}} = 0.5 \times 9.66 \times 10^{-3} = 4.8 \times 10^{-3} \, \frac{\text{Sv}}{\text{h}} \quad \left(0.48 \, \frac{\text{rad}}{\text{h}}\right).$$

Medical Internal Radiation Dose Methodology

To account for the partial absorption of gamma-ray energy in organs and tissues, the Medical Internal Radiation Dose (MIRD) Committee of the Society of Nuclear Medicine developed a formal system for calculating the dose to a "target" organ or tissue (T) from a "source" organ (S) (Fig. 6-10) containing a uniformly distributed radioisotope. S and T may be either the same organ or two different organs bearing any of the possible relationships to each other shown in Figure 6-10. The MIRD system separates the dose calculation into two basic components: the physical factors dealing with the radiation and the fraction of energy radiated by the deposited activity that is absorbed by the tissue, and the biological factors that are derived from physiologically based biokinetic models of the radionuclide. The fraction of the radiated energy that is absorbed by the target tissue is calculated by the application of Monte Carlo methods to the interactions and fate of photons following their emission from the deposited radionuclide.

Monte Carlo methods are useful in the solution of problems where events such as the interaction of photons with matter are governed by probabilistic rather than deterministic laws. In Monte Carlo solutions, individual simulated photons (or other corpuscular radiation) are "followed" in a computer from one interaction to the next. The radioisotope is assumed to be uniformly distributed throughout a given volume of tissue. Since radioactive transformation is a random process occurring at a mean rate that is characteristic of the given radioisotope, we can start the process by randomly initiating a radioactive transformation. For any of these transformations, we know the energy of the emitted radiation, its starting point, and its initial direction. We also know the probability of each possible type of interaction within the organ and the energy transferred during each interaction. A situation is simulated by starting with a very large number of such nuclear transformations, following the history of each particle as it traverses the target tissue, and summing the total amount of energy that the particles dissipate within the target tissue. For a concentration of

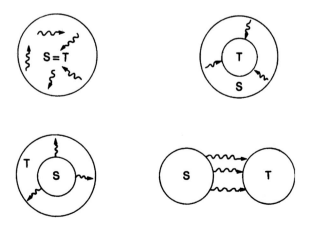

Figure 6-10. Possible relationships between source organ and target organ.

TABLE 6-5. Absorbed Fractions for Uniform Distribution of Activity in Small Spheres[a] and Thick Ellipsoids[a]

MASS (kg)	0.020 (MeV)	0.030 (MeV)	0.040 (MeV)	0.060 (MeV)	0.080 (MeV)	0.100 (MeV)	0.160 (MeV)	0.364 (MeV)	0.662 (MeV)	1.460 (MeV)	2.750 (MeV)
						φ					
0.3	0.684	0.357	0.191	0.109	0.086	0.085	0.087	0.099	0.096	0.092	0.077
0.4	0.712	0.388	0.212	0.121	0.096	0.093	0.097	0.108	0.108	0.099	0.083
0.5	0.731	0.412	0.229	0.131	0.104	0.099	0.104	0.116	0.117	0.104	0.089
0.6	0.745	0.431	0.244	0.140	0.111	0.105	0.111	0.122	0.124	0.109	0.093
1.0	0.780	0.486	0.289	0.167	0.135	0.125	0.130	0.142	0.144	0.125	0.106
2.0	0.818	0.559	0.360	0.212	0.173	0.160	0.162	0.174	0.173	0.153	0.127
3.0	0.840	0.600	0.405	0.245	0.201	0.188	0.186	0.197	0.195	0.174	0.143
4.0	0.856	0.629	0.438	0.271	0.222	0.209	0.205	0.216	0.213	0.190	0.156
5.0	0.868	0.652	0.464	0.294	0.241	0.227	0.222	0.231	0.228	0.204	0.167
6.0	0.876	0.671	0.485	0.312	0.258	0.241	0.236	0.245	0.240	0.216	0.177

[a]The principal axes of the small spheres and thick ellipsoids are in the ratios of 1:1:1 and 1:0.667:1.333.

Reprinted by permission of the Society of Nuclear Medicine from Brownell GL, Ellett WH, Reddy AR. MIRD Pamphlet No. 3: Absorbed Fractions for Photon Dosimetry. *J Nuclear Med.* February 1968; 9(1 Suppl):29–39.

1 Bq/cm^3 of tissue, for example, there would be 1 such start per cm^3/s. Since the sum of the initial energies of these particles is known, the fraction of the emitted energy absorbed by the target tissue, which is called the *absorbed fraction, φ,* can be calculated:

$$\varphi = \frac{\text{energy absorbed by target}}{\text{energy emitted by source}}. \tag{6.72}$$

Since the mean free paths of photons usually are large relative to the dimensions of the organ in which the photon-emitting isotope is distributed, the absorbed fraction for photons is less than 1. For nonpenetrating radiation, the absorbed fraction usually is either 1 or 0, depending on whether the source and target organs are the same or different.

Absorbed fractions for photons of various energies for point isotropic sources and for uniformly distributed sources in tissue and in water for spheres, cylinders, and ellipsoids have been calculated and published by MIRD in several supplements to the *Journal of Nuclear Medicine.* Tables 6-5 to 6-7 show some of these absorbed fractions.

TABLE 6-6. Absorbed Fractions for Central Point Sources in Right Circular Cylinders[a]

MASS (kg)	0.040 (MeV)	0.080 (MeV)	0.160 (MeV)	0.364 (MeV)	0.662 (MeV)	1.460 (MeV)
2	0.528	0.258	0.224	0.240	0.229	0.200
4	0.645	0.336	0.290	0.295	0.288	0.253
6	0.712	0.391	0.335	0.333	0.326	0.286
8	0.757	0.435	0.370	0.363	0.354	0.311
10	0.789	0.471	0.399	0.387	0.376	0.332
20	0.878	0.593	0.501	0.472	0.453	0.401
30	0.917	0.668	0.568	0.528	0.504	0.446
40	0.940	0.721	0.618	0.571	0.543	0.480
50	0.954	0.761	0.658	0.605	0.575	0.509
60	0.964	0.792	0.691	0.633	0.602	0.533
70	0.971	0.818	0.719	0.658	0.625	0.553
80	0.977	0.838	0.743	0.679	0.646	0.572
90	0.981	0.856	0.763	0.698	0.664	0.588
100	0.984	0.871	0.781	0.714	0.680	0.603
120	0.989	0.894	0.811	0.742	0.708	0.629
140	0.992	0.911	0.834	0.765	0.730	0.651
160	0.994	0.924	0.852	0.784	0.749	0.669
180	0.994	0.933	0.866	0.800	0.765	0.685
200	0.994	0.939	0.877	0.813	0.777	0.698

[a]The principal axes of the right circular cylinders are in the ratio of 1:1:0.75.

Reprinted by permission of the Society of Nuclear Medicine from Brownell GL, Ellett WH, Reddy AR. MIRD Pamphlet No. 3: Absorbed Fractions for Photon Dosimetry. *J Nuclear Med.* February 1968; 9(1 Suppl):29–39.

TABLE 6-7. Absorbed Fractions for Central Point Sources in Spheres

MASS (kg)	φ									
	0.020 (MeV)	0.030 (MeV)	0.040 (MeV)	0.060 (MeV)	0.100 (MeV)	0.140 (MeV)	0.160 (MeV)	0.279 (MeV)	0.662 (MeV)	2.750 (MeV)
2	0.989	0.794	0.537	0.322	0.243	0.233	0.234	0.241	0.235	0.168
4	0.996	0.878	0.658	0.421	0.317	0.301	0.297	0.302	0.293	0.209
6	0.999	0.916	0.727	0.488	0.370	0.348	0.342	0.344	0.330	0.238
8	0.999	0.938	0.772	0.540	0.413	0.386	0.379	0.377	0.359	0.259
10	0.999	0.952	0.806	0.581	0.448	0.418	0.409	0.405	0.382	0.277
20	0.999	0.982	0.894	0.709	0.569	0.529	0.517	0.500	0.461	0.339
30	0.999	0.991	0.932	0.780	0.644	0.600	0.587	0.562	0.514	0.380
40	0.999	0.995	0.954	0.826	0.698	0.652	0.639	0.608	0.554	0.411
50	0.999	0.996	0.966	0.859	0.738	0.692	0.679	0.644	0.586	0.436
60	0.999	0.997	0.974	0.882	0.770	0.725	0.712	0.675	0.613	0.457
70	0.999	0.998	0.980	0.900	0.796	0.752	0.739	0.700	0.637	0.476
80	0.999	0.998	0.983	0.915	0.818	0.775	0.762	0.722	0.657	0.492
90	0.999	0.999	0.986	0.926	0.836	0.794	0.781	0.741	0.675	0.507
100	0.999	0.999	0.988	0.935	0.851	0.811	0.799	0.758	0.691	0.520
120	0.999	0.999	0.991	0.948	0.876	0.839	0.827	0.786	0.719	0.544
140	0.999	0.999	0.993	0.958	0.895	0.860	0.849	0.809	0.742	0.564
160	0.999	0.999	0.995	0.965	0.910	0.878	0.867	0.829	0.761	0.582
180	0.999	0.999	0.996	0.971	0.923	0.892	0.882	0.845	0.778	0.598
200	0.999	0.999	0.998	0.976	0.933	0.904	0.894	0.858	0.792	0.612

Reprinted by permission of the Society of Nuclear Medicine from Brownell GL, Ellett WH, Reddy AR. MIRD Pamphlet No. 3: Absorbed Fractions for Photon Dosimetry. *J Nuclear Med.* February 1968; 9(1 Suppl):29–39.

EXAMPLE 6.16

The use of these absorbed dose fractions may be illustrated by their application to calculations of the dose rate to a 0.6-kg sphere made of tissue-equivalent material in which 1 MBq of ^{131}I is uniformly distributed.

Solution

In this case, energy will be absorbed from the beta particles and from the gamma rays. Since the range in tissue of the betas is very small, we can assume that all the beta energy is absorbed. For the gammas however, only a fraction of the energy will be absorbed. The total energy absorbed from the ^{131}I is simply the sum of the emitted beta energy plus the fraction of the emitted gamma-ray energy that is absorbed by the sphere. This sum is called the effective energy per transformation. The absorbed fraction of the gamma rays depends on the size of the absorbing medium and on the photon energy.

Using the absorbed dose fractions given in Table 6-5 and interpolating for gamma-ray energies lying between those listed in the table, we calculate the absorbed gamma-ray energy per ^{131}I transformation as follows:

$$E_e(\gamma) = \sum_i E_{\gamma_i} \times n_i \times \varphi_i, \tag{6.73}$$

where

$$
\begin{aligned}
E_e(\gamma) &= \text{absorbed gamma-ray energy, MeV/transformation,} \\
E_{\gamma i} &= \text{energy of the } i\text{th gamma photon, MeV,} \\
n_i &= \text{number of photons of } i\text{th energy per transformation, and} \\
\varphi_i &= \text{absorbed fraction of the } i\text{th photon's energy.}
\end{aligned}
$$

PHOTON ENERGY, $E_{\gamma i}$ (MEV)	x	PHOTONS PER TRANSFORMATION, n_i	x	ABSORBED FRACTION, φ	=	ABSORBED ENERGY (MeV/T)
0.723		0.016		0.123		0.0014
0.637		0.069		0.124		0.0055
0.503		0.003		0.123		0.0002
0.326		0.002		0.120		0.0001
0.177		0.002		0.112		0.0000
0.365		0.853		0.122		0.0380
0.284		0.051		0.118		0.0017
0.080		0.051		0.111		0.0005
0.164		0.006		0.111		0.0001

$$E_e(\gamma) = 0.0474 \text{ MeV/t}$$

The mean beta energy per ^{131}I transformation, which corresponds to the effective energy for the betas, may be calculated by substituting the mean beta energies

INPUT DATA

Radiation	%/dis-integration	Transition energy (MeV)	Other nuclear parameters
Beta-1	1.6	0.25 *	Allowed
Beta-2	6.9	0.33 *	Allowed
Beta-3	0.5	0.47 *	Allowed
Beta-4	90.4	0.606 *	Allowed
Beta-5	0.6	0.81 *	First forbidden unique
Gamma-1	5.06	0.0802	M1, $\alpha_K = 1.7$, $\alpha_L = 0.17$
Gamma-2	0.6	0.1640	M4, $\alpha_K = 29$, K/L = 2.3
Gamma-3	0.18	0.1772	E2, $\alpha_K = 0.189$ (T), K/L = 4.0
Gamma-4	5.06	0.2843	E2, $\alpha_K = 0.052$ K/(L + M) = 4.0
Gamma-5	0.18	0.3258	M1, $\alpha_K = 0.0285$ (T), K/L = 6.0
Gamma-6	85.3	0.3645	E2 + 2% M1, $\alpha_K = 0.02$, K/L = 6.0
Gamma-7	0.32	0.5030	E2, $\alpha_K = 0.00749$ (T), $\alpha_L = 0.0011$ (T)
Gamma-8	6.9	0.6370	E2, $\alpha_K = 0.0039$, $\alpha_L = 0.000563$ (T)
Gamma-9	1.6	0.7229	M1, $\alpha_K = 0.004$, $\alpha_L = 0.000515$ (T)

Ref.: Lederer, C. M. et al, *Table of isotopes*, 6th ed.
* Endpoint energy (MeV).   (T) = Theoretical value.

OUTPUT DATA

Radiation (i)	Mean number/disintegration (n_i)	Mean energy (MeV) ($\bar{E}_i$)	$\Delta_i \left(\dfrac{\text{g-rad}}{\mu\text{Ci-h}}\right)$
Beta-1	0.016	0.0701	0.0024
Beta-2	0.069	0.0955	0.0140
Beta-3	0.005	0.1428	0.0015
Beta-4	0.904	0.1917	0.3691
Beta-5	0.006	0.2856	0.0037
Gamma-1	0.0173	0.0802	0.0030
K int. con. electron, gamma-1	0.0294	0.0456	0.0029
L int. con. electron, gamma-1	0.0029	0.0751	0.0005
M int. con. electron, gamma-1	0.0010	0.0792	0.0002
Gamma-2	0.0001	0.1640	0.0000
K int. con. electron, gamma-2	0.0037	0.1294	0.0010
L int. con. electron, gamma-2	0.0016	0.1589	0.0005
M int. con. electron, gamma-2	0.0005	0.1630	0.0002
Gamma-3	0.0014	0.1772	0.0005
K int. con. electron, gamma-3	0.0003	0.1427	0.0001
Gamma-4	0.0475	0.2843	0.0288
K int. con. electron, gamma-4	0.0025	0.2497	0.0013
L int. con. electron, gamma-4	0.0005	0.2793	0.0003
M int. con. electron, gamma-4	0.0002	0.2834	0.0001
Gamma-5	0.0017	0.3258	0.0012
Gamma-6	0.833	0.3645	0.6465
K int. con. electron, gamma-6	0.0167	0.3299	0.0117
L int. con. electron, gamma-6	0.0028	0.3594	0.0021
M int. con. electron, gamma-6	0.0009	0.3635	0.0006
Gamma-7	0.0032	0.5030	0.0034
Gamma-8	0.0687	0.6370	0.0932
K int. con. electron, gamma-8	0.0003	0.6024	0.0004
Gamma-9	0.0159	0.7229	0.0245
K α-1 x-rays	0.0252	0.0298	0.0016
K α-2 x-rays	0.0130	0.0295	0.0008
K β-1 x-rays	0.0070	0.0336	0.0005
K β-2 x-rays	0.0015	0.0346	0.0001
L x-rays	0.0078	0.0041	0.0001
KLL Auger electron	0.0042	0.0245	0.0002
KLX Auger electron	0.0018	0.0296	0.0001
KXY Auger electron	0.0003	0.0327	0.0000
LMM Auger electron	0.0486	0.0032	0.0003
MXY Auger electron	0.117	0.0009	0.0002

IODINE·131

BETA-MINUS DECAY

Figure 6-11. Transformation scheme and input data and output data for ^{131}I dosimetry. (Reprinted by permission of the Society of Nuclear Medicine from Dillman LT. MIRD Pamphlet No. 4: Radionuclide Decay Schemes and Nuclear Parameters for Use in Radiation Dose Estimation. *J Nucl Med.* March 1969; 10(2 Suppl):1–32.)

for ^{131}I listed in the output data in Figure 6-11 into Eq. (6.74):

$$E_e(\beta) = \sum_i \bar{E}_{\beta i} \times n_{\beta i} \tag{6.74}$$

$$= (0.0701 \times 0.016) + (0.0955 \times 0.069) + (0.1428 \times 0.005)$$
$$+ (0.1917 \times 0.904) + (0.285 \times 0.006) = 0.183 \frac{MeV}{t}.$$

The effective energy E_e per transformation, that is, the amount of energy absorbed by the 0.6-kg tissue-equivalent sphere per ^{131}I transformation, is

$$E_e = E_e(\gamma) + E_e(\beta) \tag{6.75}$$

$$= 0.047 + 0.183 = 0.230 \frac{MeV}{t}.$$

The daily dose rate to a mass of m kg that absorbs $E_e \frac{MeV}{t}$ from q Bq of activity within the mass is given by

$$\dot{D} = \frac{q \, \text{Bq} \times 1 \frac{t/s}{Bq} \times E_e \frac{MeV}{t} \times 1.6 \times 10^{-13} \frac{J}{MeV} \times 8.64 \times 10^4 \frac{s}{d}}{m \, \text{kg} \times 1 \frac{J/kg}{Gy}}. \tag{6.76}$$

If we substitute

$$q = 1 \times 10^6 \text{ Bq,}$$
$$E_e = 0.230 \frac{MeV}{t}, \text{ and}$$
$$m = 0.6 \text{ kg}$$

into Eq. (6.76), we find the dose rate to be

$$\dot{D} = 5.3 \times 10^{-3} \frac{Gy}{d} \left(0.53 \frac{rad}{d}\right).$$

Let us now return to the MIRD method for internal dose calculation. Let us consider two organs in the body, one that contains the distributed radioactivity and is called the *source S* and the organ of interest T, the *target*, which is being irradiated by S. S and T may be either the same organ or two different organs bearing any of the possible geometric relationships shown in Figure 6-10.

The rate of energy emission by the radionuclide in the source at any time that is carried by the ith particle is given by

$$\chi_{ei} = A_S \, \text{Bq} \times 1 \frac{t/s}{Bq} \times \bar{E}_i \frac{MeV}{particle} \times n_i \frac{particle}{t} \times 1.6 \times 10^{-13} \frac{J}{MeV} \tag{6.77}$$

$$= 1.6 \times 10^{-13} A_S \times \bar{E}_i \times n_i \frac{J}{s}, \tag{6.78}$$

where

χ_{ei} = energy emission rate, J/s,
A_s = activity in source, Bq,
$\bar{E}_i$ = mean energy of the ith particle, MeV, and
n_i = number of particles of the ith kind per decay.

If the fraction of this emitted energy that is absorbed by the target is called φ_i, then the amount of energy absorbed by the target due to emission from the source is given by

$$\chi_{ai} = \chi_{ei} \times \varphi_i = 1.6 \times 10^{-13} \times A_S \times \bar{E}_i \times n_i \times \varphi_i \text{ J/s.} \tag{6.79}$$

Since 1 Gy corresponds to the absorption of 1 J/kg the dose rate from the ith particle to a target that weighs m kg is given by

$$\dot{D} = \frac{\left(1.6 \times 10^{-13} \times A_s \times \bar{E}_i \times n_i \times \varphi_i\right) \frac{\text{J}}{\text{s}}}{1 \frac{\text{J/kg}}{\text{Gy}} \times m \text{ kg}}. \tag{6.80}$$

If we let

$$\Delta_i = 1.6 \times 10^{-13} \times n_i \times \bar{E}_i \frac{\text{kg} \cdot \text{Gy}}{\text{Bq} \cdot \text{s}} \tag{6.81}$$

then Eq. (6.80) can be written as

$$\dot{D}_i = \frac{A_S}{m} \times \varphi_i \times \Delta_i \frac{\text{Gy}}{\text{s}}. \tag{6.82}$$

Δ_i is the dose rate in an infinitely large homogeneous mass of tissue containing a uniformly distributed radionuclide at a concentration of 1 Bq/kg. Numerical values for Δ_i for each of the radiations generated by radioisotopes in infinitely large masses of tissue are included in the output data section of the decay schemes and nuclear parameters for use in radiation dose estimation that have been published by the MIRD Committee of the Society of Nuclear Medicine. Considering all types of the particles emitted from the source, the dose rate to the target organ is

$$\dot{D} = \frac{A_s}{m} \sum \varphi_i \Delta_i. \tag{6.83}$$

Since $\dot{D}$ is a function of A_s, which is a function of time, $\dot{D}$ too is a function of time. The dose commitment, that is, the total dose due to the complete decay of the deposited radionuclide, is given by integrating the dose rate with respect to time:

$$D = \int_0^\infty \dot{D}(t)\mathrm{d}t = \frac{\sum \varphi_i \Delta_i}{m} \int_0^\infty A_s(t)\, \mathrm{d}t. \tag{6.84}$$

If we call the time integral of the deposited radioactivity the cumulated activity, $\tilde{A}$,

$$\tilde{A} = \int_0^\infty A_s(t)\, \mathrm{d}t, \tag{6.85}$$

then the total dose to the target organ is given by

$$D = \frac{\tilde{A}}{m} \sum \varphi_i \Delta_i. \tag{6.86}$$

EXAMPLE 6.17

Calculate the total dose and initial dose rate to a 70-kg, 160-cm-tall reference man who is intraveneously injected with 1-MBq ^{24}NaCl. Assume the ^{24}NaCl to become uniformly distributed within a very short time and to have a biological half-life of 11 days (264 hours). The decay scheme and tables of input and output data are shown in Figure 6-12.

Solution

The decay scheme and the accompanying table of input data show one beta (actually >0.999) particle whose maximum energy is 1.392 MeV, and one 1.3685-MeV

SODIUM-24   BETA-MINUS DECAY

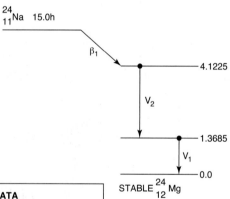

INPUT DATA

Radiation	%/disin-tegration	Transition energy (MeV)	Other nuclear parameters
Beta-1	99.9	1.392*	Allowed
All other betas	<0.1	—	—
Gamma-1	100.	1.3685	E2, αx < 0.00001 (T)
Gamma-2	99.9	2.7539	E2, αx < 0.00001 (T)
All other gammas	<0.1	—	—

Ref. Lederer, C. M. et al, *Table of isotopes*, 6th ed.
*Endpoint energy (MeV).   (T) = Theoretical value.

OUTPUT DATA

Radiation [1]	Mean number/ disinte-gration (n_i)	Mean energy (MeV) [$\bar{E}_i$]	Δ_i $\left(\frac{\text{g-rad}}{\mu\text{Ci-h}}\right)$
Beta-1	0.999	0.5547	1.1803
Gamma-1	0.999	1.3685	2.9149
Gamma-2	0.999	2.7539	5.8599

Figure 6-12. *Transformation scheme and input and output data for ^{24}Na dosimetry. (Reprinted by permission of the Society of Nuclear Medicine from Dillman LT. MIRD Pamphlet No. 4: Radionuclide Decay Schemes and Nuclear Parameters for Use in Radiation Dose Estimation.* J Nucl Med. *March 1969; 10(2 Suppl):1–32.)*

gamma per decay. The output data list the integral dose in an infinite medium, per unit of cumulated activity, in units of $\dfrac{\text{g} \cdot \text{rads}}{\mu\text{Ci} \cdot \text{h}}$ for each radiation. To convert from the old system of units found in the MIRD publications to the SI system, that is, to go from $\dfrac{\text{g} \cdot \text{rads}}{\mu\text{Ci} \cdot \text{h}}$ to $\dfrac{\text{kg} \cdot \text{Gy}}{\text{Bq} \cdot \text{s}}$, we use the following relation:

$$\frac{\text{kg} \cdot \text{Gy}}{\text{Bq} \cdot \text{s}} = \frac{\text{g} \cdot \text{rad}}{\mu\text{Ci} \cdot \text{h}} \times \frac{10^{-3} \, \dfrac{\text{kg}}{\text{g}} \times 10^{-2} \, \dfrac{\text{Gy}}{\text{rad}}}{3.7 \times 10^4 \, \dfrac{\text{Bq}}{\mu\text{Ci}} \times 3.6 \times 10^3 \, \dfrac{\text{s}}{\text{h}}}$$

$$\frac{\text{kg} \cdot \text{Gy}}{\text{Bq} \cdot \text{s}} = \frac{\text{g} \cdot \text{rad}}{\mu\text{Ci} \cdot \text{h}} \times 75.1 \times 10^{-14}. \tag{6.87}$$

To convert from SI units to traditional units:

$$\frac{\text{g} \cdot \text{rad}}{\mu\text{Ci} \cdot \text{h}} = \frac{1}{7.51 \times 10^{-14}} \times \frac{\text{kg} \cdot \text{Gy}}{\text{Bq} \cdot \text{s}} = 1.33 \times 10^{13} \times \frac{\text{kg} \cdot \text{Gy}}{\text{Bq} \cdot \text{s}}. \tag{6.88}$$

Now let us return to the problem. Since the ^{24}Na is cleared exponentially at an effective rate λ_E, the amount of activity in the source organ is given by

$$A_s(t) = A_s(0) \times e^{-\lambda_E t}, \tag{6.89}$$

where $A_s(0)$ is the initial activity in the source.

$$\tilde{A} = \int_0^\infty A_s(t)\, dt = A_s(0) \int_0^\infty e^{-\lambda_E t} dt = \frac{A_s(0)}{\lambda_E}. \tag{6.90}$$

Since

$$\lambda_E = \frac{0.693}{T_E} = \frac{0.693}{(T_R \times T_B)/(T_R + T_B)}$$

the biological half-life T_B is found in International Commission on Radiological Protection (ICRP) Publication 2 to be 264 hours, and the radioactive half-life T_R is 15 hours, therefore

$$\tilde{A} = \frac{10^6 \, \text{Bq}}{1.36 \times 10^{-5} \, \text{s}^{-1}} = 7.35 \times 10^{10} \, \text{Bq} \cdot \text{s}.$$

Now we must calculate $\Sigma \varphi_i \Delta_i$

The absorbed fractions, φ_i, in a number of target organs and tissues, for photons ranging in energy from 0.01 to 4 MeV that originate in a number of different source organs and tissues, are tabulated in Appendix A of the *Journal of Nuclear Medicine,* Supplement No. 3, August 1969.[2] Table 6-8 shows the absorbed fractions from a photon emitter that is uniformly distributed throughout the body, as in the case of ^{24}Na. The values of φ_i for the 1.369-MeV and 2.754-MeV gammas were found by interpolation between values in Table 6-8 and are listed below, together with Δ_i,

---

[2] As the MIRD system evolved, the absorbed fraction was replaced by the *specific absorbed fraction,* which is discussed in the following paragraph.

TABLE 6-8. Absorbed Fractions (and Coefficients of Variation), Gamma Emitter Uniformly Distributed Throughout the Body[a]

TARGET ORGAN	PHOTON ENERGY (MeV)												Target Organ
	0.010		0.015		0.020		0.030		0.050		0.100		
	φ	$100\sigma_\varphi$	φ	$100\sigma_\varphi$	φ	$100\sigma_\varphi$	φ	$100\sigma_\varphi$	φ	$100\sigma_\varphi$	φ	$100\sigma_\varphi$	
Adrenals	0.270E−03	35.	0.228E−03	34.	0.175E−03	37.	0.209E−03	28.	0.131E−03	23.	0.101E−03	26.	Adrenals
Bladder	0.757E−02	6.6	0.762E−02	6.5	0.683E−02	6.6	0.625E−02	6.1	0.445E−02	5.6	0.352E−02	5.2	Bladder
GI (stom)	0.570E−02	7.6	0.507E−02	8.0	0.573E−02	7.1	0.560E−02	6.4	0.391E−02	5.8	0.273E−02	5.9	GI (stom)
GI (SI)	0.254E−01	3.6	0.236E−01	3.7	0.234E−01	3.6	0.209E−01	3.4	0.163E−01	3.1	0.120E−01	3.2	GI (SI)
GI (ULI)	0.541E−02	7.8	0.561E−02	7.5	0.647E−02	6.6	0.533E−02	5.9	0.374E−02	5.4	0.262E−02	5.7	GI (ULI)
GI (LLI)	0.350E−02	9.7	0.441E−02	8.5	0.457E−02	7.7	0.285E−02	7.9	0.256E−02	6.2	0.187E−02	6.3	GI (LLI)
Heart	0.756E−02	6.6	0.804E−02	6.3	0.769E−02	6.2	0.635E−02	6.0	0.469E−02	5.4	0.420E−02	5.0	Heart
Kidneys	0.410E−02	9.0	0.446E−02	8.5	0.412E−02	8.3	0.338E−02	7.4	0.233E−02	6.4	0.183E−02	6.6	Kidneys
Liver	0.260E−01	3.5	0.244E−01	3.6	0.249E−01	3.5	0.221E−01	3.3	0.154E−01	3.2	0.120E−01	3.2	Liver
Lungs	0.127E−01	5.1	0.142E−01	4.7	0.138E−01	4.4	0.122E−01	3.8	0.808E−02	3.4	0.551E−02	3.6	Lungs
Marrow	0.560E−01	1.4	0.594E−01	1.4	0.655E−01	1.3	0.740E−01	1.1	0.613E−01	1.1	0.329E−01	1.3	Marrow
Pancreas	0.134E−02	16.	0.103E−02	18.	0.828E−03	17.	0.780E−03	14.	0.567E−03	12.	0.449E−03	12.	Pancreas
Sk. (rib)	0.168E−01	4.4	0.206E−01	3.9	0.247E−01	3.4	0.263E−01	2.9	0.176E−01	2.9	0.764E−02	3.3	Sk. (rib)
Sk. (pelvis)	0.147E−01	4.7	0.160E−01	4.51	0.163E−01	4.3	0.224E−01	3.4	0.199E−01	3.0	0.103E−01	3.3	Sk. (pelvis)
Sk. (spine)	0.186E−01	4.2	0.190E−01	4.1	0.234E−01	3.7	0.253E−01	3.3	0.229E−01	3.0	0.144E−01	3.2	Sk. (spine)
Sk. (skull)	0.103E−01	5.6	0.115E−01	5.3	0.123E−01	5.	0.128E−01	4.6	0.722E−02	5.1	0.313E−02	6.0	Sk. (skull)
Skeleton (total)	0.144	1.4	0.153	1.3	0.167	1.2	0.188	1.1	0.153	1.1	0.810E−01	1.3	Skeleton (total)
Skin	0.258E−01	3.5	0.227E−01	3.5	0.169E−01	3.7	0.116E−01	3.3	0.758E−02	2.9	0.585E−02	3.1	Skin
Spleen	0.260E−02	11.	0.237E−02	12.	0.242E−02	11.	0.223E−02	9.1	0.149E−02	8.5	0.111E−02	8.7	Spleen
Thyroid	0.265E−03	35.	0.263E−03	34.	0.602E−04	48.	0.111E−03	36.	0.114E−03	27.	0.873E−04	29.	Thyroid
Uterus	0.999E−03	18.	0.109E−02	17.	0.122E−02	15.	0.924E−03	13.	0.712E−03	12.	0.611E−03	11.	Uterus
Trunk	0.604	0.47	0.589	0.48	0.566	0.50	0.500	0.55	0.358	0.67	0.245	0.79	Trunk
Legs	0.309	0.86	0.299	0.88	0.285	0.90	0.242	0.97	0.171	1.1	0.113	1.3	Legs
Head	0.488E−01	2.5	0.474E−01	2.5	0.440E−01	2.6	0.342E−01	2.7	0.200E−01	3.1	0.127E−01	3.1	Head
Total body	0.959	0.11	0.933	0.15	0.892	0.19	0.774	0.27	0.548	0.43	0.370	0.56	Total body

(Continued)

251

TABLE 6-8. Absorbed Fractions (and Coefficients of Variation), Gamma Emitter Uniformly Distributed Throughout the Body[a] (Continued)

TARGET ORGAN	PHOTON ENERGY (MeV)												Target Organ
	0.200		0.500		1.000		1.500		2.000		4.000		
	φ	$100\sigma_\varphi$	φ	$100\sigma_\varphi$	φ	$100\sigma_\varphi$	φ	$100\sigma_\varphi$	φ	$100\sigma_\varphi$	φ	$100\sigma_\varphi$	
Adrenals	0.352E−04	36.	0.138E−03	35.	0.100E−03	42.	0.107E−03	43.	0.114E−03	43.	0.147E−02	12.	Adrenals
Bladder	0.327E−02	5.0	0.341E−02	6.6	0.274E−02	8.3	0.291E−02	8.4	0.231E−02	9.6	0.119E−02	14.	Bladder
GI (stom)	0.218E−02	7.0	0.258E−02	7.7	0.181E−02	9.8	0.199E−02	10.	0.212E−02	10.			GI (stom)
GI (SI)	0.106E−01	3.4	0.114E−01	3.8	0.109E−01	4.2	0.915E−02	4.8	0.820E−02	5.2	0.409E−02	7.3	GI (SI)
GI (ULI)	0.256E−02	6.3	0.306E−02	7.0	0.228E−02	8.9	0.209E−02	9.4	0.197E−02	10.	0.160E−02	12.	GI (ULI)
GI (LLI)	0.151E−02	7.6	0.184E−02	8.8	0.178E−02	9.7	0.181E−02	11.	0.157E−02	12.	0.673E−03	18.	GI (LLI)
Heart	0.337E−02	5.8	0.372E−02	6.6	0.301E−02	8.1	0.345E−02	7.8	0.312E−02	8.3	0.145E−02	13.	Heart
Kidneys	0.171E−02	7.4	0.142E−02	9.7	0.161E−02	10.	0.152E−02	11.	0.154E−02	12.	0.904E−03	16.	Kidneys
Liver	0.111E−01	3.4	0.101E−01	4.1	0.896E−02	4.7	0.912E−02	4.9	0.847E−02	5.1	0.560E−02	6.4	Liver
Lungs	0.507E−02	4.3	0.496E−02	5.2	0.466E−02	6.1	0.466E−02	6.5	0.427E−02	6.9	0.568E−02	6.4	Lungs
Marrow	0.221E−01	1.5	0.194E−01	1.0	0.182E−01	2.0	0.164E−01	2.2	0.156E−01	2.3	0.969E−02	3.0	Marrow
Pancreas	0.444E−03	14.	0.382E−03	17.	0.534E−03	19.	0.348E−03	22.	0.358E−03	24.	0.142E−03	39.	Pancreas
Sk. (rib)	0.505E−02	4.1	0.435E−02	5.6	0.421E−02	6.3	0.405E−02	7.0	0.350E−02	7.7	0.338E−02	8.0	Sk. (rib)
Sk. (pelvis)	0.668E−02	3.9	0.569E−02	5.0	0.562E−02	5.7	0.511E−02	6.3	0.422E−02	7.0	0.256E−02	9.3	Sk. (pelvis)
Sk. (spine)	0.910E−02	3.6	0.763E−02	4.5	0.751E−02	5.1	0.610E−02	5.7	0.606E−02	5.9	0.341E−02	8.1	Sk. (spine)
Sk. (skull)	0.277E−02	6.3	0.304E−02	7.2	0.280E−02	8.0	0.254E−02	9.0	0.292E−02	8.8	0.224E−02	10.	Sk. (skull)
Skeleton (total)	0.550E−01	1.4	0.488E−01	1.7	0.456E−01	2.0	0.413E−01	2.2	0.396E−01	2.3	0.252E−01	3.0	Skeleton (total)
Skin	0.677E−02	3.5	0.757E−02	4.2	0.745E−02	4.8	0.759E−02	5.0	0.664E−02	5.5	0.123E−01	4.3	Skin
Spleen	0.798E−03	11.	0.116E−02	11.	0.914E−03	14.	0.903E−03	16.	0.740E−03	17.	0.368E−03	24.	Spleen
Thyroid	0.418E−04	42.							0.810E−04	46.			Thyroid
Uterus	0.408E−03	15.	0.473E−03	16.	0.517E−03	18.	0.323E−03	23.	0.364E−03	25.	0.238E−03	33.	Uterus
Trunk	0.223	0.81	0.225	0.84	0.210	0.92	0.198	0.99	0.186	1.0	0.156	1.2	Trunk
Legs	0.102	1.3	0.101	1.4	0.965E−01	1.5	0.917E−01	1.6	0.846E−01	1.6	0.710E−01	1.8	Legs
Head	0.134E−01	3.2	0.147E−01	3.5	0.145E−01	3.8	0.130E−01	4.1	0.139E−01	4.1	0.127E−01	4.4	Head
Total body	0.338	0.57	0.340	0.60	0.321	0.67	0.302	0.73	0.284	0.77	0.240	0.90	Total body

[a]The digits following the symbol E indicate the powers of 10 by which each number is to be multiplied; A blank in the table indicates that the coefficient of variation was greater than 50%; Total body = head + trunk + legs.

Reprinted by permission of the Society of Nuclear Medicine from Snyder WS, Ford MR, Warner GG, Fisher HLJr. MIRD Pamphlet No. 5: Estimates of Absorbed Fractions for Monoenergetic Photon Sources Uniformly Distributed in Various Organs of a Heterogeneous Phantom. J Nucl Med. August 1969: 10(3 Suppl).

which was found in the output data listing in Figure 6-12 and was converted to $kg \cdot fGy/Bq \cdot s$, where $1\,fGy = 10^{-15}\,Gy$:

RADIATION	E_i (MeV)	φ_i	$\Delta_i, \frac{kg\text{-}fGy}{Bq\text{-}s}$	$\varphi_i\Delta_i$
Beta 1	0.555	1.000	88.64	88.64
Gamma 1	1.369	0.31	218.91	67.86
Gamma 2	2.754	0.265	440.08	116.62
				$\sum = 273.12 (kg \cdot fGy)/(Bq \cdot s)$

Substituting the values (and 10^{15} femto Gy(fGy) per Gy):

$$\tilde{A} = 7.35 \times 10^{10}\,Bq \cdot s, \quad \sum \varphi_i\Delta_i = 273.12\frac{kg \cdot fGy}{Bq \cdot s}, \quad \text{and } m = 70\,kg$$

into Eq. (6.86) yields

$$D = \frac{7.35 \times 10^{10}\,Bq \cdot s}{70\,kg} \times 273.12\,\frac{kg \cdot fGy}{Bq \cdot s}$$

$$= 2.868 \times 10^{11}\,fGy \qquad (29\,mrads).$$

The initial dose rate may be found by substituting 10^6 Bq for A_s in Eq. (6.83):

$$\dot{D} = \frac{10^6\,Bq}{70\,kg} \times 273.12\,\frac{kg \cdot fGy}{Bq \cdot s}$$

$$= 3.9 \times 10^6\,fGy/s \quad (1.4\,mrads/h).$$

The physiological kinetics, on which the calculated dose from internally deposited radioactivity is based, are contained in the term for the cumulated activity $\tilde{A}$, while the balance of the right-hand side of Eq. (6.86) deals with physical data and measurements. The absorbed fraction φ_i represents the fraction of the energy that is absorbed by the total organ or tissue. According to Eq. (6.86), we must divide the total absorbed energy, $\sum \varphi_i\Delta_i$, by the mass of the target organ m. Rather than consider the fraction of energy absorbed by the target organ and then divide by the organ weight, it may be more convenient to use the *specific absorbed fraction* Φ_i.

$$\Phi = \frac{\text{absorbed fraction}}{\text{organ mass}} = \frac{\varphi}{m}. \tag{6.91}$$

This is the fraction of the absorbed energy per unit mass of target tissue from the ith particle emitted in the source organ. Specific absorbed fractions of photons of several energies for reference person, which were calculated by Monte Carlo methods, are tabulated in Appendix D. Specific absorbed fractions for beta or alpha radiation are easily calculated. In a large medium containing a uniformly distributed beta or alpha emitter, essentially all of the emitted energy is absorbed. For the case where the target and source are the same organ and where the range of the radiation from the deposited radioisotope is less than the smallest dimension of the organ in which it is deposited, the specific absorbed fraction in an organ of mass m may be closely approximated by

$$\Phi = \frac{\varphi}{m} = \frac{1}{m}. \tag{6.92}$$

When the target organ is widely separated from the source organ, that is, when the distance between them is greater than the range of beta or alpha particles, then the target absorbs no energy from the source, and $\Phi = 0$. For the case where the target tissue is a region surrounded by the source, the specific absorbed fraction in the target is

$$\Phi = \frac{1}{m \, (\text{source})}. \tag{6.93}$$

For example, if a beta emitter is uniformly distributed throughout the body, then the specific absorbed fraction to the liver from the radioactivity outside the liver, if the liver weighs 1.8 kg and the person weighs 70 kg, is

$$\Phi = \frac{1}{70 - 1.8} = 1.47 \times 10^{-2} \, \text{kg}^{-1}.$$

When the specific absorbed fraction is used, the absorbed dose is given by

$$D = \tilde{A} \sum_i \Delta_i \Phi_i. \tag{6.94}$$

Since every organ in the body is a target for radiation from the source organ, the exact target–source relationship is identified explicitly by the symbol

$$(r_k \leftarrow r_h),$$

where r_k represents the target organ and r_h represents the source organ. Thus, the dose to target organ r_k from activity $\tilde{A}_h$ in source organ r_h is written as

$$D(r_k \leftarrow r_h) = \tilde{A}_h \sum_i \Delta_i \Phi_i (r_k \leftarrow r_h). \tag{6.95}$$

Using the specific absorbed fraction, we can define the quantity

$$S(r_k \leftarrow r_h) = \sum_i \Delta_i \Phi_i (r_k \leftarrow r_h). \tag{6.96}$$

Since S depends only on physical factors, such as the geometrical relationship between the source and the target, we can calculate the value of S for all of the target–source relationships of interest and for any radioisotope in the source organ. The dose to any target organ r_k from a source organ r_h is then

$$D(r_k \leftarrow r_h) = \tilde{A}_h \times S(r_k \leftarrow r_h). \tag{6.97}$$

Furthermore, since the radioactivity is usually widespread within the body, a target organ may be irradiated by several different source organs. The dose to the target, therefore, is

$$D(r_k) = \sum_h D(r_k \leftarrow r_h). \tag{6.98}$$

Tables of $S(r_k \leftarrow r_h)$, per unit cumulated activity for numerous target and source organs and for numerous radionuclides of interest, are published in MIRD Pamphlet No. 11. Tables 6-9 and 6-10, which are excerpted from Pamphlet No. 11, give the

TABLE 6-9. *S*, Absorbed Dose per Unit Cumulated Activity (rad/μCi · h) Mercury-203 (Half-Life 1.12E−03 h)

TARGET ORGANS	Adrenals	Bladder Contents	INTESTINAL TRACT				Kidneys	Liver	Lungs	Other Tissue (Muscle)
			Stomach Contents	SI Contents	ULI Contents	LLI Contents				
Adrenals	1.6E−02	3.6E−07	4.2E−06	2.7E−06	1.7E−06	8.4E−07	1.9E−05	9.0E−06	4.4E−06	2.7E−06
Bladder wall	2.1E−07	6.6E−04	5.0E−07	5.0E−06	3.8E−06	1.1E−05	5.9E−07	3.6E−07	1.0E−07	3.2E−06
Bone (total)	2.9E−06	1.3E−06	1.3E−06	1.8E−06	1.6E−06	2.3E−06	2.1E−06	1.6E−06	2.1E−06	1.9E−06
GI (stom. wall)	5.3E−06	5.2E−07	5.1E−04	6.5E−06	6.7E−06	3.2E−06	6.1E−06	3.5E−06	3.3E−06	2.5E−06
GI (SI)	1.6E−06	5.1E−06	4.7E−06	3.2E−04	3.0E−05	1.7E−05	5.1E−06	3.0E−06	3.9E−07	2.8E−06
GI (ULI wall)	1.7E−06	4.2E−06	6.3E−06	4.2E−05	5.5E−04	7.7E−06	5.2E−06	4.5E−06	4.9E−07	2.9E−06
GI (LLI wall)	4.6E−07	1.3E−05	2.3E−06	1.3E−05	5.4E−06	8.7E−04	1.5E−06	4.6E−07	1.8E−07	3.1E−06
Kidneys	2.1E−05	5.5E−07	6.3E−06	5.5E−06	5.0E−06	1.7E−06	8.1E−04	6.9E−06	1.7E−06	2.5E−06
Liver	8.9E−06	4.1E−07	3.6E−06	3.3E−06	4.6E−06	5.3E−07	7.0E−06	1.6E−04	4.4E−06	2.0E−06
Lungs	4.4E−06	5.6E−08	3.1E−06	4.8E−07	5.2E−07	1.6E−07	1.6E−06	4.5E−06	2.4E−04	2.4E−06
Marrow (red)	5.2E−06	3.0E−06	2.3E−06	5.8E−06	5.0E−06	6.9E−06	5.3E−06	2.3E−06	2.7E−06	2.9E−06
Other tissues (musc.)	2.7E−06	3.2E−06	2.5E−06	2.8E−06	2.7E−06	3.1E−06	2.5E−06	2.0E−06	2.4E−06	1.0E−05
Ovaries	1.0E−06	1.3E−05	8.1E−07	1.8E−05	2.1E−05	3.4E−05	2.2E−06	7.6E−07	2.3E−07	3.6E−06
Pancreas	1.5E−05	5.2E−07	3.2E−05	3.7E−06	4.1E−06	1.3E−06	1.2E−05	7.4E−06	4.7E−06	3.2E−06
Skin	1.1E−06	1.1E−06	9.0E−07	8.5E−07	8.6E−07	9.8E−07	1.1E−06	9.8E−07	1.1E−06	1.5E−06
Spleen	1.2E−05	3.3E−07	1.8E−05	2.8E−06	2.5E−06	1.5E−06	1.6E−05	1.7E−06	4.1E−06	2.6E−06
Testes	9.2E−08	8.4E−06	9.9E−08	6.3E−07	6.5E−07	3.7E−06	2.2E−07	1.6E−07	2.8E−08	2.1E−06
Thyroid	3.0E−07	9.0E−09	2.3E−07	4.8E−08	5.2E−08	2.0E−08	1.3E−07	3.8E−07	1.7E−06	2.4E−06
Uterus (nongrvd)	3.3E−06	2.8E−05	1.5E−06	1.7E−05	8.5E−06	1.2E−05	1.8E−06	7.2E−07	1.7E−07	4.0E−06
Total body	6.0E−06	3.7E−06	4.1E−06	6.0E−06	4.9E−06	5.2E−06	6.0E−06	6.1E−06	5.6E−06	5.5E−06

(Continued)

TABLE 6-9. *S*, Absorbed Dose per Unit Cumulated Activity (rad/μCi · h) Mercury-203 (Half-Life 1.12E–03 h) (Coninued)

| TARGET ORGANS | Ovaries | Pancreas | SKELETON | | | Skin | Spleen | Testes | Thyroid | Total Body |
			Red Marrow	Cort. Bone	Tra. Bone					
Adrenals	7.7E–07	1.5E–05	4.4E–06	2.5E–06	2.5E–06	1.4E–06	1.2E–05	9.2E–08	3.0E–07	6.5E–06
Bladder wall	1.2E–05	3.0E–07	1.4E–06	9.3E–07	9.3E–07	1.0E–06	2.9E–07	8.8E–06	9.1E–09	6.2E–06
Bone (total)	2.1E–06	2.0E–06	1.0E–05	4.9E–05	4.0E–05	1.6E–06	1.6E–06	1.4E–06	1.5E–06	6.0E–06
GI (stom. wall)	1.4E–06	3.3E–05	1.9E–06	1.0E–06	1.0E–06	1.0E–06	1.7E–05	1.2E–07	1.1E–07	6.4E–06
GI (SI)	2.1E–05	3.3E–06	4.7E–06	1.4E–06	1.4E–06	9.0E–07	2.5E–06	8.0E–07	2.4E–08	6.6E–06
GI (ULI wall)	2.0E–05	4.0E–06	3.8E–06	1.3E–06	1.3E–06	8.9E–07	2.3E–06	6.4E–07	2.0E–08	6.3E–06
GI (LLI wall)	2.6E–05	1.0E–06	5.3E–06	1.9E–06	1.9E–06	9.4E–07	1.2E–06	5.1E–06	1.6E–08	6.2E–06
Kidneys	1.8E–06	1.1E–05	4.1E–06	1.6E–06	1.6E–06	1.2E–06	1.6E–05	1.2E–07	7.3E–08	6.1E–06
Liver	1.1E–06	7.8E–06	1.8E–06	1.2E–06	1.2E–06	1.1E–06	1.9E–06	7.7E–08	2.3E–07	6.0E–06
Lungs	1.4E–07	4.5E–06	2.2E–06	1.8E–06	1.8E–06	1.2E–06	4.0E–06	2.2E–08	1.8E–06	5.6E–06
Marrow (red)	7.2E–06	3.8E–06	1.3E–04	6.5E–06	3.5E–05	1.5E–06	2.5E–06	1.1E–06	1.7E–06	6.4E–06
Other tissues (musc.)	3.6E–06	3.2E–06	2.3E–06	1.9E–06	1.9E–06	1.5E–06	2.6E–06	2.1E–06	2.4E–06	5.5E–06
Ovaries	2.1E–02	6.0E–07	4.7E–06	1.4E–06	1.4E–06	8.0E–07	1.2E–06	0.0	1.9E–08	6.3E–06
Pancreas	9.1E–07	2.5E–03	3.0E–06	1.9E–06	1.9E–06	1.0E–06	3.4E–05	1.2E–07	1.8E–07	6.7E–06
Skin	1.5E–07	8.1E–07	1.2E–06	1.4E–06	1.4E–06	8.4E–05	9.6E–07	2.7E–06	1.5E–06	4.5E–06
Spleen	1.0E–06	3.5E–05	1.6E–06	1.3E–06	1.3E–06	1.1E–06	1.4E–03	8.6E–08	2.2E–07	6.2E–06
Testes	0.0	1.3E–07	6.1E–07	1.1E–06	1.1E–06	1.8E–06	1.3E–07	6.6E–03	2.8E–09	5.3E–06
Thyroid	1.9E–08	2.9E–07	1.4E–06	1.7E–06	1.7E–06	1.4E–06	2.2E–07	2.8E–09	1.1E–02	5.3E–06
Uterus (nongrvd)	3.7E–05	1.1E–06	4.0E–06	1.1E–06	1.1E–06	7.8E–07	7.4E–07	0.0	1.8E–08	6.7E–06
Total body	6.7E–06	6.6E–06	5.9E–06	5.6E–06	5.6E–06	4.5E–06	6.1E–06	5.5E–06	5.3E–06	5.6E–06

Reprinted by permission of the Society of Nuclear Medicine from Snyder WS, Ford MR, Warner GG, Watson SB. MIRD Pamphlet No. 11: "S" Absorbed Dose per Unit Cumulated Activity for Selected Radionuclides and Organs. Reston, VA: Society of Nuclear Medicine; 1975.

TABLE 6-10. S, Absorbed Dose Per Unit Cumulated Activity, (rad/μCi · H) Technetium-99M (Half-Life, 6.03 h)

| TARGET ORGANS | Adrenals | Bladder Contents | INTESTINAL TRACT | | | | Kidneys | Liver | Lungs | Other Tissue (Muscle) |
			Stomach Contents	SI Contents	ULI Contents	LLI Contents				
Adrenals	3.1E−03	1.5E−07	2.7E−06	1.0E−06	9.1E−07	3.6E−07	1.1E−05	4.5E−06	2.7E−06	1.4E−06
Bladder Wall	1.3E−07	1.6E−04	2.7E−07	2.6E−06	2.2E−06	6.9E−06	2.8E−07	1.6E−07	3.6E−08	1.8E−06
Bone (Total)	2.0E−06	9.2E−07	9.0E−07	1.3E−06	1.1E−06	1.6E−06	1.4E−06	1.1E−06	1.5E−06	9.8E−07
GI (Stom Wall)	2.9E−06	2.7E−07	1.3E−04	3.7E−06	3.8E−06	1.8E−06	3.6E−06	1.9E−06	1.8E−06	1.3E−06
GI (SI)	8.3E−07	3.0E−06	2.7E−06	7.8E−05	1.7E−05	9.4E−06	2.9E−06	1.6−06	1.9E−07	1.5E−06
GI (ULI Wall)	9.3E−07	2.2E−06	3.5E−06	2.4E−05	1.3E−04	4.2E−06	2.9E−06	2.5E−06	2.2E−07	1.6E−06
GI (LLI Wall)	2.2E−07	7.4E−06	1.2E−06	7.3E−06	3.2E−06	1.9E−04	7.2E−07	2.3E−07	7.1E−08	1.7E−06
Kidneys	1.1E−05	2.6E−07	3.5E−06	3.2E−06	2.8E−06	8.6E−07	1.9E−04	3.9E−06	8.4E−07	1.3E−06
Liver	4.9E−06	1.7E−07	2.0E−06	1.8E−06	2.6E−06	2.5E−07	3.9E−06	4.6E−05	2.5E−06	1.1E−06
Lungs	2.4E−06	2.4E−08	1.7E−06	2.2E−07	2.6E−07	7.9E−08	8.5E−07	2.5E−06	5.2E−05	1.3E−06
Marrow (red)	3.6E−06	2.2E−06	1.6E−06	4.3E−06	3.7E−06	5.1E−06	3.8E−06	1.6E−06	1.9E−06	2.0E−06
Other Tissues (Musc.)	1.4E−06	1.8E−06	1.4E−06	1.5E−06	1.5E−06	1.7E−06	1.3E−06	1.1E−06	1.3E−06	2.7E−06
Ovaries	6.1E−07	7.3E−06	5.0E−07	1.1E−05	1.2E−05	1.8E−05	1.1E−06	4.5E−07	9.4E−08	2.0E−06
Pancreas	9.0E−06	2.3E−07	1.8E−05	2.1E−06	2.3E−06	7.4E−07	6.6E−06	4.2E−06	2.6E−06	1.8E−06
Skin	5.1E−07	5.5E−07	4.4E−07	4.1E−07	4.1E−07	4.8E−07	5.3E−07	4.9E−07	5.3E−07	7.2E−07
Spleen	6.3E−06	6.6E−07	1.0E−05	1.5E−06	1.4E−06	8.0E−07	8.6E−06	9.2E−07	2.3E−06	1.4E−06
Testes	3.2E−08	4.7E−06	5.1E−08	3.1E−07	2.7E−07	1.8E−06	8.8E−08	6.2E−08	7.9E−09	1.1E−06
Thyroid	1.3E−07	2.1E−09	8.7E−08	1.5E−08	1.6E−08	5.4E−09	4.8E−08	1.5E−07	9.2E−07	1.3E−06
Uterus (Nongrvd)	1.1E−06	1.6E−05	7.7E−07	9.6E−06	5.4E−06	7.1E−06	9.4E−07	3.9E−07	8.2E−08	2.3E−06
Total Body	2.2E−06	1.9E−06	1.9E−06	2.4E−06	2.2E−06	2.3E−06	2.2E−06	2.2E−06	2.0E−06	1.9E−06

SOURCE ORGANS

(Continued)

257

TABLE 6-10. *S*, Absorbed Dose Per Unit Cumulated Activity. (rad/μCi · H) Technetium-99M (Half-Life, 6.03 h) *(Continued)*

TARGET ORGANS	Ovaries	Pancreas	SKELETON			Skin	Spleen	Testes	Thyroid	Total Body
			Red Marrow	Cort. Bone	Tra. Bone					
Adrenals	3.3E–07	9.1E–06	2.3E–06	1.1E–06	1.1E–06	6.8E–07	6.3E–06	3.2E–08	1.3E–07	2.3E–06
Bladder Wall	7.2E–06	1.4E–07	9.9E–07	5.1E–07	5.1E–07	4.9E–07	1.2E–07	4.8E–06	2.1E–09	2.3E–06
Bone (Total)	1.5E–06	1.5E–06	4.0E–06	1.2E–05	1.0E–05	9.9E–07	1.1E–06	9.2E–07	1.0E–06	2.5E–06
GI (Stom Wall)	8.1E–07	1.8E–05	9.5E–07	5.5E–07	5.5E–07	5.4E–07	1.0E–05	3.2E–08	4.5E–08	2.2E–06
GI (SI)	1.2E–05	1.8E–06	2.6E–06	7.3E–07	7.3E–07	4.5E–07	1.4E–06	3.6E–07	9.3E–09	2.5E–06
GI (ULI Wall)	1.1E–05	2.1E–06	2.1E–06	6.9E–07	6.9E–07	4.6E–07	1.4E–06	3.1E–07	1.1E–08	2.4E–06
GI (LLI Wall)	1.5E–05	5.7E–07	2.9E–06	1.0E–06	1.0E–06	4.8E–07	6.1E–07	2.7E–06	4.3E–09	2.3E–06
Kidneys	9.2E–07	6.6E–06	2.2E–06	8.2E–07	8.2E–07	5.7E–07	9.1E–06	4.0E–08	3.4E–08	2.2E–06
Liver	5.4E–07	4.4E–06	9.2E–07	6.6E–07	6.6E–07	5.3E–07	9.8E–07	3.1E–08	9.3E–08	2.2E–06
Lungs	6.0E–08	2.5E–06	1.2E–06	9.4E–07	9.4E–07	5.8E–07	2.3E–06	6.6E–09	9.4E–07	2.0E–06
Marrow (Red)	5.5E–06	2.8E–06	3.1E–05	4.1E–06	9.1E–06	9.5E–07	1.7E–06	7.3E–07	1.1E–06	2.9E–06
Other Tissues (Musc.)	2.0E–06	1.8E–06	1.2E–06	9.8E–07	9.8E–07	7.2E–07	1.4E–06	1.1E–06	1.3E–06	1.9E–06
Ovaries	4.2E–03	4.1E–07	3.2E–06	7.1E–07	7.1E–07	3.8E–07	4.0E–07	0.0	4.9E–09	2.4E–06
Pancreas	5.0E–07	5.8E–04	1.7E–06	8.5E–07	8.5E–07	4.4E–07	1.9E–05	5.5E–08	7.2E–08	2.4E–06
Skin	4.1E–07	4.0E–07	5.9E–07	6.5E–07	6.5E–07	1.6E–05	4.7E–07	1.4E–06	7.3E–07	1.3E–06
Spleen	4.9E–07	1.9E–05	9.2E–07	5.8E–07	5.8E–07	5.4E–07	3.3E–04	1.7E–08	1.1E–07	2.2E–06
Testes	0.0	5.5E–08	4.5E–07	6.4E–07	6.4E–07	9.1E–07	4.8E–08	1.4E–03	5.0E–10	1.7E–06
Thyroid	4.9E–09	1.2E–07	6.8E–07	7.9E–07	7.9E–07	6.9E–07	8.7E–08	5.0E–10	2.3E–03	1.5E–06
Uterus (Nongrvd)	2.1E–05	5.3E–07	2.2E–06	5.7E–07	5.7E–07	4.0E–07	4.0E–07	0.0	4.6E–09	2.6E–06
Total Body	2.6E–06	2.6E–06	2.2E–06	2.0E–06	2.0E–06	1.3E–06	2.2E–06	1.9E–06	1.8E–06	2.0E–06

Reprinted by permission of the Society of Nuclear Medicine from Snyder WS, Ford MR, Warner GG, Watson SB. MIRD Pamphlet No. 11: "S" Absorbed Dose per Unit Cumulated Activity for Selected Radionuclides and Organs. Reston, VA: Society of Nuclear Medicine; 1975.

values of S for ^{203}Hg and ^{99m}Tc. The use of the "S" tables in calculating internal dose is illustrated by Example 6.18.

EXAMPLE 6.18

An accidental inhalation exposure to ^{203}Hg-tagged mercury vapor led to a deposition of 0.5 MBq (13.5 μCi) ^{203}Hg ($T_R = 47$ days) in the kidneys. Calculate the dose commitment to the kidneys from this exposure.

Solution

The ICRP biokinetic model for inorganic mercury (ICRP Publication 30/2, 1980) assumes that after transfer from the blood, 8% of the absorbed Hg is in the kidneys and 92% is uniformly distributed throughout the body. Of all the body's Hg content, whether in the kidneys or elsewhere, 95% is assumed to be cleared with a biological half-life of 40 days and 5% with a biological half-life of 10,000 days.

The decay scheme for ^{203}Hg (Fig. 6-13) shows that the mercury emits a single group of beta particles whose maximum energy is 0.213 MeV and whose mean energy

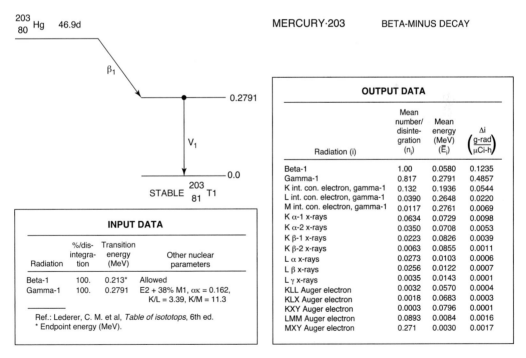

Figure 6-13. Transformation scheme and input and output data for ^{203}Hg dosimetry. (Reprinted by permission of the Society of Nuclear Medicine from Dillman LT. MIRD Pamphlet No. 4: Radionuclide Decay Schemes and Nuclear Parameters for Use in Radiation Dose Estimation. *J Nucl Med.* March 1969; 10(2 Suppl):1–32.

is listed in the output data as 0.058 MeV. A 0.279-MeV gamma ray is emitted after each beta transformation. The gamma ray, however, is internally converted in 18.3% of the transformations, thus leading to conversion electrons from the K, L, or M energy levels and, therefore, effective gamma-ray emission occurs in only 81.7% of the transformations.

Table 6-9 lists the absorbed dose per unit cumulated ^{203}Hg activity. For the kidneys as the source, S (kidneys ← kidneys) = 8.1×10^{-4} rad/μCi · h, and for the total body as the source, the dose to the kidney, S (kidneys ← total body) = 6.1×10^{-6} rad/μCi · h. The total dose to the kidneys is the sum of the doses due to the ^{203}Hg deposited in the kidneys, and also of the radiomercury in the rest of the body. If 0.5 MBq (13.5 μCi) in the kidneys represents 8% body burden of Hg, then the total activity in the body is

$$\frac{0.5\,\text{MBq}}{0.08} = 6.25\,\text{MBq}\ (168.9\,\mu\text{Ci}).$$

Since 0.5 MBq is in the kidneys, the amount of ^{203}Hg distributed throughout the rest of the body is $6.25 - 0.5 = 5.75$ MBq.

Of the 6.25 MBq deposited in the body, 95%, or 5.938 MBq, will be eliminated with an effective half-life, T_E, from Eq. (6.54):

$$T_E = \frac{T_R \times T_B}{T_R + T_B} = \frac{47\,\text{days} \times 40\,\text{days}}{47\,\text{days} + 40\,\text{days}} = 21.6\,\text{days},$$

and the remaining 5% of the deposited ^{203}Hg will have an effective half-life of 47 days. The corresponding effective clearance rate constants are

$$\lambda_1 = \frac{0.693}{21.61\,\text{days}} = 3.2 \times 10^{-2}\,\text{d}^{-1}$$

and

$$\lambda_2 = \frac{0.693}{47\,\text{days}} = 1.47 \times 10^{-2}\,\text{d}^{-1}.$$

The cumulated activity in the kidney is given by extending Eq. (6.90) to several compartments, $c_1, c_2, \ldots, c_n$, within an organ or a tissue is given as

$$\tilde{A} = \frac{A_{c_1}(0)}{\lambda_{E_1}} + \frac{A_{c_2}(0)}{\lambda_{E_2}} + \cdots + \frac{A_{c_n}(0)}{\lambda_{E_n}}. \tag{6.99}$$

From Table 6-9, we find S (kidneys ← kidneys) to be 8.1×10^{-4} rad/μCi · h. To convert rad/μCi · h to Gy/Bq · d:

$$\frac{\text{Gy}}{\text{Bq} \cdot \text{d}} = \frac{\text{rad}}{\mu\text{Ci} \cdot \text{h}} \times \frac{1\,\text{Gy}}{100\,\text{rad}} \times \frac{1\,\mu\text{Ci}}{3.7 \times 10^4\,\text{Bq}} \times \frac{24\,\text{h}}{\text{d}}$$

$$\frac{\text{Gy}}{\text{Bq} \cdot \text{d}} = \frac{\text{rad}}{\mu\text{Ci} \cdot \text{h}} \times 6.5 \times 10^{-6}. \tag{6.100}$$

Using the conversion factor in Eq. (6.100) we find that

$$S\text{ (kidney} \leftarrow \text{kidney)} = 8.1 \times 10^{-4} \frac{\text{rad}}{\mu\text{Ci} \cdot \text{h}} \times 6.5 \times 10^{-6} = 5.27 \times 10^{-9} \frac{\text{Gy}}{\text{Bq} \cdot \text{d}}.$$

The dose to the kidney from the mercury within the kidney is calculated from Eq. (6.97):

$$D(r_k \leftarrow r_h) = \tilde{A}_h \times S(r_k \leftarrow r_h)$$

$$D\text{ (kidney} \leftarrow \text{kidney)} = 1.65 \times 10^7 \text{ Bq} \cdot \text{d} \times 5.27 \times 10^{-9} \frac{\text{Gy}}{\text{Bq} \cdot \text{d}} = 8.7 \times 10^{-2} \text{Gy}.$$

The contribution of the ^{203}Hg distributed throughout the rest of the body to the kidney dose is now calculated by multiplying the cumulated body activity, $\tilde{A}$, by the value $S(\text{kidney} \leftarrow \text{body})$ from Table 6-9. The cumulated activity in the body is

$$\tilde{A}(\text{body}) = \frac{A_{b_1}(0)}{\lambda_{E_1}} + \frac{A_{b_2}(0)}{\lambda_{E_2}}$$

$$\tilde{A}(\text{body}) = \frac{0.95 \times 5.75 \times 10^6 \text{ Bq}}{3.2 \times 10^{-2} \text{d}^{-1}} + \frac{0.05 \times 5.75 \times 10^6 \text{ Bq}}{1.47 \times 10^{-2} \text{ d}^{-1}} = 1.903 \times 10^8 \text{ Bq} \cdot \text{d}.$$

The S (kidney $\leftarrow$ body) value from Table 6-9 is 6.1×10^{-6} rad/μCi $\cdot$ h. This value is converted to SI units with Eq. (6.100)

$$\frac{\text{Gy}}{\text{Bq} \cdot \text{d}} = \frac{\text{rad}}{\mu\text{Ci} \cdot \text{h}} \times 6.5 \times 10^{-6}$$

$$= 6.1 \times 10^{-6} \times 6.5 \times 10^{-6} = 3.97 \times 10^{-11} \frac{\text{Gy}}{\text{Bq} \cdot \text{d}}.$$

The dose to the kidney from the mercury distributed throughout the rest of the body is calculated from Eq. (6.97):

$$D(r_k \leftarrow r_h) = \tilde{A}_h \times S(r_k \leftarrow r_h)$$

$$D(\text{kidneys} \leftarrow \text{body}) = \tilde{A}\text{ (body)} \times S\text{ (kidneys} \leftarrow \text{body)}$$

$$= 1.903 \times 10^8 \text{ Bq} \cdot \text{d} \times 3.97 \times 10^{-11} \frac{\text{Gy}}{\text{Bq} \cdot \text{d}}$$

$$= 7.555 \times 10^{-3} \text{Gy}.$$

The total dose to the kidneys is the sum of the dose from each of the two sources:

$$D(\text{kidneys}) = D(\text{kidneys} \leftarrow \text{kidneys}) + D(\text{kidneys} \leftarrow \text{body})$$

$$D\text{ (kidneys)} = 8.72 \times 10^{-2} \text{ Gy} + 7.555 \times 10^{-3} \text{ Gy} = 9.48 \times 10^{-2} \text{ Gy (9.48 rads)}.$$

Equation (6.99) tells us that the cumulated activity in an organ or tissue is given by

$$\tilde{A} = \frac{A_{s_1}(0)}{\lambda_{E_1}} + \frac{A_{s_2}(0)}{\lambda_{E_2}} + \cdots + \frac{A_{s_n}(0)}{\lambda_{E_n}}$$

and Eq. (6.97) tells us that the dose to any organ is given by the product of the cumulated activity in the source organ and the appropriate S factor:

$$D(r_k \leftarrow r_h) = \tilde{A}_h \times S(r_k \leftarrow r_h).$$

If we substitute the expression for $\tilde{A}$ from Eq. (6.99) into Eq. (6.97), we get

$$D(r_k \leftarrow r_h) = \left(\frac{A_{hc_1}(0)}{\lambda_{E_{c_1}}} + \frac{A_{hc_2}(0)}{\lambda_{E_{c_2}}} + \cdots + \frac{A_{hc_n}(0)}{\lambda_{E_{c_n}}} \right) \times S(r_k \leftarrow r_h)$$

$$= \sum \frac{A_{c_i}}{\lambda_{E_{c_i}}} \times S(r_k \leftarrow r_h). \tag{6.101}$$

In Chapter 4, we showed that the average life of a radioisotope is simply the reciprocal of the transformation rate constant. Since the clearance of internally deposited radionuclides follows the same kinetics as radioactive transformation, it follows that the mean residence time of an internally deposited radionuclide is given by the reciprocal of the effective clearance rate constant, or its equivalent, 1.44 times the effective half-life:

$$\tau = \frac{1}{\lambda_E} = 1.44 \, T_E. \tag{6.102}$$

If the expression for $1/\lambda_E$ from Eq. (6.102) is substituted into Eq. (6.101), we obtain

$$D(r_k \leftarrow r_h) = \sum \tau_{hci} A_{hi}(0) \times S(r_k \leftarrow r_h), \tag{6.103}$$

where τ_{hci} is the residence time in the ith compartment of organ h.

The use of the mean residence time may be illustrated by the example that follows below.

 EXAMPLE 6.19

Calculate the dose from an accidental intake of ^{137}Cs that led to an initial body burden of 1 MBq (which was determined by whole-body counting).

Solution

The retention curve for ^{137}Cs is given by Eq. (6.59) as

$$q(t) = 0.1 \, q_0 \, e^{-(0.693t/2 \, \text{days})} + 0.9 \, q_0 \, e^{-(0.693t/110 \, \text{days})},$$

and MIRD Pamphlet No. 11 gives the $S(\text{body} \leftarrow \text{body})$ value for ^{137}Cs together with its very short-lived daughter $^{137\text{m}}\text{Ba}$ as 1.4×10^{-5} rad/μCi-day (3.8×10^{-6} Gy/MBq-day).

The mean residence time τ_1 in compartment 1 is calculated as follows:

$$\tau_1 = 1.44 \times 2\,\text{days} = 2.88\,\text{days}.$$

Since compartment 1 contained 10% of the activity, the cumulated activity in compartment 1 is

$$\tilde{A}_1 = 0.1 \times 1\,\text{MBq} \times 2.88\,\text{d} = 0.288\,\text{MBq} \cdot \text{d}.$$

The dose due to compartment 1 is calculated with Eq. (6.97):

$$D_1 = 0.288\,\text{MBq} \cdot \text{d} \times 3.8 \times 10^{-6}\ \text{Gy}/\left(\text{MBq} \cdot \text{d}\right) = 1.09 \times 10^{-6}\,\text{Gy}.$$

For compartment 2, the mean residence time, $\tau_{2,}$ is

$$\tau_2 = 1.44 \times 110\,\text{days} = 158.4\,\text{days}$$

and

$$\tilde{A}_2 = 0.9 \times 1\,\text{MBq} \times 158.4\,\text{days} = 142.6\,\text{MBq} \cdot \text{d}.$$

The dose from the radiocesium in compartment 2 is

$$D_2 = 142.6\,\text{MBq} \cdot \text{d} \times 3.8 \times 10^{-6}\,\text{Gy}/\left(\text{MBq} \cdot \text{d}\right) = 5.42 \times 10^{-4}\,\text{Gy}.$$

The total dose is the sum of the doses from the two compartments:

$$D = D_1 + D_2 = 1.09 \times 10^{-6}\,\text{Gy} + 5.42 \times 10^{-4}\,\text{Gy} = 5.43 \times 10^{-4}\,\text{Gy}$$
$$= 0.543\,\text{mGy}\ (54.3\,\text{mrads}).$$

ICRP Methodology

The MIRD methodology was developed to calculate doses from radionuclides that are administered for medical purposes. The ICRP methodology was developed to calculate doses from internally deposited radionuclides for health physics purposes. Since the objective for both methods is the same, namely to calculate a dose from an internal emitter, it is not surprising that the two methods are essentially the same. However, although they come to the same end point, the two computational methodologies use different terminology in constructing their formulations. Another difference between the two, which in most cases is trivial, is that the MIRD formulation calculates the dose in gray by integrating the dose rate over an infinitely long time after intake of the radionuclide, while the ICRP formulation calculates the equivalent dose in sievert (or rems when the traditional units are used) accumulated during 50 years after the intake.

The dose to a single target from a single radionuclide in a single source organ (for multiple sources and multiple radionuclides, we merely sum the contributions of each source and each radionuclide.) is given by MIRD, Eq. (6.97) as

$$D(r_k \leftarrow r_h) = \tilde{A}_h \times S(r_k \leftarrow r_h).$$

The ICRP formulation is given as

$$H_{50,T}(T \leftarrow S) = U_S \text{ transf.} \times SEE (T \leftarrow S) \frac{\text{Sv}}{\text{transf.}}, \qquad \textbf{(6.104)}$$

where

$H_{50,T}(T \leftarrow S)$ is the equivalent dose accumulated during 50 years after intake,
U_S is the total number of disintegrations during 50 years after intake, and
$SEE (T \leftarrow S)$ is the specific effective energy absorbed per gram of target tissue from each radiation, R, emitted from activity in the source organ.

It is calculated from the following equation:

$SEE (T \leftarrow S)$

$$= \sum_R \frac{Y_R \dfrac{\text{particles}}{\text{trans.}} \times (E \times w_R) \dfrac{\text{effectiveMeV}}{\text{particle}} \times 1.6 \times 10^{-13} \dfrac{\text{J}}{\text{MeV}} \times AF(T \leftarrow S)_R}{m_T \text{ kg}} \times \dfrac{1\text{Sv}}{\dfrac{\text{eff.J}}{\text{trans}}}$$

$$= \frac{\text{Sv}}{\text{trans}}, \qquad \textbf{(6.105)}$$

where

Y_R is the fractional yield, per disintegration, of the radiation under consideration,
w_R is the radiation weighting factor (formerly symbolized by Q),
$w_R = 1$ for gamma and beta radiation, and 20 for alphas,
$AF(T \leftarrow S)_R$ is the absorbed fraction from radiation R in T per transformation in S, and[3]
m_T is the mass of T, in kg.

Comparison of Eqs. (6.97) and (6.104) shows that the MIRD and ICRP equations are essentially the same. There are two differences between them: One is that the MIRD is the total lifetime dose, expressed in Gy (or rads in traditional units) while the ICRP dose is the effective dose, expressed in Sv (or rems in traditional units) for

[3]Tables of specific absorbed fractions may be found in Cristy and Eckerman, ORNL/NUREG/TM 8381.

the 50-year period following intake. The equations show that the ICRP analogs of the MIRD formulation are the following:

MIRD	ICRP
$D(r_k \leftarrow r_h)$, Total lifetime dose, Gy $\tilde{A}$, Cumulated activity, Bq-d	$H_{50,T}$ $(T \leftarrow S)$ 50-yr equivalent dose, Sv U_S, Total number of transformations in 50 yrs.
$S(r_k \leftarrow r_h)$, $\dfrac{\text{Sv}}{\text{Bq} \cdot \text{d}}$	$SEE(T \leftarrow S)$, $\dfrac{\text{Sv}}{\text{trans.}}$

The application of the ICRP notation is illustrated by the following example:

EXAMPLE 6.20

Fifty percent of the activity in inhaled soluble ^{210}Po particles is transferred to the blood. Of the polonium transferred to the blood, fractions of 0.1, 0.1, 0.1, and 0.7 are assumed to go to the liver, kidney, spleen, and all the other tissues, respectively. Having entered these tissues, the polonium is assumed to be retained with a biological half-life of 50 days. Calculate the dose to the spleen ($m = 150$ g) due to the inhalation of 1 Bq ^{210}Po particles.

Solution

^{210}Po emits one 5.3-MeV alpha particle per transformation, in which 5.4 MeV are dissipated (5.3 MeV plus 0.1 MeV ^{206}Pb daughter recoil energy).
   The effective half-life of ^{210}Po is

$$T_E = \frac{T_B \times T_R}{T_B + T_R} = \frac{50 \text{ days} \times 138 \text{ days}}{50 \text{ days} + 138 \text{ days}} = 36.7 \text{ days},$$

and the effective clearance rate constant is $\lambda_E = 0.693/T_E = 0.019$ per day.
   Inhalation of 1 Bq ^{210}Po leads to a deposition in the spleen of

$$q \text{ (spleen)} = 0.5 \times 1 \text{ Bq} \times 0.1 = 0.05 \text{ Bq}.$$

The total number of transformations in the spleen, U_s, is found with the aid of Eq. (6.90):

$$U_S = \frac{A_S(0)}{\lambda_E} = \frac{0.05 \text{ Bq} \times 1 \dfrac{\text{tps}}{\text{Bq}} \times 8.64 \times 10^4 \dfrac{\text{s}}{\text{d}}}{0.019 \text{ d}^{-1}} = 2.3 \times 10^5 \text{ transformations.}$$

Since we are dealing with alpha particles, the absorbed fraction (AF) is equal to 1. The equivalent dose to the spleen due to the ^{210}Po in the spleen is calculated with Eq. (6.105):

$$H_{50}(T \leftarrow S)_R = U_S \frac{Y_R \times (E \times w_R)\, \mathrm{AF}(T \leftarrow S)_R}{m_T} \times 1.6 \times 10^{-13} \times \frac{1\,\mathrm{Sv}}{\mathrm{effective\,J/kg}}.$$

$H_{50}(\text{spleen} \leftarrow \text{spleen})$

$$= 2.3 \times 10^5 \text{trans.} \times \frac{\left(5.4\,\dfrac{\mathrm{MeV}}{\alpha} \times 20\right) \times 1\,\dfrac{\alpha}{\mathrm{trans.}} \times 1.6 \times 10^{-13}\,\dfrac{\mathrm{J}}{\mathrm{MeV}}}{0.15\,\mathrm{kg}} \times \frac{1\,\mathrm{Sv}}{\mathrm{J/kg}}$$

$$= 2.6 \times 10^{-5}\,\mathrm{Sv}.$$

The committed equivalent dose to the spleen is thus found to be 2.6×10^{-5} Sv Bq^{-1} ^{210}Po inhaled.

EXTERNAL EXPOSURE: NEUTRONS

Exposure to neutrons is always from an external source. However, because one aspect of neutron-dose calculation simulates the dose from a uniformly distributed radionuclide, discussion was deferred until this point in the chapter.

Fast Neutrons

The absorbed dose from a beam of neutrons may be computed by considering the energy absorbed by each of the tissue elements that react with the neutrons. The type of reaction, of course, depends on the neutron energy. For fast neutrons up to about 20 MeV, the main mechanism of energy transfer is elastic collision. Thermal neutrons may be captured and initiate nuclear reactions. In cases of elastic scattering of fast neutrons, the scattered nuclei dissipate their energy in the immediate vicinity of the primary neutron interaction. The radiation dose absorbed locally in this way is called the *first collision dose* and is determined entirely by the primary neutron flux; the scattered neutron is not considered after this primary interaction. For fast neutrons, the first collision dose rate from neutrons of energy E is

$$\dot{D}_n(E) = \frac{\phi(E)\,E\,\sum_i N_i \sigma_i\, f}{1\,\mathrm{J/kg/Gy}}, \tag{6.106}$$

where

$\phi(E) =$ flux of neutrons whose energy is E, in neutrons per cm^2 per second,

$N_i =$ number of atoms per kilogram of the ith element,

$\sigma_i =$ scattering across section of the ith element for neutrons of energy E, in barns $\times 10^{-24}$ cm^2, and

$f =$ mean fractional energy transferred from neutron to scattered atom during collision with the neutron.

TABLE 6-11. *Synthetic Tissue Composition*

ELEMENT	% MASS	n (Atoms/kg)	f
Oxygen	71.39	2.69×10^{25}	0.111
Carbon	14.89	6.41×10^{24}	0.142
Hydrogen	10.00	5.98×10^{25}	0.500
Nitrogen	3.47	1.49×10^{24}	0.124
Sodium	0.15	3.93×10^{22}	0.080
Chlorine	0.10	1.70×10^{22}	0.053

(Reprinted by permission of the Society of Nuclear Medicine from Brownell GL, Ellet WH, Reddy AR. MIRD Pamphlet No. 3: Absorbed Fractions for Photon Dosimetry. *J Nuclear Med.* February 1968; 9(1 Suppl):29–39.)

For isotropic scattering, the average fraction of the neutron energy transferred in an elastic collision with a nucleus of atomic mass number M is

$$f = \frac{2M}{(M+1)^2}. \tag{6.107}$$

The composition of soft tissue, for the purpose of radiation dosimetry is given in Table 6-11. The table also lists the average fraction of the neutron energy transferred to each of the tissue elements.

EXAMPLE 6.21

What is the absorbed dose rate to soft tissue in a beam of 5-MeV neutrons whose intensity is 2000 neutrons/cm²/second?

Solution

The scattering cross sections of each of the tissue elements for 5-MeV neutrons are listed below:

ELEMENT	σ, $\times 10^{-24}$ cm²	$N_i\sigma_i f_i$
O	1.55	4.628
C	1.65	1.502
H	1.50	4.485×10^{1}
N	1.00	1.848×10^{-1}
Na	2.3	7.231×10^{-3}
Cl	2.8	2.523×10^{-3}

$$\sum N_i \sigma_i f_i = 5.117 \times 10^1 \, \frac{cm^2}{kg}$$

Substituting the appropriate values into Eq. (6.106) yields

$$\dot{D}_n = \frac{2 \times 10^3 \, \dfrac{\text{neutrons}}{\text{cm}^2/\text{s}} \times 5 \, \dfrac{\text{MeV}}{\text{(neutron)}} \times 1.6 \times 10^{-13} \, \dfrac{\text{J}}{\text{MeV}} \times 51.17 \, \dfrac{\text{cm}^2}{\text{kg}}}{1 \, \text{J/kg/Gy}}$$

$$= 8.19 \times 10^{-8} \, \frac{\text{Gy}}{\text{s}} \left(8.19 \times 10^{-6} \, \frac{\text{rad}}{\text{s}} \right),$$

or

$$8.19 \times 10^{-8} \frac{Gy}{s} \times 10^6 \frac{\mu Gy}{Gy} \times 3.6 \times 10^3 \frac{s}{h} = 295 \ \mu Gy/h \, (29.5 \ \text{mrads/h}).$$

In the example above, the neutron beam was monoenergetic and thus only one neutron energy was considered. If a beam contains neutrons of several energies, then the calculation must be carried out separately for each energy group.

Thermal Neutrons

For thermal neutrons, two reactions are considered, namely, the $^{14}N(n, p)^{14}C$ reaction and the $^1H(n, \gamma)^2H$ reaction. For the former reaction, the dose rate may be calculated from the equation

$$\dot{D}_{n,p} = \frac{\phi N_N \sigma_N Q \times 1.6 \times 10^{-13} \frac{J}{MeV}}{1 \frac{J/kg}{Gy}}, \tag{6.108}$$

where

ϕ = thermal flux, neutrons/cm^2/s,
N_N = number of nitrogen atoms per kg tissue, 1.49×10^{24},
σ_N = absorption cross section for nitrogen, 1.75×10^{-24} cm^2, and
Q = energy released by the reaction = 0.63 MeV.

The latter reaction, $^1H(n, \gamma)^2H$ is equivalent to having a uniformly distributed gamma-emitting isotope throughout the body and results in an auto-integral gamma-ray dose. The specific activity of this distributed gamma emitter, the number of reactions per second per gram, is governed by the neutron flux and is given by Eq. (6.109)

$$A = \phi N_H \sigma_H \frac{"Bq"}{kg}, \tag{6.109}$$

where

ϕ = thermal flux, neutrons/cm^2/s,
N_H = number of hydrogen atoms per kg tissue = 5.98×10^{25}, and
σ_H = absorption cross section for hydrogen = 0.33×10^{-24} cm^2.

EXAMPLE 6.22

What is the absorbed dose rate to a 70-kg person from a whole body exposure to a mean thermal flux of 10,000 neutrons/cm^2/s?

Solution

The dose rate due to the n, p reaction is calculated from Eq. (6.108).

$$\dot{D}_{n,p}$$

$$= \frac{10^4 \frac{\text{neutrons}}{\text{cm}^2/\text{s}} \times 1.49 \times 10^{24} \frac{\text{atoms}}{\text{kg}} \times 1.75 \times 10^{-24} \frac{\text{cm}^2}{\text{atom}} \times 0.63\,\text{MeV} \times 1.6 \times 10^{-13} \frac{\text{J}}{\text{MeV}}}{1 \frac{\text{J/kg}}{\text{Gy}}}$$

$$= 2.628 \times 10^{-9} \frac{\text{Gy}}{\text{s}},$$

or, the close rate per hour $= 2.628 \times 10^{-9}$ Gy/s $\times 3.6 \times 10^3$ s/h

$$\dot{D}_{n,p} = 9.5\,\frac{\mu\text{Gy}}{\text{h}} \quad \left(0.95\,\frac{\text{mrad}}{\text{h}}\right).$$

The auto-integral gamma-ray dose rate is calculated with Eq. (6.82). The gamma-ray "activity," from Eq. (6.109) is

$$A = 10^4\,\frac{\text{neutrons}}{\text{cm}^2/\text{s}} \times 5.98 \times 10^{25}\,\frac{\text{atoms}}{\text{kg}} \times 3.3 \times 10^{-25}\,\frac{\text{cm}^2}{\text{atom}}$$

$$= 1.973 \times 10^5\,\text{''}\frac{\text{Bq}''}{\text{kg}}.$$

The dose rate from this uniformly distributed gamma ray emitter is calculated from Eq. (6.82):

$$\dot{D}_\gamma = \frac{A_S}{m} \times \varphi \times \Delta\frac{\text{Gy}}{\text{s}}.$$

The absorbed fraction, φ, for the 2.23-MeV gamma ray is found, by interpolating in Table 6-8 between the 2.000 and 4.000 MeV values, to be 0.278, and Δ, the dose rate in an infinitely large mass whose specific activity is $1\,\frac{\text{Bq}}{\text{kg}}$, is calculated from Eq. (6.81):

$$\Delta = 1.6 \times 10^{-13} \times 2.23\,\frac{\text{MeV}}{\gamma} = 3.57 \times 10^{-13}\,\frac{\text{Gy/s}}{\text{Bq/kg}}.$$

The auto-integral gamma-ray dose rate, therefore, is

$$\dot{D}_\gamma = 1.973 \times 10^5\,\frac{\text{Bq}}{\text{kg}} \times 0.278 \times 3.57 \times 10^{-13}\,\frac{\text{Gy/s}}{\text{Bq/kg}}$$

$$= 1.96 \times 10^{-8}\,\frac{\text{Gy}}{\text{s}} \quad (1.96 \times 10^{-6}\,\text{rad/s})$$

or

$$71\,\mu\,\frac{\text{Gy}}{\text{h}} \quad \left(7.1\,\frac{\text{mrad}}{\text{h}}\right).$$

We cannot, in this case, add the auto-integral gamma-ray dose to the dose from the *n, p* reaction because an absorbed dose of 1 Gy of gamma radiation is not biologically equivalent to 1 Gy from proton radiation. This point, which deals with the relative biological effectiveness of the various radiations, is discussed in the next chapter.

SUMMARY

When ionizing radiation interacts with any medium (air, tissue, water, plastic, etc.), energy is transferred from the radiation field to the medium. The quantity that describes this energy transfer is the absorbed dose and is measured by the concentration of absorbed energy. Traditionally, this quantity was called a *rad*, and 1 rad was defined as the *absorption of 100 ergs of energy per gram of irradiated medium*. In the SI system, the quantity for absorbed dose is the *gray* (Gy); 1 gray is defined as an *absorption of one joule of energy per kilogram*: 1 Gy = 100 rads. Absorbed dose is a macroscopic quantity, and it applies to the average amount of energy absorbed per unit mass of absorbing medium.

The first quantitative unit that was used for radiation dose was the roentgen (R). Technically, the roentgen was a dose unit *only for air*; hence, it is a measure of X- or gamma-ray exposure, not radiation dose. However, it continues to be useful in radiation protection because an exposure of 1 R leads to a dose of approximately 1 rad to soft tissue. In SI units, exposure to X- or gamma radiation is measured in coulombs of ions produced by the radiation per kilogram of air: 1 R = 2.58×10^{-4} C/kg.

Absorbed dose is defined in the same way for external radiation as it is for the dose from internally deposited radioisotopes. For external radiation, the dose can be measured. For internally deposited radionuclides, the dose cannot be measured. The dose from an internally deposited radionuclide is calculated with the aid of a physiologically based biokinetic dosimetric model for that radionuclide that considers the radiation characteristics of the nuclide and the biological characteristics of the deposited radionuclides. This method is formalized in the MIRD system for *medical internal radiation dosimetry*, where the calculation is based on the fraction of the energy emitted by the radionuclide that is absorbed in the tissue of interest and the mean residence time of the radioactivity in the organs or tissues. A parallel computational methodology for calculating internal dose for health physics purposes was developed by the ICRP. The ICRP formulation is based on calculating the energy absorbed per kg of irradiated target tissue from one decay of a radionuclide deposited in a source organ and then multiplying this by the total number of decays in the source organ during the 50-year period following intake of the radionuclide.

 PROBLEMS

6.1. A 50-μC/kg ($\sim$200 mR) pocket dosimeter with air-equivalent walls has a sensitive volume with the dimensions 0.5 in. (diameter) and 2.5 in. (length); the volume is filled with air at atmospheric pressure. The capacitance of the dosimeter is 10 pF. If 200 V are required to charge the chamber, what is the voltage across the chamber when it reads 50 μC/kg ($\sim$200 mR)?

6.2. An air ionization chamber whose volume is 1 L is used as an environmental monitor at a temperature of $27°C$ and a pressure of 700 torr. What is the exposure rate, in $\mu C/kg/h$ and in mR/h, if the saturation current is 10^{-13} A?

6.3. A beam of 1-MeV gamma rays and another of 0.1-MeV gamma rays each produce the same ionization density in air. What is the ratio of 1:0.1 MeV photon flux?

6.4. Assuming that the specific heat of the body is 1 cal/g/$°C$, calculate the temperature rise due to a total body dose of 5 Gy.

6.5. Compute the exposure rate, in mGy/h, at a distance of 50 cm from a small vial containing 10 mL of an aqueous solution of

(a) 2-GBq (54.1-mCi) ^{51}Cr

(b) 2-GBq (54.1-mCi) ^{24}Na, based on the transformation schemes shown below:

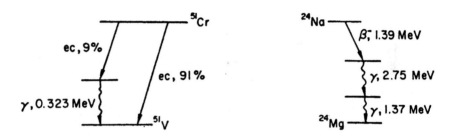

6.6. What is the soft tissue dose rate during exposure to 25.4 $\mu C/kg/h$ (100 mR/h) of 0.5-MeV gamma radiation?

6.7. A collimated beam of 0.3-MeV gamma radiation whose energy flux is 5 J/m^2/s is shielded by 2-cm Pb.

(a) What is the photon flux incident on the shield, in photons cm^{-2} s^{-1}?

(b) What is the exposure rate, mR/h and C/kg/h, in the incident and emergent beams?

(c) What is the tissue dose rate, mGy/h, in the incident and emergent beams?

6.8. The exposure rate in a beam of 100-keV gamma rays is 25.8 $\mu C/kg$ (100 mR) per hour. What is the

(a) photon flux, in photons/cm^2/s?

(b) power density, in W/m^2 and mW/cm^2?

6.9. In an experiment, a 250-g rat is injected with 10-μCi ^{203}Hg in the form of $Hg(NO_3)_2$. The rat was counted daily in a total-body counter and the following equation was fitted to the whole-body-counting data

$$Y = 0.55e^{-0.346t} + 0.45e^{-0.0346t}$$

where Y is the fraction of the injected dose retained t days after injection. If the long-lived component of the curve represents clearance from the kidneys while the short-lived component represents clearance from the rest of the body, calculate the radiation absorbed dose to the whole body and the kidneys if each kidney weighs 0.7 g. Assume the mercury to be uniformly distributed in the whole body and in the kidneys. Base the calculation on the transformation scheme given in Figure 6-13.

6.10. Iodine is deposited in the thyroid at a rate of 0.139 h^{-1}. If the radioactive half-life of ^{123}I is 13 hours, what is the effective deposition half-life?

6.11. A patient with cancer of the thyroid has been found to have a thyroid iodine uptake of 50%. How much ^{131}I must be injected to deliver a dose of 15 Gy (1500 rads) in 3 days to the thyroid which weighs 30 g?

6.12. The mean concentration of potassium in seawater is 380 mg/kg. What is the dose rate, in milligrays per year and in millirads per year, in the ocean depths due to the dissolved ^{40}K?

6.13. Calculate the annual radiation dose to a reference person from the ^{40}K and from the ^{14}C deposited in his body. The specific activity of carbon is 0.255 Bq (6.9 pCi)/g. Assume, in both instances, that the radioisotopes are uniformly distributed throughout the body.

6.14. A thin-walled carbon-wall ionization chamber, whose volume is 2 cm^3, is filled with standard air at 0°C and 760 torr and is placed inside a tank of water to make a depth–dose measurement. A 24-MeV betatron beam produces a current of 0.02 μA in the chamber. What was the absorbed dose rate?

6.15. An aluminum ionization chamber containing 10 cm^3 air at 20°C and 760 torr operates under Bragg–Gray conditions. After a 1-hour exposure to ^{60}Co gamma rays, 3.6×10^{-9} C of charge is collected. If the relative mass stopping power of Al for the electrons generated by the ^{60}Co gammas is 0.875, what was the dose to the aluminum?

6.16. An ion chamber made of 50 g copper has a 10-cm^3 cavity filled with air at STP. The temperature of the copper rose 0.002°C after exposure to ^{60}Co gamma rays. If the mass stopping power of Cu is 0.753 relative to air and if the specific heat of Cu is 0.092 cal/g/C, calculate

   (a) the absorbed dose to the copper and

   (b) the amount of charge (in coulombs) formed by ionization in the cavity during the exposure.

6.17. An aqueous suspension of virus is irradiated by X-rays whose half-value layer is 2-mm Cu. If the exposure was 335 C/kg (1.3×10^6 R), and if the depth of the suspension is 5 mm, what was the absorbed dose and what was the mean ionization density?

6.18. A child drinks 1 L of milk per day containing ^{131}I at a mean concentration of 33.3 Bq (900 pCi)/L over a period of 30 days. Assuming that the child has no other intake of ^{131}I, calculate the dose to the thyroid at the end of the 30-day ingestion period and the dose commitment to the thyroid.

6.19. A patient who weighs 50 kg is given an organic compound tagged with 4-MBq (108-μCi) ^{14}C. On the basis of bioassay measurements, the following whole-body retention data were inferred:

Day	0	1	2	3	4	5	6	8	10	12	14
MBq	4	2.94	2.32	1.9	1.6	1.4	1.2	0.9	0.8	0.6	0.5

    (a) Plot the retention data and write the equation for the retention curve as a function of time.

    (b) Assuming the ^{14}C to be uniformly distributed throughout the body, calculate the absorbed dose to the patient at day 7 and day 14 after administration of the drug.

    (c) What is the dose commitment from this procedure?

6.20. A 2-MeV electron beam is used to irradiate a sample of plastic whose thickness is 0.5 g/cm^2. If a 250-μA beam passes through a port 1 cm in diameter to strike the plastic, calculate the absorbed dose rate.

6.21. Calculate the average power density, in watts per kilogram, of an aqueous solution of ^{60}Co, at a concentration of 10 MBq/L, in

    (a) an infinitely large medium.

    (b) a 6-L spherical tank.

6.22. A 20-L sealed polyethylene cylinder contains 3700-MBq (100 mCi) ^{137}Cs waste uniformly dispersed in concrete. Neglecting absorption by the cover, estimate the dose rate at the top of the container, and at 1 m over the center of the top.

6.23. A nuclear bomb is exploded at an altitude of 200 m. Assuming 10^{18} fissions in the explosion resulting in 6 fission gammas of 1 MeV each and 2 prompt neutrons of 2 MeV each, estimate the dose from the gammas and from the neutrons at 1500 m from ground zero. Neglect the shielding effect of the air and scattering from the ground.

6.24. An unmarked, unshielded vial containing 370-MBq (10-mCi) ^{24}Na is left in a hood. A radiochemist, unaware of the presence of the ^{24}Na, spends 8 hours at his bench, which is 2 m from the ^{24}Na. Based on the ^{24}Na transformation scheme shown in problem 6.5, calculate

    (a) the dose rate at 2 m from the 370 MBq source,

    (b) the dose commitment from the 8-hour exposure.

6.25. Chlormerodrin tagged either with ^{197}Hg or ^{203}Hg is used diagnostically in studies of renal function. Calculate the dose to the kidneys, for the case of normal uptake, 35%, from injection of 3.7 MBq (100 μCi) of each of the radioisotopes. Assume very rapid kidney deposition, followed by elimination with a biological half-time of 6.5 hours.

6.26. A nuclear medicine procedure used to evaluate pulmonary perfusion uses intravenously injected ^{99m}Tc-tagged microspheres that are rapidly taken up by the lungs, where they are temporarily trapped in a small fraction of the capillaries. Absence of radioactivity in a part of the lung means decreased perfusion of that part and suggests a possible pulmonary embolism. If 60% of the ^{99m}Tc activity is transferred out of the lung with a biological half-time of 1.8 hours, and the other 40% has a biological clearance half-time of 36 hours.

    (a) What is the mean intrapulmonary residence time of the ^{99m}Tc?

    (b) What is the dose to the lung from the intrapulmonary activity per megabecquerel injected?

6.27. Three millicuries (111 MBq) ^{99m}Tc-labeled sulfur colloid is injected to visualize the liver. Sixty percent of the injectate is deposited in the liver, 30% in the spleen, and 10% in the red bone marrow. Calculate the absorbed dose to the

(a) liver,

(b) spleen, and

(c) red marrow.

6.28. A patient is treated for Graves' disease with 111-Mbq (3-mCi) ^{131}I. Uptake studies with a tracer dose of ^{125}I showed a thyroid uptake of 60% and a biological half-time of 2 days. Assuming a very rapid uptake in the thyroid, calculate the dose to the thyroid from this treatment.

6.29. A well-insulated water sample is irradiated with gamma rays at a rate of 10-Gy (1000 rads)/h. What is the rate of temperature rise in the water, in °C/h?

6.30. A laboratory worker who weighs 70 kg was accidentally exposed for several hours in an atmosphere containing tritiated water vapor. Urine analyses for tritium were made for 7 weeks, starting 1 day after exposure, and the following data were obtained on 24-hour urine samples:

Day	1	2	3	5	7	10	14	21	28	35	42	49
Bq	524	485	450	402	342	293	227	147	94	60	40	26

According to reference man, 47% of the daily water output is via the urine. Assuming that the tritium is uniformly distributed throughout the body's water,

(a) plot the data and write the equation for the clearance curve and

(b) calculate the worker's dose commitment from this accidental exposure.

6.31. Three millicuries (111 MBq) of a ^{99m}Tc tagged colloid is injected into a patient to visualize the liver. In vivo bioassay finds that 40% of the injected activity is deposited in the liver and that it is cleared out of the liver at a rate of 0.231/h. Given that

- the liver weighs 1.8 kg
- $T_{1/2}$ of ^{99m}Tc = 6 hours
- ^{99m}Tc emits only a 0.14 MeV gamma in decay
- the absorbed fraction of the gamma ray energy in the liver = 0.25, calculate the

(a) effective half-time of the ^{99m}Tc in the liver,

(b) biological half-time of the ^{99m}Tc in the liver,

(c) mean residence time of the ^{99m}Tc in the liver, and

(d) dose to the liver from the activity deposited there.

6.32. In a diagnostic examination of a patient's thyroid, the patient, who weighs 70 kg, is given a capsule containing 10-μCi (0.37 MBq) ^{131}I. Thirty percent of the radioiodine is rapidly taken up by the thyroid, whose weight is estimated as 30 g. Given that

- the biological half-life of iodine in the thyroid is 120 days,
- the radiological half life of ^{131}I is 8 days, and

- the average absorbed energy in the thyroid is 0.21 MeV (disintegration)$^{-1}$, calculate the:

   (a) effective half life of the radioiodine in the thyroid, in days,

   (b) effective turnover rate of the radioiodine in the thyroid, in percent day^{-1},

   (c) mean residence time of the radioiodine in the thyroid, in days,

   (d) time for 90% of the radioiodine to be cleared from the thyroid, and

   (e) committed dose to the thyroid, in cGy.

6.33. The tissue dose rate in a beam of 500 keV gammas is 1 Gy/min. What is the photon flux, in photons/cm^2/min?

6.34. A man swallows 1-MBq ^{210}Po. Ten percent of ingested ^{210}Po is absorbed into the blood and the balance is excreted. Of the polonium transferred to the blood, fractions of 0.1, 0.1, 0.1, and 0.7 are assumed to go to the liver, kidney, spleen, and all the other tissues respectively. Having entered these tissues, the polonium is assumed to be retained with a biological half-life of 50 days. Using the values for the reference male, 5.3 MeV per alpha, and 0.1 MeV per ^{206}Pb recoil atom, calculate

(a) the dose to each of the 4 compartments and

(b) the 50-year committed effective dose equivalent, in Sv and in rems, using the ICRP 60 tissue weighting factors.

SUGGESTED READINGS

Attix, F. A. *Introduction to Radiological Physics and Radiation Dosimetry.* John Wiley & Sons, New York, 1986.

Attix, F. H., Roesch, W. C., and Tochikin, E., eds. *Radiation Dosimetry*, Vol. I, *Fundamentals.* Academic Press, New York, 1968.

Berger, M. J. *Distribution of Absorbed Dose Around Point Sources of Electrons and Beta Particles in Water and Other Media.* MIRD Pamphlet No, 7. Society of Nuclear Medicine, New York, 1971.

Brodsky, A., ed. *Handbook of Radiation Protection and Measurement*, Vol. I, *Physical Science and Engineering Data.* CRC Press. West Palm Beach, FL, 1978.

Brodsky, A., ed. *Handbook of Radiation Protection and Measurement*, Vol. II, *Biological and Mathematical Information.* CRC Press, Boca Raton, FL, 1982.

Cristy, M., and Eckerman, K.F. *Specific Absorbed Fractions at Various Energies at Various Ages from Internal Photon Sources.* ORNL/NUREG/TM-3881, Vols. 1–7. Oak Ridge National Laboratory, TN, 1987.

Faw, R., and Shultis, J. K. *Radiological Assessment.* Prentice-Hall, Englewood Cliffs, NJ, 1993.

Fisher, D.R., ed. *Current Concepts in Lung Dosimetry.* National Technical Information Service, Springfield, VA, 1983.

Fitzgerald, J. J., Brownell, G. L., and Mahoney, F. J. *Mathematical Theory of Radiation Dosimetry.* Gordon and Breach, New York, 1967.

Greening, J. R. *Fundamentals of Radiation Dosimetry*, 2nd ed. Adam Hilger, Ltd., Bristol, England, 1985.

Hendee, W. R. *Medical Radiation Physics.* Yearbook Medical Publishers, Chicago, IL, 1970.

Hendee, W. R., Ibbott, G.S., and Hendee, E.G. *Radiation Therapy Physics*, 3rd ed. John Wiley & Sons, New York, 2005.

Howe, D. B. "Staff and patient dosimetry in a hospital health physics program," in Eicholz, G. G., and Shonka, J. J., eds. *Hospital Health Physics.* Proceedings of the 1993 Health Physics Society Summer School, Research Enterprises, Richland, WA, 1993.

International Commission on Radiation Units and Measurements (ICRU), Washington, DC
   No. 10b. *Physical Aspects of Irradiation*, 1964.
   No. 10d. *Clinical Dosimetry*, 1963.

No. 13. *Neutron Fluence, Neutron Spectra, and Kerma,* 1969.

No. 14. *Radiation Dosimetry: X-rays and Gamma Rays with Maximum Photon Energies between 0.6 and 50 MeV,* 1969.

No. 16. *Linear Energy Transfer,* 1970.

No. 17. *Radiation Dosimetry: X-rays Generated at Potentials of 5 to 150 kV,* 1970.

No. 21. *Radiation Dosimetry: Electrons with Initial Energies Between 1 and 50 MeV,* 1972.

No. 23. *Measurement of Absorbed Dose in a Phantom Irradiated by a Single Beam of X- or Gamma Rays,* 1973.

No. 24. *Determination of Absorbed Dose in a Patient Irradiated by Beams of X- or Gamma Rays in Radiotherapy Procedures,* 1976.

No. 26. *Neutron Dosimetry for Biology and Medicine,* 1977.

No. 28. *Basic Aspects of High Energy Particle Interactions and Radiation Dosimetry,* 1978.

No. 29. *Dose Specification for Reporting External Beam Therapy with Photons and Electrons,* 1978.

No. 30. *Quantitative Concepts and Dosimetry in Radiobiology,* 1979.

No. 32. *Methods of Assessment of Absorbed Dose in Clinical Use of Radionuclides,* 1979.

No. 34. *The Dosimetry of Pulsed Radiation,* 1982.

No. 35. *Radiation Dosimetry: Electron Beams with Energies Between 1 and 50 MeV,* 1984.

No. 36. *Microdosimetry,* 1983.

No. 37. *Stopping Powers for Electrons and Positrons,* 1983.

No. 44. *Tissue Substitutes in Radiation Dosimetry and Measurements,* 1989.

No. 45. *Clinical Neutron Dosimetry—Part I: Determination of Absorbed Dose in a Patient Treated by External Beams of Fast Neutrons,* 1989.

No. 46. *Photon, Electron, Proton, and Neutron Interaction Data for Body Tissues,* 1992.

No. 46d. *Photon, Electron, Proton, and Neutron Interaction Data for Body Tissues with Data Disk,* 1992.

No. 48. *Phantom and Computational Models in Therapy, Diagnosis, and Protection,* 1992.

No. 51. *Quantities and Units in Radiation Protection Dosimetry,* 1993.

No. 57. *Conversion Coefficients for use in Radiological Protection Against External Radiation,* 1998.

International Commission on Radiological Protection (ICRP). Pergamon Press, Oxford, England:

No. 10. *The Assessment of Internal Contamination Resulting from Recurrent or Prolonged Uptake,* 1971.

No. 23. *Reference Man: Anatomical, Physiological, and Metabolic Characteristics,* 1975.

International Commission on Radiological Protection (ICRP). *Annals of the ICRP,* Pergamon Press, Oxford, England or NY:

No. 26. *Recommendations of the International Commission on Radiological Protection.* Vol. 1, No. 3, 1977.

No. 30. *Limits for Intakes of Radionuclides by Workers.*
  Part 1, Vol. 2, Nos. 3/4, 1977.
  Part 2, Vol. 4, Nos. 3/4, 1980

No. 38. *Radionuclide Transformations: Energy and Intensity of Emissions.* Vols. 11–13, 1983.

No. 42. *A Compilation of Major Concepts and Quantities in Use by the ICRP.* Vol. No. 4, 1984.

No. 53. *Radiation Dose to Patients from Radiopharmaceuticals.* Vol. 18, Nos. 1–4, 1988.

No. 60. *1990 Recommendations of the International Commission on Radiological Protection.* Vol. 21, Nos. 1–3, 1991.

No. 80. *Radiation Doses to Patients from Radiopharmaceuticals, Addendum to ICRP 53.* Vol. 28, No. 3, 1998.

No. 88. *Doses to the Embryo and Fetus from Intakes of Radionuclides by the Mother.* Vol. 31, Nos. 1–3, 2001.

No. 95. *Doses to Infants from Ingestion of Radionuclides in Mothers' Milk,* Vol. 34, Nos. 3–4, 2004.

Johns, H. E., and Cunningham, J. R. *The Physics of Radiology,* 4th ed. Charles C. Thomas, Springfield, IL, 1983.

Kase, K. R., and Nelson, W. R. *Concepts of Radiation Dosimetry.* Pergamon, New York, 1978.

Killough, G. G., and Eckerman, K. F. "Internal dosimetry", in Till, J. E., and Meyer, H. R., eds. *Radiological Assessment.* NUREG/CR-3332, USNRC, Washington, DC, 1983.

Kocher, D. C. "External dosimetry," in Till, J. E., and Meyer, H. R., eds. *Radiological Assessment.* NUREG/CR-3332, USNRC, Washington, DC, 1983.

Loevinger, R., Budinger, T. F., and Watson, E. E. *MIRD Primer for Absorbed Dose Calculations.* Society of Nuclear Medicine, New York, 1988.

Medical Internal Dose Committee (MIRD) Committee, Society of Nuclear Medicine, New York.

No. 1. Loevinger, R., and Berman, M. *A Scheme for Absorbed-Dose Calculations for Biologically Distributed Radionuclides,* 1976.

No. 5 (revised). Snyder, W.S., Ford, M. R., and Warner, G. G. *Estimates of Specific Absorbed Fractions for Photon Sources Uniformly Distributed in Various Organs of a Heterogeneous Phantom,* 1978.

No. 7. Berger, M. J. *Distribution of Absorbed Dose Around Point Sources of Electrons and Beta Particles in Water and Other Media*, 1971.

No. 8. Ellett, W. H., and Humes, R. M. *Absorbed Fractions for Small Volumes Containing Photon Emitting Radioactivity*, 1971.

No. 10. Dillon, L. T., and Von Der Laage, F. C. *Radionuclide Decay Schemes and Nuclear Parameters for Use in Radiation Dose Estimation*, 1975.

No. 11. Snyder, W. S., Ford, M. R., Warner, G. G., and Watson, S. B. *"S," Absorbed Dose per Unit Cumulated Activity for Selected Radionuclides and Organs*, 1975.

No. 12. Berman, M. *Kinetic Models for Absorbed Dose Calculations,* 1977.

No. 13. Coffey, J.L., Cristy, M., and Warner, G.G. *Specific Absorbed Fractions for Photon Sources Uniformly Distributed in the Heart Chambers and Hart Wall of Heterogeneous Phantom*, 1981.

Morgan, K. Z., and Turner, J. E., eds. *Principles of Radiation Protection*. Krieger, New York, 1973.

National Council on Radiation Protection and Measurements (NCRP), Bethesda, MD.

No. 25. *Measurement of Absorbed Dose of Neutrons, and of Mixtures of Neutrons and Gamma Rays*, 1961.

No. 27. *Stopping Powers for Use With Cavity Chambers*, 1961.

No. 69. *Dosimetry of X-Ray and Gamma-Ray Beams for Radiation Therapy in the Energy Range 10 keV to 50 MeV*, 1981.

No. 82. *SI Units in Radiation Protection and Measurements*, 1985.

No. 83. *The Experimental Basis for Absorbed-Dose Calculations in Medical Use of Radionuclides*, 1985.

No. 84. *General Concepts for the Dosimetry of Internally Deposited Radionuclides*, 1985.

No. 87. *Use of Bioassay Procedures for Assessment of Internal Radionuclide Deposition*, 1987.

No. 106. *Limit for Exposure to "Hot Particles" on the Skin*, 1989.

No. 108. *Conceptual Basis for Calculations of Absorbed Dose Distributions*, 1991.

Paic, G. *Ionizing Radiation, Protection and Dosimetry*. CRC Press, Boca Raton, FL, 1988.

Polig, E. Modeling the distribution and dosimetry of internal emitters: A review of mathematical procedures using matrix methods. *Health Phys,* **81:**492–501, 2001.

Potter, C. A. Internal dosimetry—A review. *Health Phys,* **87:**455–468, Nov, 2004.

Radiological Health Handbook, Rev. ed. U.S. Public Health Service, Bureau of Radiological Health, Rockville, MD, 1970.

Reed, G. W., ed. *Radiation Dosimetry*. Academic Press, New York, 1964.

Sgouros, G. Dosimetry of internal emitters. *J Nucl Med,* **46:**18S–27S, 2005.

Sowby, F. D. Statement and recommendations of the 1980 Brighton meeting of the ICRP. *Annals of the ICRP,* Vol. 4, Nos. 3/4, 1980.

Spiers, F. W. *Radioisotopes in the Human Body*. Academic Press, New York, 1968.

Wang, Y., ed. *Handbook of Radioactive Nuclides*. Chemical Rubber Co., Cleveland, OH, 1968.

Watson, E. E. "The MIRD method of internal dose methodology," in Raabe, O. G., *Internal Radiation Dosimetry*. Medical Physics Publishing, Madison, WI, 1994.

Whyte, G. N. Chap. VI, *Principles of Radiation Dosimetry*. Academic Press, New York, 1959.

7

BIOLOGICAL BASIS FOR RADIATION SAFETY

Radiation ranks among the most thoroughly investigated etiologic agents associated with disease. Contrary to the popular belief that our experience with radiation bioeffects started with the nuclear weapons project during World War II, our experience actually goes back to the very earliest days of radiation use. As early as 1906, two French physiologists published the results of their studies on the sensitivity of various tissues and organs to radiation. They found that "the sensitivity of cells to irradiation is in direct proportion to their reproductive activity and inversely proportional to their degree of differentiation." This observation is as valid today as it was then, and is one of the bases for cancer treatment with radiation. Since then, an enormous database on radiation bioeffects has been built up from observations on the occupational exposure of workers including scientists, medical personnel, uranium miners, radium-dial painters, atomic-energy workers, and industrial radiographers. Patients who were exposed to radiation for diagnosis and therapy constitute a second source of information. The most thoroughly studied large population group, which still is supplying information for our radiation database, is the surviving population from the nuclear bombings in Japan. Included in this population group are about 280,000 persons who had received a wide range of doses, from slightly higher than background to several grays (several hundred rads), depending on their location at the time of the bombing. To study the long-term effects of nuclear radiation, the Atomic Bomb Casualty Commission (ABCC) was established in 1945 under a directive by President Truman and funded by the United States. In 1948, the ABCC became a binational agency as Japan joined the United States, both scientifically and financially, in the study of the long-term biomedical sequelae of the atom bombs. In 1975, the ABCC became the Radiation Effects Research Foundation and now operates as a not-for-profit organization funded jointly by the governments of the United States and Japan. Dose–response data for delayed radiogenic effects from the acute exposure from the atom bomb are being gathered from the Radiation Effects Research Foundation's "Life Span Study." This study is being carried out on a group of 86,572 bombing survivors whose doses are known. About 65% of the group received doses less than 100 mGy (10,000 mrads) of low linear energy transfer (LET)

279

radiation, and the balance of this population received high doses, that is, doses of 100 mGy (10 rads) or more.

In 1994, the United States and the Russian Federation established the Joint Coordinating Committee for Radiation Effects Research to study radiation effects on persons working in or living near nuclear weapons production facilities. This study population includes nuclear workers whose doses were very much greater than those of the American and Canadian workers, and the villagers who live downstream of the Mayak Production Association in the former Soviet Union and are exposed externally and internally to the very large quantities of long-lived radioactive waste that was discharged into the Techa River during the years of 1949–1956. This population group differs from the Japanese bombing survivors in one significant aspect. While the Japanese population suffered an acute high-dose radiation exposure, the Soviet nuclear workers and the Techa River population suffered continuous high-level doses, on the order of tens of mGy/yr (rads/yr), over a long period of time. Furthermore, both the external and internal doses for this population have been determined with a reasonable degree of accuracy, thus enabling the determination of a dose–response curve for chronic high-level doses.

In 1955, the United Nations General Assembly created the United Nations Scientific Committee on the Effects of Atomic Radiation (UNSCEAR) in order to report on radiation levels throughout the world and to assess the effects of exposure to ionizing radiation. UNSCEAR consists of scientists from 21 member states. Population groups under study include those exposed to radiation from fallout of nuclear weapons debris, accidents involving nuclear reactors, such as the Windscale accident in England in 1956 and Chernobyl in 1986 (there was no exposure of the public during the Three Mile Island accident) as well as numerous serious accidents from sealed sources that resulted in fatalities and radiation injuries. There also have been 60 criticality accidents that resulted in 21 deaths and numerous cases of radiation injury. Last but not least are populations living in environments with low and high natural radiation. Average annual doses from the natural background in populated areas range over a factor of about ten from low-dose to high-dose regions. The results of these studies serve to strengthen the scientific basis for radiation risk evaluation and the establishment of radiation safety standards.

Although much still remains to be learned about the interaction between ionizing radiation and living matter, more is known about the mechanism of radiation effects on the molecular, cellular, and organ system levels than is known for most other environmental stressing agents. Indeed, it is precisely this vast accumulation of quantitative dose–response data that enables health physicists to specify environmental radiation levels and engineering controls so that medical, scientific, and industrial applications of nuclear technology may continue at levels of risk no greater than, and frequently less than, those associated with other applications of science and technology that are generally accepted by society as safe.

DOSE–RESPONSE CHARACTERISTICS

Observed radiation effects (or effects of other noxious agents) may be broadly classified into two categories, namely, *stochastic* (Effects that occur randomly, and whose probability of occurrence rather than the severity of the effect, depends on the size of the dose. Stochastic effects, such as cancer, are also seen among persons with no known exposure to the agent associated with that effect.) and *nonstochastic,* or *deterministic* effects. Most biological effects fall into the category of deterministic effects. Deterministic effects are characterized by the three qualities stated by the Swiss physician and scientist Paracelsus about 500 years ago when he wrote "the size of the dose determines the poison." (A corollary to this is the old adage that there are no harmful chemicals [or radiation], only harmful uses of chemicals [or radiation]):

1. A certain minimum dose must be exceeded before the particular effect is observed.
2. The magnitude of the effect increases with the size of the dose.
3. There is a clear, unambiguous causal relationship between exposure to the noxious agent and the observed effect.

For example, a person must exceed a certain amount of alcoholic intake before he or she shows signs of drinking. After that, the effect of the alcohol depends on how much the person drank. Finally, if this individual exhibits drunken behavior, there is no doubt that the behavior is the result of drinking. For such nonstochastic effects, when the magnitude of the effect or the proportion of individuals who respond at a given dose is plotted as a function of dose in order to obtain a *quantitative relationship* between dose and effect, the dose–response curve A, shown in Figure 7-1, is obtained. Because of the minimum dose that must be exceeded before an individual shows the effect, nonstochastic effects are called *threshold effects.* Threshold radiation doses for some clinically significant deterministic effects are shown in Table 7-1.

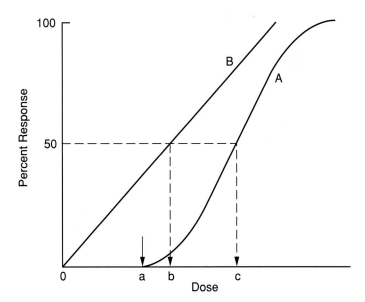

Figure 7-1. Dose–response curves. Curve A is the characteristic shape for a biological effect that exhibits a threshold dose—point *a.* The spread of the curve from the threshold at point *a* until the 100% response is thought to be due to "biological variability" around the mean dose, point *c,* which is called the *50% dose.* Curve B represents a zero-threshold, linear response. Point *b* represents the 50% dose for the zero-threshold biological effect being studied.

TABLE 7-1. Estimated Threshold Doses for Several Clinically Significant Detrimental Deterministic Effects

ORGAN	INJURY AT 5 YRS	1–5% DOSE (Gy)	25–50% DOSE (Gy)
Liver	Failure	35	45
Kidney	Nephrosclerosis	23	28
Bladder	Ulcer	60	80
Testes	Permanent sterilization	5–15	20
Ovaries	Permanent sterilization	2–3	6–12
Thyroid	Hypothyroidism	45	150
Breast	Atrophy	<50	<100

Source: Upton AC. Nonstochastic effects of ionizing radiation. In: *Some Issues Important in Developing Basic Radiation Protection Recommendations: Proceedings of the 20th Annual Meeting.* Bethesda, MD: National Council on Radiation Protection & Measurement; 1985. NCRP Proceedings 6.

In an experiment to determine the dose–response curve, the 50% dose—that is, the dose to which 50% of those who are exposed respond—is statistically the most reliable. For this reason, the 50% dose is most frequently used as an index of relative effectiveness of a given agent in eliciting a particular response. When death is the biological end point, the 50% dose is called the LD_{50} *dose.* The time required for the noxious agent to act is important and is always specified with the dose. Thus, if 50% of a group of experimental animals die within 30 days, we refer to it as the $LD_{50/30\text{-day}}$ dose. This index, the $LD_{50/30\text{-day}}$ dose, is widely used by toxicologists to designate the relative toxicity of an agent.

When the frequency of occurrence of a stochastic effect is plotted against the size of the dose (curve B in Fig. 7-1), a linear dose relationship is observed rather than the S-shaped curve that is characteristic of agents associated with a threshold response. The biological model that is compatible with this linear dose–response relationship and with our knowledge of molecular biology postulates that cancer can be initiated or a genetic change be wrought by scrambling the genetic information encoded in a single DNA molecule. Thus, carcinogenesis and mutagenesis are merely different manifestations of the same basic molecular phenomenon. According to this postulated model, a cancer is initiated by damaging the information stored in the chromosomes of a somatic cell, whereas (heritable) genetic change results from damage to the information stored in the chromosomes of a germ cell (a sperm or an ovum). This postulated model predicts a zero threshold for stochastic effects. That is, the model assumes that even the smallest amount of carcinogen or mutagen, a single molecule in the case of chemicals or a single photon in the case of X-rays, can produce the effect if the molecule or photon should happen to interact with the appropriate base pair in the DNA molecule. For these reasons, stochastic effects are assumed to lie on a *linear, zero-threshold dose–response curve.* According to the linear, zero-threshold model (which is also known as the LNT model), every increment of radiation, no matter how small, carries with it a corresponding increased probability of the stochastic effect.

Since epidemiological and laboratory data on observed stochastic radiation effects are based on relatively high doses, biologically based mathematical models are constructed to assess the stochastic effects of low doses. Several alternative models have been proposed. However, despite the fact that much, but not all, DNA damage is repaired and that the information contained in the DNA molecule is replicated, the LNT model has been adopted, in the interest of conservatism, as the basis for setting radiation safety standards. In the most recent analysis of all relevant data, the National Academy of Science in its BEIR (biological effects of ionizing radiation) VII committee report concluded that "the current scientific evidence is consistent with the hypothesis that there is a linear, no-threshold dose–response relationship between exposure to ionizing radiation and development of cancer in humans." However, this conclusion is followed by the statement that uncertainties in this judgment are recognized and noted. The LNT model is inherently unverifiable at low doses (<100 mGy or <10 rads) because the postulated number of stochastic effects from such doses is less than the statistical variability of the natural occurrence of these effects.

A parallel study by the French Academy of Sciences and the National Academy of Medicine (the Joint Report) arrived at an opposite conclusion from the BEIR VII committee. The Joint Report concluded that the LNT model was not justifiable because the BEIR committee did not sufficiently consider either the repair of the DNA damaged at low radiation doses or the elimination by cellular death of cells that suffered lethal damage by the radiation or by genetically programmed cellular death (apoptosis). The Joint Report also points out that its analysis of animal data and the lack of a carcinogenic effect in subjects contaminated with alpha emitters is not consistent with the LNT hypothesis. The Joint Report concludes that the basic radiobiological assumptions of the LNT hypothesis are not in accordance with recent data and that use of the LNT for assessing risks below 20 mSv (2,000 mrems) is not justified and should be discouraged.

Initiating Mechanisms of Radiogenic Effects

Direct Action

The gross biological effects resulting from overexposure to radiation are the sequelae of a long and complex series of events that are initiated by ionization or excitation of relatively few molecules in the organism. For example, the $LD_{50/30\text{-day}}$ dose of gamma-rays for man is about 4 Gy (400 rads). Since 1 Gy corresponds to an energy absorption of 1 J/kg, or 6.25×10^{18} eV/g, and since about 34 eV is expended in producing a single ionization, the lethal dose produces, in tissue,

$$\frac{4 \text{ Gy} \times 6.25 \times 10^{18} \, \dfrac{\text{eV/kg}}{\text{Gy}}}{34 \dfrac{\text{eV}}{\text{ion}}} = 7.35 \times 10^{17}$$

ionized atoms per gram tissue. If we estimate that about nine other atoms are excited for each one ionized, we find that about 7.35×10^{18} atoms/kg of tissue are directly affected by a lethal radiation dose. In soft tissue, there are about 9.5×10^{25} atoms/kg. The fraction of directly affected atoms, therefore, is

$$\frac{7.35 \times 10^{18}}{9.5 \times 10^{25}} \approx 1 \times 10^{-7},$$

or about 1 atom in 10 million.

Effects of radiation for which a zero-threshold dose is postulated are thought to be the result of a direct insult to a molecule by ionization and excitation and the consequent dissociation of the molecule. Point mutations, in which there is a change in a single gene locus, is an example of such an effect. The dissociation, due to ionization or excitation, of an atom on the DNA molecule prevents the information originally contained in the gene from being transmitted to the next generation. Such point mutations may occur in the germinal cells, in which case the point mutation is passed on to the next individual; or it may occur in somatic cells, which results in a point mutation in the daughter cell. Since these point mutations are thereafter transmitted to succeeding generations of cells (except for the highly improbable instance where one mutated gene may suffer another mutation), it is clear that for those biological effects of radiation that depend on point mutations, the radiation dose is cumulative; every little dose may result in a change in the gene burden, which is then continuously transmitted. When dealing quantitatively with such phenomena, however, we must consider the probability of observing a genetic change among the offspring of an irradiated individual. For radiation doses down to about 250 mGy (25 rads), the magnitude of the effect, as measured by frequency of gene mutations, is proportional to the dose. Below doses of about 250 mGy, the mutation probability is so low that enormous numbers of animals must be used in order to detect a mutation that could be ascribed to the radiation. For this reason, no reliable experimental data are available for genetic changes in the range 0–250 mGy.

Indirect Action

Direct effects of radiation, ionization, and excitation are nonspecific and may occur anywhere in the body. When the directly affected atom is in a protein molecule or in a molecule of nucleic acid, then certain specific effects due to the damaged molecule may ensue. However, most of the body is water, and most of the direct action of radiation is therefore on water. The result of this energy absorption by water is the production, in water, of highly reactive free radicals that are chemically toxic (a free radical is a fragment of a compound or an element that contains an unpaired electron) and which may exert their toxicity on other molecules. When pure water is irradiated, we have

$$H_2O \rightarrow H_2O^+ + e^-; \tag{7.1}$$

the positive ion dissociates immediately according to the equation

$$H_2O^+ \rightarrow H^+ + OH, \tag{7.2}$$

while the electron is picked up by a neutral water molecule:

$$H_2O + e^- \rightarrow H_2O^-, \tag{7.3}$$

which dissociates immediately:

$$H_2O^- \rightarrow H + OH^-. \tag{7.4}$$

The ions H^+ and OH^- are of no consequence, since all body fluids already contain significant concentrations of both these ions. The free radicals H and OH may combine with like radicals, or they may react with other molecules in solution. Their most probable fate is determined chiefly by the LET of the radiation. In the case of a high rate of LET, such as that which results from passage of an alpha particle or other particle of high specific ionization, the free OH radicals are formed close enough together to enable them to combine with each other before they can recombine with free H radicals, which leads to the production of hydrogen peroxide,

$$OH + OH \rightarrow H_2O_2, \tag{7.5}$$

while the free H radicals combine to form gaseous hydrogen. Whereas the products of the primary reactions of Eqs. (7.1) through (7.4) have very short lifetimes, on the order of a microsecond, the hydrogen peroxide, being a relatively stable compound, persists long enough to diffuse to points quite remote from their point of origin. The hydrogen peroxide, which is a very powerful oxidizing agent, can thus affect molecules or cells that did not suffer radiation damage directly. If the irradiated water contains dissolved oxygen, the free hydrogen radical may combine with oxygen to form the hydroperoxyl radical as follows:

$$H + O_2 \rightarrow HO_2. \tag{7.6}$$

The hydroperoxyl radical is not as reactive as the free OH radical and therefore has a longer lifetime than it. This greater stability allows the hydroperoxyl radical to combine with a free hydrogen radical to form hydrogen peroxide, thereby further enhancing the toxicity of the radiation.

Radiation is thus seen to produce biological effects by two mechanisms, namely, directly by dissociating molecules following their excitation and ionization and indirectly by the production of free radicals and hydrogen peroxide in the water of the body fluids. The greatest gap in our knowledge of radiobiology is the sequence of events between the primary initiating events on the molecular level described above and the gross biological effects that may be observed long after irradiation.

THE PHYSIOLOGICAL BASIS FOR INTERNAL DOSIMETRY

The determination of radiation dose from radionuclides within the body and the calculation of amounts that may be safely inhaled or ingested depend on the knowledge of the fate of these radionuclides within the body. Specifically, we need to know the pathways that the radionuclides follow, the organs and systems that make up these pathways, the rates at which they travel along these pathways, and the rates at which they are eliminated from the body.

Physiologically based pharmacokinetic models are used to mathematically describe the kinetics of metabolism of a radionuclide. If we know the quantitative relationships among exposure, intake, uptake, deposition, and excretion of a radionuclide, we can calculate the radiation dose from a given exposure. Knowledge of the kinetics of metabolism can also be used to infer the radiation dose from bioassay measurements and to set maximum acceptable concentrations in the environment. The same methodology is also used for the control of nonradioactive environmental contaminants. These underlying quantitative relationships are based on the biochemical and biophysical principles that govern physiological processes.

Biokinetic Processes

Physiological activity encompasses four vital processes:

- transport of materials,
- transport of information,
- tissue building, and
- energy conversion.

Physiological Transport

Transport of materials is accomplished by two different mechanisms:

- bulk transport due to pressure differences and
- diffusion due to concentration differences.

An example of bulk transport is the flow of air into and out of the lungs. This flow of air is passive and is due to pressure differences caused by the expansion and relaxation of the chest cavity. Inhalation occurs when the chest cavity is expanded and its volume increases. This leads to a decrease in the intrathoracic pressure of several millimeters of mercury, and air flows into the lungs. During exhalation, the muscles that control the volume of the chest cavity relax and the thoracic volume decreases, thereby increasing the intrathoracic pressure and forcing the air out of the lungs.

Other examples of bulk flow include the circulation of blood due to pressure differences from the pumping action of the heart and the passage of food along the gastrointestinal (GI) tract due to the squeezing action, called *peristalsis*, of the walls of the GI tract.

The second mechanism of transport of material is based on differences of concentration of the constituents of a solution and the diffusion of molecules from the region of higher concentration to the region of lower concentration. This net transfer of molecules continues until the concentration is uniform or until some other equilibrium condition is reached. For example, if we have a U tube filled with water and we add a solute to one side of the U tube, the solute molecules, though originally concentrated in one place, will diffuse throughout the water until they are uniformly dispersed across both arms of the U tube.

If we divide the U tube into two halves by a semipermeable barrier that allows only water molecules to pass through (Fig. 7-2) and we add a solute to one side, we will observe the process called osmosis. Because of the presence of the dissolved material on the solution side, the water is less concentrated on that side than on the

Figure 7-2. Schematic illustration of osmosis, the consequence of membrane semipermeability. Only water molecules pass through the membrane, the salt ions on the left side of the membrane do not. The result of this unidirectional movement of water is called the osmotic pressure.

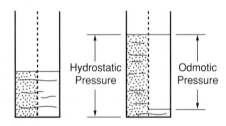

pure-water side. Water will therefore flow through the semipermeable barrier from the pure-water side into the solution side by osmosis, and the water in the solution arm will rise. Water will continue to flow through the barrier, and the solution column will continue to rise, until the hydrostatic pressure due to the increased height of the column of water is great enough to prevent further inflow of water through the semipermeable barrier. The hydrostatic pressure needed to prevent further flow through the barrier is called the *osmotic pressure* of the solution. Osmotic pressure is determined by the concentration of the solution and increases with increasing concentration.

Biological membranes may be selectively permeable to various different molecules. This selective permeability, which allows only certain ions to pass, is responsible for the electrical potential differences that form the basis for the operation of the nervous system and muscles, including the cardiac muscle. Consider the arms of a U tube that are separated by a membrane that allows only K^+ ions to pass through, as in Figure 7-3. Let us pour a solution containing a relatively high concentration of KCl and a low concentration of NaCl into one arm of the U tube, and a KCl–NaCl solution that is relatively more concentrated in Na^+ than in K^+ into the other arm. The solutions on both sides of the membrane are electrically neutral. However, since the membrane is permeable to K^+ ions, the K^+ ions will diffuse through the membrane from the more to the less concentrated K^+ solution. This transfer of K^+ ions results in a net loss of positive ions on one side of the membrane and a net gain of positive ions on the other side, thus upsetting the electrical neutrality. Since one side will now have a net positive charge and the other a net negative charge, these opposite charges will attract each other and will migrate to the membrane separating the two solutions. This accumulation of positive ions on one side and negative ions on the other side of the membrane leads to an electrical potential difference across the membrane. This potential difference continues to increase as more K^+ ions move through the membrane until the built-up positive potential is great enough to prevent more positively charged K ions from passing through the membrane. Passage of ions from a region of high to low concentration is accomplished without the expenditure of energy. However, transfer of ions against a concentration gradient, which is called *active transport,* requires the expenditure of energy.

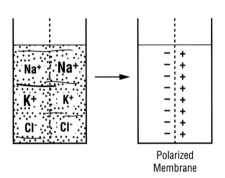

Polarized
Membrane

Figure 7-3. Schematic illustration of ionic transport, in which the membrane is permeable only to the K^+ ion. The accumulation of positive charges on one side of the membrane and negative ions on the other side leads to a potential difference across the membrane.

Information, too, is transferred by two different mechanisms: by the nervous system, in which electrical impulses pass along nerves at a rate of meters per second, and by hormones that are secreted by endocrine (ductless) glands, such as the thyroid, directly into the blood and are carried by the blood to the specific receptor organs that respond to these hormones.

Metabolism: Tissue Building and Energy Conversion

Cells, from which all tissues and organs are made, go through life cycles of their own. They are born from relatively undifferentiated progenitor cells—such as the basal layer in the skin and the stem cells in the bone marrow—go through a period of maturation, grow old, die, and are sloughed off. The time for cellular death, called *apoptosis,* and the instructions for the synthesis of new tissue is contained in the information encoded in the DNA molecules within the cells. In addition to building tissue, the body also synthesizes protein molecules such as enzymes and hormones that serve specific functions. These undifferentiated cells are much more sensitive to radiation damage than the mature cells that develop from them. The raw materials used in this tissue-building process comes from the food and water we consume. The energy necessary to drive these vital processes comes from the release of the intramolecular bonding energy that is stored in the chemical bonds of the food. The processes by which the complex food molecules are disassembled and then reassembled into cellular material and specialized proteins, and by which energy that is stored in the food is converted into useful energy are collectively called *metabolism.*

The food and drink that we consume—proteins, carbohydrates, fats, and water—supply the materials for the manufacture of new tissue and for the synthesis of specialized molecules. In the process called metabolism, the foodstuffs are broken down into their constituent subunits—amino acids, sugars, fatty acids, and glycerols—and then these units are reassembled into the cellular constituents needed for building tissues and organs. Metabolic processes include a number of oxidation–reduction reactions that result in the transfer of energy stored in the intramolecular bonds of the foodstuffs into energy-consuming reactions that drive all the vital processes. Oxygen for these oxidation reactions is brought into the body through the respiratory system. Useful energy is supplied mainly by the carbohydrates and fats, while the proteins supply most of the material for the synthesis of new protein. Whereas the initial steps in the metabolism of the different nutrients differ, eventually all the subunits are integrated into a common metabolic pool from which new molecules are synthesized.

All the chemical reactions in the metabolic process can occur only in solution. To this end, the human body is about 60% water by weight (about 42 L water in the reference person), of which about two-thirds is contained within the cells of the body and is therefore called intracellular fluid. The remaining one-third is outside the cells and is called extracellular fluid. About one-third of the extracellular fluid is in the blood and the remainder is in the interstices between the cells, thereby providing the cells with an aquatic environment. These various spaces can be thought of as compartments. Thus, we have the vascular compartment, which contains the blood; the interstitial compartment; and the intracellular compartment. Water enters the system via the GI tract and leaves by way of the kidneys as urine, by way of the GI tract as one of the constituents of feces, by way of the skin as perspiration, and via the lungs as exhaled water vapor.

Organ Systems

The body is an integrated assembly of organ systems whose structures are in accord with their functions. These organ systems include the following:

- the circulatory system,
- the respiratory system,
- the digestive system,
- the skeletal system,
- the muscular system,
- the integumentary system (skin),
- the urinary system,
- the nervous system,
- the endocrine system,
- the reproductive system, and
- sensory organs and tissues.

The organ systems are made up of several different types of tissues, and each tissue comprises specialized cells that perform specific functions. The principal types of tissues include:

- Epithelial tissue, which forms the surface of many organs and the outside surface of the body. Epithelial tissues are characterized by a basement membrane that lies beneath the lowest layer of cells. The cells in the basement membrane are the critical cells for radiation damage.
- Connective tissue, which forms the bones, cartilage, ligaments (which join two bones together), and tendons (which connect muscles to bones).
- Muscle.
- Nervous tissue.

The Circulatory System

The circulatory system (Fig. 7-4), which consists of a network of tubes called *blood vessels*, through which blood is pumped by the heart, serves several different purposes, including the

- transport of oxygen and carbon dioxide,
- transport of nutrient and metabolites from the GI tract to the various organs,
- transport of hormones and antibodies,
- transport of metabolic waste products to the kidneys for elimination, and also
- serving as a water reservoir to maintain fluid balance in the several fluid compartments and constant temperature within the body.

All these functions are carried out by the blood. As a result of pressure due to the pumping action of the heart, blood flows through the blood vessels, called *arteries*, *veins*, and *capillaries*, which carry blood to and from organs. The capillaries, a very fine network of vessels, are dispersed throughout the organs and are the functional

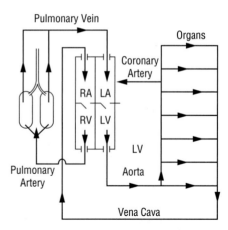

Figure 7-4. Schematic illustration of the circulatory system and the chambers of the heart.

units through which gases and all other molecules are transferred to and from the cells within the organs.

Blood consists of a liquid portion, called *plasma*; blood cells, which are suspended in the plasma; and proteins and electrolytes, which are dissolved in the plasma. Blood cells make up about 44% of the total volume of the blood. All these blood cells are made in the red bone marrow by a process called *hemopoiesis*, and they all arise from a single, undifferentiated cell type called a *stem cell*. The radiosensitivity of the hemopoietic tissue is due to the highly undifferentiated stem cells.

There are three major categories of blood cells, each serving specific functions:

- Erythrocytes, or red blood cells (RBC)
- Leukocytes, or white blood cells (WBC)
- Thrombocytes, or platelets

The main function of the RBCs is the transport of oxygen and carbon dioxide. These gases diffuse across the cell membrane and form a loose combination with hemoglobin, an iron-containing compound within the RBC. Another important function of the erythrocytes is the production of the enzyme carbonic anhydrase, which catalyzes the interaction between carbon dioxide and water and plays an important role in the maintenance of acid–base balance in the blood. There are about 5–7 million RBCs per cubic millimeter of blood, and the lifetime of an RBC is in the range of 3–4 months.

WBCs are part of the immune system, and their main role is to fight infection. There are about 4000–8000 WBCs per cubic millimeter of blood. These WBCs are grouped into two major categories: about 70% are granulocytes and about 30% are lymphocytes; there are several subcategories within each of these major groupings. The exact lifetimes of the cells depend on their category. However, in all cases their lifetime is on the order of about 1 day.

The third group of cells, the platelets, form part of the system that clots the blood. A shortage of platelets, therefore, leads to hemorrhage in case of an injury. We normally find about 200,000–400,000 platelets per cubic millimeter of blood. The lifetime of the thrombocytes is about 8 days.

The heart, which supplies the pressure that causes the blood to flow, can be thought of as two pumps combined in one organ. One of these pumps, the right heart, pumps oxygen-depleted air into the lungs. Here the carbon dioxide carried by the blood diffuses out of the blood into the pulmonary air spaces, and oxygen diffuses from the pulmonary air spaces, called the *alveoli*, into the blood. From the lungs, the newly reoxygenated blood flows into the left side of the heart, to be pumped to the various organs and tissues, including the cardiac muscle itself. Each side of the heart—that is, each of the two pumps—consists of two chambers separated by one-way valves that allow the blood to flow only in one direction. The first chamber, which receives the blood that enters into the pump, is called the *atrium*. Contraction of the atrium forces the blood into the second chamber, called the *ventricle*. Powerful contractions of the ventricle supply the pressure that drives the blood to the various organs and tissues (left heart) or to the lungs (right heart).

Blood flows into the atrium of the left heart through the *pulmonary vein* and into the atrium of the right heart through the *vena cava*. Blood flows into the atria when the heart is resting, and into the arteries that supply the organs and tissues when the ventricles contract. The beating of the heart is due to the alternating contraction and relaxation of the atria and the ventricles. Normally, this cycle is repeated about 70–80 times per minute. During periods of excitement or physical demand, the heart rate increases significantly. The cycle begins with the simultaneous contraction, called atrial systole, of both atria, which forces the blood into the relaxed ventricles. This atrial pumping action lasts about 0.1 seconds. The one-way valves immediately close, and contraction of the ventricles, called *ventricular systole*, begins; it lasts about 0.3 seconds. Total systole thus lasts for about 0.4 seconds. The resulting blood pressure, due to the systolic contractions, is normally about 120–140 mm Hg. The atria relax during ventricular contraction and remain relaxed for about 0.7 seconds. The ventricles relax for about 0.5 seconds. after contraction. These periods of relaxation are called *diastole*. During diastole, the blood pressure is normally about 60–80 mm Hg.

The Respiratory System

The respiratory system (Fig. 7-5) is the site for the exchange of oxygen from the outside environment with carbon dioxide from the blood. The respiratory system consists of three major sections whose structures are related to their function, the *nasopharyngeal* (NP), *tracheobronchial* (TB), and *pulmonary* (P), which is also called the *alveolar* (Al), regions.

The lungs, which consist of three lobes on the right side and two lobes on the left side, and the trachea, or windpipe, lie within the thoracic cavity. The trachea is connected to the outside air via the mouth and nose—the NP region. Air enters through the NP region and flows into the trachea, a tube about 16 mm in diameter and 10 cm long. From the trachea, the air flows into the lobes of the lungs through short connecting tubes, about 1 cm in diameter, called the *primary (main) bronchi* (the singular is *bronchus*). Within the lungs, the bronchi bifurcate; they then bifurcate again and again into successively smaller-diameter tubes until a size of about 0.5-mm diameter is reached. These tubes, which number several hundred thousand, are called the *terminal bronchioles*. This system of ducts, from the trachea through the terminal bronchioles, is called the *upper respiratory tract*, or the TB region. It should be pointed out that the term "upper respiratory tract" is a functional definition,

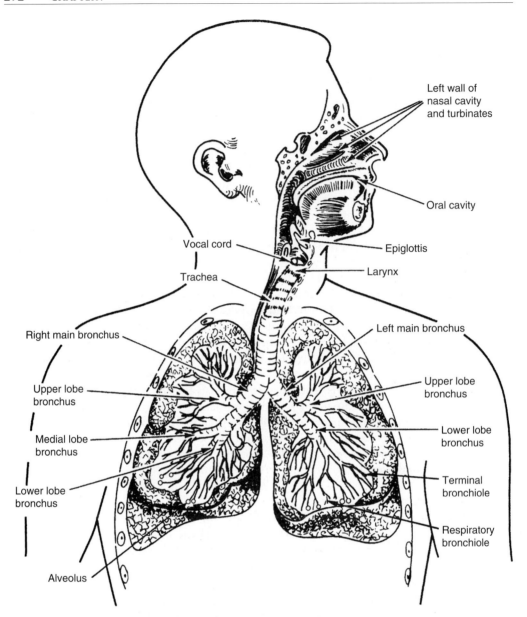

Figure 7-5. Schematic representation of the human respiratory airways. (Reproduced with permission from Raabe OG. Deposition and clearance of inhaled aerosols. In Witschi HR, Nettesheim P, eds. *Mechanisms in Respiratory Toxicology.* Vol 1. 5th ed. Boca Raton, FL: CRC Press, Inc; 1982.)

since the bronchi and bronchioles are uniformly distributed throughout the lungs. Structurally, the TB region is characterized by a unique structure on the inside surface of the airways. The lining, or epithelial, cells have hairlike filaments about 50 μm long that project into the airways. These filaments are called *cilia,* and the cells are called *ciliated epithelium.* Structures of another type, called *goblet cells,* are interspersed among the ciliated cells. These goblet cells secrete mucus that blankets the upper respiratory tract to a thickness of about 60 μm. The cilia move in a synchronized beating motion resembling a quick-return mechanism. This motion pushes the blanket of mucus upward toward the throat, with a velocity in the trachea that reaches about 1 cm/min. This ciliary "escalator" is the main method by means of which particles that are deposited in the TB region are cleared out of the lung. Generally, clearance from the TB region is fast, on the order of hours. The TB region is a system of ducts carrying air to the functional part of the respiratory system, where gas exchange occurs.

The part of the lungs where gas exchange occurs is called the *deep respiratory tract—* the P or AI region. The P region starts with the respiratory bronchioles, which arise from the bifurcation of the terminal bronchioles. The lining cells of the respiratory bronchioles are not ciliated and do not contain the mucus-secreting goblet cells. The respiratory bronchioles bifurcate to form alveolar ducts. Gas exchange takes place in the alveoli (the singular is *alveolus*), as shown in Figure 7-6, which are spherical outpouchings, on the order of 100–200 μm in diameter, of the alveolar ducts. There are several hundred million alveoli, which lead to a total surface area available for gas exchange of about 50–200 m^2. This alveolar surface is the interface between the outside environment and the body's internal milieu. Because of this large interfacial area, inhalation is considered to be the main pathway for the entry of noxious substances into the body. Each alveolus is wrapped in a network of capillaries whose walls are only one-cell thick. The alveolar wall, too, is one-cell thick. Gases thus have only two cell walls through which to diffuse to get into the blood from the lungs.

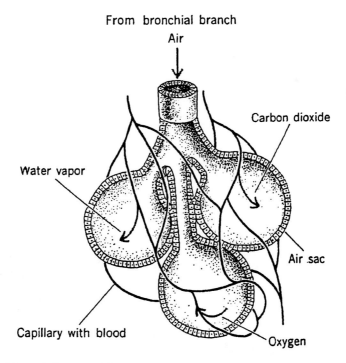

Figure 7-6.   Schematic illustration of the alveoli, or air sacs, where gas exchange occurs. (Reproduced with permission from Lessing MS. *Review Text in Life Science.* Intermediate Level. New York, NY: Amsco School Publications; 1967.)

Breathing, the flow of air into and out of the lungs, is a passive process due to changes in the volume of the thoracic (chest) cavity. During inhalation, the combined action of the intercostal muscles and the diaphragm increases the thoracic volume, thereby decreasing the air pressure in the lungs to several millimeters Hg below atmospheric pressure. This pressure difference causes air to flow into the lungs. During exhalation, the process is reversed. Relaxation of the chest muscles and the diaphragm decreases the volume of the thoracic cavity, thereby increasing the intrathoracic pressure and forcing the air out of the lungs.

Respiratory physiologists deal with several different air volumes and lung capacities:

- Tidal volume, TV—Volume of air inhaled in a single breath under ordinary conditions.
- Inspiratory reserve volume, IRV—Maximum volume of air that can be inhaled after the normal (tidal) inhalation.
- Expiratory reserve volume, ERV—Maximum volume of air that can be forcefully expelled after a normal (tidal) exhalation.
- Inspiratory capacity—Maximum volume of air that can be inhaled from the resting exhalation.
- Vital capacity, VC—The maximum volume of air that can be forcefully expelled from the lungs following a maximum inhalation.
- Reserve volume, RV—Volume of air remaining in the lungs after a maximum exhalation.
- Functional residual capacity, FRC—Volume of air remaining in the lungs after a normal (tidal) exhalation.
- Total lung capacity, TLC—Volume of air in the lung after a maximum inhalation.
- Breathing frequency, f_R—Number of respirations per minute.
- Minute volume—Volume of air inhaled in 1 minute $= f_R \times TV = 18 - 22$ L/min.

The relationships among these volumes are shown graphically in Figure 7-7, and nominal values for an adult male are listed in Table 7-2.

The Digestive System

The digestive system includes a continuous pathway through the trunk that starts at the mouth and ends at the anus. In addition, the digestive system includes several auxiliary organs that supply enzymes and other substances necessary for digestion and where metabolism occurs. This continuous pathway is called the GI tract; it includes the mouth, esophagus, stomach, small intestine, and large intestine. The large intestine terminates in the rectum, which communicates with the outside environment via the anus. The auxiliary organs include the salivary glands, which are located in the mouth; the pancreas, which is found behind the lower end of the stomach; the liver, a very large organ located in the upper right quadrant of the abdomen; and the gallbladder, which is found under the liver.

The digestive process begins in the mouth, where an enzyme called *ptyalin* is secreted by the salivary glands to convert starch into sugar. The mouthful of food is then swallowed and passes through the pharynx into the esophagus, where the process called *peristalsis* moves the food forward into the stomach. In peristalsis, involuntary contractions of the muscles in the walls of the GI tract move down the GI tract, thereby squeezing the contents ahead of the contractions. These rhythmic

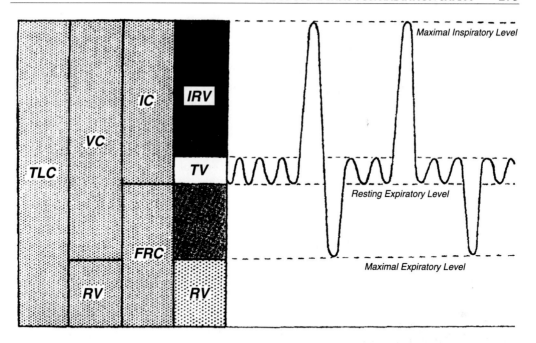

Figure 7-7. Lung volumes as they appear on a spirogram. *Abbreviations:* TLC, total lung capacity; VC, vital capacity; RV, reserve volume; FRC, functional residual capacity; TV, tidal volume; RV, reserve volume; IC, inspiratory capacity. (Reproduced with permission from Forster RE II, BuBois AB, Briscoe WA, Fisher AB. *The Lung: Physiologic Basis of Function Tests.* 3rd ed. Chicago, IL: Year Book Medical Publishers, Inc; 1986. Copyright © 1986, with permission from Elsevier.)

peristaltic contractions are coordinated by the autonomic nervous system. In this manner, a bolus of food is pushed along from the esophagus into the stomach, where the food is mixed with hydrochloric acid, mucus, and digestive enzymes. A total of about 3 L/d of these fluids is secreted by the interior lining of the stomach. The contents of the stomach are thoroughly mixed by peristaltic contractions of the stomach walls to produce a relatively homogeneous fluidized mass called *chyme*. The mean residence time of the gastric contents is about 1 hour. The chyme is propelled to the small intestine by these peristaltic contractions. Passage from the stomach to the intestine is through an opening called the *pylorus*. The size of the pyloric opening is controlled by a circumferential muscle called the *pyloric sphincter*. Chyme

TABLE 7-2. Aeration of the Lung

VOLUME	NORMAL VALUES (L)
Tidal volume (TV)	0.6
Inspiratory reserve volume (IRV)	2.0
Expiratory reserve volume (ERV)	1.5
Inspiratory capacity (IC)	3.6
Vital capacity (VC) = TV + IRV + ERV	4.1
Residual volume (RV)	1.6
Total lung capacity (TLC) = VC + RV	5.7
Respiration rate (f_R) = 18–22 min^{-1}	
Minute volume = TV × f_R	

is pushed into the intestine intermittently, as the pyloric sphincter opens and closes at a frequency determined by the gastric contents.

The small intestine is a tube approximately 6 m long, where digestion occurs and where nutrients and other materials from the chyme are absorbed into the blood. The epithelial tissue that lines the inside surface of the small intestine is covered with millions (20–40 per mm^2) of fingerlike projections called *villi* (the singular is *villus*). The epithelial tissue that covers the villi is contiguous with the epithelial cells that line the inside surface of the small intestine. These epithelial cells grow out of a basement membrane consisting of the germinal cells from which the epithelial cells develop. The basement membrane is the critical tissue for radiation damage to the small intestine, and destruction of the basement membrane with doses on the order of about 750 or more rads leads to the "GI syndrome." Nutrient molecules are transferred from the gut into the blood by diffusion across the walls of the villi and into the blood vessels within each villus. The large number of villi increases the surface area of the small intestine enormously, thus facilitating transfer of nutrient material to the blood. It should be noted that materials in the GI tract are not really in the internal milieu of the body. The GI tract is continuous at both ends with the outside environment, and material may pass through without being taken up or absorbed into the internal milieu of the body. The liver, pancreas, and intestinal mucosa secrete digestive juices into the small intestine. Peristaltic contractions mix the chyme and propel it along toward the large intestine. After a residence time of about 4 hours, many of the nutrient materials have been absorbed into the blood. The remaining contents of the small intestine enter into the large intestine.

The large intestine, or colon, is the final major division of the GI tract. The colon is about 1 m long and is called "large" because its diameter is greater than that of the small intestine. The small intestine joins the large intestine at the cecum, and passage of chyme into the large intestine is controlled by the ileocecal valve. Peristaltic contractions continue to squeeze the intestinal contents toward the rectum. The chyme entering the large intestine contains a large proportion of water. In this first part of the colon, the upper large intestine, a large fraction of the water as well as sodium and other minerals are resorbed into the blood, thus leaving a residue called feces. Passage through the upper large intestine takes about half a day. After a passage through the lower large intestine of about a day's duration, the feces enter into the rectum, where they remain until eliminated from the body during the act of defecation.

The Skeletal System

The skeleton, which accounts for about 10% of the body weight (exclusive of the bone marrow, which accounts for about another 4%) consists of 206 bones that are joined together by cartilages. Like many other organs, the skeleton serves several different functions:

- It provides the load-bearing framework for the support of all the other organs and tissues.
- It provides a protective shield for vital organs.
- It contains the bone marrow, including the red marrow, where blood cells are made.
- It is the repository for the body's store of calcium.

Bone is listed as the critical organ for many radionuclides. This suggests that bone is a single tissue. However, bone is a complex organ consisting of several different tissues whose radiosensitivities and metabolic kinetics differ. Two major types of bone are readily recognizable. These are the *cortical bone*, which is dense and compact, and the *trabecular bone*, which is soft and spongy and consists of thin walls of bone tissue forming the spaces that house the marrow. Compact bone consists of layers of cells arranged coaxially around a small cylindrical opening called a *haversian canal*. The blood vessels that supply the bone run through the haversian canals. Both cortical and trabecular bone consist of cells (called *osteoblasts*) embedded in a matrix containing collagenous fibers. This matrix is held together by the mineral hydroxyapatite, $Ca_{10}(PO_4)_6(OH)_2$. Divalent radium, strontium, and lead ions can exchange with the calcium in the mineral matter, thereby making bone a critical organ for these elements. The outside surface of the bone is covered with a layer of tissue called the *periosteum*, and the inside surfaces of bone, including the walls of the trabecular bone, are covered with a lining called the *endosteum*. Because of the large surface area in the trabecular bone, there is much more endosteal tissue than periosteal tissue. Both these linings are involved with bone growth and are therefore called *osteogenic* tissue. Whereas radium and strontium are deposited within the mineralized bone, thorium and plutonium are deposited in the linings of the bones, the periosteum and the endosteum. The skeletal cells at risk of radiogenic cancer are the osteogenic cells in the bone surfaces, particularly the endosteal cells, and the blood-forming cells in the bone marrow. DNA damage and proliferation of these damaged cells are believed to evolve into osteosarcoma.

The Muscular System

Muscle is a specialized tissue whose unique property is contractility. Muscles are made up of groups of muscle fibers that are bundled together by a wrapping of connective tissue. We find three different types of muscle tissue:

- *Skeletal (or striated) muscle.* These muscles, which are attached to the bones, contract when they are stimulated by a nerve pulse and thereby control movement. Since these movements are under our control, the skeletal muscles are also called *voluntary* muscles.
- *Cardiac muscle.* This is a specialized muscle found only in the heart. It contracts rhythmically but is not under our control. Cardiac muscle, therefore, is called *involuntary* muscle.
- *Visceral muscle.* These are involuntary muscles that are found in the GI tract, the walls of blood and lymph vessels, and the uterus. Peristalsis is caused by the contraction of these muscles, which form the walls of the GI tract.

The Skin

The skin (Fig. 7-8), which forms the outer covering of the body, is a multifunctional and hence a complex organ. The average surface area of the skin is about 1.8 m^2. Its functions include the following:

- covering the body,
- providing a protective barrier against harmful substances, such as microbes and chemicals,

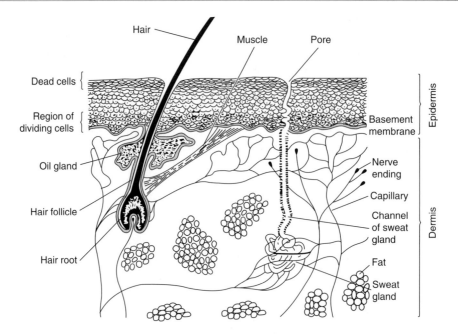

Figure 7-8. Cross-sectional representation of the skin. (Reproduced with permission from Lessing MS. *Review Text in Life Science.* Intermediate Level. New York, NY: Amsco School Publications; 1967.)

- excretion of body wastes,
- heating and cooling the body, and
- regulating the blood flow.

The skin consists of two layers, an outer layer called the *epidermis* and an inner layer called the *dermis.* At the border between these two layers is the basement membrane. This membrane, which consists of the biologically active progenitor cells that give rise to the cells in the outer surface of the skin, is the critical tissue for limiting dose to the skin. When a cell in the basement membrane divides, one of the two cells starts to migrate toward the outer surface of the skin and one remains as part of the basement membrane. As the daughter cell migrates, it undergoes progressive changes that lead to the highly differentiated cells that perform the skin's protective function. In these changes, the cell's cytoplasm is transformed into a dense substance called *keratin.* During this process, the nucleus is crushed by the increasing keratinization and eventually disappears. By this time, the cell is biologically dead and will be sloughed off after it reaches the surface. Since the epidermis consists of dead cells, its only radiobiological significance is to attenuate the energy of beta or alpha rays before they reach the basement membrane, which is the radiosensitive layer of the skin. The basement-membrane boundary between the dermis and the epidermis is an undulating layer whose distance from the outer surface varies significantly, from about 30 μm on the eyelids to about 1400 μm on the soles of the feet. Despite the actual variability in the depth, for dosimetry purposes we consider the depth of the basement membrane to be 70 μm (0.007 cm) below the surface, and we therefore define the *shallow dose* as the dose at a depth of 7 mg per cm^2. The epidermis is readily repaired following an injury because of the availability of basement cells at the margin of the injury, from which new tissues can be formed.

The structure of the dermis, the lower layer of the skin, is quite different from that of the epidermis. The dermis consists of connective tissue, elastic fibers, water, and fat. Embedded in the dermis are the sweat glands and sebaceous glands (oil glands), hair follicles, blood vessels, and nerves. The sweat glands serve as both excretory organs and as part of the body's cooling system, while the sebaceous glands secrete an oily substance that lubricates the skin's surface and at the same time acts as a barrier against penetration of the skin by water. The nerve endings in the dermis give us the sense of touch and allow us to sense the temperature of whatever substance is in contact with the skin.

The Urinary System

The urinary system plays a major role in elimination of waste products from the metabolism of food and from the intake of noxious substances—such as chemicals or radionuclides—and in maintaining water, electrolyte, and acid–base homeostasis. Included in the urinary system are two kidneys, where urine is formed; two ureters, through which the urine flows from the kidneys into the bladder; the bladder, where the urine is collected; and the urethra, through which the urine leaves the body. The function of the kidney, which is one of the boundary organs between the internal milieu of the body and the outside environment, is to selectively filter water, electrolytes, metabolic wastes, and other noxious molecules from the blood into the urine. These activities are carried out in about 1 million nephrons, which are the functional units of the kidney. The *nephron* (Fig. 7-9) is a long, convoluted tube with a cuplike structure (called *Bowman's capsule*) on one end; it joins other

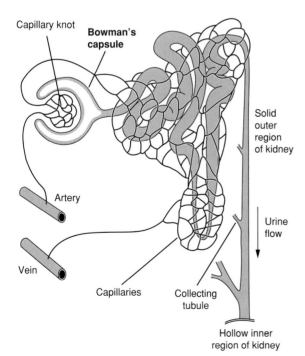

Capillary knot

Bowman's capsule

Solid outer region of kidney

Artery

Urine flow

Vein

Capillaries

Collecting tubule

Hollow inner region of kidney

Figure 7-9. Major components of the nephrons of a mammalian kidney. (Reproduced with permission from Lessing MS. *Review Text in Life Science*. Intermediate Level. New York, NY: Amsco School Publications; 1967.)

nephrons at the other end, where the urine is collected and eventually flows into the ureter. Inside Bowman's capsule is a clump of capillaries (called the *glomerulus*) from which the several substances diffuse into the tubular portion of the nephron. The rate of filtration is determined by blood pressure and by the osmotic pressure of the blood. About 1 L of blood per minute passes through the kidneys. From this, about 125 mL/min, corresponding to 180 L/d, are filtered by the glomeruli. Since the daily urinary output is about 2.2 L, it is clear that most of the glomerular filtrate is resorbed by the nephron structure downstream of Bowman's capsule. The resorption of water and sodium and potassium ions from the glomerular filtrate is regulated by hormones that are secreted by the pituitary gland (the antidiuretic hormone) and by the adrenal cortex (aldosterone). The normal pH of the blood is in the range of 7.35–7.45. Depending on the direction of deviation from the normal, the nephron will secrete or resorb acidic or basic ions. The control of pH is based mainly on shifting the plasma concentrations of carbonic acid and sodium bicarbonate in the direction that will decrease the deviation from the normal value.

The Nervous System

The nervous system is a communications network that functions to

- sense the external environment and control bodily motor responses to environmental stimuli,
- regulate the operation of internal organ systems, and
- learn and store information.

To achieve these ends, the nervous system consists of a central processing unit called the *brain*; the main trunk line that carries signals from the brain, called the *spinal cord*; and a distribution system of nerve cells, called *neurons*. The brain and the spinal cord constitute the central nervous system (CNS). Except for the category of nerves called the *cranial nerves*, which go directly from the brain to the organs that they activate (there are 12 cranial nerves), all the nerves in the network can be traced back to the spinal cord. The network of nerve fibers may be classified into two major subcategories: the voluntary nervous system, which is under our control to move our arms and legs, eyes, and so on, and the *involuntary*, or *autonomic*, nervous system, which controls our internal organs, such as the heart and stomach. The autonomic nervous system is further subclassified into two categories: the *sympathetic* and the *parasympathetic* nervous systems. The sympathetic and parasympathetic nervous systems operate in opposite directions—signals from the sympathetic nervous system stimulate the receptor organs to increase activity, while signals from the parasympathetic nervous system inhibit the activity of the receptor organs. Thus, increased heart rate and contractions in our stomach when we are agitated are due to signals from the sympathetic nervous system.

The fundamental cell in the nervous system is the neuron (Fig. 7-10). A neuron consists of a *cell body* and a long fiber called an *axon*. The cell body has several fiberlike projections called *dendrites*, and the axon terminates with several fiberlike tails called *telodendria*. Nerve impulses are transmitted from one axon to another at a junction of telodendria and dendrites called a *synapse*. At the synaptic junction, a substance called a *neurotransmitter* is secreted by the telodendria and its action on receptor sites on the dendrites initiates a nerve pulse that travels down the axon to

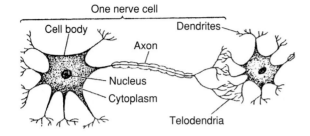

Figure 7-10. *Structure of a neuron. The picture also shows a synapse, which is the connection between two neurons that allows the nerve impulse to progress along the nervous system. (Reproduced with permission from Lessing MS.* Review Text in Life Science. *Intermediate Level. New York, NY: Amsco School Publications; 1967.)*

the next synapse. This action continues until a neuromuscular junction is reached, where the electrical impulse stimulates the muscle. The nerve pulse itself consists of a momentary depolarization of the wall of the neuron that travels along the neuron at a rate on the order of meters per second. When the nerve cell is at rest, a potential difference of about 80 mV is built up across the inside of the axon and the outside because of the difference in concentration of Na^+ and K^+ ions. The depolarization is caused by a momentary change in the permeability of the wall of the neuron that allows free passage of Na^+ and K^+ ions, thereby leading to a decreased potential difference. This change in permeability lasts about a millisecond and is followed immediately by a repolarization of the nerve cell wall.

The nervous system is considered to be the least sensitive system to radiation effects—the threshold for somatic damage is high, on the order of 10–20 Gy.

The Endocrine System

The endocrine system comprises a group of separate glands that are located in various parts of the body and secrete specific substances called *hormones* into the blood. These hormones are carried by the blood to specific sites, where they produce certain specific effects. We call the endocrine glands a system because, in many instances, they interact with each other, and the action of one may depend on interaction with a hormone secreted by another gland. A hormone that stimulates another gland is identified by a name whose prefix is the name of the gland that it stimulates and whose suffix is "tropin." Thus, the hormone called *thyrotropin* stimulates the secretion of thyroxine by the thyroid gland. The various glands in the endocrine system and their hormones include the following:

Pituitary. The pituitary gland, which is located in the base of the skull, above the roof of the mouth, is called the *master gland* because it secretes a number of different hormones, including:

- Adrenocorticotropic hormone, which regulates the growth and hormonal secretion of the adrenal cortex.
- Gonadotrophic hormones, which stimulate the production of sex hormones in the male and in the female.
  - Follicle-stimulating hormone—In the female, this hormone stimulates the production of the female hormone estrogen and the development of the ovarian follicles.

- ○ Luteinizing hormone—It stimulates the testes to secrete the male sex hormone testosterone and, in the female, stimulates the development of the corpus luteum and the production of progesterone.
  - ○ Luteotrophic hormone—It stimulates the start of lactation following the birth of a baby.
- Growth hormone (somatotropin), which stimulates growth, and thus is secreted mainly during the period of active growth. Hypersecretion during childhood leads to gigantism and hyposecrertion leads to dwarfism. Overproduction of growth hormone during adulthood leads to acromegaly, in which the bones of the head and the limbs are abnormally enlarged.
- Thyrotropic hormone, which stimulates the thyroid gland to secrete its own hormone, thyroxin.
- Oxytocin, which stimulates the milk-filled ducts in the breast of a lactating woman to contract, thereby squeezing out the milk.
- Vasopressin (antidiuretic hormone), which helps maintain fluid balance by responding to the osmotic pressure in the blood.

Thyroid. The thyroid consists of two ellipsoidal lobes, about 10–15 g each, that straddle the Adam's apple. The two lobes are connected by a narrow strip of tissue called the *isthmus*. The main role of the thyroid gland is the regulation of metabolism. To do this, the thyroid gland secretes two iodine-containing hormones that are synthesized within the thyroid, thyroxine (T4) and tri-iodothyronine (T3). The iodine used in the synthesis of these hormones comes from foods, including iodized salt, seafood, and milk. Once in the blood, they combine with a plasma protein and circulate as protein-bound iodine. Thyroxine concentration is about 10 mg per 100 mL serum, while the concentration of tri-iodothyronine is about 0.1 μg per 100 mL serum. These thyroid hormones regulate cellular metabolic rates. It is believed that they act as catalysts to increase the rate of oxidation reactions within the cells.

The release of thyroid hormones is under the indirect control of the hypothalamus, a regulatory region of the brain that modulates the activity of the pituitary gland. When the blood level of thyroid hormones falls, the hypothalamus signals the pituitary by secreting thyrotropin-releasing hormone, which causes the pituitary to release thyroid-stimulating hormone (TSH) into the blood. This hormone, in turn, stimulates the thyroid gland to release thyroid hormones. It should be pointed out that the thyroid hormones are not made on an "as needed" basis. A large amount of the hormone is made and is then stored within the thyroid gland; it is released as needed. The retention time of iodine in the thyroid gland is quite long. For the reference worker, the mean retention time of iodine is about 173 days. The release of too little or too much thyroid hormone causes pathological conditions. Hypothyroidism leads to a low basal metabolic rate, which results in decreased mental and physical capacity. In children, severe hypothyroidism can lead to a condition known as cretinism. In the adult, hypothyroidism is called myxedema and may be associated with goiter. Hyperthyroidism, overproduction of thyroid hormones, leads to the condition called thyrotoxicosis, in which a person is very nervous and excitable and has an enlarged thyroid.

The thyroid is of importance to the field of radiation safety because ^{131}I is a high-yield fission product. If ingested or inhaled, it will be incorporated into the thyroid hormones and may lead to high radiation doses (depending on the quantity of radioiodine in the thyroid) to the thyroid gland. This, in turn, may lead to cancer of the thyroid. A large increase in the thyroid cancer rate, predominantly among youngsters, was observed following the release of massive quantities of radioiodine during the nuclear reactor accident in Chernobyl in 1986.

Parathyroids. The parathyroids consist of two pea-sized glands located on the posterior surface of each of the two lobes of the thyroid. They secrete the parathyroid hormone, which controls plasma levels of calcium and phosphorus.

Adrenals. The adrenal glands sit on top of the kidneys. Each adrenal is made up of two different endocrine tissues. An outer tissue, called the *adrenal cortex*, surrounds an inner tissue, called the *adrenal medulla*. The medulla secretes a group of hormones called *catecholamines*, the most prominent one being *adrenaline* (epinephrine). The adrenal cortex secretes the steroidal hormones. One group of steroidal hormones, called the *glucocorticoids*, contains mainly hydrocortisone and is involved in metabolism of carbohydrates, proteins, fats, and electrolytes. Another major group of adrenocortical hormones is the *mineralocorticoids*, which consist mainly of aldosterone. Aldosterone regulates the retention of sodium and chloride ions and elimination of potassium and hydrogen ions; thus, it is involved in control of blood pressure and blood volume.

Islets of Langerhans. The islets of Langerhans are widely distributed within the pancreas. They contain two hormone-producing cells: alpha cells, which produce glucagon, and beta cells, which produce insulin. The function of a third islet cell, called the delta cell, is presently not known. Insulin is essential to carbohydrate metabolism. In the disease known as insulin-dependent diabetes mellitus, or Type 1 diabetes, the beta cells are destroyed through an autoimmune mechanism and insulin must be injected if the patient is to remain alive. In Type 2, or non-insulin-dependent diabetes mellitus, an insufficient amount of insulin is produced. This disease is treated either with a medicine that stimulates insulin production or by decreasing the quantity of insulin needed through dietary restriction. Glucagon is secreted from the alpha cells and is then carried by the blood to the liver, where it stimulates the liver to produce glucose. The action of glucagon is opposite to that of insulin. As a result, the coordinated release of insulin and glucagon provides a sensitive means for the control of blood glucose.

Gonads. The gonads—the ovaries in the female and the testes in the male—produce the sex hormones. The female sex hormones include the estrogens and progesterone. The androgenic or male sex hormones consist mainly of testosterone. The sex hormones determine the characteristics that distinguish males from females and regulate sexual activity and reproduction.

The Reproductive System

In the male, the reproductive system includes the penis, testicles, ducts through which semen passes into the urethra and from whence it is ejaculated during orgasm, the prostate gland, and Cowper's gland, which produce the seminal fluids. The testicles produce the male sex hormone, testosterone, as well as the sperms that are carried by the seminal fluid. Inside each of the testes is a number of convoluted seminiferous tubules whose inner surfaces are lined with a basement membrane consisting of the germinal cells from which the sperm eventually develop. The germinal cells give rise to the spermatogonia, which develop into primary spermatocytes. The primary spermatocytes undergo a meiotic division that decreases their chromosomes from the diploid number of 46 to the haploid number of 23 to become secondary spermatocytes. These secondary spermatocytes undergo a second meiotic division to become spermatids, which then develop into mature male gametes called spermatozoa. Thus, four spermatozoa evolve from a single spermatocyte, and every one of these spermatozoa is capable of fertilizing the female egg. The sole purpose of the male reproductive system is to produce the male gametes, which are designed to fertilize the female gametes. The germinal tissue in the seminiferous tubules forms the most radiosensitive tissue in the male reproductive system. Sterility can result from a dose of about 6 Gy (600 rads) to the basement membrane in the convoluted seminiferous tubules. Male potency, however, is related to the testosterone levels in the blood. A dose to the testes of about 30 Gy (3000 rads) or more is required in order to shut down testosterone production in the testes.

The reproductive system in the female consists of two ovaries; the uterus, where the fertilized egg develops into an embryo and then into a fetus; two fallopian tubes, which lead from each ovary to the uterus; and the vagina. The ovaries contain several thousand immature eggs, called *oocytes*, which are all present at the time of a female infant's birth. However, only several hundred will develop into mature eggs. The oocytes undergo two meiotic divisions, as in the case of spermatogenesis. However, in the case of oogenesis, only one mature ovum, the female gamete, is produced. In contrast to the production of male gametes, which is a continuously ongoing process, oogenesis is a cyclical process that is repeated about every 28 days. Whereas the male reproductive system has finished its task with the production and ejaculation of sperm, the female reproductive system is also designed to nurture and protect the developing conceptus until it is ready to be born. The hormone progesterone is secreted by the *corpus luteum*, which is formed in the ovary during the menstrual cycle.

Sensory Organs and Tissues

The sensory organs and tissues include the eyes, ears, olfactory nerve endings in the nose, the taste buds in the tongue, and the sensory nerve endings in the skin for tactile sensations and for monitoring temperature. The eyes, skin, and ears are of great interest in the practice of health physics and industrial hygiene because of ionizing and nonionizing radiation, and noise-regulatory requirements.

Eye. The structure of the eye is shown in Figure 7-11. The optical system of the eye includes those tissues that act together to focus a real image of the object on the retina. The system includes the following:

1. The cornea—A transparent layer about 0.5 mm thick with a mean index of refraction of 1.376. The anterior surface has a radius of curvature of about 7.7 mm, while the radius of curvature of the posterior surface is about 6.8 mm.
2. The aqueous humor—A clear, transparent, dilute solution (>99% water) of albumin, globulin, and sugar; its index of refraction is 1.336.

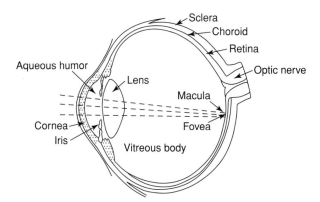

Figure 7-11. The gross structure of the human eye.

3. The lens—A biconvex, clear, transparent semisolid tissue encased in a transparent membrane called the *capsule*; its index of refraction is 1.413. Focusing of the eye is accomplished through a process called *accommodation* by thickening or elongating the lens, thus changing the radii of curvature.

4. The vitreous humor—A soft, jellylike, clear, transparent substance that fills the eye between the crystalline lens and the retina. It consists of about 99% water and has an index of refraction of 1.336.

When the eye is illuminated, the light incident on the cornea is concentrated by the eye's optical system to form an image on the retina of a much greater light intensity than that on the cornea. The light enters through the pupil, whose diameter is varied by the iris diaphragm according to the intensity of the light and the age of the person. This age dependency is shown in Table 7-3. After passing through the pupil, the light is focused by the lens on the retina, where the light is transduced to nerve impulses. These impulses are transmitted to the brain via the optic nerve (second cranial nerve) to give the sensation of sight.

The retina is a complex structure that is, in fact, an extension of the *optic disk*, its point of entry into the interior of the eyeball. On the visual axis, the retina is formed into a slightly elevated yellow spot, about 0.6 mm in diameter, called the *macula lutea*; in the center of the macula is a small, depressed area called the *fovea centralis*.

TABLE 7-3. Mean Pupil Diameter

AGE (yrs)	DAYLIGHT (mm)	NIGHT TIME (mm)	DIFFERENCE (mm)
20	4.7	8.0	3.3
30	4.3	7.0	2.7
40	3.9	6.0	2.1
50	3.5	5.0	1.5
60	3.1	4.1	1.0
70	2.7	3.2	0.5
80	2.3	2.5	0.2

Reproduced from Luckiesh M. Moss FK. *The Science of Seeing.* New York, NY: Van Nostrand; 1937.

Sharp vision is dependent on the formation of a real image on the macula. Two types of photoreceptor nerve endings are found in the retina: the *rods* and the *cones*. The cones are concentrated mainly in the fovea and serve to resolve fine details and to discriminate among the various hues of color. However, they are relatively insensitive and function only under conditions of good illumination. The rods, on the other hand, are much more light-sensitive than the cones and thus are useful in dim illumination and for "night vision." However, the rods neither resolve fine details nor discriminate among hues. At low levels of illumination, therefore, things tend to appear fuzzy and grayish regardless of their color. The retina is transparent through the layers of photoreceptors; the last layer consists of opaque, pigmented epithelium. Behind the pigmented epithelium is a layer of highly vascularized (rich in blood vessels) tissue called the *choroid,* which serves as the source of nutrition for the retina and carries away the cytometabolic wastes from the retinal cells. The retina itself is not vascular. Heat energy absorbed in the retina must therefore be conducted to the choroid before it can be transferred to the heat-exchange medium, the blood, for removal.

Ear. The ear (Fig. 7-12) is a transducer that converts the mechanical energy carried by sound waves into electrical pulses that are sent, via the auditory (eighth cranial) nerve, to the brain, where they are processed. Structurally and functionally, the ear can be thought of as having three major subassemblies. The outer ear, which includes the ear lobe (pinna), and the auditory canal, capture sound waves and conduct them to the eardrum (tympanic membrane), which is the beginning of the air-filled middle

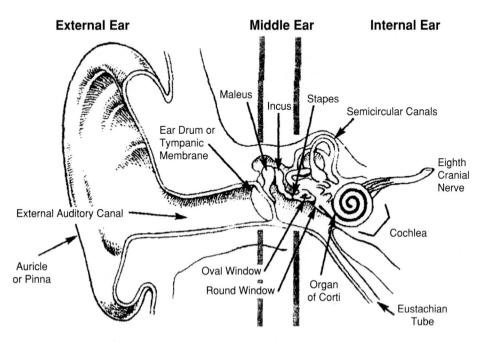

Figure 7-12. The gross structure of the human ear. (From Fleeger A, Lillquist D. *Industrial Hygiene Reference & Study Guide.* 2nd ed. Fairfax, VA: American Industrial Hygiene Association; 2006. Reproduced with permission from Elliott Berger, Aero Technologies.)

ear. The sound pressure on the eardrum activates a mechanical linkage of three tiny bones (hammer, anvil, and stirrup) collectively called the ossicles. The function of the middle ear is to mechanically amplify the sound-pressure-induced vibrations of the eardrum and to transmit these vibrations to the oval window, which is the beginning of the inner ear. The inner ear is filled with a fluid called the *perilymph.* Immersed in the perilymph are two separate systems of ducts that are filled with another physiological fluid called *endolymph.* One of these systems, the semicircular canals, is concerned with regulation of balance. The other one is the *cochlea,* a spiral-shaped structure in which the mechanical motions of the sound wave are converted into electrical impulses that are sent to the brain. The oval window is joined to the stirrup and vibrates due to the forces transmitted via the ossicles. This causes the endolymph to move back and forth. Immersed in the endolymph is a membrane (called the *organ of Corti*) from which numerous hairs project into the endolymph along the entire length of the membrane. These hairs are parts of the auditory nerve. The oscillatory motion of the endolymph causes the hairs to bend back and forth, and this bending generates the electrical impulses that are sent to the brain and are recognized as sound. The organ of Corti responds to the frequency and pressure level of the sound waves.

Radiation at levels of interest in the practice of health physics does not lead to any decrement in hearing acuity. However, loud noise, in excess of 90 dB, does lead to hearing loss. Noise control therefore is important in areas where loud noises may be generated, such as the turbine floor in a nuclear power plant.

Unity of the Body

The description of the physiological basis for radiation dosimetry sounds as if the various organ systems were independent entities. Nothing, however, could be further from the truth. The body can be thought of as a system of integrated negative feedback loops that operate together to keep its internal milieu constant. The total activity of these integrated systems is called *homeostasis.* In this manner, all the systems function together in a highly coordinated manner to produce a unified individual.

RADIATION EFFECTS: DETERMINISTIC

Acute Effects

Acute whole-body radiation overexposure affects all the organs and systems of the body. However, since not all organs and organ systems are equally sensitive to radiation, the pattern of response, or disease syndrome, in an overexposed individual depends on the magnitude of the dose. To simplify classification, the acute radiation syndrome is subdivided into three classes. In order of increasing severity, these are (1) the hemopoietic syndrome, (2) the GI syndrome, and (3) the CNS syndrome (Table 7-4). Certain effects are common to all categories; these include the following:

- nausea and vomiting
- malaise and fatigue
- increased temperature
- blood changes

In addition to these effects, numerous other changes are seen.

TABLE 7-4.   Doses Associated with the Acute Radiation Syndromes Following Whole-Body Exposure to Acute Low-LET Whole-Body Radiation

DOSE (gy)	PRINCIPAL CONTRIBUTING TO DEATH	EFFECT TIME TO DEATH (d)
3–5	Damage to bone marrow (LD$_{50/60}$)	30–60
5–15	Damage to gastrointestinal tract and lungs	10–20
>15	Damage to nervous system	1–5

Abbreviations: LET, linear energy transfer; LD, lethal dose to 50% of a population at 60 days.

Reproduced with permission from ICRP Publication 60. *Ann ICRP.* 1991; 21(1–3):105. Copyright ©1991 International Commission on Radiological Protection.

Hemopoietic Syndrome

A syndrome is a collection of signs and symptoms characteristic of a given disease state. In the case of the hemopoietic syndrome, the effects are mainly on the blood-forming tissues. Changes in the blood count have been seen in individuals with whole-body gamma-ray doses as low as 140 mGy (14 rads). However, in most cases of overexposure, changes in the blood count are seen when the dose is in the range of 250–500 mGy (25–50 rads). Blood count changes are almost certain to appear when the dose is greater than about 500 mGy (50 rads).

The hemopoietic syndrome appears after a whole-body gamma dose of about 2 Gy (200 rads) and encompasses the LD$_{50/60\text{-day}}$ dose. This disease state is characterized by depression or ablation of the bone marrow and the physiological consequences of this damage. After an acute sublethal radiation dose, there is a transitory sharp increase in the number of granulocytes, followed within a day by a decrease that reaches a minimum several weeks after exposure and then returns to normal after a period of several weeks to several months. The lymphocytes drop sharply after exposure and remain depressed for a period of several months. In contrast to the very rapid response of the WBC to radiation overexposure, the RBC count does not reflect overexposure until about a week after exposure. Depression in the erythrocyte count continues until a minimum is reached between 1 and 2 months after exposure, followed by a slow recovery over a period of weeks. The platelet count falls steadily until a minimum is reached about a month after exposure; recovery is very slow and may take several months. In all cases, the degree of change in the blood count, as well as the rate of change, is a function of the radiation dose. Figure 7-13 shows the trends and degree of blood changes following a nonlethal accidental overexposure.

The onset of the hemopoietic syndrome is rather sudden and is heralded by nausea and vomiting within several hours after the overexposure. Malaise and fatigue are felt by the victim, but the degree of malaise does not seem to be correlated with the size of the dose. Epilation (loss of hair), which is almost always seen, appears during the second or third week after exposure. Death may occur between 1 and 2 months after exposure if medical intervention is not successful. The chief effects to be noted are in the bone marrow and blood. Marrow depression is seen at 2 Gy (200 rads); at about 4–6 Gy (400–600 rads), almost complete ablation of the marrow occurs. Spontaneous regrowth of the marrow is possible if the victim survives the physiological effects of the denuding of marrow. An exposure of about 7 Gy (700 rads) or greater leads to irreversible ablation of the marrow. The LD$_{50/60\text{-day}}$ dose

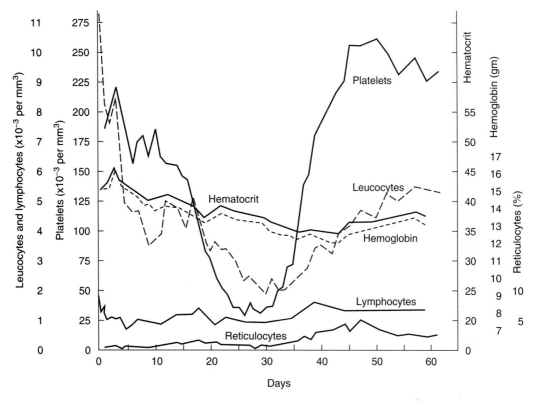

Figure 7-13. Hematologic effects of radiation overexposure. Average values for five patients who were exposed to 236–365 rads (estimated) during a criticality accident at the Y-12 plant in Oak Ridge on June 16, 1958. (Reproduced with permission from Andrews GH, Sitterson BW, Kretchmar AL, Brucer M. Criticality accident at the Y-12 plant. In: *Diagnosis and Treatment of Acute Radiation Injury*. Geneva, Switzerland: World Health Organization; 1961:27–48.)

for most mammals, including humans, falls within this range. The blood picture reflects damage to the marrow; the changes noted above are seen, and the magnitude of the change is roughly correlated with the dose. A very low lymphocyte count, 500 per mm³ or less within the first day after exposure, suggests that death will probably ensue.

GI Syndrome

The GI syndrome follows a total body dose of about 10 Gy (1000 rads) or greater and is a consequence of the destruction of the intestinal epithelium in addition to the complete destruction of the bone marrow. All the signs and symptoms of the hemopoietic syndrome are seen, but severe nausea, vomiting, and diarrhea begin very soon after exposure. Death within several weeks after exposure is the most likely outcome despite heroic medical efforts.

CNS Syndrome

A total-body gamma dose in excess of about 20 Gy (2000 rads) damages the CNS as well as all the other organ systems in the body. Unconsciousness follows within minutes after exposure and death in a matter of hours to several days; the rapidity of onset of unconsciousness is directly related to dose. In one instance, in which a 200-ms burst of mixed neutrons and gamma rays delivered a mean total-body dose of about 44 Gy (4400 rads), the victim was ataxic and disoriented within 30 seconds. Within 10 minutes, he was unconscious and in shock. Thirty-five minutes after the accident, analysis of fecal fluid from an explosive watery diarrhea showed a copious passage of fluids into the GI tract. Vigorous symptomatic treatment kept the patient alive for 34 hours after the accident. Postmortem examination showed that the victim's neuronal nuclei were about one-third the diameter of those found in normal unirradiated brains.

Other Acute Effects

Skin. Because of its physical location, the skin is subject to more radiation exposure, especially in the case of low-energy X-rays and beta rays, than most other tissues. A dose of about 3 Gy (300 rads) of Grenz rays or low-energy diagnostic X-rays may result in erythema (reddening of the skin); higher doses may lead to changes in pigmentation, epilation, blistering, necrosis, and ulceration. Radiation dermatitis of the hands and face was a relatively common occupational disease among radiologists who practiced during the early years of the twentieth century. The principal stochastic risks associated with radiation of large areas of the skin are the nonmelanoma skin cancers, basal-cell carcinoma, and squamous-cell carcinoma.

Of special interest is the radiation effect of alpha or beta radiation emitted from discrete radioactive particles, or hot particles, which may be found in nuclear reactor and in nuclear material facilities. Most hot particles range in size from about 10 μm to about 250 μm, and in activity from about 400 Bq (10 nCi) to about 200 kBq (5 μCi). These particles may consist of fission products due to tramp uranium (uranium contamination) on the outside of fuel rods or leakage from microscopic imperfections in the fuel rods (fewer than 0.1% of fuel rods are "leakers"), and neutron-activation products, such as ^{60}Co from the ^{59}Co alloys used in Stellite valve seats in the reactor coolant circulation piping system that form in the cooling water. These particles may be released into the environment during maintenance work on the coolant recirculating system. Once released into the environment, they may be deposited on the skin or inhaled.

Special concern about hot particles arises because the extremely nonuniform spatial distribution of radiation absorbed dose from hot particles (which are effectively point sources) deposited on the skin is uniquely different from that due to large area irradiation. The tissue in contact with the surface of the particle suffers a relatively high dose, whose exact magnitude is dependent on the radionuclides in the hot particle. The radiation dose decreases very rapidly with increasing distance from the particle because of dispersion due to the inverse square effect and absorption by the tissue. As a consequence of this steep gradient of absorbed energy, the radiation absorbed dose varies greatly from cell to cell in the cone of tissue that is within the range of the radiations emitted from the hot particle on the surface of the skin (or embedded in the tissue in the case of an inhaled or ingested hot particle). This extreme variation in the spatial distribution of absorbed dose leads to uncertainty regarding biologically meaningful dosimetry of hot particles. Physically, the radiation dose can be expressed in three different ways:

- By the quantitative relationship between dose rate and distance from the particle (Table 7-5).

TABLE 7-5. Tissue Dose Rate vs. Distance from a 1-μCi Particle

DISTANCE (microns)	DOSE RATE (rads/h)		
	^{14}C	^{90}Sr–^{90}Y	^{32}P
10	2,000,000	800,000	380,000
100	1500	7700	3700
200	40	1780	930
400	0.03	360	230
600		130	100
1000		36	30
2000		7	7
4000		1	0.7
6000		0.3	0.1
8000			0.01

- By the tissue mean dose, which is the mean dose to the sphere of tissue whose radius is equal to the range of the alphas or betas emitted from the hot particle. The tissue mean dose is calculated by dividing the mass of the irradiated tissue by the total amount of energy absorbed by the tissue (Table 7-6).
- In the case of a hot particle on the skin, by the mean dose to the basement layer, at a depth of 0.007 cm below the surface, averaged over 10 cm^2.
- By the organ mean dose, which is the mean dose to the entire organ calculated by dividing the total amount of energy absorbed in the organ by the total weight of the organ. This is equivalent to the radioactivity being uniformly distributed throughout the organ instead of being concentrated in a discrete point source.

It had been thought that the steep gradient of absorbed energy around the hot particle would be particularly toxic to the cells within the range of the particulate (alpha or beta) radiation. Those cells very close to the radioactive particles would be killed by the high radiation dose, while cells further away would get a sublethal dose, but a dose large enough so that the initiation of an oncogenic lesion was likely. Numerous laboratory studies and human experiences showed that this was not the case. The NCRP, in Report No. 106, *Limit for Exposure to "Hot Particles" on the Skin*, conservatively estimated the risk of fatal cancer from a discrete radioactive particle on the skin to be about 1×10^{-9} Gy^{-1} (1×10^{-11} rad^{-1}).

If an area of the skin is damaged by radiation, the damage is then repaired by regeneration of surviving cells within the damaged area and around the periphery of the damaged area. As the size of the damaged area decreases, the role of the

TABLE 7-6. Tissue Mean Dose Rate (rads/h) for a 1-μCi Particle

RADIUS OF SPHERE (cm)	TISSUE VOLUME (cm^3)	^{14}C	^{32}P	^{90}Sr–^{90}Y
0.01	4.2×10^{-6}	21,000	9400	24,000
0.1	0.0042	25	110	166
0.62	1.0	0.096	1.4	2.13
1.0	4.2	0.023	0.36	0.58

Reproduced from *Effects of Inhaled Particles: Report of the Subcommittee on Inhalation Hazards, Committee on Pathologic Effects of Atomic Radiation.* Washington, DC: National Academy Press; 1961. Publication 848.

peripheral cells in the healing process increases. If the damaged area is very small, the cells within the area may all have been killed, but healing can be complete, with little or no permanent injury because of the regeneration of the cells around the perimeter. If the area of total cellular destruction exceeds the ability of the peripheral cells to repopulate this area, then ulceration can result. There is a threshold area and a threshold dose to the basal cells in the skin, both of which must be exceeded before an ulcer can result. No ulceration will occur at any dose, no matter how great, unless the irradiated area exceeds 0.05 mm^2 (diameter = 0.25 mm); and at any irradiated area, no matter how great, unless the dose to the basal cells exceeds 20 Gy (2000 rads). For an area of 1 cm^2, the calculated threshold dose for ulceration is about 30 Gy (3000 rads).

Gonads. The gonads are particularly radiosensitive. A single dose of only 300 mGy (30 rads) to the testes may result in temporary sterility among men; for women, a 3-Gy (300-rad) dose to the ovaries may lead to temporary sterility. Higher doses increase the period of temporary sterility. One man, whose exposure to the gonads was less than 4.4 Gy (440 rads), was aspermatic for a period of several years. In women, temporary sterility is evidenced by a cessation of menstruation for a period of 1 month or more, depending on the dose. Irregularities in the menstrual cycle, which suggest functional changes in the gonads, may result from local irradiation of the ovaries with doses smaller than required for temporary sterilization.

Eyes. Much higher incidence rates of cataracts were found among physicists in cyclotron laboratories whose eyes had been exposed intermittently over long periods of time to mixed neutron and gamma radiation. Among nuclear bomb survivors whose eyes had been exposed to a single high-radiation dose, it was found that both chronic and acute overexposure of the eyes could lead to cataracts. Radiation may injure the cornea, conjunctiva, iris, and lens of the eye. In the case of the lens, the principal site of damage is the proliferating epithelial cells of the lens capsule on the anterior surface of the lens. This results in abnormal lens fibers, which eventually disintegrate to form an opaque area, thus preventing light from reaching the retina. The opacity is called a cataract when it is large enough to interfere with vision. The cataractogenic dose to the lens of the eye is on the order of 2 Gy (200 rads) of beta or gamma radiation. Cataracts have been observed among survivors of the nuclear bombings whose doses to the eyes are believed to have been in the range of 0.6–1.5 Gy (60–150 rads) of mixed neutron and gamma radiation.

Not all radiations are equally cataractogenic. Neutrons are much more efficient in producing cataracts than beta or gamma rays. The cataractogenic dose has been found, in laboratory experiments with animals, to be a function of age; young animals are more sensitive than old animals. On the basis of occupational exposure data, it is estimated that the fast-neutron threshold dose for cataracts in humans lies between about 0.15 and 0.45 Gy (15 and 45 rads). No radiogenic cataracts resulting from occupational exposure to X-rays have been reported. From patients who suffered irradiation of the eyes in the course of X-ray therapy and developed cataracts as a consequence, the cataractogenic threshold dose is estimated at about 2 Gy (200 rads). In cases, either of occupationally or iatrogenically induced radiation cataracts, a long latent period, on the order of several years, usually elapsed between exposure and the appearance of the cataract.

Birth Defects (Teratogenesis)

Teratogenic effects can result from radiation overexposure of an embryo or fetus (conceptus). The type of radiogenic damage depends on the age of the conceptus at the time of the radiation overexposure. The 9-month gestation period can be divided into three identifiable phases:

1. Weeks 1 and 2—Preimplantation, when fertilization occurs, and implantation of the fertilized egg in the wall of the uterus. Fertilization occurs in the Fallopian (uterine) tube, and the zygote (fertilized egg) migrates into the uterus. About 8–10 days after fertilization, the zygote is implanted in the wall of the uterus and the primary embryonic tissues are formed. During this phase, the cells are growing rapidly and are not well differentiated. In accordance with the Law of Bergonié and Tribondeau, these cells are very sensitive to the lethal effects of radiation. Thus, embryonic cells in this phase tend to be killed rather than survive a teratogenic radiation dose.

2. Weeks 3–7—Period of organogenesis. The embryonic tissues differentiate into the major organs. Radiation doses of ≥ 0.15 Gy (15 rads) to the embryo may lead to death of the embryo or to birth defects.

3. Weeks 8–birth—This is called the fetal period, and is characterized by rapid growth of the fetus. The fetus is sensitive to mental retardation following a fetal dose $\gtrsim 0.25$ Gy (25 rads). Studies of children who had been irradiated in utero and survived the nuclear bombings in Japan have shown a dose-related increase in mental retardation. This effect was especially pronounced among those who had been exposed during the 8th through the 17th week of pregnancy. During this part of the gestation period, the number of neurons in the developing brain increases rapidly and the neurons move into the specific part of the brain where they will permanently reside. After the 17th week, the brain cells continue to differentiate and to form synaptic junctions, but they do not undergo any further cell division. Thus, a baby is born with all the brain cells it will ever have. The high rate of mitotic activity during the 8th to the 17th week is the basis for the high degree of radiosensitivity of the CNS and thus is the explanation for the mental impairment observed among the nuclear bombing survivors who had been irradiated in utero, as shown in Table 7-7. In utero irradiation later than the 25th week of gestation did not affect the IQ of the child.

Treatment of Acute Overexposure

Medical treatment of an acutely overexposed person is directed mainly at the alleviation of symptoms. Since severe depression of the WBC (leukopenia) compromises the immune system, the patient is treated with antibiotics and kept in reverse isolation—that is, in a relatively aseptic environment—in order to prevent infection. Thrombocytopenia (low platelet count) affects blood clotting and therefore leads to hemorrhage. The 3–4-month lifetime of the erythrocytes precludes an immediate decrease in RBCs. However, anemia develops within 1–2 weeks because the extremely radiosensitive undifferentiated stem cells, which give rise to all the blood cells, are severely depleted. One of the first steps in combating these effects is a blood transfusion. In cases of very severe bone-marrow depression, bone-marrow transplants have

TABLE 7-7. Mental Retardation Among Atomic Bomb Survivors Following in Utero Exposure

MEAN DOSE (RADS)	DOSE RANGE (RADS)	ALL GESTATIONAL AGES			10–17 WKS		
		Number	No. Retarded	%	Number	No. Retarded	%
0	Control	1085	9	0.8	257	2	0.8
4	1–9	292	4	1.4	69	3	4.3
23	12–49	169	4	2.4	50	4	8.0
72	50–99	34	6	17.6	13	4	30.8
131	100–199	15	5		6	5	
274	200+	4	2	37[a]	3	1	67[a]

[a]Because of the small numbers, the data of the two highest doses were combined.

Reprinted with permission from Otake M, Schull WJ. *Mental Retardation in Children Exposed in-utero to Atomic Bombs: A Reassesment.* Hiroshima, Japan: Radiation Effects Research Foundation; 1983. RERF TR 1–83.

been used. However, there is a good deal of uncertainty about the exact indications for bone-marrow transplants. Because of the difficulties and complications associated with the procedure, this treatment modality is being either supplemented with or replaced by a treatment that uses human granulocyte macrophage colony stimulating factor. This agent stimulates the bone marrow to produce granulocytes after severe depression of the red marrow activity. Vomiting and diarrhea lead to dehydration and electrolyte imbalance. Accordingly, fluids and electrolytes are administered via the diet and by intravenous infusion.

Severe overexposure by external radiation also damages the skin. Swelling, epilation (loss of hair), and dry and wet desquamation (peeling and blistering of the skin) are seen. The degree to which these effects occur depends on the size of the dose. These skin lesions are treated medically with topical analgesics, antiseptics, and antibiotics. When necessary, the skin lesions are surgically debrided. Eventually, the wounds heal. In the case of hands and feet that are very severely overexposed, a serious complication may develop when the radiation burns seem to be healed. The arterioles (very small blood vessels) that supply the extremities may overcompensate in the healing process. Instead of regenerating enough cells to rebuild the damaged arteriolar walls to their proper thickness, the wall thickness continues to increase until the entire lumen of the arteriole is solidly filled. When this happens, the blood supply to the tissue is cut off, gangrene develops, and the affected parts of the hands or feet must be amputated.

Medical treatment in cases of acute whole-body overexposure is successful only for doses within the range of the hemopoietic syndrome. For doses in the range of the GI syndrome, there is no effective medical treatment that will prevent death.

In the case of overexposure from radioactive material taken into the body through inhalation, ingestion, transcutaneously, or through a wound, immediate actions may be taken in some instances to block deposition of the radionuclide in the critical organ. For example, iodine, when administered within 2 hours or less following intake of radioiodine will effectively saturate the thyroid with iodine and thus block the further deposition of the radioiodine. In case of an accidental overexposure to iodine, regardless of the portal of entry into the body, the NCRP recommends that the overexposed person be immediately given a 300-mg tablet of either KI or NaI. For overexposure to radiocesium, the most effective treatment is with Prussian blue (ferric ferrocyanide), which binds to the cesium. The bound cesium is not absorbed into the blood, and is excreted via the feces. Chelation with the calcium or zinc salts of DPTA (diethylenetriaminepentaacetate) is useful in the removal of transuranics from the body. Chelation therapy must be administered within several hours of exposure to be effective. Chelation is not without its own risk, and the benefits of removal of the contaminant must be weighed against the risks of chelation.

Delayed Effects

The delayed effects of radiation may be due either to a single large overexposure or continuing low-level overexposure.

Continuing overexposure can be due to exposure to external radiation fields or can result from inhalation or ingestion of a radioisotope which then becomes fixed in the body through chemical reaction with the tissue protein or, because of the chemical similarity of the radioisotope with normal metabolites, may be systemically absorbed within certain organs and tissues. In either case, the internally deposited radioisotope may continue to irradiate the tissue for a long time. In this connection, it should be pointed out that the adjectives "acute" and "chronic," as ordinarily used by toxicologists to describe single and continuous exposures, respectively, are not directly applicable to inhaled or ingested radioisotopes since a single or "acute" exposure may lead to continuous or "chronic" irradiation of the tissue in which the radioactive material is located.

Among the delayed consequences of overexposure that were seen among the Japanese atomic bomb survivors, in addition to cancers and cataracts, is decreased life span (2.6-year median decrease in longevity for those who survived doses of 1 Gy [100 rads] or more and a median loss of about 4 months for all members of the cohort whose dose exceeded zero). Because a dose-related 2–3-year reduction in the age of onset of menopause has been found among the survivors and because the decreased life span among the Japanese survivors cannot be attributed to any single medical cause, it is reasonable to infer radiation-related, accelerated physiological aging. Other delayed effects that were seen include heart disease, stroke, and diseases of the blood-forming, digestive, and respiratory systems. Although statistically significant, there were not enough data to establish a quantitative dose–response curve whose threshold that may be as high as 0.5 Gy (50 rads).

RADIATION EFFECTS: STOCHASTIC

Genetic Effects

No genetic (heritable) effects of radiation have ever been observed in any human population irradiated at any dose ranging from that due to the natural background to that received by the Japanese survivors of the nuclear bombings.

Genetic information necessary for the production and functioning of a new organism is contained in the chromosomes of the germ cells—the sperm and the ova. The normal human somatic cell contains 46 chromosomes; the mature sperm and

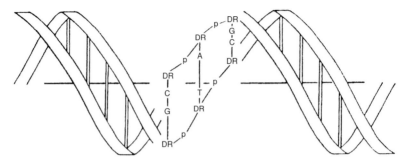

Figure 7-14. Structure of the DNA molecule. The nucleotides, the strands of the double helix, consist of alternating deoxyribose (DR) and phosphate (p) units. Two pairs of complementary bases, adenine (A) and thymine (T), and guanine (G) and cytosine (C) join the two nucleotide chains.

ova each carry 23 chromosomes. When an ovum is fertilized by a sperm, the resulting cell, called a *zygote*, contains the full complement of 46 chromosomes. During the 9-month gestation period, the fertilized egg, by successive cellular divisions and differentiation, develops into a new individual. In the course of the cellular divisions, the chromosomes are exactly duplicated, so that all the cells in the body contain the same genetic information. The units of information in the chromosomes are called *genes*. Each gene is an enormously complex macromolecule called *deoxyribonucleic acid* (DNA), in which the genetic information is coded according to the sequence of certain molecular subassemblies called *bases*. The DNA molecule (Fig. 7-14), whose molecular mass is on the order of 10^7 Da, consists of two long chains composed of pentose sugars (deoxyribose) and phosphates that wind around each other in a double helix. The two long, intertwined strands are held together by a pair of bases that are hydrogen-bonded to each other. The base pairs form cross-links between the long strands in a manner similar to the treads of a stepladder (Fig. 7-14). There are four different bases: two purines, adenine (A) and guanine (G), and two pyrimidines, cytosine (C) and thymine (T). The base cross-links are formed when two of these bases, one of which is joined to each long strand, attach to one another. The cross-linked bond is specific, with adenine coupling only with thymine (A–T) and cytosine coupling only with guanine (C–G). The bits of information are coded in triplets of various combinations of A–T and C–G cross-links, and the sequence of these triplets determines the genetic information contained in the DNA molecule.

The genetic information can be altered by many different chemical and physical agents, called mutagens, that disrupt the sequence of bases in a DNA molecule. If this information in a somatic cell is scrambled, then its descendants may show some sort of an abnormality. If the information in a germ cell is jumbled and that cell is subsequently fertilized, then the new individual may carry a genetic defect, or a mutation. Such a mutation is often called a *point mutation*, since it results from damage to one point on a gene. Most geneticists believe that the majority of such mutations in people are undesirable or harmful.

In addition to point mutations, genetic damage can arise through chromosomal aberrations. Certain chemical and physical agents, including ionizing radiation, can cause chromosomes to break. In most of these breaks, the fragments reunite. In a small fraction of breaks, however, the broken pieces do not reunite. When this happens, one of the broken fragments may be lost when the cell divides, and the daughter cell does not receive the genetic information contained on the lost fragment. The other possibility following chromosomal breakage, especially if two or more chromosomes suffer double stranded beaks, is the interchange of fragments among the broken chromosomes and the production of aberrant chromosomes. Cells with such aberrant chromosomes usually have impaired reproductive capacity as well as other abnormalities. About 200 double-stranded breaks occur per cell per year due to various reasons, including background radiation, chemicals, and spontaneous breaks due to intramolecular vibration. A whole-body dose of 10 rads (0.1 Gy) leads to about 4 double-stranded breaks per cell.

The mutagenic properties of ionizing radiation were discovered by Herman J. Muller in 1927 (for which he won the Nobel Prize in medicine in 1946). He studied the genetic effects of X-rays on fruit flies. Since then, laboratory studies of a number of different irradiated organisms have confirmed the mutagenicity of all forms of ionizing radiation.

Point mutations are changes on the molecular level. However, many biochemical events that can modify the dose–response relation that occur between molecular changes on a gene and the somatic expression of that molecular change. For example, if the genetic damage renders a germ cell or a zygote nonviable, then no living organism that carries that mutation will be born. Empirically, therefore, no detrimental effect is observed. Although the biological model used to explain genetic effects postulates a zero threshold for genetic effects of radiation, studies on dose–rate effects imply that there is a repair mechanism to correct genetic lesions. Animals exposed at low dose rates show mutation rates that are one-fifth to one-tenth the mutation rate observed at high dose rates. This dose–rate dependence implies a repair mechanism that is overwhelmed at high dose rates.

What is the quantitative relationship between radiation dose and probability of mutation? The doubling dose—that is, the gonadal radiation dose that would eventually lead to a doubling of the spontaneous mutation rate—was calculated by the BEIR VII committee from animal data, and was found to be 0.82 ± 0.29 Gy (82 ± 29 rads). The committee suggested 1 Gy (100 rads) as the estimated doubling dose. Doubling the equilibrium genetic load in a population requires the irradiation of successive generations with the doubling dose. If only one generation receives the doubling dose, then the equilibrium genetic load in the population will asymptotically approach the preirradiation value (Table 7-8). These numbers are theoretical calculations based on animal experiments. No increased mutation rate has yet been observed among any irradiated population.

Cancer

The carcinogenic effects of doses of 1 Gy (100 rads) or more of gamma radiation at high dose rates are well documented and consistent. Table 7-9 lists the BEIR VII committee's estimated excess relative risk (EER) of several solid cancers and leukemia per Sv (100 rems) of whole-body radiation. The ERRs are based on the mortality data during the period 1950–2000, among 86,572 Japanese atomic-bomb survivors whose radiation doses are reasonably known. The ERR is a prospective metric of the increased likelihood of developing cancer as a result of exposure to

TABLE 7-8. Effects of a Single or Permanent Doubling Dose of the Mutation Rate on Mutant Gene Frequency, p, and Disease Frequency, P, for a Hypothetical Autosomal Dominant Disease

| | PERMANENT DOUBLING DOSE | | SINGLE DOUBLING DOSE | |
GENERATION	p($\times 10^{-5}$)	P($\times 10^{-5}$)	p($\times 10^{-5}$)	P($\times 10^{-5}$)
Initial	2.0	4.0	2.0	4.0
1	3.0	6.0	3.0	6.0
2	3.5	7.0	2.5	6.0
3	3.8	7.5	2.3	4.5
4	3.9	7.8	2.1	4.3
5	3.9	7.9	2.1	4.1
New equilibrium	4.0	8.0	2.0	4.0

Reprinted with permission from the National Academies Press from BEIR VII: *Health Risks from Exposure to Low Levels of Ionizing Radiation*. Washington, DC: National Academies Press; 2005. Copyright © 2005, National Academy of Sciences.

a carcinogen (ionizing radiation in this case) and is dependent on several factors, including age, sex, and dose history. It is defined by

$$\text{ERR} = \frac{\text{Cancer incidence in exposed population}}{\text{Cancer incidence in unexposed population}} - 1. \tag{7.7}$$

Another metric used to estimate radiation risk to a population from a given radiation dose is the excess absolute risk (EAR). The EAR is a measure of the postulated

TABLE 7-9. Cancer Incidence Among 86,572 Atomic-Bomb Survivors with Known Radiation Dose

| | | EXCESS RELATIVE RISK (per Sv[a]) | |
CANCER SITE	NUMBER OF CASES	Male	Female
Stomach	3602	0.21 (0.11–0.40)[a]	0.48 (0.31–0.73)
Colon	1165	0.63 (0.37–1.1)	0.43 (0.19–0.96)
Liver	1146	0.32 (0.16–0.64)	0.32 (0.10–1.0)
Lung	1136	0.32 (0.15–0.70)	1.40 (0.94–2.11)
Breast	952	—	0.51 (0.28–0.83)
Prostate	281	0.12 (0–0.69)	—
Uterus	875	—	0.055 (0–0.22)
Ovary	190	—	0.38 (0.10–1.4)
Bladder	352	0.50 (0.18–1.4)	1.65 (0.69–4.0)
Other solid cancers	2969	0.27 (0.15–0.50)	0.45 (0.27–0.75)
Thyroid	243	0.53 (0.14–2.0)	1.05 (0.28–3.9)
Leukemia (Except CLL)	296	1.1 (0.1–2.6)	1.2 (0.1–2.9)

[a]ERR per Sv for exposure at age 30+ and attained age 60. The numbers in the parentheses are the 95% confidence intervals for the ERRs.

Abbreviations: CLL, chronic lymphocytic leukemia; ERR, excess relative risk.

Reprinted with permission from the National Academies Press from BEIR VII: *Health Risks from Exposure to Low Levels of Ionizing Radiation*. Washington, DC: National Academies Press; 2005. Copyright © 2005, National Academy of Sciences.

TABLE 7-10.   BEIR VII's Estimated Number of Increased Cases and Deaths for All Solid Tumors and for Leukemia[a]

	ALL SOLID CANCERS		LEUKEMIA	
	Males	**Females**	**Males**	**Females**
Number of cases in absence of exposure	45,500	36,900	830	590
Excess cases from a 0.1-Gy dose	800 (400–600)	1300 (690–2500)	100 (30–300)	70 (20–250)
Number of deaths in absence of exposure	22,100	17,500	710	530
Excess deaths from a 0.1-Gy dose	410 (200–830)	610 (300–1200)	70 (20–220)	50 (10–190)

[a]This study was conducted in a population of 100,000 persons, with an age distribution similar to that of the entire United States, who had been exposed to 0.1 Gy (10 rads).

[b]The numbers in the parentheses are the 95% confidence intervals of the lifetime attributable risks.

Reprinted with permission from the National Academies Press from BEIR VII: *Health Risks from Exposure to Low Levels of Ionizing Radiation.* Washington, DC: National Academies Press; 2005. Copyright © 2005, National Academy of Sciences.

increase in the number of cases or deaths in a population that had been exposed to a given dose—that is, the EAR tells us how many cases or deaths may be attributed to the exposure. It is therefore also called the *attributable risk* (Table 7-10). EAR is defined by

$$EAR = \text{exposed population incidence rate} - \text{control population incidence rate.}$$

$$(7.8)$$

Cancer is believed to be the culmination of a multiphase sequence of events that may be spread over many years. First is an initiating event in a single cell. This event is thought to be damage to a DNA molecule by ionizing radiation or by a chemical interaction. Additionally spontaneous damage may occur because of the Maxwell–Boltzman distribution of intramolecular vibrational energy. A break in some part of the DNA molecule occurs when the vibrational energy exceeds the bonding energy. The initiating event is followed by what is called tumor promotion, a preneoplastic phase in which the damaged cell proliferates. If natural defense mechanisms fail, the damaged clone undergoes a malignant transformation, which may progress into a clinical cancer. Because of the numerous defense mechanisms in every step of this sequence, only a very small fraction of the initiated cells actually develop into a cancer.

Although any organ or tissue may develop neoplasia after overexposure to radiation, certain organs and tissues seem to be more sensitive in this respect than others. Radiation-induced cancer is observed most frequently in the hemopoietic system, the thyroid, the bone, and the skin. In all cases, the tumor-induction time in humans is relatively long—on the order of 5–20 years after exposure. Carcinoma of the skin was the first type of malignancy associated with exposure to X-rays. Early X-ray workers, including physicists and physicians, had a much higher incidence of skin cancer than could be expected from random occurrence of the disease. Well over 100 cases of skin cancer associated with overexposure to radiation are documented in the literature. As early as 1900, a physician who had been using X-rays in his practice described the irritating effects of X-rays. He recorded erythema and itching that progressed to hyperpigmentation, ulceration, and finally to neoplasia. The entire disease process spanned a period of 9 years until his death from metastatic carcinoma. An occupational disease among dentists, before the carcinogenic properties of X-rays were well understood, was cancer of the fingers that were used to hold dental X-ray film in the mouths of patients while X-raying their teeth.

Although overexposure to radiation increases the likelihood of cancer, *it is impossible to definitely identify any particular cancer with any given exposure.* No physician, no matter how expert he or she is in pathology, can say with certainty that any particular cancer would not have occurred if the patient had not been exposed to radiation. Association of cancer with radiation exposure can be made only statistically through epidemiologic studies. Epidemiologic data relative to the carcinogenicity of low-level radiation gathered from numerous sources are contradictory and inconclusive; some even show negative correlations between the induction of cancer and dose in the low-dose range, as reported by the International Commission on Radiological Protection (ICRP) in 1991, in its Publication No. 60. For purposes of setting criteria for the management of radiation risks, therefore, the ICRP considered it prudent to estimate the risk from low-level radiation by extrapolation from the high-dose cases.

Probability of Causation

Stochastic effects, as the name implies, are those effects that occur by chance; they occur among unexposed as well as exposed individuals. Stochastic effects are therefore not unequivocally related to exposure to a noxious agent, as drunkenness is to alcohol consumption or sunburn to overexposure to the sun. In the context of radiation safety, stochastic effects mean cancer and heritable (genetic) effects. The result of exposure to a carcinogen or to a mutagen is an increase in the probability of occurrence of the effect, with the increase in probability being proportional to the size of the dose. Thus, people develop cancer whether or not they are exposed to carcinogens. However, exposure to a carcinogen increases the likelihood of cancer, and the greater the exposure, the greater the likelihood. At no time, however, regardless of the size of the dose, is it certain that cancer will result from the exposure. If cancer does develop after exposure to a carcinogen, we cannot be certain, as we are in the case of alcohol consumption and drunkenness, that the cancer was caused by the carcinogen. No pathologist can say with certainty that the cancer would not have occurred if the person had not been exposed to the carcinogen. The best we can do is to estimate the probability, based on the exposure history and dose, that the cancer was caused by the carcinogen. For example, we find lung cancer among a much higher proportion of cigarette smokers than among nonsmokers; and among smokers, lung cancer is seen in a greater proportion of heavy smokers than light smokers. Most cigarette smokers do not develop lung cancer, while some nonsmokers develop this disease. Smoking, even heavy smoking, does not ensure that the smoker will develop lung cancer; it merely increases the likelihood of developing the disease. The probability of causation of the cancer, PC, is defined as

$$PC = \frac{ERR}{1 + ERR}.$$ (7.9)

EXAMPLE 7.1

A female nuclear medicine technician accumulates 0.15 Gy (15 rads) over a 30-year working period starting at age 25. At age 60, she is diagnosed with colon cancer. She is a nonsmoker, and knows of no exposure to other risk factors for colon cancer. The lifetime risk of spontaneous colon cancer in women is 4.2% (BEIR VII), and the ERR for colon cancer in women is listed in BEIR VII as 0.43 per Gy, with a 95% confidence interval of 0.19–0.96 per Gy. What is the estimated probability that her colon cancer is due to her radiation dose?

Solution

Substituting the values for the spontaneous risk and for the ERR into Eq. (7.9), we find

$$PC = \frac{0.43 \text{ Gy}^{-1} \times 0.15 \text{ Gy}}{1 + (0.43 \text{ Gy} \times 0.15 \text{ Gy})} = 0.061 = 6.1\%.$$

After substituting the 95% confidence limits into Eq. (7.9), we find the 95% confidence interval of the PC to be 2.8–12.6%.

Leukemia

Leukemia, especially acute myelogenous leukemia and to a lesser extent chronic myelogenous or acute lymphocytic leukemia, is among the most likely forms of malignancy resulting from whole-body overexposure to radiation. Chronic lymphocytic leukemia does not appear to be related to radiation exposure.

Radiologists and other physicians who used X-rays in their practices before strict health physics practices were common showed a significantly higher incidence rate of leukemia than did their colleagues who did not use radiation. Among American radiologists, the doses associated with the increased rate of leukemia were on the order of 1 Gy (100 rads)/yr. With the increased practice of health physics, the difference between the leukemia incidence rates of radiologists and other physicians gradually disappeared. An increased incidence rate of leukemia was also seen among patients who had been treated with X-rays for ankylosing spondylitis (rheumatoid arthritis of the joints in the spine).

Among the survivors of the nuclear bombings in Japan, there was a significantly greater incidence of leukemia in those who had been within 1500 m of the hypocenter than among those who had been further away from ground zero at the time of the bombing (Fig. 7-15). The first increase in the leukemia incidence rate among

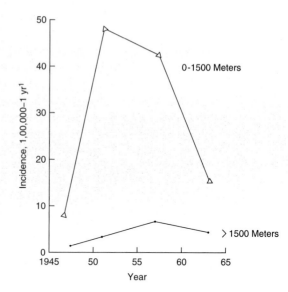

Figure 7-15. Incidence rate of leukemia among the survivors of the nuclear bombings in Hiroshima and Nagasaki.

the survivors was seen about 3 years after the bombings, and it continued to increase until it peaked about 7 years after the bombings. Since then, the leukemia incidence rate has slowly declined, until it eventually reached the same value as that in the unexposed population.

The questions regarding the leukemogenicity of low-level radiation and of the existence of a nonzero threshold for leukemia induction remain unanswered and are the subjects of controversy. A clear dose–response relationship was seen in Hiroshima and Nagasaki. The atomic bomb data show increased leukemia mortality among those whose dose was 0.4 Gy (40 rads) or more, but no increased mortality at doses less than 0.4 Gy. No radiation-induced leukemia was found among people who had been exposed in utero to radiation from the bombs. However, a study in Great Britain found that children who had been irradiated in utero during medical X-ray examinations of the mother had a significantly higher leukemia rate than did children who had not been irradiated in utero. On the basis of these studies, it was inferred that a dose to the fetus of as little as 5–50 mGy (0.5–5 rads) of X-rays might lead to leukemia.

In other studies involving in utero X-ray exposures that were made for routine pelvimetry rather than for some medical indication, no evidence of any radiation effect was seen. The difference between these two divergent observations is thought to be due to the medical factors that required the diagnostic X-rays. Thus, although all the available data show ionizing radiation to be leukemogenic at high doses, the results of studies on the leukemogenic effects of low doses are inconclusive and controversial. Because the results from low-dose studies are conflicting, however, it is reasonable to infer that the low-level radiation at doses associated with most diagnostic X-ray procedures, occupational exposure within the recommended limits, and natural background radiation is, at worst, a very weak leukemogen, and that the attributive risk of leukemia from low-level radiation is probably extremely small. The risk for leukemia per unit dose was found by the BEIR VII committee to increase at

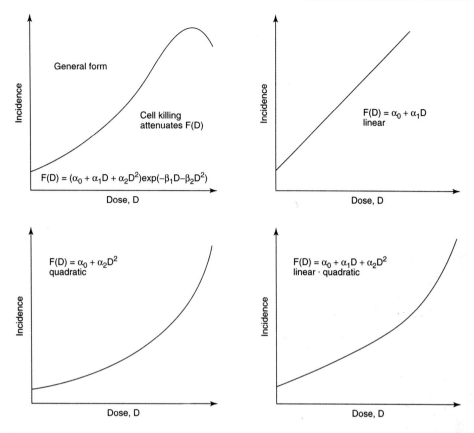

Figure 7-16. Alternative dose–response curves. (Reproduced from BEIR III: *The Effects on Populations of Exposure to Low Levels of Ionizing Radiation: 1980.* Washington, DC: National Academy Press; 1980.)

high doses. Accordingly, the BEIR VII model for estimating the radiogenic risk for leukemia is linear-quadric (Fig. 7-16).

Bone Cancer

Historically, cancers of the bone and of the lung, induced by occupational radiation, are important in studying the carcinogenicity of internally deposited radioisotopes. Although the carcinogenic properties of radium were known within several years after its discovery by Pierre and Marie Curie in 1902, little or no effort was made to protect people from the harmful effects of radium. One of the first industrial uses to which radium was put was in the manufacture of luminous paint. When powdered radium is mixed with ZnS crystals, the crystals glow owing to absorption of energy from the alpha particles emitted by the radium. Luminous paint made in this way was soon used to paint instrument and clock dials. This application of radium received a great impetus when World War I began. In order to paint fine lines, the girls who were employed as dial painters pointed their brushes between their lips. Minute amounts of radium and mesothorium were swallowed each time that a brush was pointed. In the early 1920s, several women who had worked as dial painters suffered degeneration of the jawbones and died from anemia. A dentist who was treating one of the dial painters suspected the occupational etiology of the disease. Further investigation revealed more cases of bone damage, including osteogenic sarcoma, and definitely established radium as the etiologic agent. Follow-up studies on radium-dial painters and on patients who had received radium injections therapeutically confirmed this finding. They also showed that radium is tenaciously retained in the bones. Significant deposits of radium were found 25–35 years after exposure. Further experimental work with laboratory animals revealed a number of "bone-seeking" radioisotopes that produced the same type of damage as radium.

Radiostrontium and barium, as well as radium, are chemically similar to calcium and are therefore incorporated into the mineral structure of the bone and into the epiphysis. The bone-seeking rare-earth fission products, such as ^{144}Ce–^{144}Pr, also tend to accumulate in the mineral structure. Plutonium is found to accumulate in the periosteum, endosteum, and trabeculae of the bone. All bone seekers are considered toxic because small amounts can damage the radiosensitive bone cells and hemopoietic tissue in the bone marrow; all the bone seekers produce bone cancer when they are injected into laboratory animals in sufficient quantity.

Lung Cancer

The susceptibility of the lung to radiation-induced carcinoma has been known for a long time. As early as the sixteenth century, it was noted that a large proportion of miners in the Schneeberg and Joachimsthal regions in the Carpathian Mountains died from a lung disease that was called *Bergkrankheit* (miner's disease). About 100 years ago, it was realized that *Bergkrankheit* was lung cancer. However, it was not until 1924 that the radioactive gas radon was thought to be the etiologic agent responsible for the very high death rate from lung cancer. Although these mines were worked for other minerals, mainly cobalt, the ground was particularly rich in uranium and radium. As a consequence of the high radium content of the soil, radon gas, the radioactive daughter of radium, is produced and diffuses out of the ground into the air of the mine shafts, thus leading to a high concentration of radon and radon daughters in the mine air. It is estimated that the concentration of radon in the mine air was on the order of 10 μCi/m^3 (3.7×10^5 Bq/m^3). This estimated concentration may be compared to the 1000 Bq m^{-3} maximum recommended by the International Atomic Energy Agency. Although radon is a gas, its radioactive daughters (Table 4-3) are particulate in nature and attach themselves to dust particles that are suspended in the air. In the dusty atmosphere of mines, radon gas is usually in equilibrium with its daughter RaA (^{218}Po), while the concentrations of the three successive progeny—RaB (^{214}Pb), RaC (^{214}Bi), and RaC' (^{214}Po)—have been found to be present in the mine air at about one-half the equilibrium value. There are high concentrations of radon and its daughters in the uranium mines in the United States, Canada, Australia, and France, in iron mines in Malmberget, Sweden, in tin mines in China, and in fluorspar mines in Newfoundland. In all cases, high radon and radon progeny were found to be associated with an increased incidence of lung cancer, as shown in Table 7-11. The ERR was found to depend on several other factors, such as age at exposure, attained age, exposure rate, and smoking habits, in addition to the total dose. The unweighted mean ERR was found to be 1.19% per WLM, with a range of 0.16–5.06% per WLM. The ICRP estimate the ERR to be 1 ± 0.5% per WLM. The WLM, or working level month, is a measure of exposure to airborne radon and its daughters. Working level (WL) is a measure of the atmospheric concentration

TABLE 7-11. Lung Cancer Among Miners Occupationally Exposed to Radon and Radon Daughters

STUDY	DATES OF FOLLOW-UP	PERSON-YRS AT RISK	MEAN WLM	LUNG CANCER DEATHS	ERR % PER WLM[a]
China	1976–1987	134,842	286.0	936	0.16 (0.1–0.2)
Czech Republic	1952–1990	102,650	196.8	701	0.34 (0.2–0.6)
Colorado	1950–1990	79,556	578.6	334	0.42 (0.3–0.7)
Ontario	1955–1986	300,608	31.0	285	0.89 (0.5–1.5)
Newfoundland	1950–1984	33,795	388.4	112	0.76 (0.4–1.3)
Sweden	1951–1991	32,452	80.6	79	0.95 (0.1–4.1)
New Mexico	1943–1985	46,800	10.9	68	1.72 (0.6–6.7)
Beaverlodge, Canada	1950–1980	67,080	21.2	56	2.21 (0.9–5.6)
Port Radium, Canada	1950–1980	30,454	243.0	39	0.19 (0.1–0.6)
Radium Hill, Australia	1948–1987	24,138	7.6	31	5.06 (1.0–12.2)
France	1948–1986	29,172	59.4	45	0.36 (0.0–1.2)

[a]Numbers in parentheses are 95% confidence intervals. Estimates are adjusted for age (all studies), other mine exposures (China, Colorado, Ontario, New Mexico, and France), an indicator of Rn exposure (Beaverlodge), and ethnicity (New Mexico).

Abbreviations: WLM, working level month; ERR, excess relative risk.

Reprinted with permission from the National Academies Press from BEIR VI: *Health Effects of Exposure to Radon.* Washington, DC: National Academies Press; 1999. Copyright © 1999, National Academy of Sciences.

of radon and its progeny. One WL is defined as *any combination of short-lived radon daughters in 1 L of air that will result in the ultimate emission of 1.3 × 10⁵ MeV of alpha energy.* This corresponds to an atmospheric concentration of 100 pCi of ^{222}Rn per liter (3700 Bq/m^3) in equilibrium with its daughters. One WLM is the exposure resulting from inhalation of air with a 1-WL concentration for a period of 1 working month (170 hours). An exposure of 1 WLM under conditions in a mine results in an alpha dose to the lung of about 1200 mrads (12 mGy) to the critical target cells in the lung.

When estimating the lung-cancer risk from inhaled radon daughters based on data on uranium miners, it should be understood that the uranium miners had been exposed to other noxious agents and potential carcinogens, such as diesel engine exhaust and inhaled mine dust that contained uranium and other minerals, including silica. These other agents, which may have contributed to the increased lung-cancer incidence found among the uranium miners, were accounted for in calculating the ERRs in Table 7-11.

Airborne radioactivity may be inhaled either as gaseous matter, soluble particles, or relatively insoluble particles. Inhaled gas is assumed to be uniformly distributed throughout the lung. The deposition of particles within the lung depends mainly on the particle size of the dust, while the retention in the lung depends on the physical and chemical properties of the dust as well as on the physiological status of the lung. The radionuclide in an inhaled soluble particle may, after dissolving in the lung, be absorbed into the body fluids and translocated to a tissue or organ where it may be deposited. Depending on the chemical form of the inhaled radionuclide, the radionuclide from the dissolved particle may also bind to the protein in the lung. Relatively insoluble particles that are deposited in the upper respiratory tract are rapidly cleared from the lung and swallowed. Those insoluble particles that are deposited in the deep respiratory tract remain there for relatively long periods of time and may subject the pulmonary tissue to a severe local radiation insult due to the very steep gradient of absorbed dose around a radioactive particle. Those cells very close to the radioactive particles would be killed by the high radiation dose, while those cells further away would get a sublethal dose, but a dose large enough to initiate an oncogenic lesion. Numerous laboratory studies showed that this was not the case. Particulate radioactivity in the lungs was found to be no greater hazard than the same amount of radioactivity distributed throughout the lungs. Accordingly, the lung models used for setting radiation safety standards for inhaled radioactivity, including particulate matter, are based on mean doses to the radiosensitive tissues in the respiratory tract.

Lung cancer is also associated with overexposure to external radiation. Among 4111 patients who had received X-ray therapy for ankylosing spondylitis, 88 deaths from lung cancer were observed, while only 59 deaths were expected. A similar increase in lung-cancer incidence was found among a very large population of women who had undergone radiation therapy for cancer of the uterine cervix. An increased incidence of lung cancer was also seen among the Japanese survivors of the nuclear bombings who had been exposed to high doses of radiation. According to the data, a dose of 1 Gy (100 rads) is estimated to increase the likelihood of dying from lung cancer by about 32% for males and about 140% for females (Table 7-9).

Thyroid Cancer

Increased incidence rates of thyroid cancer in children and adolescents following radiation overexposure have been well documented. An increased incidence rate was seen among children who had been therapeutically treated with X-rays for enlarged thymus glands, ringworm of the scalp, and acne. Radiogenic thyroid cancer was also seen among children who had been overexposed to both internal radiation from inhaled radionuclides of iodine and external radiation from the fallout from the BRAVO nuclear bomb test in the Marshall Islands. Thyroid cancer was the first of the solid tumors observed at a higher than expected incidence rate among Japanese survivors of the nuclear bombings. In all these cases, the latency period between exposure and the appearance of the excess thyroid cancers was measured in years.

A relatively large number of children were exposed to radioiodine in the fallout from the nuclear weapons testing program in Nevada. A total of 1378 children who had been exposed to the fallout were followed for 14 years, through 1971. No difference was found between the thyroid cancer incidence rate of the exposed children and that of unexposed controls. However, the data suggested a greater incidence rate of other thyroid abnormalities in the exposed group than in the control groups.

More recently, a sharp rise in the incidence rate of thyroid cancers was reported among young people in the Ukraine following the Chernobyl nuclear power plant disaster in April 1986. In 1986, only 15 confirmed thyroid cancers were reported among Ukrainians who were 18 years of age or less at the time of the reactor accident. In 1989, this figure increased to 36, and it reached 108 during 1992 and 101 in 1993. In this case, there seems to be little doubt that the increased thyroid cancer incidence rate is probably due to the exposure received as a result of the Chernobyl accident.

During the years 1944–1957, about 740,000 Ci (2.7×10^{16} Bq) ^{131}I were released to the atmosphere at the Hanford Laboratories. A study of 3190 persons who had been born during the years 1940–1946 were studied when they reached the ages of 46–57. Most of them still resided in the Hanford region. The thyroid doses were estimated to range from 0.0008 mGy to 2842 mGy (0.08 mrad–284,200 mrads), with a median value of 104 mGy (10,400 mrads). The study was sensitive enough to detect, at the 95% confidence level, a 2.5% per Gy increase in thyroid cancer, and a 5% per Gy increase in benign nodules. However, the study found no relationship between radiation dose and thyroid cancer or any other thyroid abnormality.

Epidemiologic studies on people who had received thyroid doses on the order of 0.5 Gy (50 rads) from diagnostic procedures using radioiodine showed no increased thyroid cancer.

Risk Coefficient Estimates: BEIR VII

Standards that are used for risk management are set on the basis of the magnitude of the risk. Public policy in managing potential risks from technological innovation is often determined more by perceived risk than by the real risk. As used in the common vernacular, "risk" usually implies an immediate threat to life or limb. In the context of health physics, the term "risk" refers to the probability of occurrence of a harmful effect, and a risk coefficient is the numerical value for the probability of occurrence of the harmful effect per unit dose. Not all harmful effects are equally harmful. Those effects that lead to death are clearly more harmful than those that lead to a manageable condition or to a curable illness (such as a cancer that is cured). For this reason, the ICRP, in its Publication No. 60, introduced the concept of *detriment*. The detriment is a coefficient that includes not only the probability of occurrence, per unit dose, of the harmful effect, but also a weighting factor that represents the severity of the effect. For the case of stochastic effects, the ICRP recommended the nominal values listed in Table 7-12.

According to these ICRP risk estimates, the probability that a nuclear worker whose mean dose over a 30-year working career was 300 mrems (3.0 mSv) per year, for a total of 9000 mrems (90 mSv), will die from a radiogenic cancer after the end of his career is

$$5 \times 10^{-4}\, \frac{1}{\text{rem}} \times 9 \times 10^3 \text{ mrems} \times \frac{1 \text{ rem}}{10^3 \text{ mrems}} = 45 \times 10^{-4},$$

or 45 chances out of 10,000. This means that he increased his "normal" chance of dying from cancer from about 24% by 0.45 percentage points.

In the case of risks from low-level exposure to ionizing radiation, the stochastic nature of the adverse effects of exposure, together with their extremely low probability of occurrence, implies that the magnitude of the risk and the calculation of the

TABLE 7-12. Nominal Probability Coefficients for Stochastic Effects

EXPOSED POPULATION	DETRIMENT ($\times 10^{-2}\text{Sv}^{-1}$)			
	Fatal Cancer	Nonfatal Cancer	Severe Hereditary Effects	Total
Adult workers	4.0	0.8	0.8	5.6
Entire population	5.0	1.0	1.3	7.3

associated risk coefficients can be determined only by epidemiological studies, that is, findings from observations of very large population groups that had been exposed to the study agent in comparison to similar studies on a population group that had not been exposed. The ICRP recommendations are based mainly on studies made on the survivors of the atomic bombings in Japan. The U.S. National Academy of Sciences Committee in the Biological Effects of Ionizing Radiation (BEIR committee) reported on the health effects of low-level ionizing radiation. The Committee reviewed the latest findings from the survivors of the Japanese bombings as well as studies on radiation workers, persons who had been treated medically with radiation, populations living in high-background areas, and relevant laboratory studies, and presented its conclusions in what is known as the BEIR VII Report, *Health Risks From Exposure to Low Levels of Ionizing Radiation* (2005).

In the BEIR VII report, which deals with somatic effects—mainly cancer—and genetic effects of low-level radiation exposure, the committee members agreed on the dose–response relationship at doses on the order of 0.1 Gy (10 rads) or more delivered at high dose rates. They also found that health effects from low doses would be difficult to evaluate because the "noise" from other factors would impose statistical limitations that would make it difficult to separate radiogenic effects from spontaneous effects. Therefore, estimates of risk coefficients must be made from interpolations, based on a suitable dose–response model, between zero dose and the lowest dose at which the effect has been seen.

The functional form of a generalized dose–response curve (Fig. 7-16) is

$$F(D) = (\alpha_0 + \alpha_1 D + \alpha_2 D^2) e^{(-\beta_1 D - \beta_2 D^2)}, \tag{7.10}$$

where $F(D)$ is the incidence rate of the effect under consideration (e.g., cancer) at dose D; α_0, α_1, α_2, β_1, and β_2 have positive values; and α_0 is the "spontaneous" or "natural" incidence rate of the effect. β_1 and β_2 are significant only at high doses. Depending on which of these coefficients becomes insignificant, the generalized curve reduces to the three simple curves shown in Figure 7-16—namely the linear, the pure quadratic, and the linear–quadratic curves.

Cancer Risk Estimates

In estimating the risk of radiogenic cancers, the committee found that the data supported a dose-related increase in the relative risk of a radiogenic cancer. Despite this relationship, the available empirical data did not allow the committee to choose decisively among the several dose–response models shown in Figure 7-16. However, the BEIR VII committee found that for all cancers except leukemia and also for the genetic effects observed in laboratory studies, the data were not incompatible with the LNT model. The committee concluded that "the current scientific evidence is consistent with the hypothesis that there is a linear, no-threshold dose–response relationship between exposure to ionizing radiation and the development of cancer in humans." (Note that this conclusion does not agree with that in the French Joint Report, which was discussed earlier in this chapter.) The LNT model, therefore, was chosen as the basis for estimating the risk coefficients for solid tumors from low-dose radiation. The linear–quadratic model was chosen for estimating risk coefficients for leukemia. Using these models, together with modifying factors to account for age and sex (these modifying factors are described in the BEIR VII report), the committee

TABLE 7-13. BEIR VII Committee's Estimates of Lifetime Excess Cancer (Solid Cancers and Leukemia) Mortality per 100,000 Exposed Persons of Same Age and Sex distribution as the U.S. Population

DOSE SCENARIO	EXCESS CANCER MORTALITY	
	Number	**Percent**
0.1 Gy (10 rads) acute dose	572	2.8
1 mGy/yr (100 mrads/yr) continuous exposure	416	2.0
10 mGy/yr (1 rad/yr) continuous exposure over working lifetime, 18–65 yrs of age	2048	10.0

Adapted from BEIR VII: *Health Risks from Exposure to Low Levels of Ionizing Radiation.* Washington, DC: National Academies Press; 2005.

estimated the number of increased cancer deaths in a population of 100,000 whose age and sex distribution is representative of the U.S. population, if everyone were to receive a radiation dose of 0.1 Gy (10 rads) (Table 7-13).

There is a good deal of uncertainty in the estimation of risk coefficients for low-level irradiation. One source of these uncertainties is the statistical uncertainty in the collection of data and the estimation of modeling parameters. Statistical uncertainty is quantified by the mathematical statement of the confidence interval and accordingly is easily dealt with. The second major source of uncertainty is based on our limited knowledge of carcinogenic mechanisms and therefore of which of the postulated dose–response models most accurately represents the actual dose–response situation. In regard to this second source of uncertainty and effects at very low doses, the BEIR V committee said the following:

> "Derivation of risk estimates for low doses and low dose rates through the use of any type of risk model involves assumptions that remain to be validated . . . . Epidemiological data cannot rigorously exclude the existence of a threshold in the millisievert (hundreds of millirems) dose range. Thus, the possibility that there may be no risks from exposures comparable to the external natural background radiation cannot be ruled out . . . . The lower limit of the range of uncertainty in the risk estimates extends to zero."

With these caveats in mind, the BEIR VII committee calculated the excess cancer mortality for three different scenarios: a single exposure to 10 rems (0.1 Sv), continuous exposure to 100 mrems/yr (1 mSv/yr), and continuous occupational exposure to 1 rem/yr (10 mSv/yr) over a working lifetime from 18 to 65 years of age. The results of these calculations are given in Table 7-13.

We can estimate the crude cancer risk per centisievert (rem) from the cancer mortality data on the life span study cohort of nuclear bomb survivors (Table 7-14). The doses to the members of the cohort are reasonably well-known, and their collective dose is 1.11×10^6 person-cSv (person-rems). The crude cancer risk per centisievert (rem) can be calculated from these data.

For low and for protracted doses, the committee applied a dose and dose–rate effectiveness factor of 1.5. Therefore, the crude (without consideration of age at exposure and sex) cancer risk coefficient is estimated:

$$\frac{491 \text{ fatal cancers}}{1.1 \times 10^6 \text{ person-cSv} \times 1.5} = 3 \times 10^{-4} \text{ fatal cancer per cSv.}$$

TABLE 7-14. Mortality Experience of Life-Span Study Cohort of Nuclear Bombing Survivors

STUDY GROUP	NUMBER	NUMBER OF DEATHS	RATE (%)
Cancer deaths			
Exposed population	49,114	5502	11.2
Control population	37,458	3833	10.2
Excess deaths	$(0.112 - 0.102) \times 49,114 = 491$		
Noncancer deaths			
Exposed population		18,049	36.8
Control population		13,832	36.9

Adapted from BEIR VII: *Health Risks from Exposure to Low Levels of Ionizing Radiation.* Washington, DC: National Academies Press; 2005.

Genetic Risk Estimates

Estimates of genetic-risk coefficients were based entirely on the results of animal studies, since no radiation-induced genetic effects in humans have ever been observed. Risk coefficients are estimated by the *doubling dose method.* Radiation-induced mutation rates observed in animal experiments are compared with spontaneous rates of genetic disorders in people, and the dose needed to double that spontaneous rate is calculated from the experimental data. The BEIR VII committee estimate of the doubling dose is 0.82 ± 0.29 Gy (82 ± 29 rads), and recommends that we use 1 Gy (100 rads), which corresponds to risk of 0.41–0.64 per million progeny per Gy (0.41×10^{-8}–0.64×10^{-8} rad^{-1}) in the first generation. The new equilibrium, at double the present mutation rate, is attained only after many generations, perhaps as many as 10 generations, who have had the gonads of the breeding population irradiated with the doubling dose. Presently, the incidence rate (spontaneous and from causes other than the additional radiation) of human genetic disorders is approximately 88,000 per million live births.

Quality Factor and Radiation Weighting Factor

Not only have neutrons been found more effective than X-rays in producing cataracts, but alpha radiation too has been found to be more toxic per unit absorbed dose than beta or gamma radiation. In comparing the relative toxicity or damage-producing potential of a given absorbed dose of various radiations, it has been found that the higher the rate of LET of the radiation, the more effective it is in producing biological damage. The ratio of the amount of energy from 200-keV X-rays required to produce a given biological effect to the amount of energy from any other radiation to produce the same effect is called the *relative biological effectiveness* (RBE) of that radiation. The RBE of any specific radiation depends on the exact biological effect on a given species of organism under a specific set of experimental conditions. For example, the RBE for 14-MeV neutrons for killing American cockroach embryos is 16, since the lethal dose from the neutrons is only one-sixteenth that from X-rays. For lethality in rats, on the other hand, the RBE of fast neutrons is only about 2. The term "RBE" is thus restricted in application to radiobiology.

For health physics purposes, a conservative upper limit of the RBE for the biological effect of greatest interest to humans due to a radiation other than the reference X-rays is used as a normalizing factor in adding doses from different radiations. This

TABLE 7-15. Quality (Q) and Radiation Weighting Factors (w_R) for Various Radiations

RADIATION	Q	w_R
X, gamma, beta—all energies	1	1
Neutrons		
Thermal	2	5
0.01 MeV	2.5	10
0.1 MeV	7.5	10
0.5 MeV	11	20
>0.1–2 MeV		20
>2–20 MeV		10
>20 MeV		5
Unknown energy	10	
High-energy protons	10	5
Alpha particles, fission fragments, heavy nuclei	20	20

Q: Adapted from NRC Regulations (10 CFR Part 20).
w_R: Adapted with permission from ICRP Publication 92. *Ann ICRP.* 2003;33(4):1–121. Copyright © 2003 International Commission on Radiological Protection.

normalizing factor is called the *quality factor* and is symbolized by the letter Q by the U.S. Nuclear Regulatory Commission (NRC). The ICRP renamed the quality factor the *radiation weighting factor*, symbolized by w_R. Values assigned to Q by the NRC and to w_R by the ICRP are given in Table 7-15.

RADIATION-WEIGHTED DOSE UNITS: THE SIEVERT AND THE REM

Radiation-weighted dose units are used for radiation safety purposes, radiological-engineering design criteria, and regulatory and administrative purposes. The ICRP calls its unit of radiation-weighted dose the *equivalent dose*, symbolized by the letter H, and has named it the *Sievert* (Sv). All its recommendations for dose limits are in units of sieverts. The equivalent dose H_T, Sv, in tissue or organ T, is defined by the ICRP as

$$H_T = \sum_R w_R \times D_{T,R}, \qquad (7.11)$$

where $D_{T,R}$ is the absorbed dose, expressed as grays, averaged over the tissue or organ T, due to radiation R. If the organ or tissue is irradiated by only one type of radiation, then Eq. (7.11) reduces to

$$H_T = w_R \times D_T. \qquad (7.12)$$

According to Eq. (7.12) and the values for w_R in Table 7-13, an absorbed dose of 1 mGy of X-, beta, or gamma radiation corresponds to an equivalent dose of 1 mSv, while an absorbed dose of 1 mGy of 5 MeV neutrons gives an equivalent dose of 10 mSv. Dose limits—the maximum allowable radiation dose—are expressed in the

SI system as sieverts or millisieverts. The use of the equivalent dose in routine health physics practice is illustrated in the example below:

EXAMPLE 7.2

The dose rates outside the shielding of a cyclotron are found to be 5 μGy/h (0.5 mrad/h) for gammas, 2 μGy/h (0.2 mrad/h) for thermal neutrons, and 1 μGy/h (0.1 mrad/h) for fast neutrons with energies greater than 2 MeV. What is the equivalent dose rate of the combined radiations according to the ICRP values for w_R?

Solution

If we multiply the absorbed dose rate by the appropriate radiation weighting factor, as shown in the table below, and sum the products, we find the equivalent dose rate to be 25 μSv/h.

	$D \times w_R = H$
Gamma rays	5 μGy/h $\times$ 1 = 5 μSv/h
Thermal neutrons	2 μGy/h $\times$ 5 = 10 μSv/h
Fast neutrons	1 μGy/h $\times$ 10 = 10 μSv/h
	Equivalent dose rate, $H = 25 \mu$Sv/h

The U.S. NRC, whose regulations are written in the traditional radiation units, refers to the radiation-weighted unit as the *dose equivalent*, also symbolized by the letter H, and calls it by its traditional name, the *rem*. In traditional units, where the dose is expressed in rads, the dose equivalent H_T to a tissue or organ T, that receives a dose of D_T rads from a radiation whose quality factor is Q_R is defined as

$$H_T(\text{rems}) = D_T(\text{rads}) \times Q_R. \tag{7.13}$$

To avoid unnecessary words when the context is used is clear, we frequently use the generic term *dose* when we refer to the radiation-weighted dose.

SUMMARY

Although it is widely believed by the lay public that relatively little is known about the biological effects of radiation, we probably know more about radiation bio-effects than the effects of most other noxious agents in our environment. Sources of information include studies of large populations who were exposed either occupationally or medically, atomic bomb victims and survivors, persons who were exposed as a result of accidents, and populations who were exposed to natural radiation as a result of living in regions of high background radiation.

Generally, radiation bioeffects fall into one of two categories: deterministic effects and stochastic effects. Deterministic effects result from exposure to very large doses of radiation. These effects have a threshold dose and their severity increases with increasing dose. Examples are the acute radiation syndromes that have a threshold in the range of 1–2 Gy (100–200 rads) whole-body X- or gamma radiation, skin burns in the range of 2–3 Gy (200–300 rads), and skin ulceration in the range of 20 Gy (2000 rads). The $LD_{50/60\text{-day}}$ dose for whole-body X- or gamma radiation is believed to lie in the range of 3–4 Gy (300–400 rads). Deterministic effects are clearly and unequivocally causally associated with the radiation exposure.

Stochastic effects occur by chance and are seen in unexposed individuals as well as in exposed individuals and therefore are not unequivocally associated with a radiation exposure. Stochastic effects include cancer and genetic mutations. Exposure to radiation increases the probability of a stochastic effect, and this probability increases with increasing dose. Whereas increased incidence of cancer has been documented among certain heavily exposed populations—such as the early radiologists, atomic bomb survivors, and patients who had received radiotherapy—no increased incidence of heritable changes has ever been observed among any human population exposed at any dose.

The stochastic effects, either in humans or in animals, that have been observed are no different in kind from those observed in unirradiated populations. The difference lies only in the frequency of occurrence. Thus, it is impossible for even the most highly skilled pathologist to definitely attribute any cancer in an exposed individual to the exposure. The only thing that can be done is to estimate the probability—based on the patient's exposure history—that the cancer can be attributed to the radiation exposure. Of the several possible models that have been postulated to infer the stochastic effects of low doses from high-dose cases, the zero-threshold, linear dose–response relationship, because it is believed to be the most conservative of all the proposed models, was chosen as the basis for setting radiation safety standards.

This brief overview shows that we know enough about the biomedical effects of radiation to enable us to set radiation safety standards with a very high level of confidence that adherence to these safety standards will allow the safe use of radiation and its sources.

SUGGESTED READINGS

Annals of the ICRP. Pergamon, Elsevier Science, Oxford, U.K.
  No. 26. *Recommendations of the International Commission on Radiological Protection*, **1:**(3), 1977.
  No. 31. *Biological Effects of Inhaled Radionuclides*, **4:**(1/2), 1979.
  No. 41. *Nonstochastic Effects of Ionizing Radiation*, **14:**(3), 1984.
  No. 42. *A Compilation of the Major Concepts and Quantities in Use by the ICRP*, **14:**(4), 1984.
  No. 48. *The Metabolism of Plutonium and Related Elements*, **16:**(2/3), 1986.
  No. 49. *Developmental Effects of Irradiation on the Brain of the Embryo and Fetus*, **16:**(4), 1986.
  No. 50. *Lung Cancer Risk from Indoor Exposures to Radon Daughters*, **17:**(1), 1986.
  No. 59. *The Biological Basis for Dose Limitation in the Skin*, **20:**(4), 1992.
  No. 60. *1990 Recommendations of the International Commission on Radiological Protection*, **21:**(1–3), 1991.
  No. 66. *Human Respiratory Tract Model for Radiological Protection*, **24:**(1–3), 1994.
  No. 68. *Dose Coefficients for Intakes of Radionuclides by Workers*, **24:**(4), 1994.
  No. 70. *Basic Anatomical and Physiological Data for use in Radiological Protection: The Skeleton*, **25:**(2), 1996.
  No. 79. *Genetic Susceptibility to Cancer*, **28:**(1/2), 1998.

No. 84. *Pregnancy and Medical Radiation*, **30:**(1), 2000.

No. 89. *Basic Anatomical and Physiological Data for Use in Radiological Protection Reference Values*, **32:**(3–4), 2002.

No. 90. *Biological Effects after Prenatal Irradiation (Embryo and Fetus)*, **33:**(1–2), 2003.

No. 92. *Relative Biological Effectiveness (RBE), Quality Factor (Q), and Radiation Weighting Factor (w_R)*, **33:**(4), 2003.

No. 100. *Human Alimentary Tract Model for Radiological Protection*, **26:**(4), 2006.

Supporting Guidance 3. *Guide for the Practical Application of the ICRP Human Respiratory Tract Model*, **32:**(1–2), 2002.

Supporting Guidance 5. *Analysis of the Criteria Used by the International Commission on Radiological Protection to Justify the Setting of Numerical Protection Level Values*, **36:**(4), 2006.

Ansari, A. Dirty bomb pills, shots, weeds, and spells. *Health Physics News*, **31:**1–17, November, 2004.

Bacq, Z. M., and Alexander, P. *Fundamentals of Radiobiology*. Pergamon Press, Oxford, U.K., 1967.

Baverstock, K. F., and Stather, J. W., eds. *Low Dose Radiation: Biological Bases of Risk Assessment*. Taylor and Francis, Bristol, PA, 1989.

Beir III. *The Effects on Populations of Exposure to Low Levels of Ionizing Radiation*. Report of the advisory committee on the biological effects of ionizing radiation. National Academy Press, Washington, DC, 1980.

Beir IV. *Health Risks of Radon and Other Internally Deposited Alpha Emitters*. Report of the advisory committee on the biological effects of ionizing radiations. National Academy Press, Washington, DC, 1988.

Beir V. *Health Effects of Exposure to Low Levels of Ionizing Radiation*. Report of the advisory committee on the biological effects of ionizing radiations. National Academy Press, Washington, DC, 1990.

Beir VII. *Health Risks From Exposure to Low Levels of Ionizing Radiation*. Report of the advisory committee on the biological effects of ionizing radiations. National Academies Press, Washington, DC, 2005.

Bergonié, J., and Tribondeau, L. De quelques resultats de la radiotherapie et assai de fixation d'une technique rationale. *Compt Rend Acad Sci*, **143:**983, 1906. English translation in *Radiat Res*, **11:**32, 1960.

Billen, D. Spontaneous DNA damage and its significance for the "negligible dose" controversy in radiation protection. *Radiat Res*, **124:**242–245, 1990.

Bolch, W. E. Physical and chemical interactions of radiation with living tissues, in Raabe, O., ed. *Internal Radiation Dosimetry*. Medical Physics Publishing, Madison, WI, 1994.

Bolch, W. E. The anatomical and physiological basis for internal dosimetry, in Bolch, W. E., ed. *Practical Applications of Internal Dosimetry*. Medical Physics Publishing Madison, WI, 2002.

Bond, V. D., Fliedner, T. M., and Archambeau, J. O. *Mammalian Radiation Lethality*. Academic Press, New York, 1965.

Brent, R., Meistrich M., and Paul, M. Ionizing and nonionizing radiations, in Paul M., ed. *Occupational and Environmental Reproductive Hazards: A Guide for Clinicians*. Williams and Wilkins, Baltimore, MD, 1993.

Brodsky, A. *Radiation Risks & Uranium Toxicity*. RSA Publications, Hebron, CT, 1996.

Carnes, B. A., Gavrilova, N., and Grahn, D. Pathology effects at radiation doses below those causing mortality. *Radiat Res*, **158:**187, 2002.

Charles, M. W. Skin, eye, and testis: Current exposure problems and recent advances in radiobiology. *J Soc Radiol Prot*, **6:**69–81, 1986.

Cronkite, E. P., Bond, V. P., and Dunham, C. L. *Some Effects of Ionizing Radiation on Human Beings*. U.S. Atomic Energy Commission, TID 5358, U.S. Govt. Printing Office, Washington, DC, 1956.

Eckerman, K. F., Leggett, R. W., Nelson, C. B., Puskin, J. S., and Richardson, A. C. B. *Cancer Risk Coefficients for Environmental Exposure to Radionuclides*. Federal Guidance Report No. 13. (EPA 402-R-99-001), 1999.

EPA. *Radionuclide Carcinogenicity Slope Factors* http://epa.gov/radiation/heast/index.html, 2002.

EPA. *Radiation Risk Assessment—Workshop Proceedings*. U.S. Environmental Protection Agency, Washington, DC, 2001.

Fabrikant, J. I. *Radiobiology*. Medical Publishers, Chicago, IL, 1972.

Fiorino, D. J. Technical and democratic values in risk analysis. *Risk Anal*, **9:**293–299, 1989.

Grosch, D. S., and Hopwood, L. E. *Biological Effects of Radiations*. Academic Press, New York, 1979.

Guilmette, R. A. Biokinetics of inhaled, ingested, and percutaneously deposited radionuclides, in *Practical Applications of Internal Dosimetry*. Medical Physics Publishing, Madison, WI, 2002.

Hall, E. J. *Radiation and Life*. Pergamon Press, Oxford, U.K., 1984.

Hall, E. J. *Radiobiology for the Radiologist*, 4th ed. Lippincott, Philadelphia, PA, 1994.

Hendee, W. R. *Health Effects of Low Level Radiation*, Institute of Physics, London, England, 1996.

Hobbie, R. K. *Intermediate Physics for Medicine and Biology*, 4th ed. Wiley and Sons, New York, 2001.

Holaday, D. A., Rushing, D. E., Coleman, R. D., et al. *Control of Radon and Daughters in Uranium Mines and Calculations on Biologic Effects*. Public Health Service Publication 494, Washington, DC, 1957.

International Atomic Energy Agency (IAEA), Vienna.
 The Radiological Accident in San Salvador. IAEA, 1990.
 The Radiological Accident in Soreq, 1993.
 The Radiological Accident in Goiania, 1988.
 The International Chernobyl Project, Technical Report, 1991.

International Commission on Radiation Units and Measurements (ICRU), Bethesda, MD.
 The Quality Factor in Radiation Protection. Report 40, 1986.
 Quantities and Units in Radiation Protection Dosimetry. Report 51, 1993.

International Commission on Radiological Protection (ICRP). Publication No. 23. *Reference Man: Anatomical, Physiological, and Metabolic Characteristics*. Pergamon Press, Oxford, U.K., 1975.

James, A. Dosimetric applications of the new ICRP lung model, in Raabe, O. G., ed. *Internal Radiation Dosimetry*. Medical Physics Publishing, Madison, WI, 1994.

Jones, R. R., and Southwood, R., eds. *Radiation and Health: The Biological Effects of Low-Level Exposure to Ionizing Radiation*. Wiley, Chichester, U.K., 1987.

Karam, P. A., Leslie, S. A., and Anbar, A. The effects of changing atmospheric oxygen concentrations and background radiation levels on radiogenic DNA damage rates. *Health Phys*, **81:**545–553, 2001.

Kleinbaum, D. G., Kupper, L. L., and Morgenstern, H. *Epidemiologic Research*. Van Nostrand Reinhold, New York, 1982.

Kopecky, K. J., Davis, S., Hamilton, T. E., Saporito, M. S., and Onstad, L. Estimation of thyroid radiation doses for the Hanford thyroid disease study: Results and implications for the statistical power of the epidemiological analyses. *Health Phys*, **87:**15–32, 2004.

Lea, D. *Actions of Radiations on Living Cells*. Cambridge University Press, Cambridge, U.K., 1955.

Little, J. B. Nontargeted effects of radiation: Implications for low dose exposures. *Health Phys*, **91:**416–426, 2006.

Lorentz, E. Radioactivity and lung cancer: A critical review of lung cancer in the miners of Schneeberg and Joachimsthal. *J Natl Cancer Inst*, **5:**1, 1944.

McLean, F. C., and Budy, A. M. *Radiation, Isotopes, and Bone*. Academic Press, New York, 1964.

Mettler, F. A. Jr., Kelsey, C. A., and Ricks, R. C., eds. *Medical Management of Radiation Accidents*. CRC Press, Boca Raton, FL, 1990.

Mills, W.A. Estimates of human cancer risks associated with internally deposited radionuclides, in Raabe, O.G., ed. *Internal Radiation Dosimetry*. Medical Physics Publishing, Madison, WI, 1994.

Mokrov, Y., Glagolenko, Y., and Napier, B. Reconstruction of radionuclide contamination of the Techa River caused by liquid waste discharge from radiochemical production at the Mayak Production Association. *Health Phys*, **79:**15–23, 2000.

Mossman, K. L., and Mills, W. A., eds. *The Biological Basis of Radiation Protection Practice*. Williams & Wilkins, Baltimore, MD, 1992.

National Council on Radiation protection and Measurements (NCRP), Bethesda, MD.
 No. 44. *Krypton-85 in the Atmosphere—Accumulation, Biological Significance, and Control Technology*, 1975.
 No. 46. *Alpha Emitting Particles in the Lungs*, 1975.
 No. 60. *Physical, Chemical, and Biological Properties of Radiocerium Relevant to Radiation Protection Guidelines*, 1978.
 No. 64. *Influence of Dose and Its Distribution in Time on Dose–Response Relationships for Low-LET Radiations*, 1980.
 No. 65. *Management of Persons Accidentally Contaminated with Radionuclides*, 1980.
 No. 80. *Induction of Thyroid Cancer by Ionizing Radiation*, 1985.
 No. 89. *Genetic Effects from Internally Deposited Radionuclides*, 1987.
 No. 96. *Comparative Carcinogenicity of Ionizing Radiation and Chemicals*, 1989.
 No. 104. *The Relative Biological Effectiveness of Radiations of Different Quality*, 1990.
 No. 109. *Effects of Ionizing Radiations on Aquatic Organisms*, 1991.
 No. 110. *Some Aspects of Strontium Radiobiology*, 1991.
 No. 115. *Risk Estimates for Radiation Protection*, 1993.
 No. 121. *Principles and Application of Collective Dose in Radiation Protection*, 1995.
 No. 126. *Uncertainties in Fatal Cancer Risk Estimates Used in Radiation Protection*, 1997.

No. 128. *Radionuclide Exposure of the Embryo/Fetus,* 1998.

No. 130. *Biological Effects and Exposure Limits for "Hot Particles,"* 1999.

No. 135. *Liver Cancer Risk from Internally-Deposited Radionuclides,* 2001.

No. 136. *Evaluation of the Linear, Non-Threshold Dose–Response Model for Ionizing Radiation,* 2001.

Oecd/Nea. *CHERNOBYL, Ten Years On, Radiological and Health Impact.* Organization for Economic Co-Operation and Development, Paris, 1996.

Ottoboni, M. A. *The Dose Makes the Poison,* Vincente Books, Berkeley, CA, 1984.

Pizzarello, D. J., and Witcofski, R. I. *Basic Radiation Biology.* Lea & Febiger, Philadelphia, PA, 1975.

Preston, R. J. Radiation biology: Concepts for radiation protection. *Health Phys,* **87**:3–14, 2004.

Raabe, O. G. Deposition and clearance of inhaled aerosols, in Witschi, H. R. and Nettesheim, P., eds. *Mechanisms in Respiratory Toxicology.* CRC Press, West Palm Beach, FL, 1982.

Raabe, O. G. Characterizations of radioactive airborne particles, in Raabe, O. G., ed. *Internal Radiation Dosimetry.* Medical Physics Publishing, Madison, WI, 1994.

Ron, E. Ionizing radiation and cancer risk: Evidence from epidemiology. *Radiat Res,* **150** (Suppl 5), S30–S41, 1998.

Sanger, E. L., ed. *Medical Aspects of Radiation Accidents.* U.S. Atomic Energy Commission, Government Printing Office, Washington, DC, 1980.

Seligman, P. The U.S.–Russian radiation health effects research program in the Southern Urals. *Health Phys,* **79**:3–8, 2000.

Semkow, T. M., and Parekh, P. P. Principles of gross alpha and beta radioactivity detection in water. *Health Phys,* **81**:567–574, 2001.

Simon, S. L., Bouville, A., and Land, C. Fallout from nuclear weapons tests and cancer risks. *Am Sci,* **94**:48, 2006.

Snipes, M. B. Biokinetics of inhaled radionuclides, in Raabe, O. G., ed. *Internal Radiation Dosimetry.* Medical Physics Publishing Co., Madison, WI, 1994.

Steinhauser, F. Epidemiological evidence of radon-induced health risks, in Nazaroff, W. W., and Nero A. V., Jr., eds. *Radon and Its Decay Products in Indoor Air.* John Wiley & Sons, New York, 1988.

Trabalka, J. R., and Kocher, D. C. Energy dependence of dose and dose rate effectiveness factor for low-let radiations: Potential importance to estimation of cancer risks and relationship to biological effectiveness. *Health Phys,* **93**:17–27, 2007.

Tubiana, M. The report of the French Academy of Science: Problems associated with the effects of low doses of ionizing radiation. *J Radiol Prot,* **18**:243–248, 1998.

Tannock, I. F., and Hill, R. P., ed. *The Basic Science of Oncology.* Pergamon Press, Oxford, U.K., 1987.

Toohey, R. E. Biokinetics of bone-seeking radionuclides, in Raabe O. G., ed. *Internal Radiation Dosimetry.* Medical Physics Publishing Co., Madison, WI, 1994.

Toppenberg, K. S., Hill, D. A., and Miller, D. P. Safety of radiographic imaging during pregnancy. *Am Fam Physician,* **59**(7):1813–1820, 1999.

United Nations Scientific Committee on the Effects of atomic radiation (UNSCEAR), United Nations, New York.

Sources and Effects of Ionizing Radiation, A Report to the General Assembly, 2000.

Hereditary Effects of Radiation, 2001.

Upton, A. C. State of the art in the 1990s: NCRP Report 136 on the scientific basis for linearity in the dose–response relationship for ionizing radiation. *Health Phys,* **85**:15, 2003.

Vargo, G. J., ed. *The Chernobyl Accident: A Comprehensive Risk Assessment.* Battelle Press, Columbus, OH, 2000.

Von Sontag, C. *The Chemical Basis of Radiation Biology.* Taylor and Francis, Philadelphia, PA, 1987.

Wakeford, R., Antell, B. A., and Leigh, W. L. A review of causation and its use in a compensation scheme for nuclear industry workers in the United Kingdom. *Health Phys,* **74**(1):1, 1998.

8

RADIATION SAFETY GUIDES

Radiation safety standards and regulations undergo continuous review and changes. These changes occur mainly as a response to a public policy based on attitudes of the public and on the philosophy of preventive conservatism, and also because of the increasing sensitivity of radiation-measuring instruments. The continual restriction of acceptable dose limits implies that earlier limits were unsafe. However, there has been no verifiable increase in radiogenic diseases among radiation workers whose radiation doses were within the limits recommended by scientific advisory committees (the International Commission on Radiological Protection [ICRP] and the National Council on Radiation Protection and Measurements [NCRP]) in 1934 and the limits established by governmental regulatory agencies after 1945.

ORGANIZATIONS THAT SET STANDARDS

The hazards of ionizing radiation became apparent almost immediately. Wilhelm Roentgen discovered X-rays in November 1895, and he announced his discovery on January 1, 1896, in a paper that he had prepared for presentation to the Physical-Medical Society of Würzburg. At about the same time, Emile Grubbe, an American physicist who was experimenting with a Crooke's tube (a cathode-ray tube) similar to the one used by Roentgen, suffered severe burns on his hands as a result of holding the energized tube in his hands. Then, in May of that same year, a man who had a diagnostic radiograph made of his head suffered skin burns and loss of hair on the side of his face that had been exposed to the X-rays. Henri Becquerel, who discovered radioactivity in 1896, developed an ulcer on the skin of his chest as a result of having kept a test tube containing a radium salt in his vest pocket. After surgical treatment, the wound healed, but it left a painful scar. The year 1899 marked the first successful use of X-rays to cure a cancer, a basal-cell carcinoma on the face of a woman. Thus, from the very beginning of the use of radiation sources for beneficial purposes, harmful effects were observed.

337

As the usefulness of radiation in medicine and science was being discovered, reports of harmful radiation effects continued, causing various practitioners to suggest a variety of radiation safety rules. The first organized action in radiation safety was taken in 1915 by the British Roentgen Society. The X-ray and Radium Protection Committee of the British Roentgen Society published further recommendations in 1921 and in 1927.

International Commission on Radiological Protection

In 1925, the radiological societies of several countries met in London at the First International Congress of Radiology. Among the main topics discussed at the meeting were radiation protection and the need for a committee to deal with questions of radiation safety. Then, in 1928, at the Second International Congress of Radiology, a committee called the International X-ray and Radium Protection Committee was established to provide guidance in these matters. At that time and for many years afterward, its main concern was regarding the safety aspects of medical radiology. Its interests in radiation protection expanded with the widespread use of radiation outside the sphere of medicine, and, in 1950, its name was changed to the International Commission on Radiological Protection (ICRP) in order to describe its area of concern more accurately. Since its inception, the ICRP has been recognized as the leading agency for providing guidance in all matters of radiation safety. In describing its operating philosophy, the ICRP states: "*The policy adopted by the Commission in preparing recommendations is to deal with the basic principles of radiation protection, and to leave to the various national protection committees the responsibility of introducing detailed technical regulations, recommendations, or codes of practice best suited to the needs of their individual countries*" (ICRP Publication 6, p. 1, Pergamon Press, Oxford, U.K., 1964). In discussing the development of its recommendations, the ICRP says: "*Since there is little direct evidence of harm at levels of annual dose at or below the limits recommended by the Commission, a good deal of scientific judgment is required in predicting the probability of harm resulting from low doses. Most of the observed data have been obtained at higher doses and usually at high dose rates.*" The ICRP goes on to say: "*The estimation of these consequences and their implications necessarily involves social and economic judgments as well as scientific judgments in a wide range of disciplines*" (ICRP Publication 60, pp. 1 and 2, Pergamon Press, Oxford, U.K., 1991). The ICRP's published reports and recommendations are listed in the Suggested Readings, at the end of this chapter.

Initially, the recommendations of the ICRP were based on the *tolerance dose*. The tolerance dose was believed to be a dose that the body can tolerate, and thus adherence to this dose limit would prevent observable harmful radiation effects. To this end, the dose to tissue deeper than 1 cm (the *deep dose*) and the skin dose to skin at a depth of 0.007 cm (the *shallow dose*) of 300 and 600 mrems per week, respectively, were recommended. When genetic damage was assumed to be the effect to be prevented, a deep-dose equivalent of 5 rems/yr was recommended in ICRP Publication 2 in 1959. By 1977, continued observation of radiation effects on the survivors of the atomic bombings in Japan, including the absence of any observable genetic effects, led the ICRP to update its radiation safety recommendations. Its new recommendations, which were published in ICRP Publication 26, are based on an *acceptable-risk* concept. This new basis for radiation safety standards recognized cancer as the main biological effect of concern. The biomathematical model for radiation carcinogenesis postulates that a single radiation-induced change in a DNA molecule can initiate an oncogenic process. According to this model, there is no dose below which cancer cannot occur. This means that every increment of radiation dose carries a proportional increase in risk of radiogenic cancer. Accordingly, radiation safety standards were recommended on the basis of a risk that would be accepted by society in exchange for the benefits resulting from radiation use at the recommended limit.

ICRP 26 also recognized that different organs and tissues have different likelihoods of developing radiogenic cancer. This fact led to the introduction of the concept of effective dose, which considers the risk of stochastic effects from nonuniform irradiation relative to the risk from uniform whole-body radiation. As a consequence, ICRP Publication 26 recommended a maximum effective dose equivalent (EDE) of 50 mSv (5000 mrems) in 1 year and also said that this limit should include the sum of external radiation dose and the dose from internally deposited radionuclides. By 1990, the continuing studies of the Japanese survivors of the atomic bombings suggested that the probability of fatal radiogenic cancer might have been underestimated by a factor perhaps as great as four in the earlier recommendations. Accordingly, in ICRP Publication 60, which was issued in 1990, the commission recommended a limit on EDE for occupational exposure of 20 mSv (2000 mrems) averaged over a 5-year period (100 mSv, or 10,000 mrems in 5 years), with a limit of 50 mSv (5000 mrems) in any single year.

International Atomic Energy Agency

The International Atomic Energy Agency (IAEA), a specialized agency of the United Nations that was organized in 1956 in order to promote the peaceful uses of nuclear energy, recommends basic safety standards that are based, to the extent practically possible, on the ICRP recommendations.

> "Under its Statute the International Atomic Energy Agency is empowered to provide for the application of standards of safety for protection against radiation to its own operations and to operations making use of assistance provided by it or with which it is otherwise directly associated. To this end authorities receiving such assistance are required to observe relevant health and safety measures prescribed by the Agency."

(From *Safe Handling of Radioisotopes.* Safety Series No. 1. IAEA, Vienna, 1962.)

The health and safety measures prescribed by IAEA are published according to subject in its *Safety Series.* The first set of recommendations was published in 1962, and a revised set of basic safety standards, which was based on ICRP Publication 26, was published in 1982. The appearance of ICRP Publication 60 in 1990 led the IAEA, in 1995, to publish a third major revision of its basic safety standards for protection against ionizing radiation and for the safety of radiation sources. These safety standards serve as the basis for the regulation of both *practices* (any human activity that may increase the likelihood of additional dose to anyone) and *interventions* (an action to mitigate the consequences of an accidental exposure or of a practice that has gone out of control).

> "The IAEA's safety standards are not legally binding on Member States but may be adopted by them, at their own discretion, for use in national regulations in respect

of their own activities. The standards are binding on the IAEA in relation to its own operations and on States in relation to operations assisted by the IAEA. Any State wishing to enter into an agreement with the IAEA for its assistance in connection with siting, design, construction, commissioning, operation, or decommissioning of a nuclear facility or any other activities will be required to follow those parts of the safety standards that pertain to the activities to be covered by the agreement. However, it should be recalled that the final decisions and legal responsibilities in any licensing procedures rest with the States."

(From IAEA Safety Standards Series. *Application of the Concepts of Exclusion,* Exemption and Clearance. Safety Guide No. RS-G-1.7, 2004).

International Labor Organization

The International Labor Organization (ILO), which was founded in 1919 and then became part of the League of Nations, survived the demise of the League to become the first of the specialized agencies of the United Nations. Its concern generally is with the social problems of labor. Included in its work is the specification of international labor standards dealing with the health and safety of workers. These specifications are set forth in the *Model Code of Safety Regulations for Industrial Establishments for the Guidance of Governments and Industries,* in the recommendations of expert committees, and in technical manuals. In regard to radiation, the model code has been amended to incorporate those recommendations of the ICRP that are pertinent to control of occupational radiation hazards, and several manuals dealing with radiation safety in the workplace have been published.

International Commission on Radiological Units and Measurements

The International Commission on Radiological Units and Measurements (ICRU), which works closely with the ICRP, has had, since its inception in 1925, as its principal objective, the development of internationally acceptable recommendations regarding the following:

1. quantities and units of radiation and radioactivity,
2. procedures suitable for the measurement and application of these quantities in clinical radiology and radiobiology, and
3. physical data needed in the application of these procedures, the use of which tends to assure uniformity in reporting.

In terms of its operating policy: "The ICRU feels it is the responsibility of national organizations to introduce their own detailed technical procedures for the development and maintenance of standards. However, it urges that all countries adhere as closely as possible to the internationally recommended basic concepts of radiation quantities and units." (ICRU Report 32, 1979.)

Nuclear Energy Agency

The Nuclear Energy Agency (NEA) is a division of the Organization for Economic Cooperation and Development (OECD), which is an international organization of 27 industrialized states that cooperate to further economic development among its members. The function of the NEA is to promote the development of scientific, engineering, and legal principles for the safe and beneficial use of nuclear energy for peaceful purposes.

International Organization for Standardization

The International Organization for Standardization (ISO) is a nongovernmental organization that is a response of industries to the globalization of commerce. Its objective is to standardize business and manufacturing practices so that customers or clients in various parts of the world will operate on a level playing field. That is, they will all adhere to the same standards. Although not explicitly radiation-related, two series of ISO standards are relevant to health physicists. The ISO 9000 series, which was adopted in 1987 in expectation of trade among the members of the European Common Market, deals with quality standards for manufactured items. ISO 9000 series includes five parts: Parts 9000 and 9004 deal with general guidelines, while parts 9001, 9002, and 9003 are well-defined quality standards that deal with all the commercial aspects of engineering, manufacturing, installing, and servicing a product. ISO 9000 certification means that the product was manufactured according to rigid standards and actually performs according to the maker's claims. The application of ISO 9000 standards to obtain uniformity among radiometric instruments made in various countries will facilitate the international interchange of radiation measurements and will add confidence in the accuracy of the measurements.

Another series, ISO 14000, was developed in order to minimize the adverse environmental impact of an organization's activities and products. General objectives of ISO 14000 are the reduction of waste and of the cost of waste management, the conservation of energy and materials, and the optimization of distribution. In addition to requiring demonstration of compliance with all applicable regulatory requirements, certification to ISO 14001 requires identifying each aspect of an operation that might have an environmental impact, prioritizing these impacts, and establishing operating procedures to eliminate or to mitigate the detrimental environmental impacts. It also requires that all employees be trained in sensitivity to the environment, the prevention of pollution, and safe practices. Of particular interest to health physicists in the context of the "NIMBY" (Not In My Back Yard) complex is ISO 14031. This part requires that the organization gives due consideration to the viewpoints of the affected public regarding any possible pollution resulting from the operations of the organization.

National Agencies

Although international scientific agencies recommend radiation safety standards and practices, legal authority for radiation safety is exercised by regulatory agencies established by national states. In almost all cases, the national agencies base their regulations on the recommendations of the international scientific agencies. In the United States of America, for example, the Environmental Protection Agency (EPA) sets radiation safety standards, while several different regulatory agencies, including the Nuclear Regulatory Commission (NRC), the Occupational Health and Safety Administration (OSHA), and the Department of Energy (DOE) promulgate radiation safety regulations, according to the EPA standards, within their areas of responsibility. In Canada, the radiation safety regulatory body is the Canadian Atomic Energy Authority; in the United Kingdom, it is the Health Protection Agency's Radiation Protection Division; and in France, the Commissiarat d'Energie Nucleaire is the national regulatory agency.

PHILOSOPHY OF RADIATION SAFETY

Public Health and Radiation Safety Practice

Public health is that responsibility which rests on the organized community for the prevention of disease and the promotion of health. Prevention of disease through community efforts is necessary as—because of the population explosion and communal living—we are no longer able to structure our own individual environments. Our environment is determined mainly by the activities of others. The objectives of public health differ significantly from those of "private" health (clinical medicine). The aim of clinical medicine is to cure sick people, while the aim of public health is to keep healthy people healthy. A comparison of public health characteristics to "private" health characteristics is shown in Table 8-1.

Radiation safety standards and public policy regarding radiation are public health concerns because (1) we cannot structure our own individual environments, and (2) the effects of low-level radiation are not unique and, if they occur, are detectable only by epidemiologic means. No verifiable, detrimental radiation health effects have ever been observed among populations exposed within the range of variability of background radiation. Until recently, no detrimental radiation effects were found among the population of radiation workers whose doses were within the limits recommended in ICRP Publication 2. However, a study in 2005 of 407,391 nuclear workers in 15 countries found a small (1–2%) excess risk of cancer.

Cancer and genetic defects are the principal radiation effects of public health concern. Both these stochastic effects are attributed to the same biological phenomenon, namely, the loss of information in a base pair by the breaking of the base-pair bond in a DNA molecule. The zero-threshold model is believed to be conservative because of base-pair repair and because the information is replicated several times within the DNA molecule. According to this model, breaking 100 base pairs in a single individual or 1 base pair each in 100 individuals leads to the same probability of initiating an oncogenic lesion or a point mutation. This leads to the concept of the *collective dose*, which was introduced by the ICRP in 1977. The collective dose, which

TABLE 8-1. Comparison of "Private" Health (Clinical Medicine) to Public Health

PRIVATE HEALTH	PUBLIC HEALTH
Patient is an individual	Patient is the community
Particular disease is either present or absent	All diseases present all the time
Health status evaluation: blood pressure, temperature, blood count, etc.	Statistical and epidemiologic data
Causes: microbial, biochemical, trauma, psychological	Ecological causes, social ills
Therapy: physical, chemical, psychological	Engineering, medical, sociopolitical
Individual pays	Society, or the community, pays

is a measure of the total amount of DNA damage in a population, is simply the sum of all the dose equivalents received by the individual members of a population and is expressed in person-rems in the traditional system of health physics units and in person-sieverts in SI units:

$$S = \sum_i n_i H_i, \tag{8.1}$$

where n_i is the number of individuals who receive a dose equivalent to H_i. For example, if, during a given year, 800 workers in a certain nuclear facility received an average dose equivalent of 0.2 rem (0.002 Sv), 199 workers averaged 0.6 rem (0.006 Sv), and 1 worker received 2.6 rems (0.026 Sv), then the collective dose equivalent would be

S = (800 persons × 0.2 rem) + (199 persons × 0.6 rem) + (1 person × 2.6 rems),

S = 282 person-rems (2.82 person-Sv).

The collective dose is the basis for calculating the stochastic impact of radiation exposure to a large group or to a population and, thus, for public health control of radiation. It should be emphasized that the collective-dose concept applies only to the postulated stochastic effects in a large population. The collective-dose concept is applied by postulating that a given collective dose will result in the same total number of detrimental effects regardless of the size of the population and the distribution of the dose. The ICRP postulates 500 excess cancer deaths among a population whose collective dose is 10^4 person-Sv (10^6 person-rems) regardless of how the collective dose is distributed among the population. Thus, 10 mSv (1 rem) among 1 million people, 1 mSv (100 mrems) among 10 million people, or 0.01 mSv (1 mrem) among 1 billion people are postulated as equivalent in their carcinogenic potential. That is, in every one of these populations, the ICRP model postulates 500 excess deaths from cancer. It should be pointed out that the model used to postulate these excess deaths is inherently unverifiable since the statistical variability in the annual number of cancer deaths is far greater than the postulated number of excess radiogenic cancer deaths. In the United States, for example, the proportion of all deaths due to cancer has remained relatively constant during the years 1999–2004, at about 23%. The number of cancer deaths during these years ranged from 549,838 to 553,888. This variability in number of cancer deaths of more than 4000 swamps any excess cancer deaths that the linear zero-threshold model may postulate based on collective-dose considerations. The linear zero-threshold model, therefore, is inherently unverifiable.

In a societal or public health context, an acceptable collective dose for a large population is determined by policy makers on the basis of societal benefits that will accrue to the population versus the postulated detrimental effects as a result of the radiation exposure. Under these conditions, the probability of a detrimental radiogenic effect in any individual is vanishingly small. The recommended risk coefficients for lifetime stochastic effects, such as ICRP's 7.3×10^{-5} per mSv (which includes fatal and nonfatal cancers and detrimental heritable effects), are intended for use in ranking radiation risk among all other public health risks for the purpose of public health decision making. It is not intended to be used as a metric for counting dead bodies or other detrimental effects that are postulated at the low radiation levels that are associated with those practices that are limited by the recommended safety standards.

Dose-Limitation System

Deterministic (Nonstochastic) Effects

Engineering control of the environment by industrial hygienists and public health personnel is usually based, in the case of nonstochastic effects, on the concept of a tolerance dose, that is, a threshold dose. If the threshold dose of a toxic substance is not exceeded, then it is assumed that the normally operating physiological mechanisms can cope with the biological insult from that substance. This threshold is usually determined from a combination of experimental animal data and clinical human data; it is then reduced by an appropriate factor of safety, which leads to the maximum allowable concentration (MAC) for the substance. The MAC is then used as the criterion of safety in environmental control. The MAC was defined by the International Association on Occupational Health in 1959 as follows: "The term maximum allowable concentration for any substance shall mean that average concentration in air which causes no signs or symptoms of illness or physical impairment in all but hypersensitive workers during their working day on a continuing basis, as judged by the most sensitive internationally accepted tests."

Stochastic Effects

A different philosophy underlies the control of environmentally based agents, such as ionizing radiation and radionuclides, that lead to increased probability of cancer and genetic effects. Although molecular biologists have found the existence of intracellular mechanisms for the repair of damaged DNA in bacteria, geneticists have observed a dose–rate dependence of radiogenic mutagenesis, and both these observations imply the existence of a threshold for stochastic effects. Although the postulated stochastic effects have not been seen in populations that had been exposed to low-dose radiation (≤ 0.1 Gy, or 10 rads), public health policy nevertheless is based on the conservative belief that absence of proof of an effect is not proof of the absence of the effect. Accordingly, *we assume, for the purpose of setting safety standards for radiation as well as for chemical carcinogens and mutagens, that the threshold dose for stochastic effects is zero dose.* The dose–response curves for carcinogenesis and mutagenesis are assumed to be linear down to zero dose. The slopes of the dose–response curves for the various stochastic effects are postulated to be the same at low doses, all the way until zero dose, as at the high doses. Since this means that every increment of dose, no matter how small, increases the probability of an adverse effect by a proportional increment, the basis for control of man-made radiation is the limitation of the radiation dose to a level that is compatible with the benefits that accrue to society and to individuals from the use of radiation.

Based on the preventive conservatism principle, it can be argued that the distinction between those agents that cause deterministic effects and those that increase the probability of stochastic effects, which is based on the existence or absence of a threshold dose, is not as clear-cut as may first appear. For those substances where a

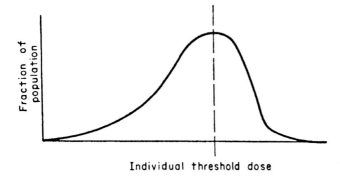

Fraction of population

Individual threshold dose

Figure 8-1. Distribution of individual thresholds among a population.

threshold has indeed been established, the threshold is for an *individual.* Different individuals have different thresholds. Thus, although the average threshold value for blood changes because of gamma radiation is taken as 0.25 Gy (25 rads), changes have been observed in persons whose doses were as low as 0.14 Gy (14 rads), while others whose doses reached as high as 0.4 Gy (40 rads) showed no blood changes. If a much larger population of exposed people were to be examined for blood changes, it is likely that changes would be seen among some whose dose was even less than 0.14 Gy (14 rads). It is not unreasonable to expect a distribution of sensitivity to most noxious agents somewhat like that shown in Figure 8-1, in which the sensitivity distribution curve is skewed to the right. The curve should actually intersect the abscissa on the high-dose end of the distribution, since we are reasonably certain that there exists some dose that will affect everyone. On the other hand, it is known that there are "hypersensitive" individuals who respond to extremely low doses, which would not affect most people. On this basis, it is reasonable to assume that the distribution curve to the left of the mode extends to the origin of the coordinate axes. In effect, the distribution of susceptibility among the individuals of a population means that the concept of a threshold dose cannot be applied to a very large population. In setting a maximum acceptable dose (MAD) for a large population group, therefore, a value judgment must be made.

Someone must decide what is an acceptable fraction of the population that may be adversely affected by the agent for which the MAD is being set in return for the benefits to be derived by that population from the use of that agent. The MAD is usually set so conservatively that an extremely large number of people would have to be exposed at that level before the hypersensitive person was found. This same type of reasoning prevails among those who are concerned with recommending radiation dose limits. For occupational exposure, the question of recommending dose limits as a guide to radiation protection is relatively simple. A vast amount of human experience was gained from the promiscuous exposures to radium and X-rays and the consequent harmful radiation effects during the first quarter of the twentieth century, from survivors of the nuclear bombings in Japan, from exposure for medical reasons, and from large population groups living in areas of high- and low-radiation background. Additionally, much more data were obtained from laboratory studies with animals. On the basis of this information, and on the assumption that every additional increment of radiation dose has a corresponding increment of risk, dose limits can be set, which, when applied to occupationally exposed radiation workers, will result in a level of risk no greater than that in other occupations that are recognized as having high safety standards and are considered to be "safe." If any uncertainty arises about where to set an acceptable limit, the uncertainty is resolved by preventive conservatism rather than by scientific realism. Dose limits for nonoccupationally exposed individual members of the general public are set at a level where the resulting postulated radiation risk is very much smaller than the risks that society already accepts in return for other technological benefits. From these societally acceptable doses, we derive annual limits of intake (ALI) and environmental concentrations of the various radionuclides that would result in radiation doses within the prescribed dose limits.

The system of dose limitation recommended by the ICRP is founded on three basic tenets stated in its Publication 26 and reiterated in its Publication 60:

1. Justification—No practice shall be adopted unless its introduction produces a net positive benefit. It should be pointed out that justification is a societal decision, not a radiation decision.
2. Optimization—All exposures shall be kept as low as reasonably achievable (ALARA), economic and social factors being taken into account.
3. Dose limitation—The dose equivalent to individuals shall not exceed the limits recommended for the appropriate circumstances by the Commission.

It should be emphasized that the second point above urges that actual operational dose limits for any radiological activity be more restrictive than the maximum recommended dose limit. This means that processes, equipment (such as shielding, ventilation, etc.), and other operational factors should be designed so that workers do not exceed the operational dose limit, which is usually much smaller than the maximum recommended dose limit. This operating philosophy is known as the ALARA concept. To apply the ALARA concept, the ICRP recommends that cost–benefit analyses of alternative lower operational dose limits be made, and then that level of radiation protection be selected that optimizes the cost of the detrimental effects of the radiation versus the benefits to be derived from the radiation practice. Since economic and social factors must be considered in implementing ALARA, it is clear that widely differing interpretations can be made by equally competent authorities on what is "as low as reasonably achievable." In the United States, the official interpretation is made by the U.S. NRC and is published in the *Regulatory Guide* series.

Societal benefits and detriments from radiological activities usually are not uniformly distributed among all members of society. Furthermore, different members and segments of society may be exposed to radiation from several different sources. The ICRP, therefore, recommends restrictions, or *constraints*, on radiation sources to try to ensure that no member of the general public will exceed the maximum dose. For example, the U.S. EPA's annual dose limit for public drinking water is 4 mrems (40 μSv), and the U.S. NRC requirement is that the annual dose to a member of the public from the entire nuclear fuel cycle may not exceed 25 mrems (250 μSv). Water treatment and operations in the nuclear fuel cycle must be designed accordingly.

The validity of the radiation safety standards was emphasized by Lauriston Taylor, the founder of the NCRP, who said, in 1980: "No one has been identifiably injured by radiation while working within the first numerical standard set by the NCRP and the ICRP in 1934." Since then, the radiation safety standards have been made about ten times more restrictive. It is, therefore, reasonable to expect that the current radiation safety standards are sufficiently restrictive to preclude identifiable radiation injury.

ICRP BASIC RADIATION SAFETY CRITERIA

For purposes of radiation safety standards, the ICRP recognizes three categories of exposure:

1. Occupational exposure to adults who are exposed to ionizing radiation in the course of their work. Persons in this category may be called radiation workers. This category contains two subgroups:

    (a) Pregnant women.
    (b) All other radiation workers.

2. Exposure of members of the general public.
3. Medical exposure. This category deals with the intentional exposure of patients for diagnostic and therapeutic purposes by technically qualified medical and paramedical personnel. It does not include exposure to the personnel involved in the administration of radiation to patients.

Occupational Exposure

For occupational exposure, the ICRP 26, in 1977, recommended the following annual dose-equivalent limits:

1. To prevent nonstochastic effects, the limit is

    (a) 0.5 Sv (50 rems) to all tissues except the lens of the eye.
    (b) 0.15 Sv (15 rems) to the lens of the eye.

    These limits applied whether the tissues were exposed singly or together with other organs.
2. To limit stochastic effects, the dose-equivalent limit from uniform whole-body irradiation is 50 mSv (5 rems) in 1 year.

Limits on intake of radioisotopes in order to meet the ICRP 26 dose limits from internal exposure are listed in ICRP 30 and its supplements.

The ICRP 26 recommendations were superseded in 1990 by the ICRP 60 recommendations for radiation safety limits. The ICRP 60 recommendations are based on a combined concept of stochastic and nonstochastic (deterministic) effects. These two categories were considered together in a single index of harm called the *detriment*, which includes consideration of both stochastic and deterministic effects. The dose limits in ICRP 60 are based on a dose, which, if exceeded, may lead to unacceptable consequences, be they either stochastic or deterministic, for an individual. These dose limits are shown in Table 8-2.

TABLE 8-2. ICRP 60 Recommended Dose Limits

APPLICATION	OCCUPATIONAL	PUBLIC
Whole body	20 mSv/yr effective dose averaged over 5 yrs., Maximum dose in any 1 yr = 50 mSv	1 mSv in 1 yr
Annual dose to		
lens of the eye	150 mSv	15 mSv
skin	500 mSv	50 mSv
hands and feet	500 mSv	—
Fetus/embryo	2 mSv	—

Effective Dose

On the principle that the risk of a stochastic effect should be equal whether the whole body is uniformly irradiated or whether the radiation dose is nonuniformly distributed, the ICRP introduced the concept of *effective dose* in the 1977 review of its radiation safety recommendations (ICRP 26).

For the purpose of setting radiation safety standards, we assume that the probability of a detrimental effect in any tissue is proportional to the dose equivalent to that tissue. However, because of the differences in sensitivity among the various tissues, the value for the proportionality factors differs among the tissues. The relative sensitivity to detrimental effects, expressed as tissue weighting factors w_T of the several organs and tissues that contribute to the overall risk, is shown in Table 8-3. If

TABLE 8-3. Tissue Weighting Factors, w_T^a

TISSUE OR ORGAN	w_T, ICRP 26	w_T, ICRP 60
Gonads	0.25	0.20
Red bone marrow	0.12	0.12
Colon	Not given	0.12
Lung	0.12	0.12
Stomach	Not given	0.12
Bladder	Not given	0.05
Breast	0.15	0.05
Liver	Not given	0.05
Esophagus	Not given	0.05
Thyroid	0.03	0.05
Skin	Not given	0.01
Bone surface	0.03	0.01
Remainder[b,c]	0.30	0.05

[a]The values are based on a reference population of equal numbers of both sexes and a wide range of ages. In the definition of effective dose, they apply to workers, to the whole population, and to either sex.

[b]For purposes of calculation, the remainder is composed of the following additional tissues and organs: adrenals, brain, upper large intestine, kidney, muscle, pancreas, spleen, thymus, and uterus. The list includes organs that are likely to be selectively irradiated. Some organs in the list are known to be susceptible to cancer induction. If other tissues and organs subsequently become identified as having a significant risk of induced cancer, they will be included either with a specific w_T or in this additional list constituting the remainder. The latter may also include other tissues or organs selectively irradiated.

[c]In those exceptional cases in which a single one of the remainder tissues or organs receives an equivalent dose in excess of the highest dose in any of the 12 organs for which a weighting factor is specified, a weighting factor of 0.025 should be applied to that tissue or organ and a weighting factor of 0.025 to the average dose in the rest of the remainder as defined above.

Abbreviation: ICRP, International Commission on Radiological Protection.

radiation dose is uniform throughout the body, then the total risk factor has a relative weight of 1. For nonuniform radiation, such as partial-body exposure to an external radiation field, or from internal exposure where the radionuclide concentrates to different degrees in the various organs, the weighting factors listed in Table 8-3 are used to calculate an EDE. The EDE, H_E, is given by

$$H_E = \sum_T w_T H_T, \tag{8.2}$$

where w_T is the weighting factor for tissue T and H_T is the dose equivalent to tissue T. Table 8-3 shows the weighting factors recommended in ICRP 26 and ICRP 60. The U.S. NRC used the ICRP 26 values for the tissue-weighting factors in Title 10 of the *Code of Federal Regulations*, Part 20, which usually is cited as 10 CFR 20, that were approved in 1991 and became effective in 1994.

 EXAMPLE 8.1

As a result of a laboratory accident, 185 kBq (5 μCi) of ^{131}I were deposited in a radioisotope technician; 37 kBq (1 μCi) were deposited in her thyroid gland and 148 kBq (4 μCi) were uniformly distributed throughout the rest of her body. Using data from bioassay measurements and body scanning, the health physicist calculated a thyroid dose equivalent of 61.5 mSv (6.15 rems) and a whole-body dose of 0.13 mSv (13 mrems).

(a) What was the technician's effective dose?

(b) Was she overexposed according to the ICRP 60 criteria?

Solution

(a) The effective dose is calculated from Eq. (8.2), using weighting factors of 0.05 for the thyroid (Table 8-3) and 0.95 for the rest of the body:

$$H_E = \sum_T w_T H_T = (0.05 \times 61.5) + (0.95 \times 0.13) = 3.2 \, \text{mSv}.$$

(b) Since the effective dose is much less than 20 mSv, the dose from this accidental exposure did not exceed the ICRP 60 dose limit. Whether her total dose for the year, after experiencing this accidental exposure, exceeds the ICRP 60 dose limits depends on her previous exposure history.

Conceptus (Embryo/Fetus)

Limits on occupational exposure for women are the same as for men. However, the ICRP has set restrictive limits on the conceptus. After pregnancy has been declared, a maximum of 2 mSv, which is the sum of external radiation and dose from internally deposited radionuclides, is recommended for the balance of the pregnancy. For external radiation, the dose assigned to the conceptus is the deep dose registered by the pregnant woman's dosimeter. The internal dose per unit intake of a radionuclide depends on the age of the conceptus. Dose coefficients (DC) from acute and chronic intakes by inhalation and by ingestion may be found in ICRP 88 (2001). For example, the DC due to an acute inhalation of elemental ^{131}I vapor during the 25th week of pregnancy is listed as 3.1×10^{-8} Sv/Bq. Thus, in the case of a nuclear technologist who accidentally inhaled 1000 Bq during her 25th week of pregnancy, her fetus would be assigned a dose of

$$3.1 \times 10^{-8} \frac{Sv}{Bq} \times 1 \times 10^3 \, Bq = 3.1 \times 10^{-5} \, Sv, \text{ or } 31 \, \mu Sv \ (3.1 \text{ mrems}).$$

If her dosimeters showed a total external dose of 100 μSv (10 mrems), then the total dose assigned to her fetus would be 31 μSv + 100 μSv = 131 μSv (13.1 mrems).

Medical Exposure

No specific dose limit was recommended by the ICRP for medical exposure. The commission, however, recommended that only necessary exposure should be made, that these exposures should be justifiable on the basis of benefits that would not otherwise have been received, and that the administered doses should be limited to the minimum dose consistent with the medical benefit to the patient.

Exposure of Individuals in the General Public

For members of the general public, the ICRP recommends an effective dose limit of 1 mSv (100 mrems) in a year. It is believed that the average dose to members of an exposed group will be less than the dose limit. The ICRP points out that the average dose to members of the public would increase if the number of sources increase, even though the dose to no single individual exceeds the 1-mSv effective dose limit. For this reason, the commission recommends that regional or national authorities should maintain surveillance over all the separate sources of exposure in order to control the collective total effective dose.

Exposure of Populations

The ICRP made no specific recommendations for the dose limit to a population. Instead, it emphasized that each man-made contribution to the population dose must be justified by its benefits, and that limits for individual members of the population refer to the total effective dose from all sources. The dose limit to a population is thus considered to be the sum of several minimum necessary contributory doses rather than a single permissible total dose limit that is available for apportionment among several sources.

Dose Coefficient

In its current (2006) recommendations, the ICRP does not list maximum acceptable concentrations of radionuclides in air or water, nor does it list the ALI as it did in ICRP 30. (The ALI is defined in the paragraph below.) Because the primary safety standard is either the dose limit to an organ (nonstochastic effect) or the effective whole-body dose (stochastic effect), the ICRP, as well as the IAEA, list the DC rather than the ALI. The DC is defined as the committed equivalent dose to an organ or tissue per unit intake, or the committed effective dose per unit intake. The ICRP lists the DC for six different age categories, from 3 months of age to adulthood, and the IAEA lists them for adult workers as Sv per Bq intake. In traditional units, the DCs are expressed as rem per μCi. The ALI for any radionuclide may be calculated, for use as a secondary safety criterion, from the dose limit and the DC for that nuclide.

Annual Limit of Intake

The ALI is defined in ICRP 30 as that quantity of activity of a radionuclide that would lead to the annual dose limit if inhaled or ingested by a "reference person."

According to ICRP 30 Criteria

ICRP 30 criteria are important in the United States because the U.S. NRC's radiation safety standards are based on the ICRP 30 recommendations. In the ICRP 30, the ALI was restricted by the basic requirements for stochastic and nonstochastic effects and was defined as the annual intake that would lead to an effective committed dose equivalent (a 50-year dose commitment) not exceeding 50 mSv (5 rems) and an annual dose equivalent to any single organ or tissue not exceeding 500 mSv (50 rems). Expressed symbolically, these requirements are

$$\sum_T w_T H_{50,T} \leq 0.05 \text{ Sv} \tag{8.3}$$

$$H_{50,T} \leq 0.5 \text{ Sv} \qquad \text{for every } T, \tag{8.4}$$

where w_T is the weighting factor shown in Table 8-3 and $H_{50,T}$ is the 50-year total committed dose equivalent in tissue T resulting from intakes of radioactive materials from all sources during the year in question. Equation (8.3) assures that the annual limit on effective whole-body dose is not exceeded in order to control stochastic effects, while Eq. (8.4) assures that the annual limit on the dose to a single tissue or organ is not exceeded in order to remain below the damage threshold for non-stochastic effects. Thus, an effective dose of 0.05 Sv (5 rems) is assigned to an intake of one ALI that is based on stochastic effects (SALI), while an organ dose of 0.5 Sv (50 rems) is assigned to an intake of one ALI based on nonstochastic effects (NALI) to the organ.

It should be noted that the intake limit is placed on the total intake of radioisotopes in any single year, and that no restrictions were placed by the ICRP on the instantaneous rate of intake. That is, the limit may be met by a single large intake or by continuing intake of small quantities. The principles involved in the application of Eqs. (8.3) and (8.4) may be illustrated by the calculation of the ALI for ingested ^{137}Cs according to ICRP 26 and 30 criteria (Example 8.2).

EXAMPLE 8.2

Calculate the ALI for ingested ^{137}Cs according to ICRP 26 and 30 criteria.

Solution

Commonly occurring cesium compounds are known to be rapidly and almost completely absorbed from the gastrointestinal (GI) tract. After absorption, cesium is uniformly distributed throughout the body. In no case is the concentration of cesium in any organ or tissue greater than it is in the muscle. The retention of cesium in the body over at least the first 1400 days is described by the two-compartment equation (Eq. [6.59])

$$q(t) = 0.1\, q_0 e^{\frac{-0.693t}{2}} + 0.9\, q_0 e^{\frac{-0.693t}{110}},$$

where q_0 is the quantity of cesium initially taken up by the body. Equation (6.59) tells us that of the cesium taken up, 10% is transferred to a tissue compartment that is cleared with a half-life of 2 days, while the remaining 90% is transferred to a tissue compartment whose residence half-time is 110 days. Since the radiological half-life of ^{137}Cs, 30 years, is very much greater than the half-times of each of the two compartments, the effective half-time for each of the compartments is essentially equal to their biological half-times. The effective clearance rates, therefore, for compartments 1 and 2, as calculated from Eq. (6.52), are

$$\lambda_{E_1} = \frac{0.693}{T_{E_1}} = \frac{0.693}{2 \text{ days}} = 0.347\, \mathrm{d}^{-1}$$

$$\lambda_{E_2} = \frac{0.693}{T_{E_2}} = \frac{0.693}{110 \text{ days}} = 6.3 \times 10^{-3}\, \mathrm{d}^{-1}.$$

The total dose from the deposited ^{137}Cs is the sum of the doses for each of the two compartments, as calculated from Eq. (6.62). To meet the stochastic-effects criterion, the EDE must not exceed 0.05 Sv (5 rems), which corresponds to a dose of 0.05 Gy (5 rads) for beta–gamma radiation.

$$D = \frac{\dot{D}_{10}}{\lambda_1} + \frac{\dot{D}_{20}}{\lambda_2} = 0.05 \text{ Gy}, \tag{8.5}$$

where $\dot{D}_{10}$ and $\dot{D}_{20}$ are the initial dose rates in compartments 1 and 2, respectively, and λ_1 and λ_2 are their effective clearance rates. These initial dose rates from the uniformly distributed ^{137}Cs may be calculated from Eq. (6.46) by using the appropriate value for the specific effective energy (SEE) of the betas plus the gammas. The SEE per transformation may be calculated with the aid of the absorbed fractions (AFs), φ, from Table 6-8, and the output data for ^{137}Cs, which are found in Figure 8-2.

If we organize the information from Table 6-8 and Figure 8-2 as shown in Table 8-4, the SEE, in MeV per transformation per kilogram, is calculated from

$$\mathrm{SEE} = \frac{\sum_i n_i E_i \varphi_i}{m}. \tag{8.6}$$

Since the radiation is absorbed uniformly throughout the entire body, m in this case is 70 kg. If we substitute this value for m and 0.4394 MeV/t from Table 8-4 into Eq. (8.6), we have

$$\mathrm{SEE} = \frac{0.4394 \, \dfrac{\mathrm{MeV}}{\mathrm{t}}}{70 \, \mathrm{kg}} = 6.28 \times 10^{-3} \, \frac{\mathrm{MeV}}{\mathrm{t/kg}}.$$

Using this value for the SEE and an activity $q = 1$ Bq in Eq. (6.46):

$$\dot{D} = \frac{q \, \mathrm{Bq} \times 1 \, \dfrac{\mathrm{tps}}{\mathrm{Bq}} \times \mathrm{SEE} \, \dfrac{\mathrm{MeV}}{\mathrm{t/kg}} \times 1.6 \times 10^{-13} \, \dfrac{\mathrm{J}}{\mathrm{MeV}} \times 8.64 \times 10^4 \, \dfrac{\mathrm{s}}{\mathrm{d}}}{1 \, \dfrac{\mathrm{J/kg}}{\mathrm{Gy}}},$$

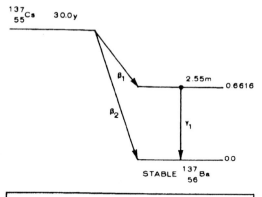

Figure 8-2 Transformation scheme: $^{137}_{55}$Cs 30.0y — CESIUM·137 — BETA-MINUS DECAY; with levels β_1, β_2, 2.55m 0.6616, γ_1, 0.0, STABLE $^{137}_{56}$Ba

INPUT DATA

Radiation	%/dis-integration	Transition energy (MeV)	Other nuclear parameters
Beta-1	93.5	0.514 *	First forbidden unique
Beta-2	6.5	1.176 *	Second forbidden
Gamma-1	93.5	0.6616	M4, $\alpha_K = 0.093$, K/L = 5.6; K/M = 25.5

Ref.: Lederer, C. M. et al, *Table of Isotopes*, 6th ed.
* Endpoint energy (MeV).

OUTPUT DATA

Radiation (i)	Mean number/disintegration (n_i)	Mean energy (MeV) ($\bar{E}_i$)	Δ_i $\left(\dfrac{\text{g-rad}}{\mu\text{Ci-h}}\right)$
Beta-1	0.935	0.1749	0.3483
Beta-2	0.065	0.4272	0.0591
Gamma-1	0.840	0.6616	1.1837
K int. con. electron, gamma-1	0.0781	0.6242	0.1038
L int. con. electron, gamma-1	0.0140	0.6560	0.0196
M int. con. electron, gamma-1	0.0031	0.6605	0.0044
K α-1 X-rays	0.0374	0.0322	0.0026
K α-2 X-rays	0.0194	0.0318	0.0013
K β-1 X-rays	0.0105	0.0364	0.0008
K β-2 X-rays	0.0022	0.0374	0.0002
L X-rays	0.0127	0.0045	0.0001
KLL Auger electron	0.0057	0.0263	0.0003
KLX Auger electron	0.0025	0.0308	0.0002
KXY Auger electron	0.0004	0.0353	0.0000
LMM Auger electron	0.0718	0.0034	0.0005
MXY Auger electron	0.173	0.0011	0.0004

Figure 8-2. Transformation scheme and input–output data for ^{137}Cs dosimetry. (Reprinted by permission of the Society of Nuclear Medicine from Dillman LT. MIRD Pamphlet No. 4: Radionuclide Decay Schemes and Nuclear Parameters for Use in Radiation Dose Estimation. *J Nucl Med.* March 1969; 10(2 Suppl):1–32.)

TABLE 8-4. Calculation of Specific Effective Energy (SEE) for Whole-Body Internal Exposure to ^{137}Cs

RADIATION	NUMBER PER DECAY, n_i	MEAN ENERGY PER PARTICLE, E_i (MeV)	ABSORBED FRACTION, φ_i	ABSORBED ENERGY (MeV/d)
β_1	0.935	0.1749	1	0.1635
β_2	0.065	0.4272	1	0.0278
γ	0.840	0.6616	0.334	0.1856
K int. con. el.	0.0781	0.6242	1	0.0488
L int. con. el.	0.0140	0.6560	1	0.0092
M int. con. el.	0.0031	0.6605	1	0.0020
$K_{\alpha 1}$ X-ray	0.0374	0.0322	0.750	0.0009
$K_{\alpha 2}$ X-ray	0.0194	0.0318	0.754	0.0005
$K_{\beta 1}$ X-ray	0.0105	0.0364	0.703	0.0003
$K_{\beta 2}$ X-ray	0.0022	0.0374	0.690	0.0001
L X-ray	0.0127	0.0045	1	0.0001
KLL Auger el.	0.0057	0.0263	1	0.0001
KXY Auger el.	0.0025	0.0308	1	0.0000
KLX Auger el.	0.0004	0.0353	1	0.0001
LMM Auger el.	0.0718	0.0334	1	0.0002
MXY Auger el.	0.173	0.0011	1	0.0002
				$\sum = 0.4394$

we find the dose rate per unit activity of ^{137}Cs to be

$$\dot{D} = 9 \times 10^{-11} \, \frac{\text{Gy/d}}{\text{Bq}}.$$

According to Eq. (6.59), the activity deposited in compartment 2 is nine times greater than the activity deposited in compartment 1. Substituting the appropriate values into Eq. (8.5) allows us to calculate the quantity of ingested ^{137}Cs that results in a dose of 0.05 Gy (5 rads), corresponding to a dose equivalent of 0.05 Sv (5 rems):

$$0.05 \, \text{Gy} = \frac{0.1 q \text{Bq} \times 9 \times 10^{-11} \dfrac{\text{Gy/d}}{\text{Bq}}}{0.347 \, \text{d}^{-1}} + \frac{0.9 q \times 9 \times 10^{-11} \dfrac{\text{Gy/d}}{\text{Bq}}}{6.3 \times 10^{-3} \text{d}^{-1}}$$

$$q = 3.9 \times 10^6 \, \text{Bq} \; = \; \text{Ingestion ALI.}$$

Since cesium is uniformly distributed throughout the body, a similar calculation for the NALI, where the annual dose equivalent limit is 0.5 Sv (50 rems), yields a much higher value than the SALI. In order to satisfy Eqs. (8.3) and (8.4), we must use the SALI. Since the ALI is rounded off to the nearest whole number, the ALI for ingested ^{137}Cs is listed in ICRP 30 as 4 MBq, and as 100 μCi in 10 CFR 20.

The calculation of the ALI for ingested ^{137}Cs was simple because of the uniform distribution of the cesium. Generally, however, an internally deposited radionuclide is not uniformly distributed, and doses contributed to the various target organs by each different source organ, with its own amount of radioactivity, must be calculated. These calculations were systematized by the ICRP for ease of programming into a computer. By substituting Eq. (6.105) into Eq. (6.104), we have for the dose equivalent to any organ or tissue, T, 50 years after intake of the radionuclide:

$$H_{50,T}\,(T \leftarrow S)$$

$$= U_S \text{ transfs.}$$

$$\times \sum_R \frac{Y_R \dfrac{\text{particles}}{\text{transf}} \times (E \times w_R)\, \dfrac{\text{effective MeV}}{\text{particle}} \times 1.6 \times 10^{-13}\, \dfrac{\text{J}}{\text{MeV}} \times \text{AF}\,(T \leftarrow S)_R}{m_T\, \text{kg}}$$

$$\times \frac{\dfrac{1\,\text{Sv}}{\text{eff.J}}}{\text{transf}}, \tag{8.7}$$

where

Y_R is the fraction of the decays in which particle R is emitted,
E_R is the energy of particle R, MeV,
w_R is the radiation weighting factor (formerly symbolized by Q),
$w_R = 1$ for gamma and beta radiation, and 20 for alphas,
$\text{AF}(T \leftarrow S)_R$ is the AF from radiation R in tissue T per transformation in S, and m_T is the mass of tissue T, in kg.

Equation (8.7) can be solved for the dose equivalent resulting from an intake of 1 Bq. An SALI can be calculated from

$$\text{SALI} = \frac{0.05\,\text{Sv}}{\sum_T w_T H_{50,T}\, \dfrac{\text{Sv}}{\text{Bq}}}. \tag{8.8}$$

To determine whether the SALI is limiting, we compare the SALI to the criterion:

$$\text{SALI}\,(\text{Bq}) \times (H_{50,T})_{\text{max}}\, \frac{\text{Sv}}{\text{Bq}} \leq 0.5\,\text{Sv}. \tag{8.9}$$

If the product of the SALI and the committed dose equivalent to the organ or tissue that receives the greatest dose equivalent from that intake, $(H_{50,T})_{\text{max}}$ exceeds 0.5 Sv (50 rems), then the SALI is too large, and an NALI must be calculated, which is given by

$$\text{NALI} = \frac{0.5\,\text{Sv}}{(H_{50,T})_{\text{max}}\, \dfrac{\text{Sv}}{\text{Bq}}}. \tag{8.10}$$

[1]Tables of specific absorbed fractions may be found in M. Cristy and K.F. Eckerman. *Specific Absorbed Fractions of Energy at Various Ages from Internal Photons Sources.* ORNL/NUREG/TM 8381/V1. Oak Ridge National Laboratories, Oak Ridge, TN, 1987.

EXAMPLE 8.3

Inhalation of 1 Bq of ^{239}Pu in the form of relatively insoluble (class Y, very long pulmonary retention half-time) particle leads to the following committed dose equivalents, $H_{50,T}$, from the ^{239}Pu and its daughters in the respective target organs: lungs, 3.2×10^{-4} Sv; red marrow, 7.6×10^{-5} Sv; bone surfaces, 9.5×10^{-4} Sv; and liver, 2.1×10^{-4} Sv. Calculate the ALI for inhalation of this solubility class of ^{239}Pu according to ICRP 30 criteria.

Solution

First, we will calculate the weighted committed dose equivalents:

TISSUE	$H_{50,T}$ (Sv)	×	w_T	=	WEIGHTED $H_{50,T}$
Lungs	3.2×10^{-4}		0.12		3.9×10^{-5}
Red marrow	7.6×10^{-5}		0.12		9.1×10^{-6}
Bone surface	9.5×10^{-4}		0.03		2.9×10^{-5}
Liver	2.1×10^{-4}		0.06		1.2×10^{-5}

$$\sum = 8.9 \times 10^{-5} \frac{\text{Sv}}{\text{Bq}}$$

The SALI is calculated from Eq. (8.8):

$$\text{SALI} = \frac{0.05\ \text{Sv}}{8.9 \times 10^{-5}\ \dfrac{\text{Sv}}{\text{Bq}}} = 5.6 \times 10^{2}\ \text{Bq}.$$

Next, let us determine whether the criterion given by Eq. (8.9) is satisfied. That is, whether the tissue receiving the greatest dose, the bone surfaces, will receive a dose equivalent exceeding 0.5 Sv from inhaling the SALI of class Y ^{239}Pu. According to Eq. (8.9), the product of the SALI and the greatest committed dose equivalent to any organ or tissue may not exceed 0.5 Sv. In this case, we have

$$5.6 \times 10^{2}\ \text{Bq} \times 9.5 \times 10^{-4}\ \frac{\text{Sv}}{\text{Bq}} = 0.53\ \text{Sv}.$$

According to ICRP 30, since 0.53 Sv exceeds the criterion of Eq. (8.8), the non-stochastic dose-equivalent limit determines the inhalation of ALI:

$$\text{NALI} = \frac{0.5\ \text{Sv}}{(H_{50,T})_{\max} \dfrac{\text{Sv}}{\text{Bq}}}$$

$$= \frac{0.5\ \text{Sv}}{9.5 \times 10^{-4} \dfrac{\text{Sv}}{\text{Bq}}} = 5.3 \times 10^{2}\ \text{Bq}.$$

Because of the uncertainties in the metabolic models, the ALIs are given to only one significant figure. Thus the ALI for inhaled "insoluble" ^{239}Pu is listed in ICRP 30, Part 1, as 5×10^{2} Bq and 0.02 μCi in 10 CFR 20.

Airborne Radioactivity

For purposes of computing concentration standards for airborne radioactivity, atmospheric contaminants may be broadly classified as gaseous and particulate. Radiation exposure from airborne radioactivity may occur via three pathways:

- *External exposure* (submersion dose) from radionuclides outside the body.
- *Internal exposure* due to radionuclides inhaled into the body.
- *Internal exposure* due to ingestion of radionuclides that had entered into the food chain as a result of fallout from the air.

The submersion dose is the limiting factor for acceptable atmospheric concentrations only for several biochemically inert gases, such as argon, krypton, and xenon. For all other airborne radionuclides, the internal dose is the limiting factor. For inhaled radioactivity, the lung is considered from two points of view: as a portal of entry for inhaled substances that are absorbed into the body from the lung and are then systematically transferred to one or more organs, and as a critical organ that may suffer radiation damage. Inhalation is a major portal of entry for noxious substances because the amount of material taken into the body by inhalation is far greater than by ingestion, as shown in Table 8-5.

The hazard from a toxicant depends mainly on two factors: its inherent toxicity and on the probability of a toxic amount reaching the site of its toxic action. The hazard from inhaled radioactive dusts—or indeed the hazard from any toxic material—must include a consideration of the likelihood that the toxic substance will reach the site of its toxic action. In the case of inhaled radioactive dusts, this site is assumed to be the bronchial epithelium, the alveolar epithelium, and the pulmonary lymph nodes. The two main factors that influence the degree of hazard from toxic airborne dusts are (1) the site in the lung where the dust particles are deposited and (2) the retention of the particles within the lung.

Particle-Size Distribution

Dusts generated by almost any process are found to be randomly distributed in size, or "diameter," around a mean value. This size distribution is found to be "log-normal." The logarithm of the particle size is found to be normally distributed, rather than the size itself. In this case, the mean size, which is called the *geometric mean*, is defined by

$$m_g = \text{antilog}\left[\frac{\sum_n \log d_n}{n}\right], \tag{8.11}$$

where d_n is the particle diameter (which most often is expressed in microns, $1 \ \mu\text{m} = 10^{-4} \ \text{cm}$) and n is the number of particles that are being sized. The

TABLE 8-5. Amounts of Material Taken into the Body via Inhalation and Ingestion

MEDIUM	VOLUME (L)	WEIGHT (kg)
Food	Not applicable	1.9
Water	2.2	2.2
Air	20,000	26

geometric standard deviation, which is the standard deviation of the distribution of the logarithms of the size distribution is defined as

$$\sigma_g = \text{antilog} \sqrt{\frac{\sum_n (\log d_n)^2}{n} - \left(\frac{\sum_n \log d_n}{n}\right)^2}. \tag{8.12}$$

The standard deviation corresponds to the inflection point of the Gaussian (normal) distribution curve, as shown in Figure 8-3A. In a normal distribution, 68.2% of the population falls within the limits bounded by plus and minus one standard deviation from the mean; 95.4% of the population is included within plus and minus two standard deviations of the mean. Because of the logarithmic nature of the distribution, the size distribution *must* be given as

$$m_g \times \sigma_g \quad \text{or} \quad m_g \div \sigma_g \tag{8.13}$$

rather than, as in the case of an arithmetic mean,

$$m_a \pm \sigma_a. \tag{8.14}$$

For example, if the log-normal size distribution of a dust is given as $(1.4 \times 2$ or $1.4 \div 2)$ μm, this means that 68% of all the particles lie between 0.7 (or $1.4 \div 2$) μm and 2.8 (or 1.4×2) μm, and that about 96% lie between 0.35 (or $1.4 \div 2^2$)μm and 5.6 (or 1.4×2^2)μm.

Particle Kinetics

A particle released into the atmosphere is buffeted from all directions by the air molecules that are in random motion and colliding with each other, at rates determined by the temperature, according to the kinetic theory of gases. These random

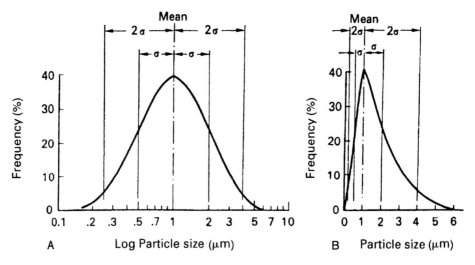

Figure 8-3. Log-normal distribution of dust particle sizes. **(A).** The logarithm of the diameter is normally distributed, thus giving a Gaussian distribution when the logarithm of the particle size is plotted against frequency. In this curve shown here, the mean size is 1 μm and the geometric standard deviation is 2. **(B).** The particle size is plotted against frequency, thus yielding a skewed distribution curve.

collisions with air molecules lead to diffusion of very small or molecule-sized particles. The released particle also falls under the influence of gravity. For particles greater than about 1 μm, the gravitational effects and inertial effects are much greater than the diffusional effects. Thus, the motion of this particle relative to the air is determined mainly by the aerodynamic properties of the particle. For particles smaller than 0.1 μm, diffusional effects predominate and particle motion relative to air is determined by thermodynamic properties of the particle. Particles between these two sizes are influenced by both aerodynamic and thermodynamic factors.

Aerodynamic Properties

When aerodynamic properties predominate, a released particle is acted upon by two forces: f_g, the downward force of gravity, and f_r, the upward retarding force due to the resistance to free fall offered by the air (Fig. 8-4). When the retarding force is equal to the gravitational force, there is no unbalanced force to accelerate the falling particle, and a constant velocity, called the *terminal velocity*, v_t, is attained by the falling particle. Equating f_r to f_g and solving for the terminal velocity, we have

$$f_r = 3\pi\eta dv = \frac{\pi d^3}{6}(\rho - \rho_{air})g = f_g \tag{8.15}$$

$$v = v_t = \frac{d^2(\rho - \rho_{air})g}{18\eta}. \tag{8.16}$$

Since the air density is very much less than the particle density, that is, $\rho_{air} \ll \rho$, Eq. (8.16) may be written as

$$v_t = \frac{d^2\rho g}{18\eta}. \tag{8.17}$$

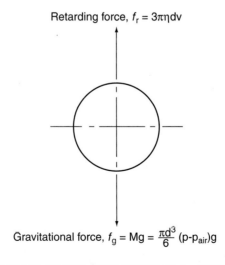

Retarding force, $f_r = 3\pi\eta dv$

Gravitational force, $f_g = Mg = \frac{\pi d^3}{6}(\rho - \rho_{air})g$

Figure 8-4. The forces acting on a particle falling through air. η = viscosity of air = 185μP at room temperature (1 P = 1 g/cm/s); d = particle diameter (cm); v = velocity of fall (cm/s); M = particle mass (g); g = acceleration due to gravity = 980 cm/s^2; ρ = particle density (g/cm^3); ρ_{air} = air density (g/cm^3).

EXAMPLE 8.4

Calculate the terminal velocities of spherical particles of U_3O_8 whose diameters are 1 μm and 20 μm. The density of U_3O_8 is 8.30 g/cm^3.

Solution

Substituting the respective values into Eq. (8.17), we have for the 1-μm particle:

$$v_t = \frac{(10^{-4}\,\text{cm})^2 \times 8.30\,\dfrac{\text{g}}{\text{cm}^3} \times 980\,\dfrac{\text{cm}}{\text{s}^2}}{18 \times 1.85 \times 10^{-4}\,\dfrac{\text{g}}{\text{cm/s}}}$$

$$v_t = 0.0244\,\frac{\text{cm}}{\text{s}} = 0.048\,\frac{\text{ft}}{\text{min}},$$

and for the 20-μm particle, the terminal velocity is calculated as

$$v_t = 9.76\,\frac{\text{cm}}{\text{s}} = 19.2\,\frac{\text{ft}}{\text{min}}.$$

The difference between the terminal settling velocities of the 1-μm- and 20-μm-diameter particles is striking. However, even the settling velocity of the 20-μm particle is less than the ambient air velocities of about 13 cm/s (25 ft/min) in occupied space. A 20-μm particle could thus be carried a relatively long distance by air currents before falling out.

Particles that differ in size and density are said to be *aerodynamically equivalent* if they have the same terminal settling velocity. If the two particles are aerodynamically equivalent, then

$$v_{t1} = v_{t2}$$

$$\frac{d_1^2 \rho_1 g}{18\eta} = \frac{d_2^2 \rho_2 g}{18\eta}$$

$$\frac{d_1}{d_2} = \sqrt{\frac{\rho_2}{\rho_1}}. \tag{8.18}$$

To normalize data for particles of different sizes and densities, we calculate the aerodynamically equivalent size of unit density particles. This normalized size is called the mass median aerodynamic diameter (MMAD). For example, with Eq. (8.18) we calculate that a U_3O_8 aerosol, $\rho = 8.3$ g/cm^3, whose *actual* mass median diameter (MMD) is 1 μm, is aerodynamically equivalent to a 2.9-μm particle whose density is 1 g/cm^3. That is, a U_3O_8 particle whose physical diameter is 1 μm has a MMAD of 2.9 μm, and behaves aerodynamically like a 2.9-μm particle whose density is 1 g/cm^3. Since the activity of a radioactive particle is directly proportional to its mass, we can describe the mean size of a radioactive aerosol by its activity mean aerodynamic diameter (AMAD) size. In radiation safety standards, particle sizes refer to the sizes of those particles whose aerodynamic behavior is equivalent to that of unit density particles.

Thermodynamic Properties

When particle sizes approach the size of air molecules, the random collisions with the air molecules impart enough energy to the aerosol particles to influence the motion of the aerosol particles. The resulting random motion of the air molecules is known as *Brownian motion,* and is the basis for the diffusion process. (The physics of Brownian motion was explained by Albert Einstein in the second of his four revolutionary papers during the annus mirabilis, the "miracle year" of 1905.) The mean thermal displacement during a time interval t, of particles suspended in a gaseous medium is independent of the particle density, and is given by

$$s = \sqrt{\frac{RT}{N} \times \frac{Ct}{3\pi\eta d}};$$
(8.19)

s is in cm when

> $R =$ gas constant $= 8.3 \times 10^7$ ergs/mol/K
> $T =$ temperature, K
> $N =$ Avogadro's number $= 6.02 \times 10^{23}$ molecules/mol
> $t =$ time interval, seconds
> $d =$ particle size, cm
> $\eta =$ viscosity of the medium $= 185 \times 10^{-6}$ g/cm/s for standard air
> $C =$ Cunningham slip correction factor. This factor corrects for the fact that the air is not a continuous medium, but consists of discrete molecules. A particle may thus "slip" between molecules. This slip factor becomes increasingly important as the particle size approaches the mean free path of the gas molecules, and
> $C = 1 + 1.7\lambda/d$, where $\lambda =$ mean free path of the gas molecules $= 6.7 \times 10^{-6}$ cm for air at 25°C.

Diffusion becomes increasingly important as a particle transport mechanism as the particle size decreases below 1 μm. The Table 8-6 shows the displacement during 1 second by gravitational settling and by diffusion of a unit density particle of 3 different sizes.

TABLE 8-6. Effect of Particle Size on Displacement Distance by Diffusion and by Gravitational Settling

PARTICLE SIZE (μm)	DIFFUSION (μm)	GRAVITATIONAL SETTLING (μm)
0.1	22.4	0.6
1.0	5.1	29.4
10.0	1.5	2940

Aerodynamic sizes are used when inertial and gravitational effects are the main determinants of a particle's behavior. For very small particles, where diffusional effects are significant, approximately ≤0.5 μm, we specify the particle size by its thermodynamic size. The thermodynamic diameter of a particle is approximately equal to the diameter of a sphere whose volume is the same as that of the particle in question. Two particles are said to be thermodynamically equivalent if their diffusion coefficients are equal. That is, if their displacement by diffusion is the same for a given time interval. The thermal size is approximately related to the aerodynamic size of a particle whose density is ρ by

$$d_{th} \approx 1.2 d_{ae} \rho^{-0.5}. \tag{8.20}$$

Inhaled Radioactive Particles

The depth of penetration of airborne particles into the respiratory tract depends on the size of the airborne particles. Large dust particles, in excess of about 5 μm, are likely to be filtered out by the nasal hair or to impact on the nasopharyngeal surface. The effect of gravitational settling becomes less pronounced as the particle size decreases. For example, a 20-μm-diameter particle of unit density settles at a velocity about 1 cm/s, while a 1-μm particle of this material settles at a rate of only 0.003 cm/s. For practical purposes, therefore, small particles may be regarded as remaining suspended in the atmosphere, and all but very large particles may be considered to be carried by moving air. In the respiratory tree, because of the relatively small cross-sectional areas of many of the air passages, the inspired air may attain relatively high velocities. Large particles that escape the hair-filter in the nose therefore have high kinetic energies as they pass through the air passages. As a consequence of the momentum of such a heavy particle, it cannot follow the inspired air around sharp curves, and strikes the walls of the upper respiratory tract. As the particle size decreases below 5 μm, this inertial impact decreases, and an increasing number of particles are carried down into the lung. The air in the alveoli is relatively still—since only a small fraction of the air there is exchanged with incoming air during a respiratory excursion. Particles that are carried into the deep respiratory tract, therefore, have the opportunity to settle out under the force of gravity. Gravitational settling, however, decreases with decreasing particle size and reaches a minimum when the particle size is about 0.5 μm. As the particle size decreases below about 0.1 μm, the effect of Brownian motion becomes significant. As the particles move randomly about, they may strike the alveolar wall and get trapped on its moist surface. The combination of these three effects—inertial impaction, gravitational settling, and Brownian motion—leads to a maximum likelihood of deposition in the deep respiratory tract for particles in the 1–2-μm size range, and a minimum deposition for particles between 0.1 and 0.5 μm, as shown in Figure 8-5.

The retention of particles in the lung depends on the area within the respiratory tract where the particles were deposited, on the physical and chemical properties of the particles, and on the physiologic properties of the lung. Retention of the inhaled particles, or its inverse—pulmonary clearance—is important in determining the degree of hazard because of its role in tissue exposure time, rate of dissolution, and total dose. Studies of pulmonary retention of various dusts show that the curve of dust remaining in the lung after cessation of exposure is fitted by a complex

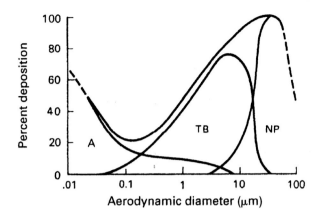

Figure 8-5. Deposition of dust in the respiratory tract. Region A represents principally alveolar deposition, region TB is mainly tracheobronchial deposition, and region NP represents mainly nasopharyngeal deposition. Total deposition is the sum of these three regions. (Reproduced with permission from Morrow PE. Evaluation of inhalation hazards based upon the respirable duse concept and the philosphy and application of selective sampling. *AIHA J.* 1964; 25(3):213–236. With permission of Taylor & Francis. http://www.informaworld.com.)

exponential curve that includes at least two components: one of half-retention time on the order of several hours, and the other on the order of days. Very often, the long-lived component is also complex, and may be resolved into two or three components. Algebraically, this curve is given by the equation

$$Q(t) = Q_1 e^{-k_1 t} + Q_2 e^{-k_2 t} + \cdots .\tag{8.21}$$

Figure 8-6 illustrates a typical two-component retention curve, which is described by the first two terms of Eq. (8.21).

In this curve, the first component represents the dust in the upper respiratory tract; Q_1 is the quantity of dust deposited there, while k_1 gives the rate at which it is cleared from the upper respiratory tract. Q_2 represents the quantity of dust deposited initially in the deep respiratory tract, and k_2 is the deep respiratory-tract clearance rate.

At least three distinct mechanisms are thought to operate simultaneously to remove foreign particles from the lung. The first of these mechanisms, ciliary clearance, can act only in the upper respiratory tract. The rhythmic beating of the cilia propels particles upward into the throat at high speeds—from whence they are swallowed. Particle velocities ranging from about 2 mm/min in the bronchi to about 3 cm/min in the trachea have been observed. The other two clearance mechanisms deal mainly with particles in the deep respiratory tract. They include solubility and absorption into the capillary bed across the alveolar membrane and removal by phagocytosis. It should be pointed out that the solubility in water of any given substance may not necessarily be a good index of solubility in the lung. For example, mercury from [203]HgS, one of the most insoluble compounds known, was found in significant quantities in the kidneys and in the urine of rats exposed to HgS particles of about 1 μm; the tagged mercury could have gotten there only after solution of the particles. On the other hand, [144]Ce intratracheally injected as CeCl₃ solution was found to be tenaciously retained in the lung for very long periods of time. In

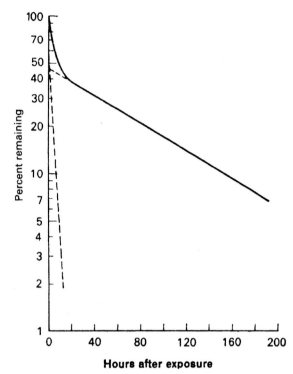

Figure 8-6. Pulmonary retention curve showing amount of BaSO$_4$ particulate activity remaining in the rat lung as a function of time after exposure. The curve shows that 53% of the dust was deposited in the upper respiratory tract; the clearance rate from the upper respiratory tract is 27% per hour. Forty seven percent of the dust was deposited in the deep respiratory tract and was cleared at a rate of 1% per hour.

this case, the Ce in solution was bound to the tissue protein in the lung; very little of the cerium found its way into the blood. The case of cerium, however, seems to be exceptional. Most inhaled soluble particles are absorbed into the blood and their chemical constituents translocated to other organs and tissues, where they may be systemically absorbed. The lung can thus be an excellent portal of entry into the body for many different radionuclides.

Phagocytosis, which is the engulfing of foreign particles by alveolar macrophages and their subsequent removal either up the ciliary "escalator" or by entrance into the lymphatic system, is a major pulmonary clearance mechanism. Phagocytes loaded with radioactive particles may be trapped in the sinuses of the tracheobronchial lymph nodes, and may remain there for long periods of time. This accumulation of radioactive dust in the lymph nodes may result in a higher radiation dose to the lymph nodes than to the lungs. The rate of phagocytosis depends to a large degree on the nature of the dust particle. Different particles have been found to be phagocytized at different rates. Furthermore, it has been found that radioactive particles are phagocytized more slowly than nonradioactive particles of the same chemical composition, physical form, and size distribution.

It is clear, from the multiplicity of factors that play a role in determining the biological effects of inhaled radioactive materials, that no simple quantitative relationship between gross atmospheric concentration of a radioisotope and lung effects can be assumed. Conservative criteria, derived from physiologically based biokinetic models of the human respiratory tract (HRT), are therefore used when setting safety standards for airborne radioactivity.

Lung Models

Radiation dosimetry and calculation of inhalation ALIs and acceptable atmospheric concentrations of radioactivity are based on dosimetric models of the respiratory tract. The first such dosimetric model was introduced by the ICRP in 1959. It was a relatively simple model that considered only aerosols and modeled the lung as a two-compartment system: the upper respiratory tract and the deep respiratory tract, and only two classes of particle solubility, "soluble" and "insoluble." The ICRP 2 recommendations for maximum permissible concentrations (MPCs) of airborne particulate radioactivity in the workplace were based on this model. These recommendations were incorporated into the IAEA's first edition of its basic safety standards (1962) and into the radiation safety regulations of the various countries, including the United States, in the Atomic Energy Commission's (AEC) Part 20 of 10 CFR.

ICRP 30 Lung Model

In 1978, in its Publication 30, the ICRP introduced a more sophisticated dosimetric model of the respiratory tract in order to account for the oversimplification and deficiencies of the earlier two-compartment model. The newer model accounted for the fact that deposition of particles in the respiratory tract is governed by airflow patterns in the respiratory tract and by the size distribution of the inhaled aerosol, and that the clearance rate of the deposited particles is governed by the deposition site as well as by chemical and physical properties of the particles. The ICRP 30 dosimetric lung model was designed to calculate the mean dose to blood-filled lungs from inhaled particles in the size range of 0.2–10 μm in size. This model was used as the basis for safety standards for inhaled radioactive aerosols that were published in ICRP 30 and again in 1990 in the revised standards published in ICRP 61. The U.S. NRC based its 1991 revision of 10 CFR 20 atmospheric concentrations on the ICRP 30 dosimetric model.

Figure 8-7 is a graphic representation of the ICRP 30 dosimetric lung model used to calculate the inhalation ALIs in ICRP 30, ICRP 61, and in the U.S. NRC's 1991 revision of its 10 CFR 20 regulations. This lung model consists of three regions where inhaled aerosols may be deposited: The nasopharyngeal region (NP), the tracheobronchial region (TB), and the pulmonary region (P) representing the deep respiratory tract where gas exchange occurs. The NP region is divided into two compartments, a and b. Compartment a represents that part in which the dust deposited in the NP region dissolves and is absorbed directly into the blood. Compartment b represents the region from which dust is cleared into the GI tract by swallowing. The TB region is also represented by two compartments, c and d, from which deposited particles are cleared by the same two mechanisms as above. Compartment c represents the region in which dissolution and absorption into the blood takes place, whereas the mechanical transfer by way of the ciliary escalator to the throat and

REGION	COMPARTMENT	CLASS					
		D		W		Y	
		T	F	T	F	T	F
NP	a	0.01	0.5	0.01	0.1	0.01	0.01
(D_{NP} = 0.30)	b	0.01	0.5	0.40	0.9	0.40	0.99
TB	c	0.01	0.95	0.01	0.5	0.01	0.01
(D_{TB} = 0.08)	d	0.2	0.05	0.2	0.5	0.2	0.99
	e	0.5	0.8	50	0.15	500	0.05
P	f	n.a.	n.a.	1.0	0.4	1.0	0.4
(D_P = 0.25)	g	n.a.	n.a.	50	0.4	500	0.4
	h	0.5	0.2	50	0.05	500	0.15
L	i	0.5	1.0	50	1.0	1000	0.9
	j	n.a.	n.a.	n.a.	n.a.	∞	0.1

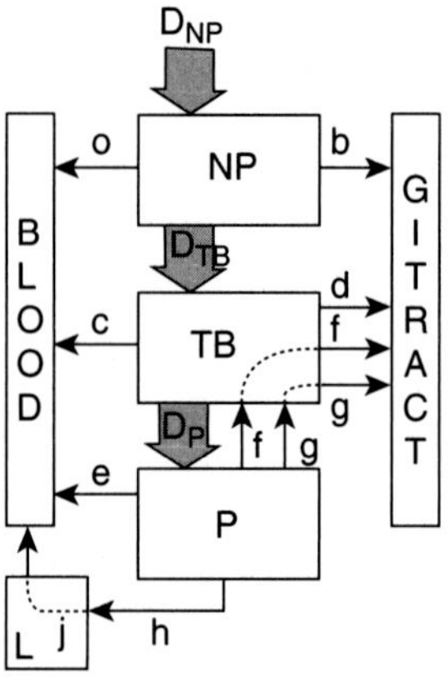

Figure 8-7. ICRP 30 respiratory tract model used to calculate inhalation limits for airborne radioactive particles. The values for removal half-times, T_{a-j}, and compartmental fractions, F_{a-j}, are given in the tabular portion of the figure for each of the three classes of retained materials. The values given for D_{NP}, D_{TB}, and D_P (left column) are the regional depositions based on an aerosol with an activity mean aerodynamic diameter (AMAD) of 1 μm. The schematic drawing identifies the various clearance pathways, a–j, in relation to the deposition D_{NP}, D_{TB}, D_P and the three respiratory regions: nasopharyngeal (NP), trachobronchial (TB), and pulmonary (P). The entry "n.a." indicates "not applicable." (From Watson SB, Ford MR. *A User's Manual to the ICRP Code: A Series of Computer Programs to Perform Dosimetric Calculations for the ICRP Committee 2 Report.* Oak Ridge, TN: Oak Ridge National Laboratory; February 1980. TM-6980.)

into the GI tract by swallowing is represented by compartment *d*. The pulmonary region, P, is modeled by four compartments. One of these compartments, *e*, represents dissolution and absorption into the blood. Compartments *f* and *g* represent transfer of undissolved particles into the GI tract via the upper respiratory tract (the TB region). Compartment *f* is cleared by mechanical transport, presumably by unbalanced forces during respiratory excursions, and compartment *g* is cleared by alveolar macrophages that migrate into the TB region. Compartment *h* empties into the pulmonary lymph nodes. The pulmonary lymph nodes are represented by two compartments, *i* and *j*. Compartment *i* empties into the bloodstream after the particles have dissolved, while compartment *j* permanently retains some highly insoluble particles.

The exact fraction of the deposited aerosol that is cleared by each route and the respective clearance rates are governed by the chemical composition of the aerosol and particle size. However, since it is not practical to determine each of these parameters for every compound of every element, the various compounds of all the elements have been assigned, to one of three classes: D, W, and Y. Class D aerosols are rapidly cleared from the deep respiratory tract with a clearance half-time on the order of a day or a fraction of a day. Class W aerosols are cleared on the order of weeks, while class Y materials are retained in the lungs on the order of years. Of the various forms of dust that may be transported to the lymph nodes, only class Y materials are permanently retained in the lymph nodes. For health physics purposes, the lung and the pulmonary lymph nodes are considered as a single organ. That is, the activity in the lung and in the lymph nodes is added together, and the total weight of the lungs and pulmonary lymph nodes is used to calculate dose from inhaled aerosols. The ICRP's recommendations for inhaled aerosols are based on inhalation and deposition of an aerosol whose AMAD is 1 μm and whose geometric standard deviation is 4. This assumed distribution leads to deposition of 30% of the inhaled dust in the NP region, 8% in the TB region, and 25% in the P region. The balance, 37% is exhaled. Deposition for other size distributions is shown in Figure 8-8.

Material brought up from the lung and swallowed enters the GI tract, from which it may subsequently be eliminated in the feces, irradiating the various parts of the GI tract and other organs during its passage. It may also undergo dissolution in the GI tract, and the dissolved portion may be absorbed into the blood and transferred to organs where it may be deposited (Fig. 8-9). Thus, for example, inorganic mercury is deposited mainly in the kidneys, iodine in the thyroid, strontium and radium in the skeleton, and plutonium in the liver and skeleton. The fraction of the activity deposited in the lung that is subsequently transferred to the blood may be calculated with the information given in the lung model. In Figure 8-8, we see that inhaled 1-μm AMAD particles are deposited in the respiratory tract with the regional distribution shown in Table 8-7.

Figure 8-7 tells us the fractions of the deposited particles that are cleared from the lung by each of the two clearance mechanisms: (1) dissolution and direct absorption into the blood and (2) physical transport to the throat followed by swallowing into the GI tract. In the case of highly soluble class D particles, for example, one-half of the 30% deposited in the NP region, 95% of the inhaled aerosol deposited in the TB region, and all of the inhaled particles (25%) deposited in the P region are transferred directly to the blood by dissolution:

$$(0.5 \times 0.3) + (0.95 \times 0.08) + (1 \times 0.25) = 0.48.$$

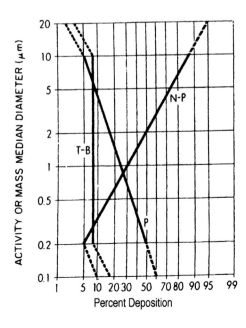

Figure 8-8. ICRP 30 particle deposition model. The radioactive or mass fraction of an aerosol which is deposited in the nasopharyngeal (NP), trachobronchial (TB), and pulmonary (P) regions is given in relation to the activity or mass median aerodynamic diameter (AMAD or MMAD) of the aerosol distribution. This model is intended for use with aerosol distributions having an AMAD or MMAD between 0.2 and 10 μm and whose geometric standard deviations are less than 4.5. Provisional deposition estimates further extending the size range are given by the dashed lines. For the unusual distribution having an AMAD or MMAD greater than 20 μm, complete NP deposition is assumed. The model does not apply to aerosols with AMAD or MMAD below 0.1 μm.

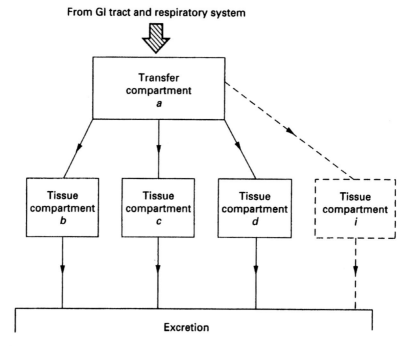

From GI tract and respiratory system

Figure 8-9. Model used to describe the kinetics of radionuclides in the body. *Abrreviation:* GI, gastrointestinal. (Reproduced with permission from ICRP Publication 30, Part 1: Limits for Intakes of Radionuclides by Workers. *Ann ICRP.* 1979; 2(3/4):17. Copyright © 1979 International Commission on Radiological Protection.)

From the particles deposited in the respiratory tract and transported to the GI tract, the activity transferred to the blood is

$$(0.5 \times 0.3 \times f_1) + (0.05 \times 0.08 \times f_1) = 0.15 f_1,$$

where f_1 represents the fraction of the radionuclide in the GI tract that is absorbed into the blood. Similar calculations can be made for class W and Y particles. The results of these calculations are given in Table 8-8.

The GI tract is modeled by four distinct regions, each with its own kinetic parameters, so that organ doses during passage of radionuclides can be calculated. Similarly, the organs where the radionuclides are deposited are also modeled by appropriate equations, usually one or more first-order linear differential equations that allow the organ doses to be calculated.

TABLE 8-7.   Pulmonary Deposition of 1-μm AMAD Particles

REGION	PERCENT DEPOSITED
NP	30
TB	8
P	25
Total	63

Abbreviations: AMAD, activity mean aerodynamic diameter; NP, nasopharyngeal; TB, tracheobronchial; P, pulmonary.

TABLE 8-8. Fractions of Activity in the Lung from Inhaled 1-μm Particles That Are Transferred to the Blood

CLASS	FRACTION
D	$0.48 + 0.15\, f_1$
W	$0.12 + 0.51\, f_1$
Y	$0.05 + 0.58\, f_1$

EXAMPLE 8.5

Inhalation ALI According to ICRP 30 Criteria

Calculate the inhalation ALI, according to ICRP 30 criteria, of ^{137}Cs particles. The AMAD of the particles is 1 μm and the geometric standard deviation less than 4.5. Table 8-7 shows that 63% of the inhaled dust is deposited in the respiratory tract and 37% is exhaled. For purposes of ALI calculations, particles of cesium compounds are assigned to clearance category D, since they are found to be cleared rapidly from the lungs. The amount of activity deposited in each of the lung compartments following an inhalation of 1 Bq, together with the corresponding removal rate, is shown in Table 8-9.

Solution

We shall calculate the committed dose equivalent from the 1-Bq intake. Then we shall determine how many becquerels may be inhaled before reaching the limiting committed dose equivalent. To do this, we shall calculate the dose to the lung from the ^{137}Cs deposited in the lung and then from the ^{137}Cs distributed in the rest of the body, which also irradiates the lungs. Next, we shall calculate the whole-body dose from the inhaled activity. In making these calculations, it should be noted that the material deposited in the NP region does not contribute to the intrapulmonary dose; it contributes to the lung dose only by virtue of its presence in the rest of the body. The intrapulmonary dose from the 1-Bq intake is due only to the 0.08-Bq ^{137}Cs deposited in the TB region and the 0.25 Bq deposited in the P region.

TABLE 8-9. Activity Deposited in the Several Compartments of the Lung after an Inhalation of 1-Bq ^{137}Cs , and the Clearance Rates for Each Compartment

COMPARTMENT	$A_S(0)$ (t/s)	$T_{1/2}$ (d)	$\lambda_E (d^{-1})$
c (TB → blood)	0.076	0.01	69.3
d (TB → GI)	0.004	0.2	3.47
e (P → blood)	0.200	0.5	1.39
f (P → LN)	0.050	0.5	1.39
LN	0.050	0.5	1.39

Abbreviations: TB, tracheobronchial; GI, gastrointestinal; P, pulmonary; LN, lymph nodes. See Figure 8.7 for values of $T_{1/2}$. Note that $A_S(0)$ is the fraction deposited in a particular compartment multiplied by the compartmental fraction listed in Figure 8.7, i.e., $A_S(0)$ for compartment c is $0.08 \times 0.95 = 0.076$.

The 50-year committed dose equivalent to a target T after deposition of 1 Bq can be calculated with Eq. (8.22):

$$H_{50,T} = \frac{1.6 \times 10^{-13} \, \frac{J}{MeV} \times \sum U_S \, \text{transf.} \times \text{SEE} \, (T \leftarrow S) \, \frac{MeV}{t/kg}}{1 \, \frac{J/kg}{Gy}}.$$

(8.22)

The SEE (lung ← lung) is calculated from the output data for ^{137}Cs (Fig. 8-2), together with the specific AFs listed in Appendix D. Table 8-10 shows the organization of the data to obtain the SEE for each of the electrons and photons and their summation to yield 0.280 MeV per transformation per kg.

$$\sum \text{SEE} \left(\text{lung} \leftarrow \text{lung}\right) = 0.28 \, \frac{MeV}{t/kg}$$

$$\sum \text{SEE}(\text{lung} \leftarrow \text{total body}) = 6.5 \times 10^{-3} \, \frac{MeV}{t/kg}.$$

Next, we calculate the cumulated number of transformation in the lung during the 50 years following the 1-Bq intake. To do this, we add the number of transformations in each compartment of the lung. The cumulated number of transformations in a

TABLE 8-10. Organization of Data for Calculation of Specific Effective Energy in the Lung from Inhaled ^{137}Cs

RADIATION	NUMBER/ TRANS, n_i	ENERGY Per Particle, E_i(MeV)	LUNG ← LUNG Specific Absorbed Fraction ϕ_i (kg^{-1})	SEE (MeV/t/kg)	LUNG ← TOTAL BODY Specific Absorbed Fraction ϕ_i (kg^{-1})	SEE (MeV/t/kg)
β_1	0.935	0.1749	1	1.64E − 01	1.43E − 02	2.34E − 03
β_2	0.065	0.4272	1	2.78E − 02	1.43E − 02	3.97E − 04
γ	0.840	0.6616	4.8E − 02	2.70E − 02	5.11E − 03	2.84E − 03
K int. con. el.	0.0781	0.6242	1	4.88E − 02	1.43E − 02	6.97E − 04
L int. con. el.	0.0140	0.6560	1	9.18E − 03	1.43E − 02	1.31E − 04
M int. con. el.	0.0031	0.6605	1	1.52E − 03	1.43E − 02	2.93E − 05
$K_{\alpha 1}$ X-ray	0.0374	0.0322	2.26E − 01	2.72E − 04	1.22E − 02	1.47E − 05
$K_{\alpha 2}$ X-ray	0.0194	0.0318	2.26E − 01	1.39E − 04	1.22E − 02	7.35E − 06
$K_{\beta 1}$ X-ray	0.0105	0.0364	2.17E − 01	8.29E − 05	1.13E − 02	4.32E − 06
$K_{\beta 2}$ X-ray	0.0022	0.0374	2.15E − 01	1.77E − 05	1.10E − 02	9.05E − 07
L X-rays	0.0127	0.0045	1	5.72E − 05	1.43E − 02	8.12E − 07
KLL Auger el.	0.0057[a]	0.0263	1	1.50E − 04	1.43E − 02	2.14E − 06
KXY Auger el.	0.0025	0.0308	1	7.70E − 05	1.43E − 02	2.02E − 07
KLX Auger el.	0.0004	0.0353	1	1.41E − 05	1.43E − 02	2.02E − 07
LMM Auger el.	0.0718	0.0034	1	2.44E − 04	1.43E − 02	3.49E − 06
MXY Auger el.	0.173	0.0011	1	1.9E − 04	1.43E − 02	2.72E − 06

[a]Auger electrons are photoelectrons that are ejected by characteristic X-rays. The first two letters give the transition that gave rise to the X-ray, and the last letter gives the electron shell from which the Auger electron was ejected. The letters X and Y represent electron shells beyond the L level.

Abbreviation: SEE, specific effective energy.

compartment after a time t is given by

$$U_S(t) = \frac{A_S(0)\, \text{Bq} \times 1\, \dfrac{\text{t/s}}{\text{Bq}}}{\lambda_E \text{s}^{-1}} (1 - e^{-\lambda_E t}), \tag{8.23a}$$

where $A_S(0)$ is the activity initially deposited in the compartment and λ_E is the effective clearance constant for the compartment. For a very long time relative to the effective half-time of the isotope (50 years for ICRP calculations), Eq. (8.23) reduces to

$$U_S(50\text{years}) = \frac{A_S(0)\, \text{Bq} \times 1\, \dfrac{\text{t/s}}{\text{Bq}}}{\lambda_E\, \text{s}^{-1}}. \tag{8.23b}$$

The total cumulated number of transformations in the lung is the sum of the cumulated transformations in each of the j compartments:

$$U = \sum_j \frac{A_{Sj}}{\lambda_{Ej}}. \tag{8.24}$$

Since 50 years is a very long time relative to the effective half-time of cesium in every one of the lung compartments, the cumulated number of transformations in the lung is calculated from Eq. (8.24) with the values listed in Table 8-9.

$$U_{\text{lungs}} = 8.64 \times 10^4 \text{ s/d}$$

$$\times \left\{ \frac{0.076 \text{ t/s}}{69.3 \text{ d}^{-1}} + \frac{0.004 \text{ t/s}}{3.47 \text{ d}^{-1}} + \frac{0.200 \text{ t/s}}{1.39 \text{ d}^{-1}} + \frac{0.050 \text{ t/s}}{1.39 \text{ d}^{-1}} + \frac{0.050 \text{ t/s}}{1.39 \text{ d}^{-1}} \right\}$$

$$U_{\text{lungs}} = 1.9 \times 10^4 \text{ transformations.}$$

The committed dose equivalent to the lung from ^{137}Cs in the lung is calculated from Eq. (8.22):

$$H_{50} = \frac{1.6 \times 10^{-13}\, \dfrac{\text{J}}{\text{MeV}} \times 1.9 \times 10^4 \text{ t} \times 0.280\, \dfrac{\text{MeV}}{\text{t/kg}} \times 1\, \dfrac{\text{Sv}}{\text{Gy}}}{1\, \dfrac{\text{J/kg}}{\text{Gy}}}$$

$$H_{50} = 8.6 \times 10^{-10} \text{ Sv.}$$

The next step is to calculate the committed dose equivalent to the lungs from the ^{137}Cs in the rest of the body. The total amount absorbed into the body includes contributions from that deposited in the NP region as well as from that deposited in the lungs. The total amount absorbed into the body is

$$0.3 + 0.08 + 0.25 - 0.63 \text{ Bq.}$$

Retention of ^{137}Cs in the body is given by Eq. (6.59). The equation tells us that 10% of the absorbed cesium, or 0.063 Bq, is transferred to the compartment whose clearance rate is 0.347 per day, while 90%, or 0.567 Bq, is transferred to the compartment that is cleared at a rate of 0.0063 per day. The total number of transformations in the body from the 0.63 Bq deposited in the respiratory tract after inhalation of 1 Bq and subsequently transferred to the body is given by Eq. (8.22):

$$U_{body} = 8.64 \times 10^4 \; \frac{s}{d} \left(\frac{0.063 \text{ t/s}}{0.347 \text{ d}^{-1}} + \frac{0.567 \text{ t/s}}{0.0063 \text{ d}^{-1}} \right)$$

$$U_{body} = 7.8 \times 10^6 \text{ transformations.}$$

Using the gamma and X-ray specific AFs for (lung←total body) obtained by interpolating between the values listed in Appendix D, and the beta-ray- and electron-specific AF of 1.43×10^{-2}, as calculated from Eq. (6.92), and then by summing the SEE of each contributing radiation as shown in Table 8-8, we find the SEE (lung←total body) to be 6.47×10^{-3} MeV per transformation per kg. The 50-year committed dose equivalent to the lung from the ^{137}Cs in the body is calculated from Eq. (8.22):

$$H_{50} = \frac{1.6 \times 10^{-13} \; \dfrac{J}{MeV} \times 7.8 \times 10^6 \text{ t} \times 6.74 \times 10^{-3} \; \dfrac{MeV}{t/kg} \times 1 \; \dfrac{Sv}{Gy}}{1 \; \dfrac{J/kg}{Gy}}$$

$$H_{50} = 8.4 \times 10^{-9} \text{ Sv.}$$

The total (50-year) committed dose equivalent to the lungs, therefore, from the inhalation of 1 Bq ^{137}Cs is

$$H_{50} = 8.6 \times 10^{-10} \; \frac{Sv}{Bq} + 8.4 \times 10^{-9} \; \frac{Sv}{Bq} = 9.3 \times 10^{-9} \; \frac{Sv}{Bq}.$$

In the calculation for the ingestion ALI, it was found that the committed dose equivalent from ^{137}Cs uniformly distributed throughout the body is

$$\frac{0.05 \text{ Sv}}{3.9 \times 10^6 \text{ Bq}} = 1.3 \times 10^{-8} \; \frac{Sv}{Bq}.$$

Since only 0.63 Bq is absorbed into the body when 1 Bq is inhaled, and using the tissue-weighting factors of 0.12 for the lung and 0.88 for the remainder of the body, we find the committed effective dose equivalent (CEDE) from 1 Bq of inhaled ^{137}Cs to be

$$\text{CEDE} = \sum_T w_T H_{50,T} = (0.12 \times 9.3 \times 10^{-9}) + 0.63(0.88 \times 1.3 \times 10^{-8})$$

$$\text{CEDE} = 8.3 \times 10^{-9} \; \frac{Sv}{Bq}.$$

The inhalation SALI is calculated according to ICRP 26 and 30 criteria from Eq. (8.8):

$$\text{SALI(inhalation)} = \frac{0.05 \text{ Sv}}{8.3 \times 10^{-9} \; \dfrac{Sv}{Bq}} = 6 \times 10^6 \text{ Bq.}$$

Now we must determine whether the SALI will lead to a committed dose equivalent greater than 0.5 Sv in any organ or tissue. Since the cesium that is transferred out of the lung to the body is uniformly distributed throughout the body, no tissue will receive a CEDE greater than the 1.3×10^{-8} Sv/Bq delivered to the whole body. The product of the SALI and the whole-body committed dose equivalent from the 0.63 Bq deposited in the body is

$$6 \times 10^6 \, \text{Bq} \times 0.63 \times 1.3 \times 10^{-8} \, \frac{\text{Sv}}{\text{Bq}} = 0.05 \, \text{Sv}.$$

Since the SALI leads to a committed dose equivalent less than 0.5 Sv, the SALI is applicable and limits the inhaled intake of ^{137}Cs to 6×10^6 Bq during 1 year.

Inhalation ALI According to ICRP 60 Criteria

Publication 60 of the ICRP recommends a primary dose limit of 100 mSv over a 5-year period, with a maximum in any 1 year of 50 mSv, or an average of 20 mSv/yr. In addition, it does away with the nonstochastic classification, and bases all its recommendations for derived limits on a committed effective dose of 20 mSv/yr. It also changed the nomenclature from "*dose equivalent*" to "*equivalent dose.*" The ALIs for ingestion and for inhalation are thus calculated by

$$\text{ALI} = \frac{0.02 \, \text{Sv}}{\sum_T w_T H_{50,T} \, \frac{\text{Sv}}{\text{Bq}}}, \tag{8.25}$$

where the denominator is the committed effective dose either by ingestion or by inhalation. For example, in the case of ^{137}Cs, we found the CEDE from ingested activity to be 1.3×10^{-8} Sv/Bq. By substituting this value into Eq. (8.25), we find the ingestion ALI to be

$$\text{ALI (ingestion)} = \frac{0.02 \, \text{Sv}}{1.3 \times 10^{-8} \, \frac{\text{Sv}}{\text{Bq}}} = 1.54 \times 10^6 \, \text{Bq} = 2 \, \text{MBq}.$$

and for inhalation, we have

$$\text{ALI (inhalation)} = \frac{0.02 \, \text{Sv}}{8.3 \times 10^{-9} \, \frac{\text{Sv}}{\text{Bq}}} = 2.41 \times 10^6 \, \text{Bq} = 2 \, \text{MBq}.$$

ICRP 66 Human Respiratory Tract Model

A still more sophisticated dosimetric model for the HRT, called the human respiratory tract model (HRTM), was recommended by the ICRP in 1994, in Publication 66. This new dosimetric model is the result of increased knowledge of the biokinetics of the respiratory processes involved in the inhalation of aerosols and gases, the radiosensitivity of the several different tissues within the respiratory tract, and the biological effects of inhaled radioactivity. This increased knowledge makes the new model applicable to all population groups, old and young, male and female, and at different levels of physical activity (heavy exercise, light exercise, resting, and sleeping), rather than only to occupationally exposed, unisexual adults at work. It accounts for the effects of other air pollutants and for smoking, and considers respiratory disease and the health status of the individual. While with the ICRP 30 model only the average dose to the lung was calculated, the ICRP 66 dosimetric model allows the calculation of the doses to the various tissues within the respiratory tract and then the weighting of the mean doses to the various tissues within the respiratory tract according to the radiosensitivity of the tissue. The ICRP 66 HRTM is used by the IAEA and by most regulatory agencies outside the United States as the basis for the safety standards and dose conversion factors (DCFs) for airborne radioactivity. At this time (2008), the United States has not yet adopted the new HRTM, and the NRC safety standards are based on the ICRP 30 lung model.

When dealing with the safety aspects of exposure to airborne radioactivity, which includes aerosols and gases or vapors, we are interested in the answers to several questions:

1. What is in the air, and what is being inhaled?
2. Which of the inhaled aerosols are exhaled and which are deposited in the respiratory tract?
3. Where in the respiratory tract are inhaled particles deposited?
4. What is the fate of the deposited particles?
5. What is the radiation dose from this inhalation exposure?
6. How much of the airborne radioactivity may be safely inhaled?

The new model of the HRT gives a more realistic response to these questions than does the previous model by dealing quantitatively with the inhalability of aerosols, the deposition of inhaled aerosols based on particle size and on airflow velocity in the various airways in the respiratory tract, and on the time-dependent decreased clearance rates from the lungs. Calculation of the lung dose with the new model is fundamentally different from the calculation with the earlier lung models. While the mean dose to uniform blood-filled lungs was calculated with the previous model, the new model considers the several different cell types in the respiratory tract, their masses, and their relative sensitivities to radiation. The dose to each of these different tissues is calculated, and then the pulmonary tissue doses are combined, through the use of appropriate weighting factors, to obtain the effective lung dose.

While the previous models were designed for the purpose of calculating secondary safety standards for occupational exposure to aerosols on the size range of 0.2–10 μm, the new model was made to be universally useful by extending its range of applicability to include

- particle sizes from 0.0006 μm to 100 μm,
- males and females,
- 3-month-old infants to adults,
- nose and mouth breathers,
- breathing rates for four different levels of exertion: sleeping, sitting, light exercise, and heavy exercise,
- the effects of smoking, air pollutants, and pulmonary diseases,

- classification of particles on the basis of the rate of absorption of the inhaled radioactivity into the blood (instead of classifying particles on the basis of their solubility as classes D, W, and Y):

  - type F (fast)—100% absorbed into blood in ≤10 minutes,
  - type M (moderate)—10% absorbed into blood in ≤10 minutes, 90% absorbed in ≤140 days, and
  - type S (slow)—0.1% absorbed in ≤10 minute, 99.9% absorbed in >140 days.

- gases as well as aerosols.

The updated HRTM is designed to calculate the DC, which is defined as the committed dose per unit intake, rem/μCi or Sv/Bq, of an airborne radionuclide. The HRTM supplies only the first part of this calculation—the dose to the lung and the rate of transfer of the inhaled radioactivity to the body fluids and to the GI tract. The biokinetic model for the particular radionuclide must then be used to complete the calculation of the DC.

The ICRP 66 model consists of five interrelated submodels: anatomical (morphometric), physiological, deposition, clearance, and dosimetry models.

Anatomical Model. The anatomical model describes the overall structure, including airway dimensions, of the HRT. ICRP 66 models the respiratory tract by four sequential anatomical regions (Fig. 8-10):

1. Extrathoracic (ET) region—the portion of the respiratory tract outside of the chest, which contains two subparts:

   - ET_1, consisting of the anterior nasal airways.
   - ET_2, consisting of the posterior nasal airways, pharynx, and larynx.

2. Bronchial (BB) region, which includes the trachea and the bronchi.
3. Bronchiolar (bb) region, consisting of bronchioles and terminal bronchioles.
4. Alveolar-interstitial (AI) region, which consists of the respiratory bronchioles, the alveoli, and interstitial connective tissue.

Each region is drained by lymphatic fluid, which flows into lymph nodes. The lymph nodes that drain the ET region are symbolized by LN_{ET}, and those that drain the 3 thoracic regions are labeled LN_{TH}. For dosimetry purposes, only LN_{TH} nodes contribute to the lung dose. The ET lymph nodes, LN_{ET}, are considered as "other tissues" when calculating the effective dose.

The physical dimensions and branching angles of the air pathways in the tracheobronchial tree are listed in ICRP 66 for the adult male. For example, the trachea is given as 1.65 cm (diameter) × 9.1 cm (length)—each of the five primary bronchi is 1.2 cm (diameter) × 3.8 cm (length)—and is at an angle of 36° (which represents the change in direction of the bulk flow of air from the trachea into the primary bronchi). Continuous bifurcation of the bronchi leads to increasing numbers of smaller airways, until the dead-ended alveoli are reached. The alveoli are the functional part of the respiratory tract, where inhaled oxygen diffuses into the blood and carbon dioxide diffuses out of the blood into the alveoli to be exhaled. The total surface area available for gas exchange in the alveoli is 140 m². These dimensions are scaled down for females and for younger persons.

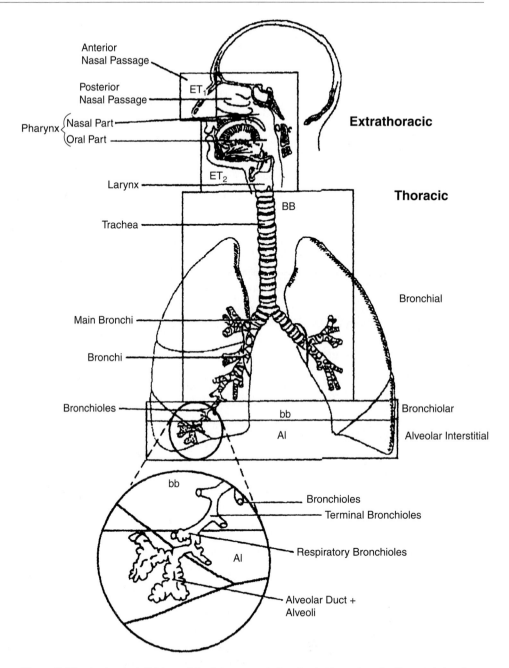

Figure 8-10. Anatomical divisions of the human respiratory tract. (Reproduced with permission from ICRP Publication 66: Human Respiratory Tract Model for Radiological Protection. *Ann ICRP.* 1994; 24(1–3). Copyright © 1994 International Commission on Radiological Protection.)

Physiological Model. The physiological model describes the functional aspects of the HRT. The kinetics of respiration, including volumes of inhaled air and inhalation rates are given for males and females of various ages and for the four different levels of physical exertion that the model considers, and for nose and for mouth breathers. Correction factors are also given for conditions that modify or impair the normal functioning of the respiratory tract, such as old age, various illnesses, and smoking.

The importance of these physiological considerations may be illustrated by comparing the velocity of inhaled air in the trachea of a male worker when he is seated and when he is engaged in heavy exercise. While sitting, he inhales air at a maximum rate of 300 mL/s. Using the default tracheal diameter of 1.65 cm, this leads to a maximum airstream velocity in the trachea of 140 cm/s. While engaged in heavy physical exertion, the worker's maximum inhalation rate is 1670 mL/s, which leads to a maximum airstream velocity of 781 cm/s. These two very different velocities lead to significant differences in deposition patterns of inhaled particles.

Deposition Model. Deposition of particles in the respiratory tract is calculated on the basis of particle size, velocity of the air, and the geometrical contours of the air path. Deposition, therefore, depends on the person's age, sex, and ventilation rate.

When the mean particle size of an aerosol distribution exceeds about 0.5 μm, deposition is determined mainly by the aerodynamic properties of the particle, and the AMAD or the MMAD is used in the description of the aerosol size. (For a solid radioactive particle, the activity is directly proportional to the particle's mass.) When the mean size is less than about 0.5 μm, diffusion is the main deposition mechanism, and the mean size is expressed as the activity median thermodynamic diameter (AMTD).

To simulate particle deposition, the respiratory tract is modeled as a prefilter followed by a successive series of filters (Fig. 8-11). The prefilter represents the nares and the anterior nasal airways. Each of the successive filters represents the successive anatomical regions in the respiratory tract. Therefore, smaller fractions of the inhaled particles pass through each successive filter. In this model, filtration occurs during both inhalation and exhalation. Using this model, and considering the simultaneous deposition mechanisms of inertial impaction, gravitational settling, and diffusion of particles in the respiratory tract, deposition fractions for each region were calculated for equivalent sizes of 0.0006–100 μm. The deposition of 0.001–100 μm particles in the respiratory tract of a male worker are plotted in Figure 8-12. Table 8-11 lists the regional depositions of a 5-μm AMAD aerosol inhaled by an adult male reference worker and the regional depositions of a 1-μm AMAD aerosol in an adult male member of the public.

Clearance Model. Radioactive particles are cleared from the HRTM by three independent processes: mechanical transfer, dissolution of particles, and radioactive decay. Actual clearance is the sum of these three processes acting simultaneously.

The clearance model deals with the transfer, to the throat, of the deposited radioactive particles up the respiratory tract from the deposition sites and then into the GI tract by swallowing. Concurrently with this mechanical transfer via the ciliary action, the model deals with dissolution of deposited particles and the absorption of the dissolved radioactivity into the blood. It also accounts for the time-dependent changing clearance rates from each of the intrathoracic regions.

Mechanical Transfer. Mechanical transfer, which accounts for the transport of particles to the GI tract and to the lymph nodes, is affected by ciliary action and phagocytosis within the lungs and by sneezing and coughing in the ET airways. The modeled mechanical clearance rates are independent of particle type, sex, and

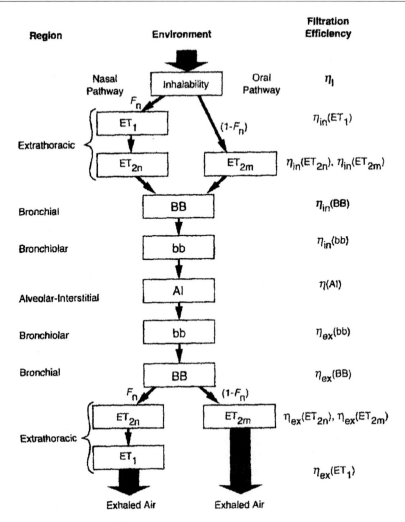

Figure 8-11. Filter model for deposition of inhaled particles in the respiratory tract of a reference worker. Two intake pathways are considered: the nasal pathway for which the fractional airflow is F_n; and the oral pathway, for which the fractional airflow is $1 - F_n$. The subscripts "in" and "ex" of the filtration efficiency, η, represent the inhalation and exhalation phases of the breathing cycle. (Reproduced with permission from ICRP Publication 66: Human Respiratory Tract Model for Radiological Protection. *Ann ICRP.* 1994; 24(1–3). Copyright © 1994 International Commission on Radiological Protection.)

age. However, in vivo laboratory studies on animals and bioassay studies on humans show a time dependence of pulmonary clearance rate. That is, initially most particles are rapidly cleared, and the remaining particles are cleared more slowly. The time dependence is modeled by dividing each region into several compartments that empty at different rates, as shown in Figure 8-13. Each region contains a compartment that is very slowly cleared. For ET_2, BB, and bb regions, the very slowly cleared compartment is subscripted "seq" (for sequestered). The fraction of each regional deposit that is assigned to the several compartments is specified by the model, and is listed in Table 8-12.

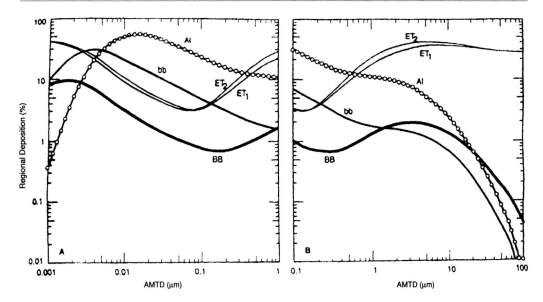

Figure 8-12. Fractional deposition in each region of the respiratory tract of a reference nose-breathing worker as functions of (**A**). activity median thermodynamic diameter, AMTD, and (**B**). the activity median aerodynamic diameter, AMAD. Deposition is expressed as a fraction of the activity present in the volume of inspired air, and the radioactive particles sizes are log-normally distributed. The particles' specific gravity is 3 and the shape factor is 1.5. *Abbreviations:* AI, alveolar-interstitial; bb, bronchiolar; ET, extrathoracic; BB, bronchial. (Reproduced with permission from ICRP Publication 66: *Human Respiratory Tract Model for Radiological Protection. Ann ICRP.* 1994; 24(1–3). Copyright © 1994 International Commission on Radiological Protection.)

For modeling purposes, the numerical values for the size-dependent parameter f_s in Table 8-12 is given for two categories of aerodynamic diameter, d_{ae}:

- if $d_{ae} \leq 2.5 \left(\dfrac{\rho}{\chi} \right)^{0.5} \mu m$,

  then $f_s = 0.5$.

- if $d_{ae} > 2.5 \left(\dfrac{\rho}{\chi} \right)^{0.5} \mu m$,

  then $f_s = 0.5 \exp\left[-0.63 \left(d_{ae} \sqrt{\tfrac{\chi}{\rho}} - 2.5 \right) \right]$.

TABLE 8-11. Regional Deposition of 5-μm and 1-μm AMAD Aerosols in Two Persons

REGION	WORKER, 5 μm (%)	ADULT MALE, 1 μm (%)
ET$_1$	33.9	16.5
ET$_2$	39.9	21.1
BB	1.8 (33%in BB$_2$)	1.2 (47% in BB$_2$)
bb	1.1 (40% in bb$_2$)	1.7 (49% in bb$_2$)
AI	5.3	11.7
Total	82.0	51.2

Abbreviations: ET, extrathoracic; BB, bronchial; bb, bronchiolar; AI, alveolar-interstitial.

Reproduced with permission from Guide for the Practical Application of the ICRP Human Respiratory Tract Model, Supporting Guidance 3. *Ann ICRP.* 2002; 32(1,2). Copyright © 2002 International Commission on Radiological Protection.

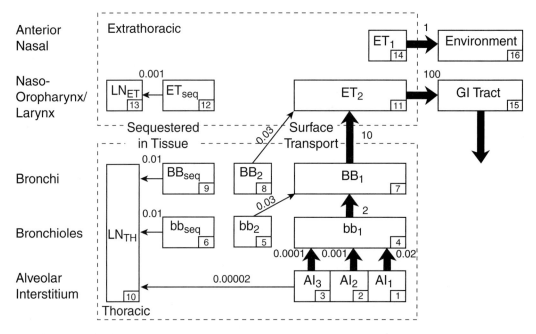

Figure 8-13. Compartmental model to represent time-dependent particle transport in the respiratory tract. The arrows show the transport pathway, and the numbers represent the compartmental clearance rates, per day. *Abbreviations:* ET, extrathoracic; LN_{ET}, lymph nodes (extrathoracic); LN_{TH}, lymph nodes (thoracic); BB, bronchial; bb, bronchiolar; AI, alveolar-interstitial; GI, gastrointestinal. (Reproduced with permission from ICRP Publication 66: Human Respiratory Tract Model for Radiological Protection. *Ann ICRP.* 1994; 24(1–3). Copyright © 1994 International Commission on Radiological Protection.)

The partitioning among the compartments in the bb and BB regions is dependent on the particle size; the partition factors for the other regions are independent of the particle size. For example, for the particles deposited in the AI region, 30% of the deposit is in the AI_1 compartment, which empties to the bb_1 compartment at a rate of 0.02 (2%) per day, 60% of the AI deposit is in the AI_2 compartment,

TABLE 8-12. Factors for Partitioning Regional Deposits Among the Regional Compartments

REGION	COMPARTMENT	FRACTION TO COMPARTMENT
ET_2	ET_2	0.9995
	ET_{seq}	0.0005
BB	BB_1	$0.993 - f_s$
	BB_2	f_s
	BB_{seq}	0.007
bb	bb_1	$0.993 - f_s$
	bb_2	f_s
	bb_{seq}	0.007
AI	AI_1	0.3
	AI_2	0.6
	AI_3	0.1

Abbreviations: ET, extrathoracic; BB, bronchial; bb, bronchiolar; AI, alveolar-interstitial.

Reproduced with permission from ICRP Publication 66: Human Respiratory Tract Model for Radiological Protection. *Ann ICRP.* 1994; 24(1–3). Copyright © 1994 International Commission on Radiological Protection.

whose clearance rate to bb_1 is 0.001 per day. Ten percent of the deposit is in the AI_3 compartment, which is cleared very slowly at a rate of 0.0001 per day to bb_1 and at a rate of 0.00002 per day to the thoracic lymph nodes, LN_{TH}. Additionally S_t per day (see paragraph below and Table 8-13) dissolves and is absorbed into the blood. The effective clearance rate for compartment AI_3 is the sum of the clearance rates for each of the three pathways: $\lambda_E(AI_3) = 0.0001 + 0.00002 + S_t$ per day. The quantity of activity in the AI region at time t days after deposition of activity Q Bq (or μCi) in region AI can be described mathematically by the three compartment retention curve:

$$Q_{AI}(t) = 0.3\, e^{-0.02t} + 0.6\, e^{-0.01t} + 0.1\, e^{-(0.00012+S_t)t}. \tag{8.26}$$

In the BB and bb regions, 0.007 of the deposit is sequestered and is cleared to LN_{TH} at a rate of 0.01 per day. The partition fractions of the regional deposits among the several different compartments are listed in Table 8-12.

Particle Dissolution. Transfer of particulate radioactivity to the blood is modeled as a two-stage process: dissolution of the particle followed by its absorption into the body fluids, including the blood. The model assumes that absorption into the body fluids occurs at the same rate from all the parts of the HRTM except ET_1, where no absorption occurs.

The rate of solubilization of a particle is a function of its size, because dissolution is a surface phenomenon. As a particle dissolves, its surface area rapidly decreases. The rate of dissolution, therefore, decreases with time as the particle continues to dissolve. The HRTM deals with this decreasing rate of dissolution in two alternate ways. In the first time-dependent alternative, a fraction of the deposited activity, f_r, dissolves rapidly and is absorbed at a rate of S_r per day. The remaining fraction, $1 - f_r$, dissolves slowly and is absorbed at a rate S_s per day. According to this model, the overall fractional dissolution rate, f_d, of the intrapulmonary deposit dissolving and being absorbed at time t days after deposition is

$$f_d(t) = f_r e^{-S_r t} + (1 - f_r)e^{-S_s t}. \tag{8.27}$$

A situation where the dissolution and absorption rates increased with time could be modeled by the second alternative through a suitable choice of values for the parameters. In the alternative model, shown in Figure 8-14, the regional deposits are said to be in an "initial" state. Some of these particles dissolve at a constant rate S_p per day, and the rest of the particles are simultaneously changed into a "transformed" state at a rate S_{pt} per day. In the transformed state, the particles dissolve and the dissolved activity is absorbed into the body fluids at a rate of S_t per day, which is different from the absorption rate of the untransformed particles. For the usual case where the dissolution and absorption rates decrease with time, both models are equivalent. The parameters of the two alternative absorption models are related by the following equations:

$$S_p = S_s + f_r(S_r - S_s), \tag{8.28}$$

$$S_{pt} = (1 - f_r)(S_r - S_s), \text{ and} \tag{8.29}$$

$$S_t = S_s. \tag{8.30}$$

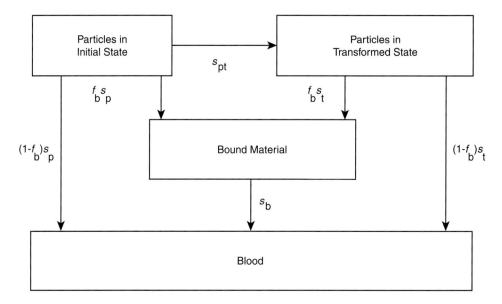

Figure 8-14. Compartmental model for time-dependent absorption into blood. *Source:* Human respiratory tract model for radiological protection. (Reproduced with permission from ICRP Publication 66: Human Respiratory Tract Model for Radiological Protection. *Ann ICRP.* 1994; 24(1–3). Copyright © 1994 International Commission on Radiological Protection.)

In the absence of material-specific absorption rates, the default values for the solubility and absorption parameters recommended by the ICRP for each of the three solubility–absorption categories are listed in Table 8-13. Both alternatives postulate that a certain fraction, f_b, of the dissolved particles is chemically bound to the tissue, and that the bound material eventually diffuses into the body fluids. This "bound" state is a special case for which specific binding data must be available. Therefore, the "bound" state is not used for setting default values, that is, $f_b = 0$ for all three solubility–absorption categories.

The model representing the overall clearance of particles from the respiratory tract is shown in Figure 8-15.

TABLE 8-13. Default Values of Absorption Parameters for Type F, M, and S Materials

PARAMETER	F	M	S
f_r	1	0.1	0.001
S_r (d^{-1})	100	100	100
S_s (d^{-1})	—	0.005	0.0001
S_p (d^{-1})	100	10	0.1
S_{pt} (d^{-1})	0	90	100
S_t (d^{-1})	—	0.005	0.0001

Reproduced with permission from ICRP Publication 66: Human Respiratory Tract Model for Radiological Protection. *Ann ICRP.* 1994; 24(1–3). Copyright © 1994 International Commission on Radiological Protection.

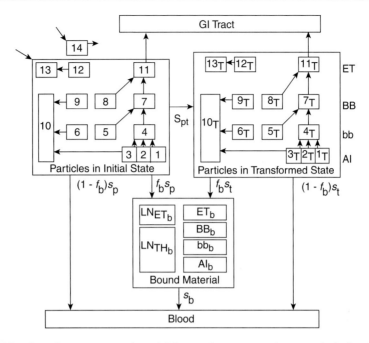

Figure 8-15. Overall compartmental model for respiratory tract clearance, including both time-dependent particle transport and absorption into the blood. *Abbreviations:* GI, gastrointestinal; ET, extrathoracic; BB, bronchial; bb, bronchiolar; AI, alveolar-interstitial; LN$_{ET}$, lymph nodes (extrathoracic); LN$_{TH}$, lymph nodes (thoracic).

Dosimetric Model. The HRT is considered as two separate organs for dosimetric purposes. The thoracic region is considered to be the lungs, and the ET region is considered as one of the "remainder" tissues when we calculate the EDE. Each of these organs consists of several different types of cells of differing radiosensitivity, and lie at different depths below the tissue–air interface (Table 8-14). Figure 8-16 shows the modeled tube that contains the tissue–air interface and the source and target tissues in airways in the ET, BB, and bb regions. For example, the sensitive target cells in the bb region are the nuclei of the secretory (Clara) cells (Fig. 8-17) that lie within the epithelial layer shown in Figure 8-16. These cells are believed to be the progenitor cells for squamous cell carcinoma, the most frequently occurring lung cancer. These depths are important because alphas, betas, and electrons that are emitted from radioactive particles that are deposited on the interface surface dissipate some of their energy in passing through the less-sensitive tissue. Thus, only a fraction of the energy of the emitted radiation is absorbed by the sensitive target cells. Figure 8-18 shows the absorbed fractions, AF (T←S) of beta particle energy that is absorbed by the target cells in the bb region. ICRP Publication 66 contains values for the AFs of all the target cells from alphas, betas, and electrons that originate in the various parts of the respiratory tract, as well as tables of the specific AFs of photon energy in various tissues and organs with the lungs as the source.

The HRTM is used to calculate the radiation dose to the lungs from an inhaled radioisotope. The dose to the rest of the body from the radioactivity transferred from the respiratory system to the blood requires knowledge of the

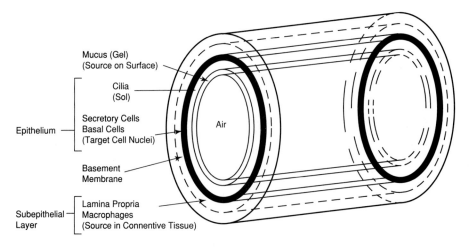

Figure 8-16. Simplified geometrical model of the tissue–air interface and the source and target tissues in dosimetry of the extrathoracic, bronchial, and bronchiolar regions. (Reproduced with permission from ICRP Publication 66: Human Respiratory Tract Model for Radiological Protection. *Ann ICRP.* 1994; 24(1–3). Copyright © 1994 International Commission on Radiological Protection.)

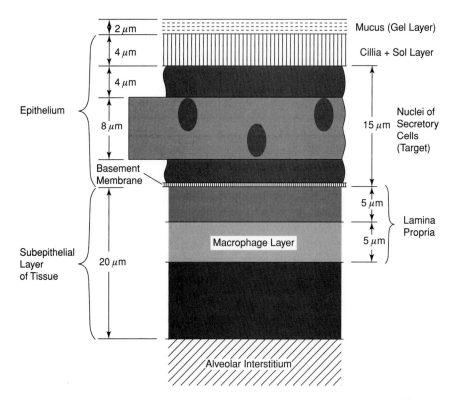

Figure 8-17. Dosimetric model of the target cells (secretory cells) in the bronchiolar wall of the bronchiolar region. (Reproduced with permission from ICRP Publication 66: Human Respiratory Tract Model for Radiological Protection. *Ann ICRP.* 1994; 24(1–3). Copyright © 1994 International Commission on Radiological Protection.)

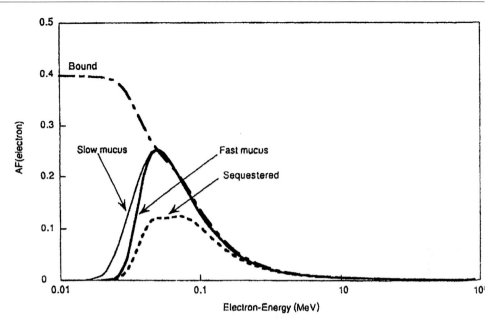

Figure 8-18. Absorbed fractions for betas emitted in the bronchiolar (bb) region. Curves are shown for emissions from the mucous gel layer (fast mucous), sol layer (slow mucous), sequestered, and bound activity. (Reproduced with permission from ICRP Publication 66: Human Respiratory Tract Model for Radiological Protection. *Ann ICRP.* 1994; 24(1–3). Copyright © 1994 International Commission on Radiological Protection.)

TABLE 8-14. Target Cells and Assigned Fraction of w_T (Lung)

REGION	COMPARTMENT	TARGET CELL	CRITICAL TISSUE DEPTH (μm)	MASS (kg)	A OF w_T
Extra thoracic airways	ET₁ (anterior nose)	Basal	40–50	2.0N5[a]	0.001
	ET₂ (posterior nose, mouth, pharynx, larynx)	Basal	40–50	4.5N4	0.998
	LN_ET (lymphatics)			1.5N2	0.001
Thoracic airways (lungs)	BB (bronchial)	Basal	35–50	4.3N4	0.333
		Secretory	10–40	8.6N4	0.333
	bb (bronchiolar)	Secretory	4–12	1.9N3	0.333
	AI (alveolar-interstitial)			1.1	0.333
	LN_TH (lymphatics)			1.5N2	0.001

[a] 2.0N5 means 2×10^{-5}, 4.5N4 means 4.5×10^{-4}, etc.

Note: Regional doses, with weighting factors A assigned for the partition of the radiation detriment, are summed to give a value of committed dose equivalent for the extrathoracic region and another for the thoracic region, as follows:

$$H_{ET} = H_{ET1} \times A_{ET1} + H_{ET2} \times A_{ET2} + H_{LN(ET)} \times A_{LN(ET)}$$
$$H_{TH} = H_{BB} \times A_{BB} + H_{bb} \times A_{bb} + H_{AI} \times A_{AI} + H_{LN(TH)} \times A_{LN(TH)}$$
H_{TH} is considered the lung, $w_f = 0.12$

When calculating effective dose equivalent, H_{ET} is considered a "remainder" tissue dose.

Reproduced with permission from ICRP Publication 66: Human Respiratory Tract Model for Radiological Protection. *Ann ICRP.* 1994; 24(1–3). Copyright © 1994 International Commission on Radiological Protection.

metabolic kinetics or a physiologically based biokinetic model for that radioisotope.) or element. To calculate the lung dose from inhaled radioactive particles we

1. determine the regional deposition of the particles,
2. apportion the deposition within the regional compartments,
3. calculate the activity in each compartment, including the activity transported into the compartment from other compartments,
4. calculate compartmental mean residence time (MRT), including activity lost from each compartment by mechanical transport, dissolution, and radioactive decay,
5. calculate the total number of disintegrations in each compartment,
6. calculate the total energy emitted in each compartment,
7. calculate the total energy absorbed by the target tissues, using values from Tables G and H in ICRP 66 (abstracted in Table 8-17),
8. divide absorbed energy by mass of target tissues (Table 8-13, which is abstracted from Table 5, ICRP 66),
9. multiply the dose absorbed in each tissue by the appropriate radiation and tissue weighting factors, w_R and w_T, and
10. calculate lung dose $= w_R \sum H_T w_T$.

Calculation of the lung dose using the ICRP 66 HRTM is a long, tedious, and complex operation that requires input of many physiological and physical parameters whose values are listed in the model. Accordingly, computer models that incorporate these many numerical values and computational methodologies have been devised. A computer program for the respiratory tract, such as LUDEP, is usually used together with an internal dosimetry program, such as CINDY or IMBA to calculate the doses to other organs and the effective dose from inhaled radionuclides.

The principles of the HRTM computational methodology may be illustrated with the following relatively simple example:

 EXAMPLE 8.6

Calculate the lung dose from the intake of 1 Bq ^{14}C tagged tungsten carbide, WC, particles whose AMAD is 5μm. The CRC *Handbook of Chemistry and Physics* lists WC as insoluble, and thus is a type S material; its specific gravity is 15.6, and the default shape factor of 1.5 will be used in the calculation.

Solution

From the regional deposition curves, we find the fraction of the intake that is deposited in each region.

REGION	FRACTION DEPOSITED
ET_1	0.34
ET_2	0.40
BB	0.018
bb	0.011
Al	0.053

Table 8-15 (17-B, ICRP 66) gives the size-dependent partition of a regional deposit into the several regional compartments. For the BB region, the slowest cleared fraction of the bronchial deposit is called BB_{seq}, and is listed as 0.007. The next more-rapidly cleared fraction is listed as f_s, and fastest cleared fraction is given $0.993 - f_s$. The value for f_s is size dependent, and is given by the following relations:

- for $d_{ae} \leq 2.5 \left(\dfrac{\rho}{\chi} \right)^{0.5} \mu m$, $f_s = 0.5$,

- for $d_{ae} > 2.5 \left(\dfrac{\rho}{\chi} \right)^{0.5} \mu m$, $f_s = 0.5 \exp \left[-0.63 \left(d_{ae} \sqrt{\dfrac{\chi}{\rho}} - 2.5 \right) \right]$.

For the case of WC we have: $2.5(15.6/1.5)^{0.5} = 8.1$. Since $d_{ae} = 5\,\mu m < 8.1$, therefore, $f_s = 0.5$. Using this value for f_s, we can calculate the activity deposited in each of the regional compartments:

The MRT in each compartment is given by

$$ \text{MRT} = \frac{1}{\lambda_E}, \tag{8.31} $$

where λ_E = effective clearance rate constant $= \lambda_{ab} + S_s + \lambda_R$.

For very long lived insoluble activity, $\lambda_R \approx 0$, therefore,

$$ \lambda_E = (\lambda_{ab} + 0.0001) \text{ per day.} $$

TABLE 8-15. *Compartmental Distribution of Deposited Activity*

REGION	REGIONAL FRACTIONAL DEPOSIT	COMPARTMENT	COMPARTMENTAL FRACTIONAL DEPOSIT	DEPOSITED ACTIVITY (Bq)
ET_1	0.34	ET_1	1	0.34
ET_2	0.40	ET_2	0.9995	0.3998
		ET_{seq}	0.0005	0.0002
BB	0.018	BB_1	$0.993 - 0.5 = 0.493$	0.22887
		BB_2	0.5	0.0090
		BB_{seq}	0.007	0.00013
bb	0.011	bb_1	$0.993 - 0.5 = 0.493$	0.00542
		bb_2	0.5	0.0055
		bb_{seq}	0.007	0.000077
Al	0.053	Al_1	0.3	0.0159
		Al_2	0.6	0.0318
		Al_3	0.1	0.0053

ET, extrathoracic; BB, bronchial; bb, bronchiolar; Al, alveolar-interstitial.

TABLE 8-16. Mean Compartmental Residence Times

REGION	COMPARTMENT	$\lambda_E(d^{-1})$	MRT (d)
ET_1	ET_1	$1 + 0.0001$	0.9999
ET_2	ET_2	$100 + 0.0001$	0.01
	ET_{seq}	$0.001 + 0.0001$	909.1
LN_{TH}	LN_{TH}	0.0001	10,000
BB	BB_1	$10 + 0.0001$	0.1
	BB_2	$0.03 + 0.0001$	33.223
	BB_{seq}	$0.01 + 0.0001$	99.01
bb	bb_1	$2 + 0.0001$	0.499975
	bb_2	$0.03 + 0.0001$	33.223
	bb_{seq}	$0.01 + 0.0001$	99.010
AI	AI_1	$0.02 + 0.0001$	49.751
	AI_2	$0.001 + 0.0001$	909.1
	AI_3	$0.0001 + 0.00002 + 0.0001$	4545.5

Abbreviations: MRT, mean residence time; ET, extrathoracic; LN_{TH}, lymph nodes (thoracic); BB, bronchial; bb, bronchiolar; AI, alveolar-interstitial.

For example, the transfer rate λ_{ab} from bb_2 to BB_1 is 0.03 per day. Therefore, MRT in compartment bb_2 is

$$MRT(bb_2) = \frac{1}{(0.03 + 0.0001)} = 33.223 \text{ days.}$$

The mean compartmental residential times for all the pulmonary compartments, as calculated above for compartment bb_2, are listed in Table 8-16.

Now, we will calculate the number of disintegrations in a compartment that contribute to the dose to that compartment. These disintegrations are from activity that had been deposited there during inhalation plus activity that had been transferred from deeper compartments. Tissues in AI_1, AI_2, and AI_3 are irradiated only, in the case of pure alpha and pure low-energy beta emitters, such as ^{14}C betas, by the activity deposited there. High-energy betas and gammas from activity in the other compartments can also irradiate the AI region. In our example, we have only the low-energy betas from ^{14}C, and thus the compartments in the AI region are irradiated only from the activity deposited there. The number of disintegrations in any P region that contribute to the dose is the sum of the contributions from the several compartments within that region: The number of disintegrations in a compartment, ci, that contribute to the dose is

$$N_{ci}(\text{dose}) = A_{ci} \frac{\text{dis}}{\text{s}} \times 8.64 \times 10^4 \frac{\text{s}}{\text{d}} \times MRT_{ci} \text{ days,} \tag{8.32}$$

and the total number of disintegrations in a region, N_{Ri}, is

$$N_{Ri} = \sum N_{ci}. \tag{8.33}$$

For the AI region, for example, the number of disintegrations in the three compartments is

$$
\begin{aligned}
N_{AI1} &= 0.0159 \text{ dps} \times 86400 \text{ s/d} \times 49.75 \text{ d} & = 68{,}346 \text{ disintegrations} \\
N_{AI2} &= 0.0318 \text{ dps} \times 86400 \text{ s/d} \times 909.1 \text{d} & = 2{,}497{,}770 \text{ disintegrations} \\
N_{AI3} &= 0.0053 \text{ dps} \times 86400 \text{ s/d} \times 4545.5 \text{ d} & = 2{,}081{,}475 \text{ disintegrations} \\
N_{AI} &= \text{Total disintegrations in AI} & = 4{,}647{,}591 \text{ disintegrations}
\end{aligned}
$$

The bb compartments are irradiated by the activity deposited there plus the activity brought up from the compartments in the AI region. Activity transferred from a given compartment is equal to the activity initially deposited there minus the sum of the dissolved activity plus the decayed activity:

Activity transferred = deposited activity − (dissolved + decayed) activity.   **(8.34)**

For long-lived activity, such as in ^{14}C, decay may be neglected. The slow dissolution rate (Table 8-13) is 0.0001 per day. For the half-day mean retention time, an insignificant amount will have dissolved, and we can ignore the decrease in activity by solution. Therefore, the number of disintegrations in bb_1 due to activity transferred from AI_1 to bb_1 ($AI_1 \rightarrow bb_1$), that contribute to the dose to bb_1 is

$$0.0159 \text{ Bq} \times \frac{1 \text{dps}}{\text{Bq}} \times 86,400 \, \frac{\text{s}}{\text{d}} \times 0.499975 \text{ d} = 687 \text{ disintegrations.}$$

Similar calculations for transfers to bb_1 from AI_2 and AI_3 plus the activity initially deposited there, yield a total of 2,318 disintegrations in compartment bb_1. In the bb_2 compartment, we calculate 15,788 and in bb_{seq}, 659 disintegrations. The number of disintegrations in each compartment that contribute to the regional dose, which was calculated by multiplying the activity in the source by the mean retention time from Table 8-16, is listed in Table 8-17.

The radiosensitive target cells within the HRT are irradiated from several different sources of radioactive particles that are located in several different parts of the respiratory system. In the ET regions, for example, the radiation sources are particles that lie directly on the surface of the skin, by particles sequestered by macrophages that are concentrated in the subepithelial tissue of the airway wall, and by radionuclides chemically bound to the epithelium.

Target cells in the BB and bb regions are irradiated by radioactive particles that are being transported by the fast-moving mucous and by the slow-moving mucous within the airways of the upper respiratory tract, by particles sequestered in macrophages, by radioactivity chemically bound to the airway wall, and by particles that are within the alveolar-interstitium. The AI region is irradiated by radioactive particles within the alveoli and by particles in the bb and BB regions. The fractions of the energy emitted from the several sources that are absorbed by the radiosensitive target cells, $AF(T \leftarrow S)$, are listed in ICRP 66 Tables H.1 to H.5. Absorbed fractions for three beta emitters: tritium, $\bar{E} = 0.0056$ MeV; ^{14}C, $\bar{E} = 0.0498$ MeV; and ^{32}P, $\bar{E} = 0.6918$ MeV, which are taken from ICRP 66 Table H.5, are shown in Table 8-18.

To calculate the dose to the lung, we will

(1) calculate the regional equivalent dose, H_R,

(2) multiply the regional doses by the appropriate fraction, A, of the tissue weighting factor, w_T, for the lung (from Tables 8-3 and 8-14), and

(3) sum the products $H_R \times A$ to calculate the equivalent dose to the lungs.

$$H(\text{lungs}) = \sum (H_R \times A) \text{ Sv (or rem).} \tag{8.35}$$

TABLE 8-17. Compartmental Disintegrations That Contribute to Regional Dose

REGION	COMPARTMENT	DEPOSITED IN	AMOUNT DEPOSITED (Bq)	NUMBER OF DISINTEGRATIONS	TOTAL NUMBER OF DISINTEGRATIONS
Al	Al_1	Al_1	0.0159	68,346	
	Al_2	Al_2	0.0318	2,497,745	
	Al_3	Al_3	0.0053	2,081,455	4,647,546
bb	bb_1	bb_1	0.00542	234	
		Al_1	0.0159	687	
		Al_2	0.0318	1374	
		Al_3	0.0053	104	2399
	bb_2	bb_2	0.0055	15,788	15,788
	bb_{seq}	bb_{seq}	0.000077	659	659
BB	BB_1	BB_1	0.01187	102	
		bb_1	0.00652	56	
		bb_2	0.0055	48	
		Al_1	0.0159	137	
		Al_2	0.0318	275	
		Al_3	0.0053	21	639
	BB_2	BB_2	0.00591	16,956	16,956
	BB_{seq}	BB_{seq}	0.000125	1072	1072
LN_{TH}	LN_{TH}	Al_3	0.0053	342,870	
		bb_{seq}	0.000077	55,250	
		BB_{seq}	0.000125	89,907	488,027
ET_2	ET_2	ET_2	0.3998	346	
		BB_1	0.01187	10	
		BB_2	0.00591	5	
		bb_1	0.00652	6	
		bb_2	0.0044	4	
		Al_1	0.0159	14	
		Al_2	0.0318	25	
		Al_3	0.0053	2	412
	ET_{seq}	ET_{seq}	0.0002	15,709	15,709
ET_1	ET_1	ET_1	0.34	29,373	29,373
LN_{ET}	LN_{ET}	ET_{seq}	0.0002	15,709	15,709

Abbreviations: Al, alveolar-interstitial; bb, bronchiolar; BB, bronchial; LN_{TH}, lymph nodes (thoracic); ET, extrathoracic; LN_{ET}, lymph nodes (extrathoacic).

The regional dose is calculated by

$$H_R = \frac{N \text{ dis} \times \bar{E} \dfrac{\text{Mev}}{\text{dis}} \times 1.6 \times 10^{-13} \dfrac{\text{J}}{\text{MeV}} \times \text{AF}(T \leftarrow S)}{m \text{ kg}}$$

$$\times 1 \frac{\text{Gy}}{\text{J/kg}} \times w_T \frac{\text{Sv}}{\text{Gy}}, \tag{8.36}$$

where

$\bar{E}$ is the average energy of the beta particle, MeV/dis. For the ^{14}C beta in this illustrative example, $\bar{E} = 0.0498$ MeV,

TABLE 8-18. Values of Absorbed Fractions, AF (T ← S), for Negatrons

T	ET₁			ET₂				BB_bas					BB_sec					BB_sec
S	Surf.	Bound	Sequ.	Fast mucous	Slow mucous	Bound	Sequ.	AI	Fast mucous	Slow mucous	Bound	Sequ.	AI	Fast mucous	Slow mucous	Bound	Sequ.	AI
$\bar{E}$																		
0.0056	0	1.82N1	2.81N5	0	0	2.50N1	1.01N6	0	0	2.18N6	5.00N1	0	0	0	1.57N1	3.98N1	0	0
0.0498	4.56N2	2.32N2	1.22N1	9.71N1	2.16N1	5.08N2	1.89N1	9.85N2	0	2.35N1	3.99N1	1.01N1	0	1.65N1	2.17N1	9.62N1	0	3.68N4
0.6918	1.13N2	8.03N3	1.32N2	1.25N2	1.56N2	1.58N2	1.81N2	1.60N2	2.37N4	3.50N2	3.67N2	3.73N2	2.98N2	9.20N3	9.25N3	1.02N2	8.26N3	1.71N3

Note: N1 = 10^{-1}, N5 = 10^{-5}, etc.

Abbreviations: T, target; S, source; ET, extrathoracic; BB, bronchial; bb, bronchiolar; AI, alveolar-interstitial.

Abstracted with permission from James AC, Akabani G, Birchall A, Jarvis NS, Briant NS, Durham JS. Annexe H: absorbed fractions for alpha, electron, and beta emissions. *Ann ICRP.* 1994; 24(1–3):459–482. Copyright © 1994 International Commission on Radiological Protection.

AF(T←S) is the fraction of the energy emitted from the source S by the target tissue T (from Table 8-17, which is abstracted from Tables H.1 to H.5, ICRP 66),

m is the mass of the target tissue (Table 8-14 from Table 5, ICRP 66), and

w_T is the tissue weighting factor (from Table 8-14).

Using the disintegration data from Table 8-15, the values of AF(T←S) from Table 8-17, the tissue weighting factor, w_T, from Table 8-3 and tissue mass, m, from Table 8-13, we can calculate the dose to each region. For example, for the basal cells in the BB region, we have

COMPARTMENT	N_C, DISINTEGRATIONS	AF(T←S)$_C$
BB_1	604	0.0508
BB_2	16,956	0.0542
BB_{seq}	1,072	0.0985
AI	4,647,546	0

$\bar{E} = 0.0498$ MeV,

$w_T = 0.1665$ (= 1/2 of 0.333), and

$m = 0.00043$ kg.

We obtain the dose to the basal cells in the BB region by summing the contributions from each of the compartments

$$H(BB)_{bas} = \frac{E \, \frac{Mev}{dis} \times 1.6 \times 10^{-13} \, \frac{J}{MeV} \times w_T \times w_R \, \frac{Sv}{Gy}}{m \text{ kg} \times 1 \, \frac{J/kg}{Gy}}$$

$$\times \sum N_C \text{ dis} \times AF(T \leftarrow S)_C, \tag{8.37}$$

Substituting the respective values from the table above, we calculate

$H(BB)_{bas} = 3.256 \times 10^{-9}$ Sv.

In a similar manner, we can calculate the doses to the other cells in the lung, the secretory cells in the BB region and in the bb region, then add the respective doses to obtain the dose to the lung. The data for making these calculations, as well as the data for the BB basal cells (which are calculated above), are listed in Table 8-19.

The weighted sum of all the doses to the various parts of the lung is the dose to the lung from the inhalation, by an adult male, of 1 Bq of ^{14}C tagged tungsten carbide, WC, (type S) whose AMAD is 5 μm, is 2.8×10^{-8} Sv. Doses to other organs depend on the fate of the activity transferred to the blood. When calculating the EDE from this inhalation, the lung dose must be multiplied by the weighting factor for the lung, 0.12.

Gases and Vapors. Inhaled gases either dissolve in the fluids of the airway surfaces and are "deposited" there, or are exhaled. Those gases that dissolve may interact

TABLE 8-19. Summary of Dose Calculation Data for Example 8.6

TARGET	m (kg)	SOURCE	DISINTEGRATIONS	AF (T ← S)	w_T	DOSE (Sv)
BB_{bas}	4.3N4	BB_1	604	0.0508	0.1665	3.256N9
		BB_2	16,956	0.0542		
		BB_{seq}	1072	0.0985		
		Al	4,647,546	0		
BB_{sec}	8.6N4	BB_1	604	0.216	0.1665	6.440N9
		BB_2	16,956	0.235		
		BB_{seq}	1072	0.101		
		Al	4,647,546	0		
bb	1.9N3	bb_1	2399	0.157	0.333	6.641N9
		bb_2	15,788	0.165		
		bb_{seq}	659	0.0962		
		Al	4,647,546	3.68N4		
Al	1.1	Al	4,647,546	1	0.333	1.121N8
LN_{TH}	0.015	LN_{TH}	488,034	1	0.001	2.592N10
						$\sum = 2.757N8$

Note: N4 = 10^{-4}.

Abbreviations: AF (T ← S), absorbed fraction (source to target); BB, bronchial; bb, bronchiolar; Al, alveolar-interstitial; LN_{TH}, lymph nodes (thoracic).

chemically with the tissue in the airway, or it may diffuse into bloodstream and be absorbed into the body, or both processes may occur simultaneously. The biological effects of an inhaled gas thus depend on its solubility and its chemical reactivity. Accordingly, all gases are assigned to one of three classes: SR-0, SR-1, and SR-2.

- Type SR-0 are gases of limited solubility and are nonreactive, such as H_2, He, Ar, Kr, and SF_6. Such gases do not interact with the pulmonary tissues, and are not significantly absorbed into the blood from the alveoli. It is reasonably assumed that all the inhaled SR-0 gas is also exhaled. Radiation dose to the lungs is due to the presence of the gas within the respiratory airways. The radiation hazard from type SR-0 gas usually is from external radiation due to immersion in the gaseous cloud. Radon is an inert gas, and would fall into this hazard category if its progeny were not radioactive. The hazard from radon is not from the gas, but from radon's radioactive daughters. These radioactive descendents attach themselves to atmospheric dust particles, as explained in Chapter 7, and these dust particles are inhaled and deposited in the lungs.
- Type SR-1 are gases that are either soluble or reactive or both, such as CO, NO_2, I_2, CH_3I, and Hg vapor. In the absence of specific data on the interaction of the gas with the airway tissues, the HRTM assumes that all the inhaled gas is deposited, with 10% in the ET_1 region, 20% in ET_2, 10% in BB, 20% in bb, and 40% in the alveoli. From the alveoli, they may be absorbed into the blood and transported to other organs and tissues where they may be metabolized or deposited.
- Type SR-2 gases are both highly soluble and reactive, such as HTO, SO_2, H_2S, HF, and Cl_2. These gases rapidly interact with the tissues in the upper respiratory tract

and do not reach the pulmonary region. Thus, they are considered to be totally deposited in the ET regions of the respiratory tract. For dosimetric calculations, the HRTM assumes that SR-2 gases are instantaneously absorbed into the body. The radiation dose then is calculated according to the biokinetic behavior of the gas in the body.

Highly reactive gases and vapors that ordinarily may not penetrate into the alveoli may be adsorbed on the surface of airborne particles, and the particles may be deposited in the alveoli. There the reactive gases may interact with the gas exchange surfaces, which may result in biological damage to the AI tissues. This was the mechanism for the lethality of the Donora, PA, smog in 1948. Highly reactive SO_2 gas was adsorbed on the surface of zinc-ammonium-sulfate particles that were of the optimum size for alveolar deposition. There, the adsorbed SO_2 was rapidly oxidized, and the resultant sulfuric acid in the alveoli caused severe pulmonary edema, which led to the excess number of deaths.

Generally, the dynamics of uptake and transfer for most gases are not precisely known (the case of CO and CO_2, whose biokinetic behaviors are reasonably well known, are notable exceptions to this generalization). Lacking specific knowledge of the uptake kinetics of a specific gas, the HRTM assumes extremely rapid, essentially instantaneous uptake of the inhaled gas. It should be noted that many airborne contaminants, including tritiated water, are absorbed through the skin as well as through the lungs. Such airborne contaminants that are regulated in the United States by the Occupational Safety and Health Administration (OSHA) are listed in Occupational Safety and Health Standards, 29 CFR 1910.1000.

Dose Coefficient

The HRTM allows us to calculate the dose *only to the lung* from inhaled radioactivity. The activity absorbed into the body fluids and swallowed into the GI tract supplies the input data to physiologically based pharmacokinetic models that allow us to calculate the doses to the other organs and tissues, and to calculate the effective dose from the inhaled activity.

Through the use of the respective physiologically based pharmacokinetic models, we can calculate the committed equivalent dose and the committed effective dose from inhalation and ingestion of 1 Bq (or 1 μCi) of every radionuclide. These calculations yield the DC for each of the radionuclides, which, when multiplied by the intake, give the estimated dose to the exposed person. DCs for all the radionuclides have been published by the U.S. EPA, the ICRP, and the IAEA. Some of these DCs are given in Table 8-20.

 EXAMPLE 8.7

A worker at a heavy-water-moderated nuclear reactor station accidentally inhaled 37 MBq (1000 μCi) ^{3}H as tritiated water vapor. What is his CEDE from this exposure?

TABLE 8-20. Dose Coefficients for Selected Radionuclides

RADIONUCLIDE/CLASS	INTAKE ROUTE	TARGET	DC (Sv/Bq)
^{3}H (water vapor)	Inhalation	Whole body (effective)	1.73N11
^{32}P	Ingestion	Red marrow	8.09N9
^{32}P	Ingestion	Whole body (effective)	2.37N9
^{90}Sr–^{90}Y/D (F)	Inhalation	Bone surface	7.27N7
^{90}Sr–^{90}Y/D (F)	Inhalation	Whole body (effective)	6.47N8
^{137}Cs/D (F)	Inhalation	Whole body (effective)	8.63N9
^{137}Cs	Ingestion	Whole body (effective)	1.35N8
^{226}Ra	Ingestion	Bone surface	6.83N6
^{239}Pu/W (M)	Inhalation	Bone surface	2.11N3

Note: N11 = 10^{-11}.

Abbreviation: DC, dose coefficient.

Source: Eckerman KF et al. Federal Guidance Report No. 11, 1988.

Solution

$$\text{CEDE} = \text{intake} \times \text{DC}$$

$$= 3.7 \times 10^7 \, \text{Bq} \times 1.73 \times 10^{-11} \frac{\text{Sv}}{\text{Bq}}$$

$$= 6.4 \times 10^{-4} \, \text{Sv} = 0.64 \, \text{mSv} \, (= 64 \text{ mrems}).$$

Derived Air Concentration

The ALI, which is a secondary standard that is based on the primary dose limit, only gives the annual intake limit; it does not deal with the rate of intake or with the atmospheric or environmental concentrations of a radionuclide that lead to the intake. It also is not amenable to direct measurement. For engineering design purposes, for control of routine operations, and for demonstration of compliance with regulations, we must know the environmental concentrations of the radionuclides with which we are dealing. To this end, the *derived air concentration* (DAC) is used by the U.S. NRC as a regulatory limit for airborne contaminants. The DAC is simply that average atmospheric concentration of the radionuclide that would lead to the ALI in a reference person as a consequence of exposure at the DAC for a 2000-hour working year. Since a reference worker inhales 20-L air per minute, or 2400 m^3 during the 2000 hours per year spent at work, the DAC is

$$\text{DAC} = \frac{\text{ALI} \dfrac{\text{Bq}}{\text{yr}}}{2400 \dfrac{\text{m}^3}{\text{yr}}}. \tag{8.38}$$

Thus, for airborne ^{137}Cs, whose inhalation ALI is listed in ICRP 30 as 6×10^6 Bq, the DAC is

$$\text{DAC} = \frac{6 \times 10^6 \dfrac{\text{Bq}}{\text{yr}}}{2400 \dfrac{\text{m}^3}{\text{yr}}} = 2.5 \times 10^3 \frac{\text{Bq}}{\text{m}^3},$$

which is rounded off to 2×10^3 Bq/m^3.

According to ICRP 60 criteria, the annual dose limit is 0.02 Sv/yr. For 5-μm AMAD, class F ^{137}Cs particles, the DC is listed as 6.7×10^{-9} Sv/Bq, the ALI is calculated as

$$\text{ALI} = \frac{0.02 \text{ Sv}}{6.7 \times 10^{-9} \dfrac{\text{Sv}}{\text{Bq}}} = 3 \times 10^6 \text{ Bq},$$

and the DAC is

$$\text{DAC} = \frac{3 \times 10^6 \text{ Bq}}{2400 \text{ m}^3} = 1.3 \times 10^3 \frac{\text{Bq}}{\text{m}^3}.$$

Gaseous Radioactivity

Immersion in a cloud of radioactive gas leads to external exposure from the activity in the surrounding air and to internal exposure due to the inhaled gas. For the case of biochemically inert gases argon, krypton, and xenon, the external submersion dose limits the atmospheric concentration, as shown by the calculations for ^{41}Ar in the following paragraphs.

Argon-41, a biochemically inert gas, is transformed to ^{41}K by the emission of a 1.2-MeV beta particle and a 1.3-MeV gamma ray. The half-life of ^{41}Ar is 110 minutes, or 0.076 days. For the case of submersion, it is assumed that a person is exposed in an infinite hemisphere of the gas. For this exposure condition, ICRP 68 lists the effective DC for ^{41}Ar as 5.3×10^{-9} Sv/d/ per Bq/m^3. The reference working year is 250 days of 8 hours each. For an effective annual dose of 0.02 Sv (2 rems), the mean concentration of ^{41}Ar is calculated by

$$0.02 \text{ Sv} = 5.3 \times 10^{-9} \frac{\text{Sv/d}}{\text{Bq/m}^3} \times 250 \text{ d} \times C \frac{\text{Bq}}{\text{m}^3} \tag{8.39}$$

$$C = 1.5 \times 10^4 \frac{\text{Bq}}{\text{m}^3} \left(4 \times 10^{-7} \frac{\mu\text{Ci}}{\text{mL}} \right).$$

When a gas is inhaled, it may dissolve in the body fluids and fat after diffusion across the capillary bed in the lung. In the case of an inert gas, absorption into the body stops after the body fluids and fat are saturated with the dissolved gas. The saturation quantity of dissolved ^{41}Ar in the body fluids due to inhalation of contaminated air at the DAC, based on submersion, must be calculated in order to determine the internal dose. The first step in this calculation is the determination of the molar concentration of ^{41}Ar that corresponds to 1.5×10^4 Bq/m^3 ($4 \times 10^{-7} \mu$Ci/mL). The specific activity of ^{41}Ar is calculated with Eq. (4.30):

$$SA_i = 3.7 \times 10^{10} \left(\frac{A_{Ra} \times T_{Ra}}{A_i \times T_i} \right) \frac{Bq}{g}$$

$$= 3.7 \times 10^{10} \left(\frac{226 \times 1.6 \times 10^3 \text{ years} \times 365\frac{d}{yr}}{41 \times 0.076 \text{ days}} \right) = 1.57 \times 10^{18} \frac{Bq}{g},$$

and the molar concentration of the ^{41}Ar is calculated as

$$\frac{1.5 \times 10^4 \frac{Bq}{m^3}}{1.57 \times 10^{18} \frac{Bq}{g}} \times \frac{1 \text{ mol}}{41 \text{ g}} = 2.33 \times 10^{-16} \frac{\text{mol } ^{41}\text{Ar}}{m^3}.$$

The molar concentration of air at standard temperature and pressure is

$$\frac{1 \text{ mol}}{22.4\frac{L}{mol} \times 10^{-3}\frac{m^3}{L}} = 44.6 \frac{\text{mol air}}{m^3}.$$

Since argon constitutes 0.94 volume percent of the air, the molar concentration of naturally occurring argon in the air is

$$9.4 \times 10^{-3} \frac{\text{mol Ar}}{\text{mol air}} \times 44.6 \frac{\text{mol air}}{m^3 \text{ air}} = 0.42 \frac{\text{mol Ar}}{m^3 \text{ air}}.$$

The amount of argon corresponding to the ^{41}Ar DAC based on submersion dose is thus seen to be insignificant relative to the argon already in the air. The molar concentration of argon in the air may therefore be assumed to be unchanged by the addition of 1.5×10^4 Bq/m^3 ($4 \times 10^{-7} \mu$Ci/mL) ^{41}Ar to the air. With this amount of ^{41}Ar in the air, the specific activity of the argon in the air is

$$\frac{1.5 \times 10^4 \frac{Bq}{m^3}}{0.42 \text{ mol}\frac{Ar}{m^3}} = 3.57 \times 10^4 \frac{Bq}{\text{mol Ar}} \left(9.65 \times 10^{-7} \frac{Ci}{\text{mol Ar}} \right).$$

Now we will calculate the concentration of argon in the body fluids when the dissolved argon is in equilibrium with the argon in the air. According to Henry's law, the amount of a gas dissolved in a liquid is proportional to the partial pressure of the gas above the liquid:

$$P_{gas} = KN = K\frac{n_g}{n_g + n_s}, \tag{8.40}$$

TABLE 8-21.   Solubility of Several Gases in Water at 38°C

GAS	K (x 10⁷)
H_2	5.72
He	11.0
N_2	7.51
O_2	4.04
Ar	3.41
Ne	9.76
Kr	2.13
Xe	1.12
Rn	0.65
CO_2	0.168
C_2H_2	0.131
C_2H_4	1.21
N_2O	0.242

Note: $K = \dfrac{\text{partial pressure of gas in mm Hg}}{\text{mole fraction of gas in solution}}$.

where

P_{gas} = partial pressure of the gas,
K = Henry's law constant,
N = mole fraction of the dissolved gas,
n_g = molar concentration of the dissolved gas, and
n_s = molar concentration of the solvent.

The solubilities of several gases in water at 38°C, expressed in terms of Henry's law constant, are given in Table 8-21. At body temperature, K for argon is 3.41×10^7, and the partial pressure of argon in the atmosphere is

$$P_{\text{Ar}} = 0.0094 \times 760 = 7.15 \text{ mm Hg.}$$

The total body water in a 70-kg reference person is 43 L. Therefore, the molar concentration of water, the solvent in Eq. (8.40), is

$$n_g = \frac{1000 \text{ g/L}}{18 \text{ g/mol}} = 55.6 \frac{\text{mol}}{\text{L}}.$$

Equation (8.40) may now be solved for the concentration of dissolved argon.

$$7.15 = 3.41 \times 10^7 \left(\frac{n_g}{n_g + 55.6} \right)$$

$$n_g = 1.17 \times 10^{-5} \frac{\text{mol}}{\text{L}}.$$

Since the specific activity of the dissolved argon is 3.57×10^4 Bq/mol (9.65×10^{-7} Ci/mol), the argon activity concentration in the body fluids is

$$3.57 \times 10^4 \frac{\text{Bq}}{\text{mol}} \times 1.17 \times 10^{-5} \frac{\text{mol}}{\text{L}} = 0.42 \frac{\text{Bq}}{\text{L}} \left(1.1 \times 10^{-5} \frac{\mu\text{Ci}}{\text{L}} \right),$$

and the total activity in the body fluids is

$$43 \, L \times 0.42 \, \frac{Bq}{L} = 18.1 \, Bq (4.9 \times 10^{-4} \, \mu Ci).$$

Argon is more soluble in fat than in water. At equilibrium, the partition coefficient, which is the concentration ratio of argon in fat to argon in water, is 5.4:1 at body temperature. The amount of argon in the 10 kg of fat in the reference worker is

$$5.4 \times 0.42 \, \frac{Bq}{kg} \times 10 \, kg = 22.7 \, Bq (6.1 \times 10^{-4} \, \mu Ci).$$

The total argon activity in the reference person is the sum of the argon in the body fluids and in the fat:

Total body burden of ^{41}Ar $= 18.1 \, Bq + 22.7 \, Bq = 40.8 \, Bq (= 1.1 \times 10^{-3} \mu Ci).$

If the argon is assumed to be uniformly distributed throughout the body, then the whole body dose from the absorbed ^{41}A is calculated from

$\dot{D}(\text{body} \leftarrow \text{body})$

$$= \frac{q \, Bq \times 1 \frac{tps}{Bq} \times E_a \frac{MeV}{t} \times 1.6 \times 10^{-13} \frac{J}{MeV} \times 3.6 \times 10^3 \frac{s}{h} \times 1 \frac{Sv}{Gy}.}{70 \, kg \times 1 \frac{J/kg}{Gy}} \qquad (8.41)$$

If we substitute $q = 40.8 \, Bq$

$$E_a = \varphi \times E_\gamma + \bar{E}_\beta = 4.53 \times 10^{-6} \times 1.3 \, \frac{MeV}{t} + \frac{1}{3} \times 1.2 \, \frac{MeV}{t} = 0.4 \, \frac{MeV}{t}$$

into Eq. (8.41), we find

$$\dot{D}(\text{body} \leftarrow \text{body}) = 1.3 \times 10^{-10} \, \frac{Sv}{h} \quad \text{or} \quad 2.6 \times 10^{-7} \, \frac{Sv}{yr}.$$

The lungs are also irradiated by the ^{41}Ar within the airways, whose volume (according to ICRP 68) is 3.862 L. Since the air concentration is 15 Bq/L, there are 57.9 Bq in the air inside the lungs. This leads to a dose rate of 2.7×10^{-5} Sv/yr. The effective annual dose due to inhaling ^{41}Ar at the concentration based on the submersion dose is

$$H = \sum w_T H_T.$$

Substituting the appropriate weighting factors, we have

$$H = 0.12 \times 2.7 \times 10^{-5} + 0.88 \times 2.6 \times 10^{-7} = 3.5 \times 10^{-6} \, Sv.$$

The inhalation dose due to an atmosphere containing the limiting concentration for submersion is thus seen to be very much less than the submersion dose. The submersion dose is therefore the limiting dose. The same thing is true for the radioisotopes of krypton and xenon. For these radionuclides, therefore, the limiting atmospheric concentrations are based on the submersion dose.

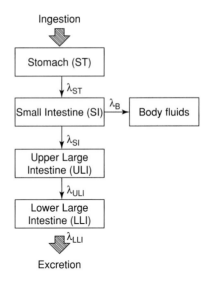

Ingestion

Stomach (ST)

Small Intestine (SI) $\xrightarrow{\lambda_B}$ Body fluids

Upper Large
Intestine (ULI)

Lower Large
Intestine (LLI)

Excretion

Section of GI Tract	Mass of Walls (g)	Mass of Contents (g)	Mean Residence Time (d)	λ (d^{-1})
Stomach (ST)	150	250	1/24	24
Small Intestine (SI)	640	400	4/24	6
Upper Large Intestine (ULI)	210	220	13/24	1.8
Lower Large Intestine (LLI)	160	135	24/24	1

Figure 8-19. *Dosimetric model of the gastrointestinal tract. The clearance rate for transfer from the small intestine into the body fluids is given by Eq. (8.42). (Reproduced with permission from ICRP Publication 30, Part 1: Limits for Intakes of Radionuclides by Workers. Ann ICRP. 1979; 2(3/4):33. Copyright © 1979 International Commission on Radiological Protection.)*

Gastrointestinal Tract

In cases of ingested radionuclides or radionuclides transferred to the GI tract from the lungs, and especially for those nuclides that are poorly absorbed from the GI tract, the GI tract or portions of it may be the tissue or organ that receives the greatest dose. The dose to the GI tract is calculated on the basis of the four-compartment dosimetric model shown in Figure 8-19. According to this model, the radionuclide enters the stomach (ST) and then passes sequentially through the small intestine (SI), from which most absorption into the body fluids occurs. It then passes through the upper large intestine (ULI) and the lower large intestine (LLI). Finally, the remaining activity is excreted in the feces. The clearance rate for transfer from the small intestine into the body fluids is given by

$$\lambda_B = \frac{f_1 \lambda_{SI}}{1 - f_1}, \tag{8.42}$$

where f_1 = fraction of the stable element reaching the body fluids after ingestion.

In making dose calculations for the purpose of calculating a DC and an ALI, we assume the radionuclide to be uniformly distributed throughout the contents of the respective segments of the GI tract and the weight of the contents of each segment to be as listed in Figure 8-19. Furthermore, the movement of the contents between compartments is assumed to follow first-order kinetics, with compartmental clearance rates as shown in Figure 8-19. The time rate of change of the contents of each of the four compartments can be calculated on the basis of mass balance. The increase or decrease in the quantity of radionuclide in any of the compartments is simply equal to the difference between what goes in and what goes out:

$$\text{Rate of change of contents} = \text{rate in} - \text{rate out}. \tag{8.43}$$

If we have a constant input rate, $\dot{I}$ per day, as in the case of continuous ingestion of radioactivity in food or continuous inhalation of a radioactive aerosol that is cleared from the lung into the GI tract, then the mass balance equation for the stomach becomes

$$\left(\frac{dq}{dt}\right)_{St} = \dot{I} - \lambda_{St} q_{St} - \lambda_R q_{St}, \tag{8.44}$$

where q may be measured either in SI units or in traditional units and λ is the turnover rate per day. When the amount of activity entering into the stomach is equal to the amount leaving, we have a steady-state condition, and $(dq/dt)_{ST}$ becomes equal to zero. Under this condition, Eq. (8.44) becomes

$$\dot{I} = \lambda_{St} q_{St} + \lambda_R q_{St}. \tag{8.45}$$

The stomach contents empty into the small intestine, whose kinetics are similar to those of the stomach. The time rate of change of the contents, therefore, is described by the difference between what enters from the stomach and what leaves the small intestine. Material is cleared from the small intestine by two pathways:

1. by peristalsis into the upper large intestine, and
2. by molecular diffusion into the blood vessels in the inner surface of the small intestine.

The difference between what goes into the small intestine and what leaves it is expressed mathematically by

$$\left(\frac{dq}{dt}\right)_{SI} = \lambda_{St} q_{St} - \lambda_{SI} q_{SI} - \lambda_R q_{SI} - \lambda_B q_{SI}, \tag{8.46}$$

where λ_B is the transfer rate of the radionuclide from the small intestine into the blood and is given by Eq. (8.42). The dosimetric model of the GI tract assumes that only water is absorbed into the bloodstream from the large intestine. The rate of change of the radioactivity in the upper large intestine, therefore, is given by

$$\left(\frac{dq}{dt}\right)_{ULI} = \lambda_{SI} q_{SI} - \lambda_{ULI} q_{ULI} - \lambda_R q_{ULI}, \tag{8.47}$$

and for the lower large intestine, from which the radioactivity leaves the body, we have

$$\left(\frac{dq}{dt}\right)_{LLI} = \lambda_{ULI} q_{ULI} - \lambda_{LLI} q_{LLI} - \lambda_R q_{LLI}. \tag{8.48}$$

With the aid of Eqs. (8.44) to (8.48) and the appropriate specific AFs, we can calculate the dose per unit intake of radioactivity to the walls of the GI tract and to other organs and tissues for steady-state conditions and thus can compute the intake that will result in the dose limit, the ALI.

Dosimetric Model for Bone

ICRP 2 Methodology

To gain an insight into the evolution of safety standards for bone seekers, it is instructive to examine the ICRP 2 recommendations for intake limits, which were based on the critical organ concept. That is, on the organ that received the greatest dose from the intake of a radionuclide. For bone-seeking radionuclides, the intake limits were based on the application of a simple dosimetric model to data derived mainly from humans. The skeleton was treated as though it were a single tissue that weighed 7 kg. Because we had a great deal of experience with human exposure to radium and because radium is a "bone seeker"—that is, it is deposited in the bone—the maximum permissible body burdens of all bone seekers were established by comparing the dose equivalent of the bone seeker with that delivered to the bone by radium. On the basis of data on humans, 0.1 μg radium, corresponding to 3.7 kBq, in equilibrium with its decay products, was recommended as the maximum permissible body burden of ^{226}Ra. Using the then quality factor of 10 for alpha particles, the calculated dose equivalent to the bone from 0.1 μg ^{226}Ra and its daughters was 0.56 rem (5.6 mSv) per week.

Radium is deposited relatively uniformly in the bone. Other bone seekers, however, were found to be deposited in a patchy, nonuniform manner that results in doses to some parts of the bone as much as five times greater than the average bone dose. For this reason, the ICRP introduced the *relative damage factor, N*, as a multiplier of the quality factor QF. This factor has a value of 5 for all corpuscular (alpha or beta) radiation except for those cases where the corpuscular radiations are due to a chain whose first member is radium. When radium is the first member of the chain, then $N = 1$, since the distribution of the radioisotope will be determined by the radium. For example, the value of the relative damage factor N for

$$^{228}\text{Th} \xrightarrow{\beta} {}^{224}\text{Ra} \xrightarrow{\alpha}$$

is 5 for each particle, while the same particles are weighted with a relative damage factor of 1 in the chain

$$^{228}\text{Ra} \xrightarrow{\beta} {}^{228}\text{Ac} \xrightarrow{\beta} {}^{228}\text{Th} \xrightarrow{\beta} {}^{224}\text{Ra} \xrightarrow{\alpha}.$$

The energy dissipated in the bone by ^{226}Ra and the daughters that remain in the bone is 11 MeV per transformation. Applying the QF value of 10 brings the effective energy to 110 MeV per transformation. Since 99% of the radium body burden is in the skeleton, ICRP 2, using data on humans as a basis, calculated a maximum permissible body burden of any other bone seeker:

$$q = \frac{3.7 \times 10^3 \text{ Bq} \times 0.99}{f_2} \times \frac{110 \frac{\text{MeV}}{\text{t}}}{E \frac{\text{MeV}}{\text{t}}} = \frac{4 \times 10^5}{f_2 E} \text{ Bq}, \tag{8.49}$$

where E is the effective corpuscular energy per transformation of any other bone seeker and f_2 is the fraction of the total body burden of the bone seeker that is in the skeleton. For the case of ^{90}Sr, for example, we have

^{90}Sr-^{90}Y are pure beta emitters whose average energy is 0.194 MeV (^{90}Sr) + 0.93 MeV (^{90}Y) = 1.12 MeV/transformation

Q (quality factor) = 1,

$N = 5$, and

$f_2 = 0.99$.

The effective energy is $5 \times 1.12 = 5.6$ MeV per transformation. From Eq. (8.49) we find the maximum permissible body burden to be

$$q = \frac{4 \times 10^5}{0.99 \times 5.6} = 7.2 \times 10^4 \text{ Bq } (2 \ \mu\text{Ci})$$

The effective half-life for ^{90}Sr in the skeleton is found in ICRP 2 to be 6400 days, which corresponds to an effective clearance rate, $\lambda_E = 1.08 \times 10^{-4}$ per day. Since 9% of the ingested Sr is deposited in the bone, the maximum permissible concentration in drinking water that will maintain the body burden at 7.2×10^4 Bq ($2 \ \mu$Ci) is found through the use of activity-balance calculations. If we assume that the drinking water is the only source of intake of ^{90}Sr and that the ^{90}Sr containing water is the person's sole source of water, then we can calculate the concentration of radiostrontium in the water that would lead to a steady-state ^{90}Sr activity of $2 \ \mu$Ci. Under steady-state conditions,

$$\text{activity deposited} = \text{activity eliminated,} \tag{8.50a}$$

that is,

$$C \ \frac{\mu\text{Ci}}{\text{mL}} \times 2.2 \times 10^3 \ \frac{\text{mL}}{\text{d}} \times f = \lambda_E \ \text{d}^{-1} \times q \ \mu\text{Ci.} \tag{8.50b}$$

In SI units, Eq. (8.50b) becomes

$$C \ \frac{\text{Bq}}{\text{mL}} \times 2.2 \times 10^3 \ \frac{\text{mL}}{\text{d}} \times f = \lambda_E \ \text{d}^{-1} \times q \ \text{Bq,} \tag{8.50c}$$

where

$\quad C$ = maximum permissible concentration (MPC, which was an ICRP 2 concept),

$\quad f$ = fraction of the intake that is deposited in the critical organ,

$\quad \lambda_E$ = effective elimination rate constant, and

$\quad q$ = steady-state activity in the critical organ.

Substituting the appropriate values into Eq. (8.50b) and solving for C yields

$$C = \frac{1.08 \times 10^{-4} \ \text{d}^{-1} \times 2 \ \mu\text{Ci}}{2.2 \times 10^3 \ \frac{\text{L}}{\text{d}} \times 9 \times 10^{-2}} = 1 \times 10^{-6} \frac{\mu\text{Ci}}{\text{mL}} \ \left(3.7 \times 10^{-2} \frac{\text{Bq}}{\text{mL}} \right).$$

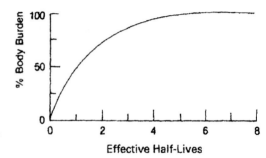

Figure 8-20. Buildup of a radioisotope in the body resulting from continuous intake.

Ingestion of water at the rate assumed in the calculation above will result in the maximum permissible body burden *when equilibrium is attained* (Fig. 8-20). Because of the very long effective half-life of ^{90}Sr in the bone, the maximum allowable body burden is not attained during the 50-year occupational exposure time assumed for the purpose of computing values for the radiation safety guide. After 50 years of continuous ingestion at the above rate, the amount of ^{90}Sr in the skeleton will be

$$q = q_{\text{equil.}}(1 - e^{-\lambda_E t})$$

$$q = 2\,\mu\text{Ci}(1 - e^{-1.08 \times 10^{-4} \times 50 \times 365})$$

$$q = 1.7\,\mu\text{Ci} \quad (6.2 \times 10^4 \text{Bq}),$$

or only 86% of the maximum body burden. It is thus clear that the average body burden, and consequently the average dose rate to the skeleton during a 50-year period of maximum permissible ingestion, will be considerably less than the maximum permissible body burden. The mean body burden during a period of ingestion, T, starting at time zero when there is no radioisotope of the species in question in the body, and assuming the effective elimination rate for the radioisotope to be λ_E, is given by

$$\bar{q} = \frac{1}{T}\int_0^T q_{\text{equil.}}(1 - e^{-\lambda_E t})\,dt. \tag{8.51}$$

Integrating Eq. (8.51), we obtain

$$\bar{q} = q_{\text{equil.}}\left[1 + \frac{1}{\lambda_E T}(e^{-\lambda_E T} - 1)\right]. \tag{8.52}$$

For ^{90}Sr, whose $\lambda_E = 0.0395$ yr^{-1}, we have for a 50-year exposure period

$$\bar{q} = 1.13\,\mu\text{Ci} \quad (4.18 \times 10^4 \text{ Bq}).$$

Several other radionuclides (Table 8-22) do not attain their equilibrium values in the body during 50 years of continuous ingestion at the maximum recommended concentrations.

TABLE 8-22. Radioisotopes That Do Not Reach Equilibrium in 50 Years

Z	ISOTOPE	T_E (yrs)	% EQUILIBRIUM AFTER 50 YRS
38	^{90}Sr	18	86
88	^{226}Ra	44	56
89	^{227}Ac	20	83
90	^{230}Th	200	16
90	^{232}Th	200	16
91	^{231}Pa	200	16
93	^{237}Np	200	16
94	^{238}Pu	62	43
94	^{239}Pu	200	16
94	^{240}Pu	190	16
94	^{241}Pu	12	94
94	^{242}Pu	200	16
95	^{241}Am	140	22
95	^{243}Am	200	16
96	^{243}Cm	30	69
96	^{244}Cm	17	87
96	^{245}Cm	200	16
96	^{246}Cm	190	16
98	^{249}Cf	140	22
98	^{250}Cf	10	97

ICRP 30 Dosimetric Model

While the ICRP 2 recommendations were based on a dosimetric model that considered the "bone" as a single tissue consisting of a homogeneous mixture of its chemical compounds, the ICRP 30 dosimetric model considers the various different tissues within the bone that are at risk. Bone is modeled as three separate tissues:

- Cortical (or compact) bone, which is the hard outer portion of the bone, is assigned a mass of 4 kg in the ICRP 30 model. (ICRP 89 lists the masses of the skeleton's components according to sex and age.)
- Trabecular bone, which is the soft spongy inside the cortical bone, is assigned a mass of 1 kg in the ICRP 30 model.
- Red (or active) marrow, which is located in the spaces within the trabecular bone, has an assigned mass of 1.5 kg.

The most radiosensitive tissues are the 120 g of endosteum that lie within the first 10 μm of the adjacent bone surfaces and the 1.5 kg of red bone marrow. Since the AF of the energy emitted by radionuclides within the bone depends on where the radionuclides are deposited, the newer bone model classifies the bone-seeking radionuclides as *volume seekers* and *surface seekers*. Whether any specific radionuclide is a volume or surface seeker is determined by the metabolism of the element. In this regard, the ICRP 30 dosimetric model established two general categories:

1. Isotopes of the alkaline earth elements whose half-lives exceed 15 days are assumed to be uniformly distributed throughout the volume of the bone.
2. Shorter-lived radionuclides are assumed to be distributed on the bone surfaces, since they are unlikely to have distributed themselves within the bone volume before they decay.

For dosimetric purposes, six nonexclusive categories of bone seekers are used in the ICRP 30 bone model:

1. photon emitters,
2. alpha-emitting volume seekers,
3. alpha-emitting surface seekers,
4. beta-emitting surface seekers whose mean beta energy is at least 0.2 MeV,
5. beta-emitting surface seekers whose mean beta energy is less than 0.2 MeV, and
6. beta-emitting volume seekers.

These categories are not mutually exclusive because a radionuclide, such as a beta–gamma emitter, belongs in two categories. In this case, each different type of radiation is considered separately. The AF for the various particle emitters are given in Table 8-23. The AFs for photons are given in Appendix D.

Using the physiologically based biokinetic model for a bone-seeking radionuclide, we can calculate the dose to the bone or bone surface and the doses to the other organs and tissues due to the intake, by ingestion or inhalation, of 1 Bq or 1 μCi of activity. Then, using either the ICRP and IAEA criterion of 0.02-Sv effective dose limit, or U.S. NRC criterion of 5-rems (0.05-Sv) effective dose limit or 50-rems (0.5-Sv) organ dose limit, or we can calculate the secondary ALI and the tertiary DAC or maximum concentration in water. If we were to use the ICRP criterion of a mean annual effective dose of 0.02 Sv and the DC of 2.4×10^{-9} Sv/Bq for 5-μm moderately soluble ^{45}Ca particles, then the inhalation ALI would be

$$\text{ALI(effective)} = \frac{0.02\,\text{Sv}}{2.4 \times 10^{-9}\,\dfrac{\text{Sv}}{\text{Bq}}} = 8.33 \times 10^6\,\text{Bq} = 225\,\mu\text{Ci}.$$

For example, the U S NRC's inhalation ALI for soluble (class D) ^{90}Sr, using the DCs for the bone surface and for whole-body effective dose listed in Table 8-20, we have

$$\text{ALI(bone surface)} = \frac{0.5\,\text{Sv}}{7.29 \times 10^{-7}\,\dfrac{\text{Sv}}{\text{Bq}}} = 6.86 \times 10^5\,\text{Bq} = 1.86 \times 10^1\,\mu\text{Ci}$$

$$\text{ALI(effective)} = \frac{0.05\,\text{Sv}}{6.47 \times 10^{-8}\,\dfrac{\text{Sv}}{\text{Bq}}} = 7.73 \times 10^5\,\text{Bq} = 2.09 \times 10^1\,\mu\text{Ci}.$$

TABLE 8-23. Recommended Absorbed Fractions for Dosimetry of Radionuclides in Bone

SOURCE	TARGET	A, Vol.	α, BS	β, Vol.	β, $\bar{E} \geq 0.2$ MeV, BS	β, $\bar{E} < 0.2$ MeV, BS
Trabecular	Surface (BS)	0.025	0.25	0.025	0.025	0.25
Cortical	Surface	0.01	0.25	0.015	0.015	0.25
Trabecular	Red Marrow	0.05	0.5	0.35	0.5	0.5
Cortical	Red Marrow	0.0	0.0	0.0	0.0	0.0

Abbreviation: BS, bone surface.

The smaller of the two ALIs is designated as the limit, and thus the dose to the bone surface is the limiting dose. Since the limits are rounded to one significant figure, the ALI for inhalation of 1-μm, class D ^{90}Sr particles is listed in 10 CFR 20 as 2×10^1, and would be applicable to both stochastic and nonstochastic cases. However, 10 CFR 20, Table 1 notes that the dose to the bone surface is the deciding criterion.

UNITED STATES NUCLEAR REGULATORY PROGRAM

National Council on Radiation Protection and Measurements

The ICRP is not a regulatory agency. It is a scientific body that makes recommendations for radiation safety standards. In accordance with the policy laid down by the ICRP, its recommendations are adapted to the needs and conditions in the various countries by national bodies. In the United States, this function is served by the NCRP. This organization, which was originally known as the Advisory Committee on X-ray and Radium Protection (founded in 1929), consists of a group of technical experts who are specialists in radiation safety and scientists who are experts in the disciplines that form the basis for radiation safety. The concern of the NCRP is only with the scientific and technical aspects of radiation safety. To accomplish its objectives, the NCRP is organized into a main council, whose members are selected on the basis of their scientific expertise, and a number of subcommittees. Each of the subcommittees is responsible for preparing specific recommendations in its field of competence. The recommendations of the subcommittees require approval of the council before they are published. Finally, the approved recommendations are published by the council, with titles such as Report No. 147, *Structural Shielding Design for Medical X-Ray Imaging Facilities*. It should be emphasized that the NCRP is not an official government agency, although its recommendations are very seriously considered by regulatory agencies.

Atomic Energy Commission

In the United States, regulatory responsibility for radiation safety in the nuclear energy program originally was given by the U.S. Congress to the United States Atomic Energy Commission (AEC) through the enactment of the Atomic Energy Act of 1946 and the Atomic Energy Act Amendments of 1954. The AEC continued to function until 1974, when its responsibilities were divided between two other agencies. The Atomic Energy Acts of 1946 and 1954 regulated the possession, use, and production of the following:

Source materials—Uranium and thorium, and their ores containing $\geq 0.05\%$ U or Th,
Special nuclear materials (SNM)—Plutonium, ^{233}U, and uranium enriched in either ^{233}U or ^{235}U,
By-product material—Originally defined by the USAEC as "any material, except SNM, produced or made radioactive incident to making or using SNM." The Energy Policy Act of 2005 expanded the definition of "by-product material" to include certain discrete sources of radium, certain accelerator-produced radioactive material, and certain discrete sources of naturally occurring radioactive material (NORM), and other radioactive material that the AEC's successor, the NRC, determines could pose a threat to public health and safety or the common defense and security.

Previously, these materials, as well as U or Th in concentrations <0.05% and radioisotopes produced by accelerators that were not on government contracts, had been regulated by the states.

The AEC exercised its regulatory authority through the issuance of radiation safety standards and regulations, the licensing of applicants who wished to use any of the materials that the AEC was authorized to regulate, a system of inspection to verify that a licensee was in fact complying with the radiation safety regulations, and a system of penalties and fines for those licensees who were found not in compliance with the regulations. The AEC's regulations were published in 10 CFR 20, and contained the standards for safe use of radiation sources. These standards, which were designed to protect radiation workers, included a dose limit called the maximum permissible dose, and maximum permissible concentrations (MPCs) of radionuclides in air and water within the context of occupational exposure. MPCs in the gaseous and aqueous emissions to the environment from licensed facilities were also published in 10 CFR 20. The permissible concentrations in the emissions were much lower than those for occupational exposure, since the emitted radionuclides could now expose the general population. The published maximum permissible doses and maximum permissible environmental concentrations were *upper limits only*. In all instances, planning for radiation protection was and still is based on radiation doses that are ALARA. Furthermore, the tabulated MPCs for radionuclides emitted from the licensed facility notwithstanding, radiation safety in any particular case was required to be based on the most sensitive segment of the exposed population and on the environmental pathway that would lead to the greatest dose to the critical population group. For example, in the case of atmospheric ^{131}I in a region where dairy cattle graze, the critical population group is the milk-drinking infant population, and the critical exposure pathway is air to grass to cow to milk to infant. These considerations lead to a reduction of the tabulated occupational MPC of ^{131}I by a factor of 700.

Environmental Protection Agency

There are numerous other sources of radiation—such as medical and industrial X-ray machines; NORMs, which include uranium and thorium and their progeny; and accelerator-produced radionuclides. The acronyms NORM and NARM (natural and accelerator-produced radioactive materials) are frequently applied to these radiation sources. These radiation sources might be injurious to health but nevertheless were not regulated under the Atomic Energy Acts of 1946 and 1954. Accordingly, the Federal Radiation Council (FRC) was formed in 1959 to provide a uniform federal policy on human exposure to radiation. The FRC was charged to "Advise the President with respect to radiation matters directly or indirectly affecting health, including guidance for all federal agencies in the formulation of radiation standards and in the establishment and execution of programs of cooperation with states. . . . " In 1970, under the terms of the Energy Reorganization Act, the FRC was abolished and its functions were transferred to the newly established U.S. EPA. In addition to its other environmental protection responsibilities, the EPA was charged with the task of setting radiation safety policy and basic standards. To accomplish these tasks, the EPA submits *Radiation Protection Guides* to the president of the United States. If the president approves, these guides then become legally binding, and all the

TABLE 8-24. U.S. Environmental Protection Agency Radioactivity Limits for Drinking Water

RADIONUCLIDE	CONCENTRATION LIMIT
Gross alpha, excluding Rn and U	15 pCi/L
Beta–gamma emitters	4 mrems/yr
Combined ^{226}Ra + ^{228}Ra	5 pCi/L
Tritium	20,000 dpm/L
^{90}Sr	8 pCi/L
Uranium, natural	30 μg/L

federal regulatory agencies that deal with radiation must issue regulations that are compatible with those in the guides. Promulgation of radiation safety regulations is the responsibility of the several regulatory agencies, including the EPA itself, which regulates radioactive discharges into the atmosphere and into waters, establishes drinking water standards, and regulates recovery and disposal of radioactive wastes not regulated under the Atomic Energy Act. EPA regulations are published in Title 40, CFR (40 CFR 9, 141, 142). The EPA limits for radioactivity in drinking water are listed above in Table 8-24.

Nuclear Regulatory Commission

According to the Atomic Energy Act, the AEC had two responsibilities. One was to develop nuclear energy and useful applications for by-product materials. The second was to regulate these activities so that they were carried out safely. Thus, a single agency was charged with the duty to develop and promote nuclear energy and also to regulate its safe use. Many persons in policymaking positions thought that these two responsibilities were mutually incompatible and that there was an inherent conflict of interest in carrying them out. To remedy this situation, the AEC was abolished in 1974 under the authority of the Energy Reorganization of 1974, and two new agencies were established in its place. The development and promotion of nuclear energy was assigned to the Energy Research and Development Administration (ERDA), which later became the Department of Energy (DOE). Responsibility for radiation safety in the use of source material, special nuclear material, and by-product material was assigned to the Nuclear Regulatory Commission (NRC). The NRC's regulations are published in 10 CFR. The standards for protection against radiation are published in Part 20 of these regulations, 10 CFR 20. A basic tenet of these safety regulations is that the licensee must maintain strict control over all licensed sources at all times.

Dose Limits

A dose limit is the upper permissible bound for radiation dose; it is a dose level that may not be exceeded. From 1957 until 1991, the AEC and then NRC radiation safety regulations published in 10 CFR 20 were based on ICRP 2 recommendations for radiation workers. To keep up with scientific and engineering advances, the original regulations were amended numerous times. The publication of ICRP 26 in 1977 and ICRP 30 in 1979, which are based on "uniform risk" concept for fatal radiogenic cancers and for serious hereditary effects rather than the "critical organ" concept of ICRP 2, led to dose limits and calculational methodologies that differed significantly from those used in 10 CFR 20. These changes in the philosophical basis for dose limitation and in calculational methodology led to a need for revisions in derived limits, such as the ALI (which was only implied in the former 10 CFR 20), and in secondary limits, such as the DAC and effluent concentrations. Furthermore, in 1987, the EPA based its guidance on ICRP 26 and 30 recommendations. Since the NRC is required to comply with the EPA's guidance, the NRC revised 10 CFR 20 to make it compatible with the EPA's guidance. In this revision, however, the use of the traditional radiation units (rads, rems, and curies) was retained. The dose limits for radiation workers and for members of the general public that are listed in the revised Part 20 are summarized in Table 8-25. It is essential to understand that when setting dose limits, the NRC assumes that licensees will design routine operations so that workers will receive substantially smaller doses than the limit. Limits were to be approached only under unusual circumstances, and that only a small fraction of the exposed population would approach this limit.

Regulatory limits of the NRC generally do not apply to medical radiation exposure. However, if X-ray tests are included in a physical examination required by an employer as a condition of employment, then the X-ray dose is considered as occupational exposure. Chest X-rays are almost always included in these physical examinations. The effective dose from such medical radiation doses must be included in the worker's occupational dose history.

Dose Constraints

A constraint is a level below the maximum limit, which may be exceeded only under certain conditions. For example, a constraint on airborne emissions [10 CFR 20.1101(d)] requires that emissions be so limited that the dose to a member of the public from the emissions be ≤10 mrems in a year. However, when it is exceeded, the NRC requires the licensee to take certain actions, including appropriate timely corrective actions and a report to the NRC.

Agreement States

Under the terms of the Atomic Energy Act of 1954, the NRC may transfer to approved states the authority to license and regulate uranium, thorium, and certain quantities of special nuclear material. To be approved by the NRC, a state must agree to promulgate and to enforce radiation safety standards that are at least as rigorous as the NRC's standards, and must also have the resources and the legal authority to exercise these responsibilities. The NRC evaluates the technical licensing and inspection of the agreement states; it also conducts training courses and workshops, involves the agreement states in NRC rulemaking and other regulatory efforts, and coordinates with agreement states in the reporting of events and responses to allegations reported to the NRC involving agreement states.

TABLE 8-25. 10 CFR 20 Annual Occupational Dose Limits

DOSE LIMIT TO	DOSE LIMIT
Whole body	5 rems effective dose
Lens of the eye	15 rems
Any other organ or tissue	50 rems
Limbs below elbow or knee	50 rems
Skin, averaged over 10 cm^2	50 rems
Minors	0.1 adult dose
Conceptus	0.5 rem
Members of the general public	0.1 rem

Kentucky became the first agreement state in 1962. By 2007, this number had grown to 34 states.

Computational Methodology

ICRP 30 Methodology

The NRC uses ICRP 30 methodology to calculate radiation dose, ALIs, and DACs for internal emitters. However, the NRC chose to use the traditional radiation units rather than the SI units. The appropriate ALI (either inhalation or ingestion, and either stochastic or nonstochastic) is calculated by the U.S. NRC from

$$\text{ALI, } \mu\text{Ci/yr} = \frac{\text{Dose limit, } \dfrac{\text{rems}}{\text{yr}}}{\text{DCF, } \dfrac{\text{rems}}{\mu\text{Ci}}}. \tag{8.53}$$

The DCF expressed in traditional units of rems/μCi is related to the DC expressed in SI units of Sv/Bq by the following:

$$\text{DCF rems}/\mu\text{Ci} = \text{DC} \frac{\text{Sv}}{\text{Bq}} \times 3.7 \times 10^4 \frac{\text{Bq}}{\mu\text{Ci}} \times 100 \frac{\text{rems}}{\text{Sv}}$$

$$= 3.7 \times 10^6 \times \text{DCF} \frac{\text{Sv}}{\text{Bq}}. \tag{8.54}$$

Thus, for ^{137}Cs, for inhalation of class D particles, we have, using the SI value for the DC from Table 8-20 in Eq. (8.54):

$$\text{DCF} = 3.7 \times 10^6 \times 8.63 \times 10^{-9} \frac{\text{Sv}}{\text{Bq}} = 3.2 \times 10^{-2} \frac{\text{rems}}{\mu\text{Ci}}.$$

The SALI for inhaled class D ^{137}Cs particles is calculated with Eq. (8.53),

$$\text{SALI (inhalation)} = \frac{5 \dfrac{\text{rems}}{\text{yr}}}{3.2 \times 10^{-2} \dfrac{\text{rems}}{\mu\text{Ci}}} = 1.6 \times 10^2 \frac{\mu\text{Ci}}{\text{yr}}.$$

Since the values published in 10 CFR 20 are rounded off to one significant figure, the SALI for inhaled class D ^{137}Cs aerosol is listed as $2 \times 10^2 \mu$Ci/yr.

The occupational DAC in traditional units is calculated from

$$\text{DAC, } \mu\text{Ci/mL} = \frac{\text{ALI(unrounded), } \dfrac{\mu\text{Ci}}{\text{yr}}}{2 \times 10^3 \dfrac{\text{h}}{\text{yr}} \times 1.25 \dfrac{\text{m}^3}{\text{h}} \times 10^6 \dfrac{\text{mL}}{\text{m}^3}}. \tag{8.55}$$

For ^{137}Cs class D aerosols, Eq. (8.55) gives the calculated DAC as

$$\text{DAC} = \frac{1.6 \times 10^2 \dfrac{\mu\text{Ci}}{\text{yr}}}{2 \times 10^3 \dfrac{\text{h}}{\text{yr}} \times 1.25 \dfrac{\text{m}^3}{\text{h}} \times 10^6 \dfrac{\text{mL}}{\text{m}^3}} = 6 \times 10^{-8} \frac{\mu\text{Ci}}{\text{mL}},$$

when rounded to one significant figure. It should be noted that the rounding to one significant figure is for listing the final value only, not for carrying out the successive calculations. If the numbers rounded to one significant figure were to be used successively, rounding errors would accumulate and might lead to erroneous final results.

Particle Size and DAC

Safety standards for radioactive aerosols that are listed in 10 CFR 20 are based on ICRP 30 criteria for occupational inhalation. That is, they are for particles of $1\text{-}\mu m$ AMAD and $\sigma_g \leq 4.5$. For particles whose AMAD differs from $1\ \mu m$, adjustment of the published DAC may be made according to the following relationship, given in ICRP 30, between the dose from the ith particle size and the dose from $1\text{-}\mu m$ particles:

$$\frac{H_{50}(i)}{H_{50}(1\mu m)} = f_{NP}\frac{D_{NP}(i)}{D_{NP}(1\mu m)} + f_{TB}\frac{D_{TB}(i)}{D_{TB}(1\mu m)} + f_P\frac{D_P(i)}{D_P(1\mu m)}, \tag{8.56}$$

where

$$H_{50} = \text{committed dose equivalents from the } 1\text{-}\mu m \text{ and } i\text{th-}\mu m \text{ AMAD particles;}$$

$$f_{NP}, f_{TB}, \text{ and } f_P = \text{fractions of the committed dose equivalent due to deposition in the NP, TB, and P respiratory compartments (these values are listed in the supplements to Parts 1 and 2 of ICRP 30. Values can also be found in Table 8.8); and}$$

$$D_{NP}, D_{TB}, \text{ and } D_P = \text{deposition fractions in the respective respiratory compartments for a given particle size.}$$

 EXAMPLE 8.8

The AMAD of UO_2 particles in one of the production departments of a uranium-processing facility was found to be $9.6\ \mu m$. The DAC given in 10 CFR 20 for class Y (UO_2 is a class Y compound) for $1\text{-}\mu m$ AMAD particles is $2 \times 10^{-11} \mu Ci/mL$ (and $7 \times 10^{-1}\ Bq/m^3$ in ICRP 30). What is the DAC corrected for the particle size?

Solution

We will calculate the size-corrected DAC with the aid of Eq. (8.56). The regional deposition probabilities for the two different size distributions, which are found in Figure 8-4, are listed below:

AMAD	D_{NP}	D_{TB}	D_P
1.0	0.30	0.08	0.25
9.6	0.87	0.08	0.05

The fraction of the committed dose equivalent due to the particles deposited in each of the respiratory compartments for class Y^{238}U compounds is found in ICRP 30, supplement to Part 1, page 378 (Figure 8.8 may also be used to estimate deposition), to be

$$f_{NP} = 0,$$
$$f_B = 0, \text{ and}$$
$$f_P = 1.$$

If we insert the respective values into Eq. (8.56), we have

$$\frac{H_{50}(9.6\,\mu\text{m})}{H_{50}(1\,\mu\text{m})} = 0 \times \frac{0.87}{0.3} + 0 \times \frac{0.08}{0.08} + 1 \times \frac{0.05}{0.25} = 0.2.$$

Since the committed dose from the 9.6-mm particle is only 20% of that from 1-mm particles, the recommended DAC may be increased by as much as a factor of 5.

Effluents Released into the Environment

Since the dose limit for members of the general public is much lower than for radiation workers, radionuclide concentrations in air and water that is discharged from NRC licensed facilities must be lower than those applied to occupational exposure. Accordingly, in addition to the secondary limits for occupational exposure that are published in Appendix B, Table 1 of 10 CFR 20, limits on the concentrations of air and water effluents from licensed facilities are published in Table 2 of Appendix B. Monthly average concentrations of radionuclides that are released to sanitary sewers are listed in Table 3 of Appendix B. The concentration values given in Table 2 are equivalent to radionuclide concentrations, which, if inhaled or ingested continuously, would result in a total effective dose equivalent (TEDE) of 0.1 rem to a member of the general public. For those airborne radionuclides whose occupational DAC is limited by submersion (external dose), the occupational DAC is divided by 219 to obtain the limiting atmospheric concentration before release to the public environment. The number 219 includes two factors: (1) a factor of 50 that relates the occupational dose limit of 5 rems/yr to the limit of 0.1 rems/yr to a member of the public and (2) a factor of 4.38 that relates the total exposure time of 8760 h/yr to the occupational exposure time of 2000 h/yr. Thus, for ^{41}Ar, whose occupational DAC is 3×10^{-6} μCi/mL, the effluent concentration is

$$\text{Effluent conc. (air, submer.)} = \frac{\text{DAC, }\dfrac{\mu\text{Ci}}{\text{mL}}}{219}; \tag{8.57}$$

substituting the given values, we obtain

$$\text{Effluent conc.}(^{41}\text{Ar}) = \frac{3 \times 10^{-6}\,\dfrac{\mu\text{Ci}}{\text{mL}}}{219} = 1 \times 10^{-8}\,\frac{\mu\text{Ci}}{\text{mL}}.$$

To calculate the effluent concentrations for those airborne nuclides that are limited by the internal dose and consequently have an ALI, the inhalation ALI is reduced by several factors. A factor of 1/50 relates the 5-rem occupational dose limit to the 0.1-rem limit for the general public, a factor of 1/3 to account for the difference in exposure time and inhalation rate between a worker and a member of the general public, and finally a factor of 1/2 to account for the age difference between workers and the general public. This reduced ALI is divided by the air inhaled by a worker during a 2000-hour working year:

$$\text{Effluent conc. (air, inhal.)} = \frac{\frac{1}{50} \times \frac{1}{3} \times \frac{1}{2} \times \text{inhalation ALI}, \frac{\mu\text{Ci}}{\text{yr}}}{2.4 \times 10^9 \ \frac{\text{mL}}{\text{yr}}}$$

$$= \frac{\text{inhalation ALI}, \frac{\mu\text{Ci}}{\text{yr}}}{300 \times 2.4 \times 10^9 \ \frac{\text{mL}}{\text{yr}}}$$

$$= \frac{\text{inhalation ALI}, \frac{\mu\text{Ci}}{\text{yr}}}{7.2 \times 10^{11} \ \frac{\text{mL}}{\text{yr}}}. \qquad (8.58)$$

For ^{137}Cs, whose unrounded occupational ALI is 156 μCi, the effluent air concentration listed in Table 2 of Appendix B is calculated as

$$\text{Effluent air conc.}(^{137}\text{Cs}) = \frac{156 \ \mu\text{Ci}}{7.2 \times 10^{11} \ \text{mL}} = 2 \times 10^{-10} \ \frac{\mu\text{Ci}}{\text{mL}}.$$

The concentration limits in 10 CFR 20 for radionuclides in liquid effluents discharged into waterways are based on two considerations:

1. The contaminated water will be the sole source of potable water for members of the general public.
2. The limiting annual dose through this exposure pathway is 0.1 rem. The occupational ALI for ingestion was therefore reduced by a factor of 50 to account for the difference between the occupational dose limit and the general public dose limit, and by a factor of 2 to account for the age difference between the working and general populations. Since the annual water intake by a reference person, is 7.3×10^7 mL, the activity concentration liquid effluents is calculated from

$$\text{Effluent conc. (water)} = \frac{\frac{1}{50} \times \frac{1}{2} \times \text{ingestion ALI}, \frac{\mu\text{Ci}}{\text{yr}}}{7.3 \times 10^5 \ \frac{\text{mL}}{\text{yr}}}$$

$$= \frac{\text{ingestion ALI}}{7.3 \times 10^7} \ \frac{\mu\text{Ci}}{\text{yr}}. \qquad (8.59)$$

For the case of ^{137}Cs, for example, Table 1 of CFR 20 says that the ingestion

ALI $= 100\ \mu$Ci. The listing in Table 2 for the effluent concentration in water is obtained as follows:

$$\text{Effluent conc. (water)} = \frac{\text{ingestion ALI}}{7.3 \times 10^7} = \frac{100\ \dfrac{\mu\text{Ci}}{\text{yr}}}{7.3 \times 10^7\ \dfrac{\text{mL}}{\text{yr}}}$$

$$= 1.4 \times 10^{-6}\ \frac{\mu\text{Ci}}{\text{mL}}.$$

Since the table's values are given to one significant figure, the effluent concentration limit is listed as $1 \times 10^{-6}\ \mu$Ci/mL.

Dose Tracking

Part 20 of 10 CFR specifies that the 5-rem EDE limit includes the sum of the external dose and the dose from internally deposited radionuclides. This means that

$$\left[\frac{\text{External dose}}{5\text{ rems}}\right] + \left[\frac{\text{intake}}{\text{ALI}}\right]_{\text{ingestion}} + \left[\frac{\text{intake}}{\text{ALI}}\right]_{\text{inhalation}} \leq 1. \qquad \textbf{(8.60)}$$

For *regulatory purposes,* in order to demonstrate compliance with the regulations, personal dosimeter measurements are used for tracking external doses, and either environmental sampling, in vitro bioassay, or whole-body counting (in vivo bioassay) methods may be used for internal dose tracking. Environmental sampling may be used for the determination of

- intakes and comparison with ALIs,
- exposure to airborne radionuclides and comparison with DAC-hour limits, and
- CEDE and comparison with dose limits.

EXAMPLE 8.9

A worker wears a personal lapel sampler for an entire 8-hour shift to monitor 1-μm AMAD ^{60}Co particles. The sampler draws 2 L/m, and the measured activity on the filter is 10,000 tpm. The ALI for class Y ^{60}Co particles is 30 μCi and the DAC is $1 \times 10^{-8}\mu$Ci/mL. Calculate the worker's

(a) intake,

(b) exposure, DAC-hours, and

(c) CEDE.

Solution

(a) Intake $=$ sample activity $\times \dfrac{\text{breathing rate}}{\text{sampling rate}},$ $\qquad \textbf{(8.61)}$

therefore,

$$\text{Intake} = 10,000 \, \frac{t}{m} \times \frac{1 \, \mu\text{Ci}}{2.22 \times 10^6 \, \frac{t}{m}} \times \frac{\dfrac{10^4 \text{L}}{8\text{h}}}{\dfrac{960\text{L}}{8\text{h}}} = 4.69 \times 10^{-2} \mu\text{Ci}.$$

(b) $\text{Exposure} = \dfrac{\text{Intake}, \mu\text{Ci}}{\text{ALI}, \dfrac{\mu\text{Ci}}{\text{yr}}} \times 2000 \, \dfrac{\text{DAC} \cdot \text{h}}{\text{yr}},$ (8.62)

therefore,

$$\text{Exposure} = \frac{4.69 \times 10^{-2} \mu\text{Ci}}{30 \, \dfrac{\mu\text{Ci}}{\text{yr}}} \times 2000 \, \frac{\text{DAC} \cdot \text{h}}{\text{yr}} = 3.13 \, \text{DAC} \cdot \text{h}.$$

(c) $\text{CEDE} = \text{DAC} \cdot \text{h} \times \dfrac{5000 \, \text{mrems}}{2000 \, \text{DAC} \cdot \text{h}},$ (8.63)

therefore,

$$\text{CEDE} = 3.13 \, \text{DAC} \cdot \text{h} \times \frac{5000 \, \text{mrems}}{2000 \, \text{DAC} \cdot \text{h}} = 7.8 \, \text{mrems} \qquad (780 \, \mu\text{Sv}).$$

If intake is by inhalation only, then regulatory requirements are met if

$$\frac{\text{Effective external dose}}{5 \, \text{rems}} + \sum_j \frac{I_j}{(\text{ALI})_j} \leq 1,$$ (8.64)

where I_j is the intake of radionuclide j by inhalation and $(\text{ALI})_j$ is the annual limit of intake of radionuclide j by inhalation.

Since the intake is given by the product of the atmospheric concentration and inhalation time and the inhalation ALI is 2000 times the DAC, we can rewrite Eq. (8.64) as

$$\frac{\text{Effective external dose}}{5 \, \text{rems}} + \sum_j \frac{\bar{C}_j}{(\text{DAC})_j} \times \frac{t \, \text{hours}}{2000 \, \text{hours}} \leq 1,$$ (8.65)

where

$\bar{C}_j$ = average air concentration of nuclide j over the total exposure time during the year,

t = annual exposure time, hours, and

$(\text{DAC})_j$ = value for radionuclide j from 10 CFR 20, Appendix B, Table 1, Col. 3.

EXAMPLE 8.10

A worker's external dose was 3000 mrems for the year. During the year, he was also exposed to airborne radioactivity. Radiation work permits and air-sampling records showed his exposure to have been as follows:

RADIONUCLIDE	EXPOSURE TIME (h)	CONCENTRATION (μCi/mL)	DAC (μCi/mL)
^{131}I	120	1E−8	2E−8
^{125}I	120	1E−8	3E−8
^{89}Sr	60	2E−7	4E−7
^{90}Sr	60	2E−9	8E−9

Was the worker's TEDE within regulatory limits?

Solution

Substituting the respective data into Eq. (8.62), we have

$$\frac{\text{External effective dose}}{5\,\text{rems}} + \sum_j \frac{\bar{C}_j}{(\text{DAC})_j} \times \frac{t\,\text{hours}}{2000\,\text{hours}}$$

$$= \frac{3}{5} + \left(\frac{1 \times 10^{-8}}{2 \times 10^{-8}} \times \frac{120}{2000}\right) + \left(\frac{1 \times 10^{-8}}{3 \times 10^{-8}} \times \frac{120}{2000}\right) + \left(\frac{2 \times 10^{-7}}{4 \times 10^{-7}} \times \frac{60}{2000}\right)$$

$$+ \left(\frac{2 \times 10^{-9}}{8 \times 10^{-9}} \times \frac{60}{2000}\right)$$

$$= 0.67.$$

Since 0.67 is less than 1, the worker's TEDE is within regulatory limits.

Respirator Use

According to ALARA principles, the TEDE must be minimized. This principle must be considered when a worker is in an area of high radiation and high airborne radioactivity. Wearing a respirator can offer protection against inhalation of the airborne activity. However, wearing a respirator decreases the worker's efficiency and increases the time necessary to complete a job by about 20–25%. Thus, the decision about whether or not to use respiratory protection depends on the actual levels of atmospheric activity and radiation. These relationships are illustrated by the following examples:

EXAMPLE 8.11

A task whose estimated duration is 3 hours is to be done in an area where the radiation level is 15 mrems/h (150 μSv/h). Air samples and spectroscopic analyses of the samples show the air to contain the following activities:

ISOTOPE	μCi/cm^3	DAC
^{54}Mn	1.5×10^{-7}	3×10^{-7}
^{60}Co	1.5×10^{-8}	7×10^{-8}
^{63}Ni	5×10^{-10}	2×10^{-9}
^{65}Zn	2×10^{-8}	1×10^{-7}

Previous experience showed that wearing a half-face respirator, protection factor = 10, increases the task time by 20%. Calculate the

(a) equivalent airborne activity concentration in units of the DAC and

(b) the worker's TEDE

(1) without a respirator and
(2) with a respirator.

Solution

(a)

$$DAC(equivalent) = \sum_i \frac{C_i}{DAC_i}$$

$$= \frac{1.5 \times 10^{-7}}{3 \times 10^{-7}} + \frac{1.5 \times 10^{-8}}{7 \times 10^{-8}} + \frac{5 \times 10^{-10}}{2 \times 10^{-9}} + \frac{2 \times 10^{-8}}{1 \times 10^{-7}} = 1.16$$

(b)

(1) For regulatory purposes, 1 DAC-hour of exposure to a radioactive atmosphere corresponds to a dose of 2.5 mrems. Therefore,

$$TEDE(without) = 3\,hours \times 1.16\,DAC \times 2.5\frac{mrems}{DAC \cdot h} + 3\,hours \times 15\,mrems/h$$

$$= 53.7\,mrems$$

(2) TEDE (with) $= (3 \times 1.2)\,hours \times (0.1 \times 1.16\,DAC) + 3\,hours \times 15\,mrems/h$

$$= 46\,mrems.$$

EXAMPLE 8.12

A worker is in an area where he is exposed to radiation and to an airborne radioactivity concentration of 1 DAC. The estimated time for completion of the job without wearing a respirator is 2 hours. Time and motion studies showed a 20% reduction in worker efficiency if the worker wears a half-face respirator but is not subject to heat stress.

For radiation fields of 5, 9, and 13 mrems/h, calculate the worker's total dose committment if he

(a) wears a respirator.

(b) does not wear a respirator.

Solution

(a) The total dose to the worker in radiation field of 5 mrems h^{-1}, while wearing a half-face respirator whose protection factor (PF) is 10 (10 CFR 20, Appendix A) and which reduces his working efficiency by 20%, is

$$\frac{1\,\text{DAC}}{10} \times \frac{2}{0.8}\,\text{hours} \times 2.5\,\frac{\text{mrems}}{\text{DAC}\cdot\text{h}} + \left(\frac{2\,\text{hours}}{0.8} \times 5\,\frac{\text{mrems}}{\text{h}}\right) = 13\,\text{mrems}.$$

(b) Without a respirator, his dose is

$$\left(1\,\text{DAC} \times 2\,\text{hours} \times 2.5\,\frac{\text{mrems}}{\text{DAC}\cdot\text{h}}\right) + \left(2\,\text{hours} \times 5\,\frac{\text{mrems}}{\text{h}}\right) = 15\,\text{mrems}.$$

By performing similar calculations for the cases where the worker is in external radiation fields of 9 and 13 mrems/h, we find the total doses as listed in the table below:

DOSE RATE (mrems/h)	TOTAL DOSE (mrems)	
	With respirator	Without respirator
5	13	15
9	23	23
13	33	31

The example above shows that the decision regarding the use of a respirator is governed by the relationship between the TEDE when wearing a respirator and when not wearing a respirator. For the condition where the TEDE is the same whether or not a respirator is used, we have

$$(\text{CEDE} + \dot{D})_{\text{with resp}} = (\text{CEDE} + \dot{D})_{\text{without resp.}} \tag{8.66}$$

where CEDE is the committed effective dose equivalent from airborne activity and $\dot{D}$ is the external radiation dose rate.

Equation (8.63) can be rewritten in terms of the atmospheric concentration of radioactivity expressed as a fraction or multiple, f DAC, of the inhalation DAC, the radiation dose rate $\dot{D}$, exposure time, and decrease in the worker's efficiency, ε, due to the respirator:

$$\left[\frac{f\,\mathrm{DAC}}{\mathrm{PF}} \times 2.5\frac{\mathrm{mrems}}{\mathrm{DAC}\cdot\mathrm{h}} + \dot{D}\frac{\mathrm{mrems}}{\mathrm{h}}\right]_{\mathrm{with\ resp}} \times \frac{t\,\mathrm{h}}{1-\varepsilon}$$

$$= \left[f\,\mathrm{DAC} \times 2.5\frac{\mathrm{mrems}}{\mathrm{DAC}\cdot\mathrm{h}} + \dot{D}\frac{\mathrm{mrems}}{\mathrm{h}}\right]_{\mathrm{without\ resp}} \times t\ \mathrm{hours}. \tag{8.67}$$

For the case of a half-face respirator whose PF is 10 and the value of ε (the reduction in the worker's efficiency) is 20%, we have

$$\left[\frac{f\,\mathrm{DAC}}{10} \times 2.5 + \dot{D}\right] \times \frac{t}{0.8} = (f\,\mathrm{DAC} \times 2.5 + \dot{D}) \times t.$$

If we divide both sides of the equation by $\dot{D}$, we have

$$0.25\frac{f\,\mathrm{DAC}}{\dot{D}} + 1 = 2\frac{f\,\mathrm{DAC}}{\dot{D}} + 0.8$$

and solving for f DAC, the atmospheric concentration expressed as a multiple or fraction of the DAC gives

$$f\,\mathrm{DAC} = 0.114 \times \dot{D}. \tag{8.68}$$

This means that a respirator is required if 0.114 times the ambient radiation level in mrems/h exceeds the atmospheric activity concentration expressed in multiples or fractions of the DAC.

EXAMPLE 8.13

Determine whether a worker should wear a half-face respirator, PF $= 10$, if the concentration of airborne $^{137}\mathrm{Cs}$ particles is $2 \times 10^{-8}\mu\mathrm{Ci/mL}$, the ambient radiation level is 5 mrems/h, the estimated time for the job at 100% worker efficiency is 2 hours, and the worker's efficiency is decreased to 80% when wearing the respirator.

Solution

The inhalation DAC for $^{137}\mathrm{Cs}$ is $6 \times 10^{-8}\mu\mathrm{Ci/mL}$. The fractional DAC, f DAC, therefore is

$$f\,\mathrm{DAC} = \frac{2 \times 10^{-8}\ \dfrac{\mu\mathrm{Ci}}{\mathrm{mL}}}{6 \times 10^{-8}\ \dfrac{\mu\mathrm{Ci}}{\mathrm{mL}}} = 0.33.$$

Substituting this value into Eq. (8.68) and solving for the dose rate gives

$$\dot{D} = \frac{f \, \text{DAC}}{0.114} = \frac{0.33}{0.114} = 2.9 \text{ mrems/h}.$$

Since the dose rate in this example exceeds 2.9 mrems/h, wearing a respirator would decrease the worker's efficiency, thereby increasing his or her total exposure time and leading to a greater TEDE than if he or she had not worn a respirator. In this case, the worker would have received a TEDE of 12.7 mrems with a respirator but only 11.7 mrems without a respirator.

ECOLOGICAL RADIATION SAFETY

Radioecology and environmental health physics evolved mainly in the context of risk assessment to humans, and thus may be considered anthropocentric. To this end, radiation-exposure pathways and potential exposure to humans from naturally occurring radioisotopes and from residual anthropogenic environmental radioactivity was extensively studied. A long-term (25 years) study of the environmental and human-health effects from a nuclear power plant that discharged liquid radioactive waste into a major river within the guidelines of the U.S. NRC found that the releases had no known environmental or human-health impact. It was believed that the environmental radiation safety standards that had been developed would also be protective of the biosphere. This belief seems reasonable, since all life evolved in a higher radiation environment than the present one. Now there is an increasing societal concern about the health of the environment. However, there is no universally accepted agreement about what we mean by the "environment." In the case of nonhuman species, for example, are we interested in protecting individual members of the species, as in the case of humans, or is our interest in protecting the species in the interests of biodiversity? To answer some of these questions, the ICRP has suggested that a framework be developed for assessing the impact of ionizing radiation on nonhuman species.

SUMMARY

The harmful effects of overexposure to ionizing radiation were seen almost immediately after the discovery of X-rays and its introduction into medicine, science, and industry. Initially, the incidence rate of cancer and other harmful effects among users of radiation was relatively high. For example, during the period 1929–1949, the death rate of radiologists from leukemia was nine times greater than the leukemia death rate among nonradiologist physicians. Today, the leukemia rate among radiologists is no greater than among their nonradiologist colleagues. Furthermore, the nuclear industry today is among the safest of all industrial enterprises. Eight different epidemiological studies of 15,674 deaths among 77,000 nuclear workers found the overall standardized mortality ratio (SMR) for all causes of death to be 82 and the SMR for cancer deaths to be 90. (An SMR of 100 means that the actual number of deaths in the study population equals the number of expected deaths. A smaller SMR means that the death rate among the study population is less than expected. The expected death rate is the age-adjusted death rate of the general population.). This change in the hazards of radiation work, from relatively hazardous to safer than average, is attributable to the evolutionary development of radiation safety standards by the ICRP and the application of these standards by the various national regulatory authorities and by the United Nations' specialized agencies.

SUGGESTED READINGS

Bair, W. J. Overview of ICRP respiratory tract model. *Radiat Prot Dosim,* **38**(1):147–152, 1991.

Beral, V., Fraser, P., Booth, M., and Carpenter, L. Epidemiological studies of workers in the nuclear industries, in Jones, R. S., and Southwood, R., eds. *Radiation and Health.* John Wiley & Sons, Chichester, U.K., 1987.

Berry, R. J. The International Commission on Radiological Protection—A historical perspective, in Jones, R. S., and Southwood, R., eds. *Radiation and Health.* John Wiley & Sons, Chichester, U.K., 1987.

Drottz-Sjoberg, B.M., and Persson, L. Public reaction to radiation: Fear, anxiety, or phobia? *Health Phys,* **64:**223, 1993.

Eckerman, K. F. Dosimetric methodology of the ICRP, in Raabe, O. G., ed. *Internal Radiation Dosimetry.* Medical Physics Publishing, Madison, WI, 1994.

Eckerman, K. F., Wolbarst, A. B., and Richardson, A. C. B. *Limiting Values of Radionuclide Intake and Air Concentration and Dose Conversion Factors for Inhalation, Submersion, and Ingestion.* Federal Guidance Report No. 11, EPA-520/1-88-020, Office of Radiation Programs, U.S. Environmental Protection Agency, Washington, DC, 1988.

Eckerman, K.F., Leggett, R.W., Nelson, C.B., Puskin, J.S., and Richardson, A.C.B. *Cancer Risk Coefficients for Environmental Exposure to Radionuclides.* Federal Guidance Report 13, U.S. Environmental Protection Agency, Washington, DC, 1999.

Fiorino, D. J. Technical and democratic values in risk analysis. *Risk Anal,* **9:**293–299, 1989.

Fritsch, P. Uncertainties in aerosol deposition within the respiratory tract using the ICRP 66 Model: A study in workers. *Health Phys,* **90:**114–126, 2006.

Gonzalez, A. Radiation safety standards and their application: International policies and current issues. *Health Phys,* **87:**258–272, 2004.

Hobbie, R.K. *Intermediate Physics for Medicine and Biology,* 4th ed. Wiley & Sons, New York, 2001.

Holm, L.E. Current activities of the International Commission on Radiological Protection. *Health Phys,* **87:**300–311, 2004.

James, A. C. Dosimetric applications of the new ICRP lung model, in Raabe, O. G., ed. *Internal Radiation Dosimetry.* Medical Physics Publishing, Madison, WI, 1994.

Jarvis, N.S., Birchall, A., James, A.C., Baily, M.R., and Dorrain, M.D. *LUDEP 2.0 Personal Computer Program for Calculating Internal Doses Using the ICRP 66 Respiratory Tract Model.* National Radiological Protection Board, Chilton, Didcot, Oxfordshire, U.K., 1996.

Jones, C.R. Radiation protection challenges facing the federal agencies. *Health Phys,* **87:**173–281, 2004.

Kase, K.R. Radiation protection principles of the NCRP. *Health Phys,* **87:**251–257, 2004.

Kathren, R. L. and Ziemer, P., eds. *Health Physics: A Backward Glance.* Pergamon Press, New York, 1980.

Leggett, R.W., and Eckerman, K.F. *Dosimetric Significance of the ICRP's Updated Guidance and Models, 1989–2003, and Implications for U.S. Federal Guidance,* ORNL 2003/207. National Information Service, Springfield, VA, 2003.

Meinhold, C. B. The evolution of radiation protection—From erythema to genetic risks to cancer. *Health Phys,* **87:**240–248, 2004.

National Council on Radiation Protection and Measurements (NCRP), Bethesda, MD, NCRP Publication No.

22. *Maximum Permissible Body Burdens and Maximum Permissible Concentrations of Radionuclides in Air and in Water for Occupational Exposure,* 1963.

46. *Alpha-Emitting Particles in Lungs,* 1975.

64. *Influence of Dose and Its Distribution in Time on Dose–Response Relationships for Low-LET Radiations,* 1980.

82. *SI Units in Radiation Protection and Measurement,* 1985.

84. *General Concepts for the Dosimetry of Internally Deposited Radionuclides,* 1985.

92. *Public Radiation Exposure from Nuclear Power Generation in the United States,* 1987.

93. *Ionizing Radiation Exposure of the Population of the United States,* 1987

94. *Exposure of the Population of the United States and Canada from Natural Background Radiation, 1987.*

95. *Radiation Exposure in the U.S. Population from Consumer Products and Miscellaneous Sources,* 1987.

96. *Comparative Carcinogenicity of Ionizing Radiation and Chemicals,* 1989.

100. *Exposure of the U.S. Population from Diagnostic Medical Radiation,* 1989.

101. *Exposure of the U.S. Population from Occupational Radiation,* 1989.

104. *The Relative Biological Effectiveness of Radiations of Different Quality,* 1990.

106. *Limit for Exposure to "Hot Particles" on the Skin,* 1989.

108. *Conceptual Basis for Calculations of Absorbed-Dose Distributions,* 1991.

115. *Risk Estimates for Radiation Protection,* 1993.

116. *Limitation of Exposure to Ionizing Radiation,* 1993.

121. *Principles and Application of the Collective Dose in Radiation Protection,* 1995.

123. *Screening Models for Release of Radionuclides to Atmosphere, Surface Water, And Ground,* 1996.

125. *Deposition, Retention, and Dosimetry of Inhaled Radioactive Substances,* 1997.

Patrick, R., Palms, J., Kreeger, D., and Harris, C. Twenty-five year study of radionuclides in the Susquehanna river via periphyton biomonitors. *Health Phys,* **92:**1–9, 2007.

Persson, L., and Shrader-Frechette, K. An evaluation of the ethical principles of the ICRP's radiation protection standards for workers. *Health Phys,* **80:**225–234, 2001.

Shrader-Frechette, K., and Persson, L. *Ethical Problems in Radiation Protection.* SSI Report 2001:11, Swedish Radiation Protection Institute, Stockholm, 2001.

Stannard, J. N. *Radioactivity and Health: A History.* DOE/RL/01830-T59 (DE 88013791), National Technical Information Service, Springfield, VA, 1988.

Taylor, L. S. *Organization for Radiation Protection.* DOE/TIC 10124, National Technical Information Service, Springfield, VA, 1979.

International Atomic Energy Agency (IAEA), Vienna. Safety Series Publication No.

6. *Regulations for the Safe Transport of Radioactive Material,* 1985. 2nd ed., 1990.

7. *Explanatory Material for the IAEA Regulations for the safe Transport of Radioactive Material,* 1985. 2nd ed., 1990.

37. *Advisory Material for the IAEA Regulations for the Safe Transport of Radioactive Material,* 1985. 3rd ed., 1990.

67. *Assigning a Value to Transboundary Radiation Exposure,* 1985.

89. *Principles for the Exemption of Radiation Sources and Practices from Regulatory Control,* 1988.

Recommendations for the Safe Use and Regulation of Radiation Sources in Industry, Medicine, Research, and Teaching, 1990.

104. *Extension of the Principles of Radiation Protection to Sources of Potential Exposure,* 1990.

115. *International Basic Safety Standards for Protection against Ionizing Radiation and for the Safety of Radiation Sources,* 1996.

RS-G-1.1. *Occupational Radiation Protection Safety Guide,* Safety Standards Series No. RS-G-1.1, 1999.

RS-G-1.2. *Assessment of Occupational Exposure Due to Intake of Radionuclides,* Safety Standards Series No. RS-G-1.2, 1999.

Assessment of Occupational Exposure Due to External Sources of Radiation, Safety Standards Series No. RS-G-1.3, 1999.

Radiological Protection for Medical Exposure to Ionizing Radiation, Safety Standards Series No. RS-G-1.5, 2002.

Effects of Ionizing Radiation on Plants and Animals at Levels Implied by Current Radiation Protection Standards, Technical Report Series No. 332, 1992.

International Commission on Radiological Protection (ICRP).

X-ray and Radium Protection. Recommendations of the 2nd International Congress of Radiology, 1928. Circular No. 374 of the Bureau of Standards, U.S. Government Printing Office (January 23, 1929). *Br J Radiol,* **1:**359, 1928.

Recommendations of the International X-ray and Radium Protection Commission. Alterations to the 1928 Recommendations of the 2nd International Congress of Radiology. 3rd International Congress of Radiology, 1931. *Br J Radiol,* **4:**485, 1931.

International Recommendations for X-ray and Radium Protection. Revised by the International X-ray and Radium Protection Commission and adopted by the 3rd International Congress of Radiology, Paris, July 1931. *Br J Radiol,* **5**:82, 1932.

International Recommendations for X-ray and Radium Protection. Revised by the International X-ray and Radium Protection Commission and adopted by the 4th International Congress of Radiology, Zurich, July 1934. *Radiology,* **23**:682–685, 1934. *Br J Radiol,* **7**:695, 1934.

International Recommendations for X-ray and Radium Protection. Revised by the International X-ray and Radium Protection Commission and adopted by the 5th International Congress of Radiology, Chicago, September 1937. British Institute of Radiology, 1938. *Radiology,* **30**:511, 1938.

International Recommendations on Radiological Protection. Revised by the International Commission on Radiological Protection at the 6th International Congress of Radiology, London, 1950. *Radiology,* **56**:431–439, March, 1951. *Br J Radiology,* **24**:46–53, 1951.

Recommendations of the International Commission on Radiological Protection (Revised December 1, 1954). *Br J Radiol,* Suppl 6, 1955.

Exposure of man to ionizing radiation arising from medical procedures. An enquiry into methods of evaluation. A report of the International Commission on Radiological Protection and on Radiological Units and Measurements. *Phys Med Biol,* **2**:No. 2, 1957.

Report on Amendments during 1956 to the Recommendations of the International Commission on Radiological Protection (ICRP). *Radiation Research,* **8**:539–42, June 1958; *Acta Radiol,* **48**:493–495, December 1957; *Radiology,* **70**:261–262, February 1958; Fortschritte *a.d. Gebiete d. Rontgenstrahlen u.d. Nuklearmedizin,* **88**:500–502, 1958.

Report on Decisions at the 1959 Meeting of the International Commission on Radiological Protection (ICRP). *Radiology,* **74**:116–19, 1960; *Am J Roentg* **83**:372–375, 1960; *Strahlentherapie,* Band 112, Heft 3, 1960; *Acta Radiol.* **53**:Fasc. 2, February 1960; *Br J Radiol,* **33**:189–192, 1960.

Report of the RBE Committee to the International Commissions on Radiological Protection and on Radiological Units and Measurements. *Health Phys,* **9**:357–384, 1963.

Radiobiological aspects of the supersonic transport: A report prepared by a task group of Committee 1. *Health Phys,* **12**:209–226, 1966.

Deposition and retention models for internal dosimetry of the human respiratory tract: A report prepared by a task group of Committee 2. *Health Phys,* **12**:173–207, 1966.

A review of the physiology of the gastrointestinal tract in relation to radiation doses from radioactive materials: A report prepared by a consultant to Committee 2. *Health Phys,* **12**:131–61, 1966.

Calculation of radiation dose from protons and neutrons to 400 MeV: A report prepared by a task group of Committee 3. *Health Phys,* **12**:227–237, 1966.

International Commission on Radiological Protection, published as ICRP Publications, by Pergamon, Elsevier Ltd., U.K. Publication No.

1. *Recommendations of the International Commission on Radiological Protection,* 1959.
2. *Report of Committee II on Permissible Dose for Internal Radiation,* (1960). [Also published in *Health Phys* **3**, June, 1960.]
3. *Report of Committee III on Protection Against X-rays up to Energies of 3 MeV and Beta and Gamma-rays from Sealed Sources,* 1960.
4. *Report of Committee IV (1953–1959) on Protection Against Electromagnetic Radiation above 3 MeV and Electrons, Neutrons, and Protons,* 1964.
5. *Report of Committee V on Handling and Disposal of Radioactive Materials in Hospitals and Medical Research Establishments,* 1965.
6. *Recommendations of the International Commission on Radiological Protection,* 1964.
7. *Principles of Environmental Monitoring Related to the Handling of Radioactive Materials,* 1966.
8. *The Evaluation of Risks from Radiation,* 1966.
9. *Recommendations of the International Commission on Radiological Protection,* 1966.
10. *Report of Committee IV on Evaluation of Radiation Doses to Body Tissues from Internal Contamination Due to Occupational Exposure,* 1968.
10a. *The Assessment of Internal Contamination Resulting From Recurrent or Prolonged Uptakes,* 1971.
11. *A Review of the Radiosensitivity of the Tissues in Bone,* 1968.
13. *Radiation Protection in Schools for Pupils up to the Age of 18 years,* 1970.
14. *Radiosensitivity and Spatial Distribution of Dose,* 1969.
15. *Protection Against Ionizing Radiation from External Sources,* 1970.

16. *Protection of the Patient in X-ray Diagnosis,* 1970.

17. *Protection of the Patient in Radionuclide Investigations,* 1971.

18. *The RBE for High LET-Radiations with Respect to Mutagenesis,* 1972.

19. *The Metabolism of Compounds of Plutonium and Other Actinides,* 1972.

20. *Alkaline Earth Metabolism in Adult Man,* 1973.

21. Data for Protection Against Ionizing Radiation from External Sources: *Supplement to ICRP Publication 15,* 1973.

22. *Implications of Commission Recommendations that Doses be kept as Low as Readily Achievable,* 1974.

23. *Report of the Task Group on Reference Man,* 1975.

The following reports of the ICRP are published in the Annals of the ICRP, Pergamon, Elsevier Ltd., Oxford, U.K.

24. *Radiation Protection in Uranium and Other Mines,* **1**(1), 1977.

25. *The Handling, Storage, Use and Disposal of Unsealed Radionuclides in Hospitals and Medical Research Establishments,* **1**(2), 1977.

26. *Recommendations of the International Commission on Radiological Protection,* **1**(3), 1977.

27. *Problems Involved in Developing an Index of Harm,* **1**(4), 1977.

28. *Statement from the 1978 Stockholm Meeting of the ICRP* and *The Principles and General Procedures for Handling Emergency and Accidental Exposures of Workers,* **2**(1), 1978.

29. *Radionuclide Release into the Environment: Assessment of Doses to Man,* **2**(2), 1979.

30-1. *Limits for Intakes of Radionuclides by Workers,* **2**(3,4), 1979.

30-1. Supplement. *Limits for Intakes of Radionuclides by Workers,* **3**(1–4), 1979.

30-2. *Statement and Recommendations of the 1980 Brighton Meeting of the ICRP* and *Limits for Intakes of Radionuclides by Workers,* **4**(3,4), 1980.

30-2. Supplement. *Limits for Intakes of Radionuclides by Workers,* **5**(1–4), 1981.

30-3. *Limits for Intakes of Radionuclides by Workers,* **6**(2,3), 1981.

30-3. Supplement. *Limits for Intakes of Radionuclides by Workers,* **7**(1–3), 1982.

30-3. Supplement B, Limits *for Intakes of Radionuclides by Workers,* **8**(1–3), 1982.

31. *Biological Effects of Inhaled Radionuclides,* **4**(1,2), 1980.

32. *Limits for Inhalation of Radon Daughters by Workers,* **6**(1), 1981.

38. *Radionuclide Transformations: Energy and Intensity of Emissions,* **11–13**, 1983.

42. *A Compilation of the Major Concepts and Quantities in Use by the ICRP,* **14**(4), 1984.

45. *Quantitative Basis for Developing a Unified Index of Harm,* **15**(3), 1986.

48. *The Metabolism of Plutonium and Related Elements,* **16**(2,3), 1986.

50. *Lung Cancer Risk from Indoor Exposures to Radon Daughters.* **17**(1), 1987.

53. *Radiation Dose to Patients from Radiopharmaceuticals,* **18**(1–4), 1988.

54. *Individual Monitoring for Intakes of Radionuclides by Workers: Design and Interpretation,* **19**(1–3), 1989.

55. *Optimization and Decision Making in Radiological Protection,* **20**(1), 1989.

56. *Age-Dependent Doses to Members of the Public from Intake of Radionuclides, Part 1,* **20**(2), 1989.

57. *Radiological Protection of the Worker in Medicine and Dentistry,***20**(3), 1990.

58. *RBE for Deterministic Effects,* **20**(4), 1990.

60. *1990 Recommendations of the International Commission on Radiological Protection,* **21**(1–3), 1991.

61. *Annual Limits on Intake of Radionuclides by Workers Based on 1990 Recommendations,* **21**(4), 1991.

62. *Radiological Protection in Biomedical Research,* **22**:No. 3, 1993.

63. *Principles for Intervention for Protection of the Public in a Radiological Emergency,* **22**(4), 1993.

64. *Protection from Potential Exposure: A Conceptual Framework,* **23**(1), 1993.

65. *Protection Against Radon-222 at Home and at Work,* **23**:No. 2, 1994.

66. *Human Respiratory Tract Model for Radiological Protection,* **24**(1–3), 1994.

67. *Age-Dependent Doses to Members of the Public from Intake of Radionuclides, Part 2,* **23**(3/4), 1993.

68. *Dose Coefficients for Intakes of Radionuclides by Workers,* **24**(4), 1994.

69. *Age-Dependent Doses to Members of the Public from Intake of Radionuclides, Part 3, Ingestion Dose Coefficients,* **25**(1), 1995.

71. *Age-Dependent Doses to Members of the Public from Intake of Radionuclides, Part 4, Inhalation Dose Coefficients,* **25**(3/4), 1996.

72. *Age-Dependent Doses to Members of the Public from Intake of Radionuclides, Part 5, Compilation of Ingestion and Inhalation Dose Coefficients,* **26**(1), 1996.

84. *Pregnancy and Medical Radiation,* **30**(1), 2000.

88. *Doses to the Embryo and Fetus from Intakes of Radionuclides by the Mother,* **31**(1–3), 2001.

89. *Basic Anatomical and Physiological Data for Use in Radiological Protection: Reference Values,* **32**(3,4), 2002.

91. *A Framework for Assessing the Impact of Ionizing Radiation on Non-human Species,* **33**(3), 2003.

92. *Relative Biological Effectiveness (RBE), Quality Factor (Q), and Radiation Weighting Factor (w_R),* **33**(4), 2003.

100. *Human Alimentary Tract Model for Radiological Protection,* **26**(4), 2006.

101. *Assessing Dose of the Representative Person for the purpose of Radiation Protection of the Public and The Optimisation of Radiological Protection: Broadening the Process,* **36**(3), 2006.

Analysis of the Criteria Used by the International Commission on Radiological Protection to Justify the Setting of Numerical Protection Level Values, ICRP Supporting Guidance 5, **36**(4), 2006.

International Commission on Radiological Units and Measurements (ICRU), Washington, DC, ICRU Publication No.

25. *Conceptual Basis for the Determination of Dose Equivalent,* 1976.

40. *The Quality Factor in Radiation Protection,* 1986.

51. *Quantities and Units in Radiation Protection Dosimetry,* 1993.

66. Determination of operational dose equivalent quantities for neutrons, *J ICRU,* **3**(3), 2001.

HEALTH PHYSICS INSTRUMENTATION

RADIATION DETECTORS

Humans do not possess any sense organs that can detect ionizing radiation. As a consequence, they must rely entirely on instruments for the detection and measurement of radiation. Instruments used in the practice of health physics serve a wide variety of purposes. It is logical, therefore, to find a wide variety of instrument types. We have, for example, instruments such as the Geiger-Müller counter and scintillation counter, which measure particles; film badges, pocket dosimeters, and thermoluminescent dosimeters, which measure accumulated doses; and ionization-chamber-type instruments, which measure dose and dose rate. In each of these categories, one finds instruments designed specifically for the measurement of a certain type of radiation, such as low-energy X-rays, high-energy gamma rays, fast neutrons, and so on.

Although there are many different instrument types, the operating principles for most radiation-measuring instruments are relatively few. The basic requirement of any such instrument is that its detector interacts with the radiation in such a manner that the magnitude of the instrument's response is proportional to the radiation effect or radiation property being measured. Some of the physical and chemical radiation effects that apply to radiation detection and measurement for health physics purposes are listed in Table 9-1.

During the last few decades, there has been relatively little change in the basic detectors that interact with radiation to produce an output signal. During this same period, there have been enormous advances in the electronic processing of the output signals from these detectors and in the subsequent treatment of the information contained in them. These advances are the result of the invention of the transistor and the integrated circuit. Since integrated circuits were introduced, the number of transistors that could be placed on a silicon chip has doubled approximately every 1.5 years. As a consequence, microprocessor technology advanced at a very rapid rate. Integrated circuits continue to become smaller and also to require ever-decreasing amounts of power. In health physics instrumentation, these advances have resulted

TABLE 9-1. Radiation Effects Used in the Detection and Measurement of Radiation

EFFECT	TYPE OF INSTRUMENT	DETECTOR
Electrical	1. Ionization chamber	1. Gas
	2. Proportional counter	2. Gas
	3. Geiger counter	3. Gas
	4. Solid state detector	4. Semiconductor
Chemical	1. Film	1. Photographic emulsion
	2. Chemical dosimeter	2. Solid or liquid
Light	1. Scintillation counter	1. Crystal or liquid
	2. Cerenkov counter	2. Crystal or liquid
	3. Opticoluminescent dosimeter	3. Crystal
Thermoluminescence	Thermoluminescent dosimeter (TLD)	Crystal
Heat	Calorimeter	Solid or liquid

in much smaller and lighter "smart" instruments. Instruments now have the capability of correcting for dead time and background, logging, manipulating, plotting, and analyzing the data and then storing the results, and identifying unknown radioisotopes from analysis of their spectra. The information recorded and stored in this fashion is available for downloading into computers and/or other instruments.

Health physics instruments are designed for a number of different applications, such as routine environmental monitoring; monitoring occupational exposure; measuring contamination of surfaces, air, and water; measuring radon and its progeny; medical radiation measurements; and nonintrusive inspection in the context of antiterrorism and homeland security. The specific operating requirements vary according to the intended use of the instruments. Standards for the design, use, and calibration of the various categories are set by the American National Standards Institute (ANSI) and the International Electrochemical Commission (IEC). Neither of these organizations are governmental agencies. However, their recommendations are frequently incorporated into the regulations of the various regulatory agencies of the federal and state governments.

PARTICLE-COUNTING INSTRUMENTS

Particle-counting instruments are frequently used by health physicists to determine the radioactivity of a sample taken from the environment, such as an air sample, or to measure the activity of a biological fluid from someone suspected of being internally contaminated. Another important application of particle-counting instruments is in portable radiation-survey instruments. Particle-counting instruments may be very sensitive—they literally respond to a single ionizing particle. They are, accordingly, widely used in searching for unknown radiation sources, leaks in shielding, and areas of contamination. The detector in particle-counting instruments may be either a gas or a solid. In either case, the passage of an ionizing particle through the detector results in energy dissipation by a burst of ionization. This burst of ionization is converted into an electrical pulse that actuates a readout device, such as a scaler or a ratemeter, to register a count.

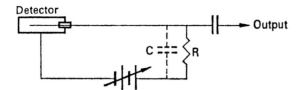

Figure 9-1. Basic circuit of a gas-filled detector.

Gas-Filled Particle Counters

Consider a gas detector system such as is shown in Figure 9-1. This system consists of a variable voltage source V, a high-valued resistor R, and a gas-filled counting chamber D, which has two coaxial electrodes that are very well insulated from each other. All the capacitance associated with the circuit is indicated by the capacitor C. Because of the production of ions within the detector when it is exposed to radiation, the gas within the detector becomes electrically conducting. If the time constant RC of the detector circuit is much greater than the time required for the collection of all the ions resulting from the passage of a single particle through the detector, then a voltage pulse of magnitude

$$V = \frac{Q}{C},$$

(9.1)

where Q is the total charge collected and C is the capacitance of the circuit, and of the shape shown by the top curve in Figure 9-2, appears across the output of the detector circuit.

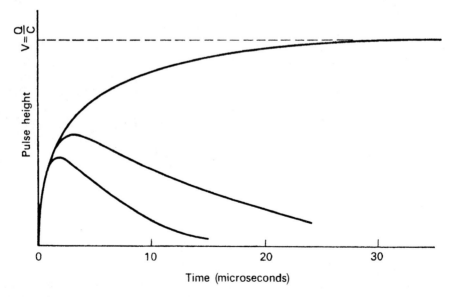

Figure 9-2. Dependence of pulse shape on the time constant of the detector circuit. The top curve is for the case where $RC = \infty$, the center curve is for the case where RC is less than the ion collection time, while the lowest curve is for the case where RC is much less than the ion collection time.

A broad output pulse would make it difficult to separate successive pulses. However, if the time constant of the detector circuit is made much smaller than the time required to collect all the ions, then the height of the developed voltage pulse is smaller, but the pulse is very much narrower, as shown by the curves in Figure 9-2. This allows individual pulses to be separated and counted.

Ionization Chamber Counter

If a constant flux of radiation is permitted to pass through the detector and the voltage V is varied, several well-defined regions of importance in radiation measurement may be identified (Fig. 9-3). As the voltage is increased from zero through relatively low voltages, the first region, known as the *ionization chamber region*, is encountered. If the instrument has the electrical polarity shown in Figure 9-1, then all the positive ions will be collected by the outer cathode, while the negative ions, or electrons, will be collected by the central anode. "Low voltages," in this case, imply a range of voltage great enough to collect the ions before a significant fraction of them can recombine yet not great enough to accelerate the ions sufficiently to produce secondary ionization by collision. The exact value of this voltage is a function of the type of gas, the gas pressure, and the size and geometric arrangement of the electrodes. In this region, the number of electrons collected by the anode will be equal to the number produced by the primary ionizing particle. The pulse size, accordingly, will be independent of the voltage, and will depend only on the number of ions produced by the primary ionizing particle during its passage through the detector. The ionization chamber region may be defined as that range of operating voltages in which there is no multiplication of ions due to secondary ionization; that is, the gas amplification factor is equal to one. The amplitude of the signal is proportional to the quantity of energy deposited in the active region of the detector. Therefore, an ionization chamber in which the average current generated by the radiation is measured is used mainly to measure radiation dose.

Proportional Counter

The fact that the pulse size from a counter operating in the ionization chamber region depends on the number of ions produced in the chamber makes it possible to use this instrument to distinguish between radiations of different specific ionization, such as alphas and betas or gammas. For example, an alpha particle that traverses the chamber produces about 10^5 ion pairs, which corresponds to 1.6×10^{-14} C. If the chamber capacitance is 10 pF and if all the charges are collected, then the voltage pulse resulting from the passage of this alpha will be

$$V = \frac{Q}{C} = \frac{1.6 \times 10^{-14}}{10 \times 10^{-12}} = 1.6 \times 10^{-3} \, \text{V}.$$

A beta particle, on the other hand, may produce about 1000 ion pairs within the chamber. The resulting output pulse due to the beta particle will be only 1.6×10^{-5} V. Amplification of these two pulses by a factor of 100 leads to pulses of 0.16 V for the alpha and 0.0016 V for the beta. With the use of a discriminator in the scaler (or other readout device), voltage pulses less than a certain predetermined size can be rejected; only those pulses that exceed this size will be counted. In the case of the example given above, a discriminator setting of 0.1 V would allow the pulses due

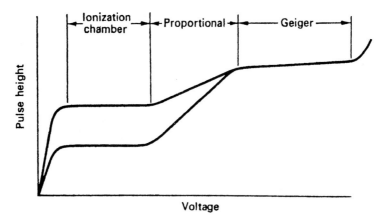

Figure 9-3. Curve of pulse height *versus* voltage across a gas-filled pulse counter, illustrating the ionization chamber, proportional, and Geiger regions.

to the alphas to be counted but would not pass any of the pulses due to the beta particles. This discriminator setting is often referred to as the input sensitivity of the scaler. Increasing the input sensitivity, in the example above, would allow both alphas and betas to be counted. This ability to distinguish between the two radiations is illustrated in Figure 9-3, which shows the output-pulse height as a function of voltage across the counting chamber.

One of the main disadvantages of operating a counter in the ionization chamber region is the relatively feeble output pulse, which requires either much amplification or a high degree of input sensitivity in the scaler. To overcome this difficulty and yet take advantage of the pulse-size dependence on ionization for the purpose of distinguishing between radiations, the counter may be operated as a proportional counter. As the voltage across the counter is increased beyond the ionization chamber region, a point is reached where secondary electrons are produced by collision. This is the beginning of the proportional region. The voltage drop across resistor R will now be greater than it was in the ionization chamber region because of these additional electrons. The gas amplification factor is greater than one. This multiplication of ions in the gas, which is called an avalanche, is restricted to the vicinity of the primary ionization. Increasing the voltage causes the avalanche to increase in size by spreading out along the anode. Since the size of the output pulse is determined by the number of electrons collected by the anode, the size of the output voltage pulse from a given detector is proportional to the high voltage across the detector. Besides the high voltage across the tube, the gas amplification depends on the diameter of the collecting electrode (the electric field intensity near the surface of the anode, which is given by Eq. [2.40], increases as the diameter of the collecting anode decreases) and on the gas pressure. Decreasing gas pressure leads to increasing gas multiplication, as shown in Figure 9-4. Because of the dependence of gas multiplication, and consequently the size of the output pulse, on the high voltage, it is important to use a very stable high-voltage power supply with a proportional counter.

An example of the use of a proportional counter to distinguish between alpha and beta radiation is shown in Figure 9-5. At point *A*, the "threshold" voltage, the

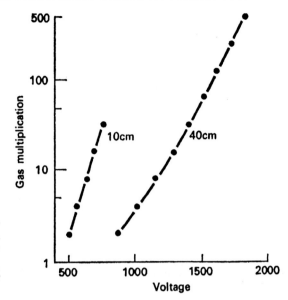

Figure 9-4. Gas multiplication *versus* voltage for gas pressures of 10-cm Hg and 40-cm Hg argon; anode diameter = 0.01 in., cathode diameter = 0.87 in. (Reproduced with permission from Rossi BB, Staub HH. *Ionization Chambers and Counters.* New York, NY: McGraw-Hill; 1949.)

pulses produced by the alpha particles that traverse the counter are just great enough to get by the discriminator. A small increase in voltage causes a sharp increase in counting rate because all the output pulses due to alphas now exceed the input sensitivity of the scaler. Further increase in high voltage has little effect on the counting rate and results in a "plateau," a span of high voltage over which the counting rate is approximately independent of voltage. With the system operating on this alpha plateau, the pulses due to beta particles are still too small to get by the discriminator. However, as the high voltage is increased, point *B* is reached, where the gas amplification is great enough to produce output pulses from beta particles that exceed the input sensitivity of the scaler. This leads to another plateau where both alpha and beta particles are counted. By subtracting the alpha count rate from the alpha–beta count rate, the beta activity may be obtained.

Geiger-Müller Counter

Continuing to increase the high voltage beyond the proportional region will eventually cause the avalanche to extend along the entire length of the anode. An avalanche across the entire length of the anode is called a *Townsend avalanche*. When this happens, the end of the proportional region is reached and the Geiger region begins. At this point, the size of all pulses—regardless of the nature of the primary ionizing particle—is the same. When operated in the Geiger region, therefore, a counter cannot distinguish among the several types of radiations. However, the very large output pulses (>0.25 V) that result from the high gas amplification in a Geiger-Müller (GM) counter means either the complete elimination of a pulse amplifier or use of an amplifier that does not have to meet the exacting requirements of high pulse amplification. Since all the pulses in a GM counter are about the same height, the pulse height is independent of energy deposition in the gas.

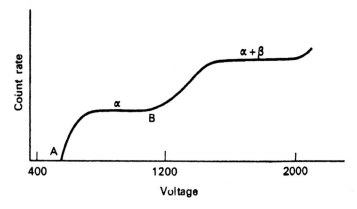

Figure 9-5. Alpha and alpha–beta counting rates as a function of voltage in a proportional counter.

Figure 9-5 shows the alpha and alpha–beta plateaus of a proportional counter. A GM counter too has a wide range of operating voltages over which the counting rate is approximately independent of the operating voltage. This plateau extends approximately from that voltage which results in pulses great enough to be passed by the discriminator to that which causes a rapid increase in counting rate that precedes an electrical breakdown of the counting gas. In the Geiger region, the avalanche is already extended as far as possible axially along the anode. Increasing the voltage, therefore, causes the avalanche to spread radially, resulting in an increasing counting rate. We therefore have a slight positive slope in the plateau, as shown in Figure 9-6. Figures of merit for judging the quality of a counter are the length of the plateau, the slope of the plateau, and the resolving time (discussed later). The slope is usually given as percentage increase in counting rate per 100 V:

$$\text{Slope} = \frac{\dfrac{(C_2 - C_1)}{C_1}}{0.01(V_2 - V_1)} \times 100. \tag{9.2}$$

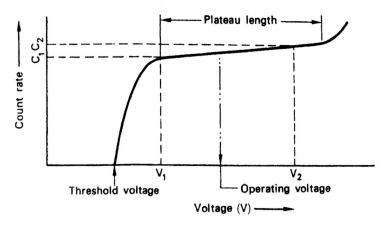

Figure 9-6. Operating characteristics of a Geiger-Müller counter.

A GM counter has a slope of about 3% per 100 V. The operating voltage for a Geiger counter is about one-third to one-half the distance from the knee of the curve of count rate versus voltage.

Quenching a GM Counter

When the positive ions are collected after a pulse, they give up their kinetic energy by striking the wall of the tube. Most of this kinetic energy is dissipated as heat. Some of it, however, excites the atoms in the wall. In falling back to the ground state, these atoms may lose their excitation energy by emitting ultraviolet (UV) photons. Since at this time the electric field around the anode is reestablished to its full intensity, the interaction of UV photons with the gas in the counter may initiate an avalanche, and thereby produce a spurious count. Prevention of such spurious counts is called *quenching.*

Quenching may be accomplished either electronically, by lowering the anode voltage after a pulse until all the positive ions have been collected, or chemically, by using a self-quenching gas. A self-quenching gas is one that can absorb the UV photons without becoming ionized. One method of doing this is to introduce a small amount of an organic vapor, such as alcohol or ether, into the tube. The energy from the UV photon is then dissipated in dissociating the organic molecule. Such a tube is useful only as long as it has a sufficient number of organic molecules for the quenching action. In practice, an organic-vapor GM counter has a useful life of about 10^8 counts. Self-quenching also results when the counting gas contains a trace of a halogen. In this case, the halogen molecule does not dissociate after absorbing the energy from the UV photon. The useful life of a halogen-quenched counter, therefore, is not limited by the number of pulses that have been produced in it.

Resolving Time

Resolving time is the minimum time interval between the arrival of two particles that the detector can recognize as two particles. If two particles enter the counter in rapid succession, the avalanche of ions from the first particle paralyzes the counter, and renders it incapable of responding to the second particle. The avalanche of ionization starts very close to the anode and spreads longitudinally along the anode because the electric-field intensity is greatest near the surface of the anode. The negative ions thus formed migrate toward the anode, while the positive ions move toward the cathode. The negative ions, being electrons, move very rapidly and are soon collected, while the massive positive ions are relatively slow-moving and therefore travel for a relatively long period of time before being collected. The collection time for positive ions formed near the surface of the anode is given by the equation

$$t = \frac{(b^2 - a^2)\, p \times \ln\left(\dfrac{b}{a}\right)}{2 \times V\mu} \text{ seconds,} \tag{9.3}$$

where

> b = radius of cathode, cm;
> a = radius of anode, cm;
> p = gas pressure in counter, mm Hg;

V = potential difference across counter, volts; and

μ = mobility of positive ions (cm/s)/(V/cm); for air, μ has a value of 1070 and for argon its value is 1040.

 # EXAMPLE 9.1

How long will it take to collect all the positive ions in a GM counter filled with argon at a pressure of 100 mm Hg if the operating voltage is 1000 V and the cathode and anode have radii of 1 cm and 0.01 cm respectively?

Solution

By substituting the appropriate numbers into Eq. (9.3), we have

$$t = \frac{(1 - 0.01^2) \times 100 \times \ln\left(\dfrac{1}{0.01}\right)}{2 \times 1000 \times 1040} = 221 \times 10^{-6} \text{ seconds.}$$

These slow-moving positive ions form a sheath around the positively charged anode, thereby greatly decreasing the electric field intensity around the anode and making it impossible to initiate an avalanche by another ionizing particle. As the positive ion sheath moves toward the cathode, the electric field intensity increases, until a point is reached when another avalanche could be started. The time required to attain this electric field intensity is called the *dead time*. After the end of the dead time, however, when another avalanche can be started, the output pulse from this avalanche is still relatively small, since the electric field intensity is still not great enough to produce a Geiger pulse. As the positive ions continue their outward movement, an output pulse resulting from another ionizing particle would increase in size. When the output pulse is large enough to be passed by the discriminator and be counted, the counter is said to have recovered from the previous ionization, and the time interval between the dead time and the time of full recovery is called the *recovery time*. The sum of the dead time and the recovery time is called the *resolving time*. Alternatively, the resolving time may be defined as the minimum time that must elapse after the detection of an ionizing particle before a second particle can be detected. The relationship between the dead time, recovery time, and resolving time is illustrated in Figure 9-7. The resolving time of a GM counter is on the order of 100 μs or more. A proportional counter is much faster than a GM counter. Since the avalanche in a proportional counter is limited to a short length of the anode, a second avalanche can be started elsewhere along the anode while the region of the first avalanche is completely paralyzed. The resolving time of a proportional counter, therefore, is on the order of several microseconds.

Measurement of Resolving Time

The resolving time of a counter may be conveniently measured by the two-source method. Two radioactive sources are counted—singly and together. If there were no resolving time loss, the counting rate of the two sources together would be equal to

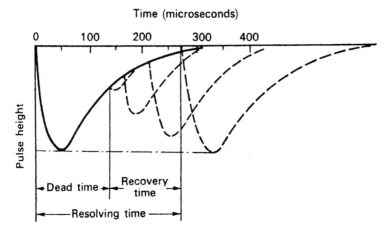

Figure 9-7. Relationship among dead time, recovery time, and resolving time.

the sum of the two single-source counting rates. However, because of the counting losses due to the resolving time of the counting system, the sum of the two single counting rates exceeds that of the two sources together. If R_1 is the counting rate of source 1, R_2 of source 2, $R_{1,2}$ of the two sources together, and R_b the background counting rate, then the resolving time is given by

$$\tau = \frac{R_1 + R_2 - R_{1,2} - R_b}{R_{1,2}^2 - R_1^2 - R_2^2}. \tag{9.4}$$

All the source counting rates above include the background. Because $R_1 + R_2$ is only slightly greater than $R_{1,2}$, all the measurements must be made with a great degree of accuracy in determining the resolving time. For the case where the resolving time is τ and the observed counting rate of a sample is R_0, the counting rate that would have been observed had there been no resolving time loss; that is, the resolving time correction to give the "true" counting rate, R, is

$$R = \frac{R_0}{1 - R_0\tau}. \tag{9.5}$$

Scintillation Counters

A scintillation detector is a transducer that changes the kinetic energy of an ionizing particle into a flash of light. Historically, one of the earliest means of measuring radiation was by scintillation counting. Rutherford, in his classical experiments on scattering of alpha particles, used a zinc sulfide crystal as the primary detector of radiation; he used his eye to see the flickers of light that appeared when alpha particles struck the zinc sulfide. Today, the light is viewed electronically by photomultiplier tubes or photodiodes whose output pulses may be amplified, sorted by size, and counted. The various radiations may be detected with scintillation counters by using the appropriate scintillating material. Table 9-2 lists some of the substances used for this purpose.

Scintillation counters are widely used to count gamma rays and low-energy beta particles. The counting efficiency of GM or proportional counters for low-energy

TABLE 9-2. *Scintillating Materials*

PHOSPHOR	DENSITY (g.cm^{-3})	WAVELENGTH OF MAXIMUM EMISSION (Å)	RELATIVE PULSE HEIGHT	DECAY TIME (μs)
NaI (Tl)	3.67	4100	210	0.25
CsI (Tl)	4.51	Blue	55	1.1
KI (Tl)	3.13	4100	50	1.0
Anthracene	1.25	4400	100	0.032
Trans-Stilbene	1.16	4100	60	0.0064
Plastic		3550–4500	28–48	0.003–0.005
Liquid		3550–4500	27–49	0.002–0.008
p-Terphenyl	1.23	4000	40	0.005

(Source: Swank R. Characteristics of scintillators. *Annu Rev Nucl Sci.* 1954; 4:111–140.)

betas may be very low due to the dissipation of the beta energy within the sample. (This phenomenon is called *self-absorption*.) This disadvantage can be overcome by dissolving the radioactive sample in a scintillating liquid. Such liquid scintillation counters result in detection efficiencies that approach 100%. They are widely used in research applications, especially in the field of biochemistry and by health physicists to measure ^{14}C and ^{3}H.

Whereas the inherent detection efficiency of gas-filled counters is close to 100% for those alphas or betas that enter the counter, their detection efficiency for gamma rays is very low—usually less than 1%. Solid scintillating crystals, on the other hand, have relatively high detection efficiencies for gamma rays. Furthermore, since the intensity of the flicker of light in the detector is proportional to the energy of the gamma ray that produces the light, a scintillation detector can, with the aid of the appropriate electronics, be used as a gamma-ray spectrometer.

For gamma-ray measurement, the scintillation detector used most frequently is a sodium iodide crystal activated with thallium, NaI(Tl), that is optically coupled to a photomultiplier tube. The thallium activator, which is present as an "impurity" in the crystal structure to the extent of about 0.2%, converts the energy absorbed in the crystal to light. The high density of the crystal, together with its high effective atomic number, results in a high detection efficiency (Fig. 9-8).

Gamma-ray photons, passing through the crystal, interact with the atoms of the crystal by the usual mechanisms of photoelectric absorption, Compton scattering, and pair production. The primary ionizing particles resulting from the gamma-ray interactions—the photoelectrons, Compton electrons, and positron–electron pairs—dissipate their kinetic energy by exciting and ionizing the atoms in the crystal. The excited atoms return to the ground state by the emission of quanta of light. These light pulses, upon striking the photosensitive cathode of the photomultiplier tube, cause electrons to be ejected from the cathode. These electrons are accelerated to a second electrode, called a dynode, whose potential is about 100-V positive with respect to the photocathode. Each electron that strikes the dynode causes several other electrons to be ejected from the dynode, thereby "multiplying" the original photocurrent. This process is repeated about ten times before all the electrons thus produced are collected by the anode of the photomultiplier tube. This current pulse, whose magnitude is proportional to the energy of the primary ionizing particle, can then be amplified and counted. Figure 9-9 illustrates schematically the sequence of events in the detection of a photon by a scintillation counter.

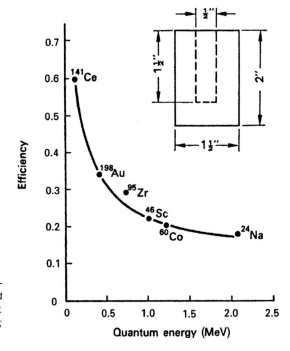

Figure 9-8. Detection efficiency *versus* gamma-ray energy for a NaI(Tl) well crystal. (Reproduced from Borkowski CJ. *ORNL Progress Report 1160.* Oak Ridge, TN: Oak Ridge National Laboratory; 1951.)

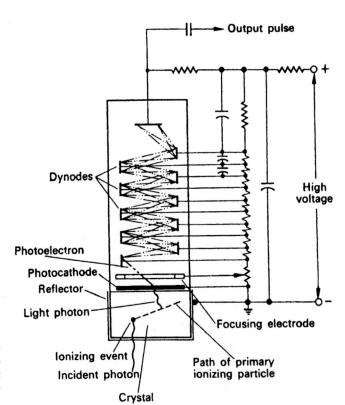

Figure 9-9. Schematic representation of the sequence of events in the detection of a gamma-ray photon by a scintillation counter. An average of about four electrons are knocked out of a dynode by an incident electron.

A photoelectric interaction within the crystal produces essentially monoenergetic photoelectrons, which, in turn, produce light pulses of about the same intensity. These light pulses, being of equal intensity, lead to current output pulses of approximately the same magnitude. In Compton scattering, on the other hand, a continuous spectrum of energy results from the Compton electron—the most energetic electron being that which results from a 180° backscatter of the incident photon. This most energetic Compton electron is called the "Compton edge" in scintillation spectrometry. The scattered photon may pass out of the crystal, or it may interact again, either by photoelectric absorption or by another Compton scattering. The most energetic Compton electron results from a 180° backscatter of the incident photon. Since photons may be scattered through angles ranging from 0° to 180°, there is a continuum of Compton electrons from the most energetic due to a 180° backscatter to electrons due to photons scattered through very small angles.

 EXAMPLE 9.2

Calculate the energy of

(a) a 0.661 MeV ^{137}Cs gamma that is backscattered 180°.

(b) the resultant Compton electron (the Compton edge).

Solution

(a) From Eq. (5.19), we find the wavelength of the 0.661-MeV gamma to be

$$\lambda = \frac{12,400}{E\ eV} = \frac{12,400}{0.661 \times 10^6\ eV} = 0.0188\ \text{Å}.$$

Equation (5.30) tells us that the increase in wavelength of a photon after scatter through an angle of θ is

$$\Delta\lambda = 0.0242\ (1 - \cos\theta)$$

$$= 0.0242\ (1 - \cos 180°)$$

$$= 0.0242\ [1 - (-1)]$$

$$= 0.0484\ \text{Å}$$

Therefore,

$$\lambda' = \lambda + \Delta\lambda = 0.0188 + 0.0484 = 0.0672\ \text{Å}.$$

The energy for this scattered photon is calculated with Eq. (5.19):

$$E' = \frac{12,400}{\lambda'} = \frac{12,400}{0.0672} = 1.85 \times 10^5\ eV = 0.185\ \text{MeV}.$$

(b) The energy of the Compton electron (Compton edge) is equal to the difference between the energy of the incident photon and the scattered photon:

$$E_{\text{Compton electron}} = E - E' = 0.661 - 0.185 = 0.476 \text{ MeV}.$$

In pair production, a flicker of light representing the original quantum energy minus 1.02 MeV is produced as the positron and negatron simultaneously dissipate their energies in the crystal. After losing its energy, the positron combines with an electron, thus annihilating the two particles and producing two photons of 0.51 MeV. Depending on the time sequence, the crystal size, and the geometric location of the initial interaction, we may have two pulses representing 0.51 MeV each—one light pulse representing 1.02 MeV, or one light pulse representing the total energy of the original photon.

Nuclear Spectroscopy

Nuclear spectroscopy is the analysis of radiation sources or radioisotopes by measuring the energy distribution of the source. A spectrometer is an instrument that separates the output pulses from a detector, usually a scintillation detector or a semiconductor detector, according to size. Since the size distribution is proportional to the energy of the detected radiation, the output of the spectrometer provides detailed information that is useful in identifying unknown radioisotopes and in counting one isotope in the presence of others. This technique has found widespread application in X-ray and gamma-ray analysis using NaI(TI) scintillation detectors and HPGe (high-purity germanium) semiconductor detectors, in beta analysis using liquid scintillation detectors or plastic scintillation detectors, and in alpha analysis using semiconductor detectors. Nuclear spectrometers are available in two types, either a single-channel instrument or a multichannel analyzer (MCA). The essentials of a single-channel spectrometer consist of the detector, a linear amplifier, a pulse-height selector, and a readout device, such as a scaler or a ratemeter (Fig. 9-10). The pulse height selector is an electronic "slit," which may be adjusted to pass pulses whose amplitude lies between any two desired limits of maximum and minimum. The output from the pulse-height analyzer is a logic pulse to a scaler or to a count ratemeter. The main use of the single-channel analyzer is to discriminate between a desired radiation and other radiations that may be considered noise. Thus, the single-channel spectrometer is used to measure one radiation in the presence of another or to optimize the signal-to-noise ratio when a low-activity source is being measured in the presence of a significant background.

An MCA (Fig. 9-11) has an analog-to-digital converter (ADC) instead of a pulse-height selector to sort all the output pulses from the detector according to height. The MCA also has a computer memory for storing the information from the ADC or from another source. This feature allows automated data-processing operations such as background subtraction and spectrum stripping. Spectrum stripping is a technique for analysis of compound spectra that is based on sequential subtraction of known gamma-ray spectra of individual isotopes from the compound spectrum

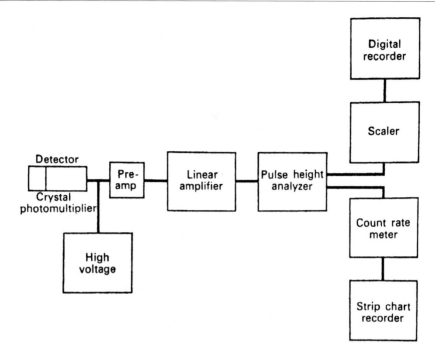

Figure 9-10. *Block diagram of a single-channel gamma-ray spectrometer.*

recorded when the sample undergoing nuclear analysis contains several different gamma emitters.

ADC conversion is accomplished by charging a capacitor to the peak voltage of the pulse to be analyzed and then discharging it. While the capacitor is being discharged, "clock" pulses from a high-frequency oscillator are counted by a scaler. The number of clock pulses counted during the capacitor discharge is proportional to the time required for the capacitor to discharge and thus is proportional to the height of the output pulse from the detector. The output from the ADC is a logic pulse that is stored in a channel whose number, or "address" is determined by the number of clock pulses that were counted during the discharge of the capacitor. Most MCAs

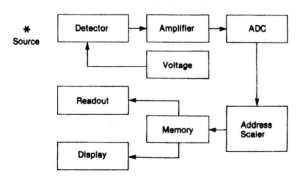

Figure 9-11. *Block diagram of a multichannel analyzer.*

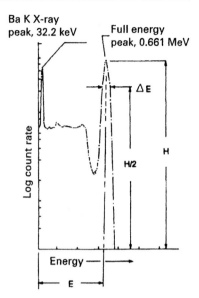

Figure 9-12. Gamma-ray spectrum of ^{137}Cs. The 0.661-MeV, full-energy peak is actually due to the isomeric transition of the 2.6-minute ^{137m}Ba daughter of ^{137}Cs. The 32.2-keV barium characteristic X-ray is due to the internal conversion of 8.5% of the 0.661-MeV photons. (Reproduced with permission from *A Handbook of Radioactivity Measurements Procedures*. 2nd ed. Bethesda, MD: National Council on Radiation Protection & Measurement; 1985. NCRP Report 58.)

are built with the number of channels varying by a factor of 2 over the range of 128–16,384, each with a storage capacity of 10^5–10^6 counts per channel, and "clock" frequencies ranging from 4 to 100 MHz. The multichannel spectrometer can print out the counts in each channel as well as visually display the gamma-ray spectrum on a flat-screen computer monitor. A typical simple gamma-ray spectrum is shown in Figure 9-12.

The basis for nuclear spectroscopy is the location of spectral lines arising from the total absorption of charged particles or photons. For this purpose, the resolution of the detector is important if spectral lines that are close together are to be separated and observed. *Resolution* is defined as the ratio of the full width at half maximum (FWHM) of the full-energy peak (often called the *photopeak* when dealing with photon detectors) to the energy midpoint of the full-energy peak (Fig. 9-12). If the FWHM is ΔE, then

$$\text{percent resolution} = \frac{\Delta E}{E} \times 100. \tag{9.6}$$

The smaller the energy spread, ΔE, the better is the ability of a detector to separate full-energy peaks that are close together. The resolution of a given detector is a function of energy and improves with increasing energy. For example, for a 100-keV photon, the resolution of a NaI(Tl) detector may be about 14%, whereas for a 1-MeV photon, it may be as good as about 7%. The resolution of semiconductor detectors is very much better than that of scintillation counters.

Cerenkov Detector

The popular photograph of a nuclear reactor core immersed in a deep pool of water (a "swimming pool" reactor) shows a blue glow that is known as *Cerenkov radiation*.

Cerenkov radiation is visible light, in the blue end of the spectrum, produced when a charged particle travels through a transparent medium faster than the speed of light in that medium. When this happens, the high-speed charged particles polarize the molecules along their path asymmetrically. Cerenkov radiation is emitted when these molecules fall back to the ground state.

The relativistic kinetic energy of a high-speed electron is given by Eq. (2.20):

$$T = m_0 c^2 \left[\frac{1}{\sqrt{1 - \dfrac{v^2}{c^2}}} - 1 \right].$$

The speed of light in a medium whose index of refraction is n is equal to c/n. The kinetic energy of the electron when its speed is equal to the speed of light in the transparent medium is the threshold energy for the Cerenkov effect in that medium. If we substitute c/n for v in Eq. (2.20) and 0.51 MeV for $m_0 c^2$, we find that the threshold energy of the high-speed electron is

$$T = 0.51 \left(\frac{1}{\sqrt{1 - \dfrac{1}{n^2}}} - 1 \right) \text{MeV}. \tag{9.7}$$

The index of refraction for water for the range of wavelengths in the visible light spectrum is about 1.33. If we substitute this value for n in Eq. (9.7), we find that the threshold energy for the Cerenkov effect of an electron or beta particle in water is 0.264 MeV. Thus, primary electrons from a gamma source or betas from a beta emitter immersed in water whose kinetic energies exceed this value will produce Cerenkov radiation. The emission of Cerenkov radiation is favored by a high index of refraction of the medium. Accordingly, solid-state Cerenkov detectors are made from high-density glass whose index of refraction for the sodium D lines is on the order of 1.6–1.7. Cerenkov radiation, after being produced in the detector, is viewed by a photomultiplier tube for measurement. Generally, Cerenkov counters find their main use in high-energy physics measurements rather than in health physics. However, the Cerenkov effect can be used in liquid scintillation counters to measure, with very high efficiency, the energetic beta particles that are emitted by radionuclides such as ^{32}P and ^{90}Y.

Semiconductor Detector

A semiconductor detector acts as a solid-state ionization chamber. The ionizing particle—beta particle, alpha particle, etc.—interacts with atoms in the sensitive volume of the detector to produce electrons by ionization. The collection of these ions leads to an output pulse. In contrast to the relatively high mean ionization energy of 30–35 eV for most counter gases, a mean energy expenditure of only 3.5 eV is required to produce an ionizing event in a semiconductor detector (silicon).

A semiconductor is a substance that has electrical conducting properties midway between a "good conductor" and an "insulator." Although many substances can be classified as semiconductors, the most commonly used semiconductor materials are silicon and germanium. These elements, each of which has four valence electrons, form crystals that consist of a lattice of atoms that are joined together by covalent bonds. Absorption of energy by the crystal leads to disruption of these bonds—only 1.12 eV are required to knock out one of the valence electrons in silicon—which results in a free electron and a "hole" in the position formerly occupied by the valence electron. This free electron can move about the crystal with ease. The hole too can move about in the crystal; an electron adjacent to the hole can jump into the hole, and thus leave another hole behind. Connecting the semiconductor in a closed electric circuit results in a current through the semiconductor as the electrons flow toward the positive terminal and the holes flow toward the negative terminal (Fig. 9-13).

The operation of a semiconductor radiation detector depends on its having either an excess of electrons or an excess of holes. A semiconductor with an excess of electrons is called an n-type semiconductor, while the one with an excess of holes is called a p-type semiconductor. Normally, a pure silicon crystal will have an equal number of electrons and holes. (These electrons and holes result from the rupture of the covalent bonds by absorption of heat or light energy.) By adding certain impurities to the crystal, either an excess number of electrons (an n region) or an excess number of holes (a p region) can be produced. Germanium and silicon both are in group IV of the periodic table. If atoms from one of the elements in group V, such as phosphorus, arsenic, antimony, or bismuth, each of which has five valence electrons, are added to the pure silicon or germanium, four of the five electrons in each of the added atoms are shared by the silicon or germanium atoms to form a covalent bond. The fifth electron from the impurity is thus an excess electron and is free to move about in the crystal and to participate in the flow of electric current. Under these conditions, the crystal is of the n type. These group V elements are called electron donors when used in this way.

A p-type semiconductor, having an excess number of holes, can be made by adding an impurity from group III of the periodic table to the semiconductor crystal. Elements from group III, such as boron, aluminum, gadolinium, or indium, have

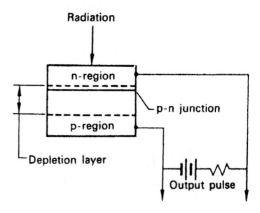

Figure 9-13. *Semiconductor junction detector. This detector is most useful for measuring electrons or other charged particles.*

three valence electrons. Incorporation of one of these elements as an impurity in the crystal, therefore, ties up only three of the four valence bonds in the crystal lattice. This deficiency of one electron is a hole, and we have p-type silicon or germanium. These group III impurities are called electron acceptors.

A p region in silicon or germanium that is adjacent to an n region is called an $n - p$ junction. If a forward bias is applied to the junction, that is, if a voltage is applied across the junction such that the p region is connected to the positive terminal and the n region to the negative terminal, the impedance across the junction will be very low, and current will flow across the junction. If the polarity of the applied voltage is reversed, that is, if the n region is connected to the positive terminal and the p region to the negative, we have the condition known as reverse bias. Under this condition, no current (except for a very small current due to thermally generated holes and electrons) flows across the junction. The region around the junction is swept free, by the potential difference, of the holes and electrons in the p and n regions. This region is called the *depletion layer*, and is the sensitive volume of the solid-state detector. When an ionizing particle passes through the depletion layer, electron–hole pairs are produced as a result of ionizing collisions between the ionizing particles and the crystal. The electric field then sweeps the holes and electrons apart, giving rise to a pulse in the load resistor as the electrons flow through the external circuit.

Semiconductor detectors are especially useful for nuclear spectroscopy because of their inherently high energy resolution. For charged-particle spectroscopy, surface-barrier-type semiconductors are used. Figure 9-14 shows the resolution obtainable with such a detector; alphas of 5.443 and 5.486 MeV are easily and clearly separated. By using an appropriate neutron-sensitive material such as ^{3}He gas, ^{6}Li, ^{10}B, ^{235}U, or a hydrogenous material together with a surface-barrier detector, either the slow or the fast neutrons can be measured.

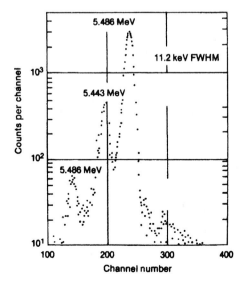

Figure 9-14. Alpha spectrum of ^{241}Am obtained with a silicon surface-barrier detector. *Abbreviation*: FWHM, full width at half maximum. (Courtesy of ORTEC Products, AMETEK, Inc.)

Detection and measurement of photons generally requires a greater sensitive volume, that is, a thicker depletion layer, than is possible with the ordinary p–n junction detectors whose depletion layers are on the order of 1 or 2 mm in thickness. For any given bias voltage, the depth of the depletion layer varies inversely with the square root of the net bulk concentration of the impurity atoms. One method of increasing the depth of the depletion layer is to decrease the effective concentration of the impurities. This is done by infusing lithium ions into the silicon or germanium crystal lattice. The Li ions compensate for the excess number of impurity atoms that are introduced during the production of n- and p-type semiconductors, thus leading to an effective smaller bulk concentration of impurities, which in turn leads to a larger depletion layer. Silicon and germanium detectors so treated are called Si(Li) or Ge(Li) detectors. Although these detectors require cryogenic temperatures at all times, whether or not they are in use, Si(Li) detectors may be stored at room temperature for several days before they deteriorate. Detectors made with very high purity germanium, on the other hand, which must be used at cryogenic temperatures, may be kept at ambient temperatures when not in use. The required low temperature is obtained by mounting the detector on a "cold finger" that is immersed in liquid nitrogen (77 K) in a Dewar flask (Fig. 9-15).

Advantages of semiconductor detectors include (1) high-speed counting due to the very low resolving time—on the order of nanoseconds; (2) high energy resolution (Fig. 9-16); and (3) relatively low operating voltage—about 25–300 V.

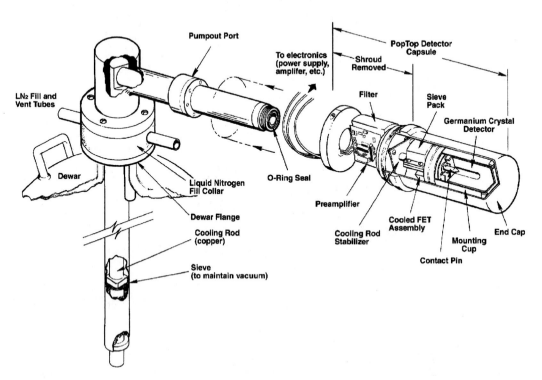

Figure 9-15. Diagram showing a HPGe detector–cryostat assembly mounted on a Dewar flask containing liquid nitrogen at 77 K (–196°C, –351°F). (Courtesy of ORTEC Products, AMETEK, Inc.)

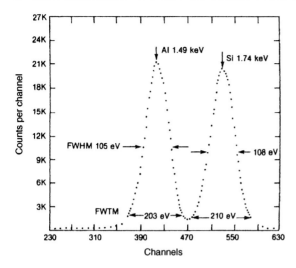

Figure 9-16. Characteristic X-ray lines from an aluminum-silicate sample. The spectrum shows the excellent resolution capability of a Si(Li) low-energy photon detector. *Abbreviations:* FWHM, full width at half maximum; FWTM; full width at one tenth maximum peak height. (Courtesy of ORTEC Products, AMETEK, Inc.)

DOSE-MEASURING INSTRUMENTS

Radiation flux (fluence rate) is only one of the several factors that determine radiation dose rate. The fact that a particle-measuring instrument does not necessarily measure dose is shown by the following example:

EXAMPLE 9.3

Consider two radiation fields of equal energy flux. In one case, we have a 0.1-MeV photon flux of 2000 photons/cm^2/s. In the second case, the photon energy is 2 MeV and the flux is 100 photons/cm^2/s. Calculate the dose rates for the two radiation fields. The energy absorption coefficients for muscle are

μ (energy, 0.1 MeV) = 0.0252 cm^2/g and
μ (energy, 2 MeV) = 0.0257 cm^2/g.

Solution

The dose rates for the two radiation fields are given by

$$\dot{D} = \frac{\phi \dfrac{\text{photons}}{\text{cm}^2/\text{s}} \times E \dfrac{\text{MeV}}{\text{photon}} \times 1.6 \times 10^{-13} \dfrac{\text{J}}{\text{MeV}} \times \mu \,(\text{energy}) \dfrac{\text{cm}^2}{\text{g}}}{10^{-3} \dfrac{\text{J/g}}{\text{Gy}}}. \tag{9.8}$$

Substituting the given values in the above equation, we obtain

$$\dot{D}(0.1 \text{ MeV}) = 8.1 \times 10^{-10} \text{ Gy/s}$$

$$\dot{D}(2.0 \text{ Mev}) = 8.2 \times 10^{-10} \text{ Gy/s}.$$

The dose rates for the two radiation fields are about the same. A particle-flux-measuring instrument, however, such as a GM counter, would register about 20 times more for the 0.1-MeV radiation than for the higher energy radiation. Since ionization chambers measure absorbed energy rather than individual particles and are reasonably energy independent (Fig. 9-17), we use ionization-chamber-type instruments when measuring radiation dose rates (unless a specific counter-type instrument is calibrated for a specific gamma-ray energy, in which case it may be used for dosimetry for that quantum energy only).

As shown in Example 9.3, particle-counting survey instruments, such as GM counters and scintillation counters, are very energy dependent when used to measure radiation dose (Fig. 9-18). The GM counter's response is *much flatter* (although still not flat) with the beta window closed than with the beta window open. The reason for this is that the thicker wall, represented by the closed beta window, absorbs more low-energy photons than does the open window. This is the basis for *energy-compensated* GM detectors. An energy-compensated GM detector has a wall thick enough to flatten the energy response to within about ±15% of the response to ^{137}Cs, yet thin enough to detect photons down to about 50 keV (Fig. 9-19).

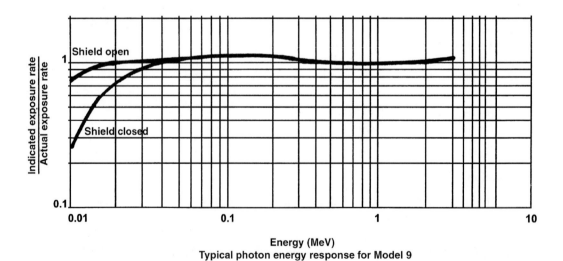

Energy (MeV)
Typical photon energy response for Model 9

Figure 9-17. Energy response curve for a general-purpose ionization-chamber-type survey meter with a 300-mg/cm²-thick retractable beta shield. (Courtesy of Ludlum Measurements, Inc, Sweetwater, TX.)

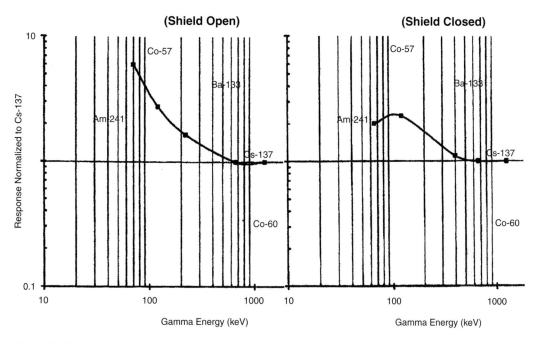

Figure 9-18. Energy response curves for a Geiger-Müller counter whose wall is 30-mg/cm²-thick stainless steel. The tube is in a cylindrical probe with a sliding beta shield. The figure on the left shows the instrument's response to photons of various energies with the shield open, and the curve on the right shows its response with the shield closed. (Courtesy of Ludlum Measurements, Inc, Sweetwater, TX.)

Personal Monitoring

The International Commission on Radiological Protection (ICRP) recommends monitoring individual radiation workers for external exposure unless it is clear that their doses will be consistently low. The International Atomic Energy Agency (IAEA), in its *Basic Safety Standards*, interprets this to mean that workers whose occupational dose may exceed 30% of the regulatory limit should be monitored. The regulations in the United States require personal monitoring if the worker's annual dose is likely to exceed 10% of the regulatory limit. Individual monitoring for external radiation is relatively simple. The worker wears a dosimeter, and the dose is tracked on the basis of the individual readings of the dosimeter. The most widely used personal monitoring devices include pocket dosimeters, film badges, thermoluminescent dosimeters, opticoluminescent dosimeters, and electronic dosimeters.

The U.S. Nuclear Regulatory Commission (NRC) not only requires the monitoring of licensees, but also that the personal dosimetry devices used to demonstrate compliance with NRC regulations be processed by laboratories or commercial services that have been accredited by the National Voluntary Laboratory Accreditation Program (NVLAP) of the National Institute of Standards and Technology (NIST). Earlier studies showed a great deal of disagreement between doses reported by various commercial and in-house monitoring organizations and the actual doses delivered to these test dosimeters. This concern about the reliability of the reported doses led to the establishment, in 1984, of the NVLAP by the National Bureau of

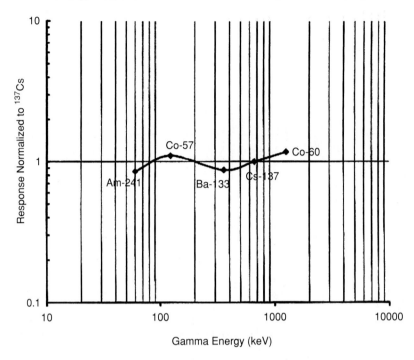

Figure 9-19. Response of an energy-compensated GM detector. (Courtesy of Ludlum Measurements, Inc, Sweetwater, TX.)

Standards (now called the NIST). Accreditation review is limited to those dosimeters that document skin dose and whole-body dose. The accreditation program does not include pocket ionization chambers, extremity dosimeters, or environmental monitors. Accreditation is granted for a 2-year period to those applicants who pass stringent proficiency testing and other rigorous requirements. To renew the accreditation for another 2-year period, the applicant must pass through the same process again. The U.S. Department of Energy requires a similar use of accredited personal dosimeters through its Department of Energy Laboratory Accreditation Program (DOELAP).

Pocket Dosimeters

To measure radiation dose, the response of the instrument must be proportional to absorbed energy. A basic instrument for doing this, the free-air ionization chamber, was described in Chapter 6. In that chapter too, it was shown that an "air wall" ionization chamber could be made on the basis of the operational definition of the exposure unit, or the roentgen, and that such an instrument could be used to measure exposure. Ionization chambers of this type, which are often called *pocket dosimeters*, have been widely used for personnel monitoring. The first type of pocket dosimeter that was in common use is the condenser type, as illustrated in Figure 6-2.

This type of pocket dosimeter is of the indirect reading type; an auxiliary device is necessary in order to read the measured dose. This device, which is, in reality, an electrostatic voltmeter that is calibrated in roentgens, is called a "charger-reader" (because it is also used to charge the chamber). Commercially available capacitor-type pocket dosimeters measure integrated X- or gamma-ray exposures up to 200 mR (μC kg^{-1}) with an accuracy of about $\pm$15% for quantum energies between about 0.05 and 2 MeV. For quantum energies outside this range, correction factors, which are supplied by the manufacturer, must be used. These dosimeters also respond to beta particles whose energy exceeds 1 MeV. By coating the inside of the chamber with boron, the pocket dosimeter can also be made sensitive to thermal neutrons. The standard type of pocket dosimeter, however, is designed for measuring X- and gamma radiation only. It is calibrated with radium, ^{60}Co, or ^{137}Cs gamma rays. Pocket dosimeters discharge slowly even when they are not in a radiation field because of cosmic radiation and because charge leaks across the insulator that separates the central electrode from the outer electrode. A dosimeter that leaks more than 5% of the full-scale reading per day should not be used. Usually, two pocket dosimeters are worn. Since a malfunction will always cause the instrument to read high, the lower of the two readings is considered as more accurate. Because of leakage and possibility of malfunction due to being dropped, pocket dosimeters are usually worn for one day. Reading the instrument erases its information content. It is therefore necessary to recharge the indirect-reading pocket dosimeter after each reading.

The capacitor-type pocket dosimeter has been superseded by a direct-reading pocket dosimeter (often called a self-reading dosimeter, SRD) that operates on the principle of the gold-leaf electroscope (Fig. 9-20). A quartz fiber is displaced electrostatically by charging it to a potential of about 200 V. An image of the fiber is focused on a scale and is viewed through a lens at one end of the instrument. Exposure of the dosimeter to radiation discharges the fiber, thereby allowing it to return to its original position. The amount discharged, and consequently the change in position of the fiber, is proportional to the radiation exposure. An advantage of the direct-reading dosimeter is that it does not have to be recharged after being read. Commonly used direct-reading dosimeters that are commercially available have a range of 0–200 mR (0–51.5 μC/kg), and read within about $\pm$15% of the true exposure for energies from about 50 keV to 2 MeV. Low-energy X- and gamma-ray dosimeters that read within $\pm$20% over the range of 20–200 keV are commercially available.

To measure thermal neutron dose with an SRD, the cavity is lined with boron. Thermal neutrons that enter into the cavity interact with the boron according to the ^{10}B$(n, \alpha)^7$Li reaction, and the dosimeter responds to the alpha particles. The X- and gamma-ray sensitivity of these dosimeters is low, the ratio of neutrons to photons is about 200:1. The operating range of thermal neutron SRDs is about 0–120 mrems (using 10 CFR 20's $Q = 2$ for thermal neutrons). Using the ICRP's $Q = 5$ for thermal neutrons, the same dosimeter would read 0–3 mSv. An auxiliary charger must be used with this dosimeter.

Film-Badge Dosimeters

Another very commonly used personal monitoring device is the film-badge dosimeter, which consists of a packet of two (for X- or gamma radiation) or three

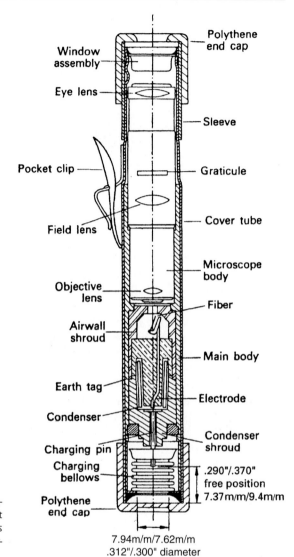

Figure 9-20. Simplified cross section of a direct-reading quartz-fiber electroscope-type pocket dosimeter. The energy dependence characteristics of this dosimeter are shown in Figure 6-4. (Courtesy of RA Stephen & Co, Ltd.)

(for X- or gamma radiation and neutrons) small pieces of film wrapped in light-proof paper and worn in a suitable plastic or metal container. The two films for X- and gamma radiation include a sensitive emulsion and a relatively insensitive emulsion. Such a film pack is useful over an exposure range of about 10 mR to about 1800 R ($2.58 \times 10^{-6} - 0.464$ C/kg) of radium gamma rays. The film is also sensitive to beta radiation, and may be used to measure beta dose from about 50 mrads (0.5 mGy) to about 1000 rads (10 Gy), given betas whose maximum energy exceeds about 400 keV. Using appropriate film and techniques, thermal neutron doses of 5 mrads (50 mGy) to 500 rads (5 Gy), and fast neutron doses from about 4 mrads (40 mGy) to 10 rads (0.1 Gy) may be measured.

Film-badge dosimetry is based on the fact that ionizing radiation exposes the silver halide in the photographic emulsion, which results in a darkening of the film.

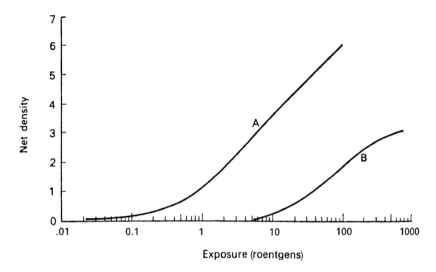

Figure 9-21. *Relationship between radiation exposure and optical density. Curve A is the response of duPont type 555 and curve B is the response of duPont type 834 dosimeter film to ^{60}Co gamma rays.*

The degree of darkening, which is called the optical density of the film, can be precisely measured with a photoelectric densitometer whose reading is expressed as the logarithm of the intensity of the light transmitted through the film. The optical density of the exposed film is quantitatively related to the magnitude of the exposure (Fig. 9-21). By comparing the optical density of the film worn by an exposed individual to that of films exposed to known amounts of radiation, the exposure to the individual's film may be determined. Small variations in emulsions greatly affect their quantitative response to radiation. Since the films used in film badges are produced in batches and slight variations from batch to batch may be expected, it is necessary to calibrate the film from each batch separately.

Films used in film-badge dosimeters are highly energy-dependent in the low-energy range, from about 0.2 MeV gamma radiation downward (Fig. 9-22). This energy dependence arises from the fact that the photoelectric cross section for the silver in the emulsion increases much more rapidly than that of air or tissue as the photon energy decreases below about 200 keV. A maximum sensitivity is observed at about 30–40 keV. Below this energy, the sensitivity of the film decreases because of the attenuation of the radiation by the paper wrapper. As a result of this very strong energy dependence, film dosimetry can lead to serious errors for X-rays less than 200 keV unless the film was calibrated with radiation of the same energy distribution as the radiation being monitored or if the energy dependence of the film is accounted for.

Correction for energy dependence is made by selective filtration. The film-badge holder is designed so that radiation may reach the film directly through an open window, or the radiation may be filtered by the film-badge holder or by one of several different filters, such as aluminum, copper, cadmium, tin, silver, and lead, which are built into the film holder. The exact design and choice of filter is governed by the type of radiation to be monitored. The evaluation of the exposure is then

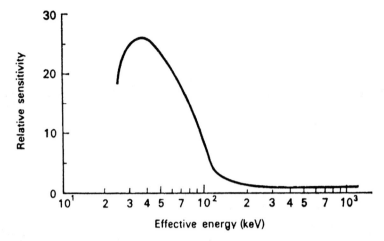

Figure 9-22. Energy dependence of a film-badge dosimeter to X-rays. (Reproduced from Ehrlich E. *Photographic Dosimetry of X- and Gamma-Rays.* Washington, DC: US Government Printing Office; 1954. NBS Handbook 57.)

made by considering the ratio of the film densities under each of the various filters. Beta dose is determined from the ratio of the open-window film reading to that behind the filters. If exposure was to beta radiation only, then film darkening is seen only in the open-window area. To help distinguish between low-energy gamma rays and beta particles, for example, comparison is made between the darkening in the open window and under two thin filters, such as aluminum and silver, which are of the same density thickness and are, therefore, equivalent beta absorbers. The different atomic numbers, however, result in much greater low-energy X-ray filtration by the silver filter than by the aluminum filter, thereby giving different degrees of darkening under the two filters. Interpretation of mixed beta–gamma radiation with a film badge is difficult because of the greatly different penetrating powers of beta and gamma radiation. For this reason, information from beta monitoring with film badges is used mainly in a qualitative or semiquantitative manner to evaluate exposure.

Fast neutrons, whose energy exceeds 1/2 MeV, can be monitored with nuclear track film, such as Eastman Kodak NTA, which is added to the film badge. Irradiation of the film by fast neutrons results in proton recoil tracks due to elastic collisions between hydrogen nuclei in the paper wrapper, in the emulsion, and in the film base. Although the n, p scattering cross section decreases with increasing neutron energy—from 13 b at 0.1 MeV to 4.5 b at 1 MeV to 1 b at 10 MeV—the recoil protons do not have sufficient energy below about 0.5 MeV to make recognizable tracks, and hence the threshold is at 0.5 MeV. Because the concentration of hydrogen atoms in the film and its paper wrapper is not very much different from that of tissue, the response of the film to fast neutrons is approximately tissue equivalent, and the number of proton tracks per unit area of the film is therefore proportional to the absorbed dose.

Fast-neutron exposure is estimated by scanning the developed film with a high-powered microscope and counting the number of proton tracks per square centimeter of film. The U.S. NRC regulatory limit of 5 rems (0.05 Sv) in a year corresponds to a mean weekly dose rate of 100 mrems (1 mSv). This corresponds to a mean proton-track density of about 2600 cm^{-2} of NTA film for neutrons from a Pu–Be source. Since the area seen by the oil immersion lens is about 2×10^{-4} cm^2, a fast neutron dose of 100 mrems corresponds to a mean track density of about one proton recoil track per two microscopic fields.

Thermal neutrons also produce proton-recoil tracks in the neutron film as a result of their capture by nitrogen in the film according to the $^{14}N(n,\ p)^{14}C$ reaction. Although the cross section for 2200 m/s neutrons for this reaction is 1.75 b, the concentration of nitrogen in the film is much less than that of hydrogen, thus making this reaction less sensitive, on a per-neutron basis, than the $n,\ p$ scattering reaction for fast neutrons. Nevertheless, because, in practice, fast neutrons are usually part of a mixed radiation field that includes thermal neutrons (and gamma radiation), and because the permissible flux for thermal neutrons is much higher than for fast neutrons, allowance must be made for the proton tracks due to thermal neutrons.

A film badge designed for use in a mixed radiation field that includes neutrons always has at least two metal filters of equal density thickness—one of cadmium and the other usually of tin. Cadmium has a very high cross section, 2500 b for the $^{113}Cd(n,\ \gamma)^{114}Cd$ for 0.025-eV neutrons, and 7400 b for 0.179-eV neutrons. The capture cross section of tin for thermal neutrons is insignificantly small. As a result, a thermal-neutron field will show a high track density under the tin filter but no tracks under the cadmium. Fast neutrons, on the other hand, will produce the same track density under both filters. Furthermore, because of the $n,\ \gamma$ reaction in cadmium, a thermal-neutron field will produce a darker area on the gamma-ray film under the cadmium filter than under tin. In the absence of any neutrons, γ radiation would expose the film under each of these filters to the same degree. By counting the tracks and measuring the gamma-ray film density, we determine the thermal-neutron flux as well as allowing for the thermal neutron background track density in the determination of the fast-neutron flux. It should be reemphasized that the ordinary neutron film badges are not sensitive to neutrons in the energy range between epithermal and 0.5 MeV. However, if the spectral distribution of the neutron field is known, then allowance for neutrons in the film-badge-insensitive range can be made.

Thermoluminescent Dosimeters

Many different crystals emit light if they are heated after having been exposed to radiation. This effect is called *thermoluminescence,* and dosimeters based on this effect are called *thermoluminescent dosimeters* (TLD). Some of these TLD crystals include LiF, $CaF_2 : Mn$ (CaF_2 containing a small amount of added Mn, which functions as an activator), $CaSO_4 : Tm$, $Li_2B_4O_7 : Cu$, and LiF : Mg,Ti. Absorption of energy from the radiation excites the atoms in the crystal, which results in the production of free electrons and holes in the thermoluminescent crystal. These are trapped by the activators or by imperfections in the crystalline lattice, thereby locking the excitation energy in the crystal. Heating the crystal releases the excitation energy as light. Measurement of the emitted-light intensity leads to a *glow curve* (Fig. 9-23). Trapped excited electrons also spontaneously fall down to the ground state even at low temperatures. At room temperatures, trapped electrons fall down to the ground state at a rate of about $10^{-8} - 10^{-7}$ percent per second. This leads to fewer trapped

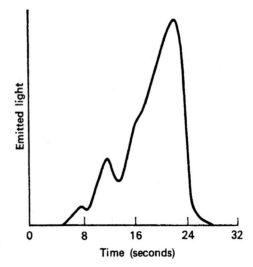

Figure 9-23. Glow curve for LiF that had been dosed with 100 rems (1 Sv) X-rays. The area under the curve is proportional to the total dose. (Reproduced with permission from Cameron JR, Zimmerman D, Kenney G, Buch R, Bland R, Grant R. Thermoluminescent dosimetry utilizing LiF. *Health Phys.* January 1964;10:25–29.)

electrons at readout, and consequently to a smaller dose at readout than originally recorded, as shown in the following example.

EXAMPLE 9.4

In a laboratory where TLD badges are changed every 4 weeks, and are read 2 days later, a radiation worker is exposed on the day that he received the dosimeter, and has no further exposure. What fraction of the actual dose will be reported if the spontaneous fading rate is 1.35×10^{-8} s^{-1}?

Solution

Since the dose is directly proportional to the number of trapped electrons, the fraction of the original measured dose remaining 30 days later is

$$\frac{D}{D_0} = e^{-kt} = e^{-1.35\times10^{-8}\frac{1}{s}\times8.64\times10^4\frac{s}{d}\times30\text{ d}} = 0.97 = 97\%.$$

Figure 9-23 shows a characteristic glow curve for LiF, which is obtained by heating the irradiated crystal at a uniform rate and measuring the emitted light as the temperature increases. The temperature at which the maximum light output occurs is a measure of the binding energy of the electron or the hole in the trap. More than one peak on a glow curve indicates different trapping sites, each with its own binding energy. The total light output is proportional to the number of trapped, excited electrons, which, in turn, is proportional to the amount of energy absorbed from the radiation. Thus, the light output is directly proportional to the radiation absorbed dose.

Thermoluminescent materials are found in the form of loose powder, disks, squares, and rods. For personal monitoring, one or more small pieces of thermoluminescent material (about 50 mg each) are placed into a small holder that is worn by the person being monitored. After being worn for the prescribed period of time, the TLD material is heated and the intensity of the resulting luminescence is measured with a photomultiplier tube whose output signal, after amplification, is applied to a suitable readout instrument, such as a digital voltmeter. The instrument is calibrated by measuring the intensity of light from thermoluminescent phosphors that had been exposed to known doses of radiation.

Neutron Dosimeters

Lithium-6, the naturally occurring isotope in lithium (7.4% natural abundance), captures thermal neutrons and undergoes an n, α reaction, and thus can be used for neutron monitoring. Thermoluminescent-dosimeter phosphors, containing lithium as LiF, are widely used because LiF is approximately tissue equivalent and almost energy independent from about 100-keV to 1.3-MeV gamma radiation, as shown in Figure 9-24. The several TLD phosphors in the TLD badge may be made of different materials and may be differently filtered in order to take advantage of the differing energy dependence of the filters and to make the TLD badge approximately energy independent. One such TLD badge, for example, contains four TLD phosphors, two each of $LI_2B_4O : Cu$ and two each of $CaSO_4 : Tm$. With appropriate filters, this dosimeter is approximately energy independent from 30-keV to 10-MeV X- or gamma radiation, 0.5-MeV to 4-MeV beta radiation, and 0.025-eV to 10-MeV neutrons. It can measure doses from ^{60}Co from 10 μSv (1 mrem) to 10 Sv (1000 rems).

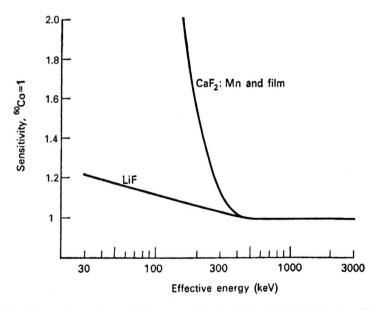

Figure 9-24. Energy dependence of LiF compared to that of unshielded dosimeters. (Reproduced with permission from Cameron JR, Zimmerman D, Kenney G, Buch R, Bland R, Grant R. Thermoluminescent dosimetry utilizing LiF. *Health Phys.* January 1964; 10:25–29.)

Albedo Neutron Dosimeter

Personnel monitoring for neutrons can be accomplished through the use of nuclear track film, wherein the neutron knocks a proton out of a molecule in the film emulsion and the proton leaves a track in the film. A major drawback of this technique, however, is the neutron energy threshold requirement. Unless the neutron energy exceeds about 0.5 MeV, the recoil protons do not have sufficient energy to make recognizable tracks in the film. This disadvantage can be overcome through the use of neutron-sensitive thermoluminescent dosimeters whose sensitivity is enhanced by neutrons that are backscattered from the body. Since the human body has many hydrogen atoms, a significant fraction of intermediate energy and fast neutrons can be slowed down to epithermal energies and backscattered and thus can interact with the neutron-sensitive thermoluminescent material. One neutron monitor of this kind is called an *albedo*-type neutron dosimeter. Albedo dosimeters of this type are especially useful in the neutron energy range from the Cd cutoff, about 0.2 eV to about 500 keV.

Since the neutron-sensitive TLD also responds to gamma radiation, and neutrons are almost always accompanied by gamma radiation, a neutron-insensitive TLD is used together with the neutron-sensitive TLD. The measured thermoluminescence due to gammas can be separately determined and subtracted from the total thermoluminescence of the neutron-sensitive detector. To distinguish between the thermoluminescence due to neutrons and gammas in this way, ^{6}LiF TLD material is used as the neutron-sensitive detector, while ^{7}LiF is used as the neutron-insensitive dosimeter. Both these TLD materials have about the same response to gamma radiation. For this reason, the gamma thermoluminescence of the ^{7}LiF chip can be subtracted from that of the ^{6}LiF chip to obtain a net luminescence that is due only to the neutrons. This differential thermoluminescence allows a measurement of 0.1 mSv(10 mrems) of neutrons in a gamma field of 2 mSv (200 mrems).

Albedo-type neutron dosimeters are highly energy-dependent. Their response changes by a factor of about 15 over the neutron energy range of 0.1–1.7 MeV. For this reason, an albedo neutron dosimeter must be calibrated with a neutron source whose spectral distribution of energy is as close as possible to the energy distribution of the neutrons to be monitored.

Optically Stimulated Luminescence

Environmental monitoring with TLDs requires phosphors that are much more sensitive than those used for monitoring radiation workers. Thermoluminescent dosimeters used to demonstrate compliance with occupational dose limits need sufficient sensitivity only for that task. Environmental radiation limits are much more restrictive than occupational limits. Dosimeter phosphors used for environmental monitoring must therefore have much greater sensitivity than those used for monitoring radiation workers. This increased sensitivity is provided by optically stimulated luminescence (OSL) dosimeters, Al_2O_3 : C (Fig. 9-25), which can measure doses as low as 0.01 mSv (1 mrem). This high degree of sensitivity is useful for environmental measurements and for monitoring pregnant workers, as well as all other radiation workers. The Al_2O_3 : C dosimeter is sandwiched in a three-element filter system for X-ray spectral determination. The dosimeter assembly is sealed inside a light-tight wrapping, which is in turn sealed inside a plastic blister pack about the

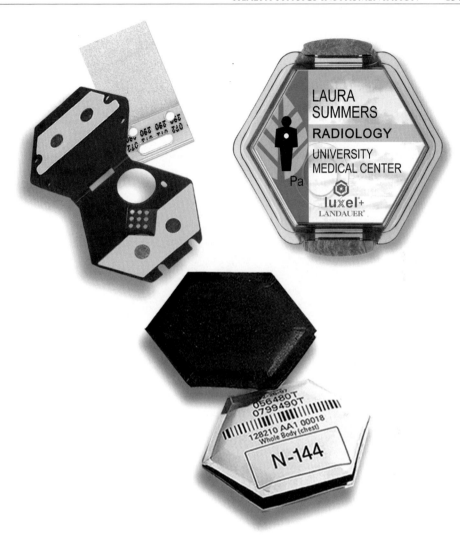

Figure 9-25. *Optically stimulated dosimeter. (Courtesy of Landauer, Inc, Glenwood, IL.)*

same size as a film badge or a TLD. After exposure to radiation, the OSL dosimeter is read after exposing it to laser light. This causes the $Al_2O_3 : C$ to luminesce, with the degree of luminescence being proportional to the radiation dose. OSL dosimeters can measure doses ≥ 1 mrem (0.01 mSv) from X-rays of quantum energies ≥ 5 keV and beta doses ≥ 10 mrems (0.1 mSv) for beta energies ≥ 150 keV. This sensitivity, together with other desirable properties, has made this the phosphor of choice for environmental monitoring and for monitoring occupationally exposed workers.

Electronic Dosimeters

The continuing evolution of solid-state electronics and electronic data processing have led to ever smaller, more reliable, and more sophisticated instruments. This miniaturization has made possible small, lightweight (about 100 g), accurate

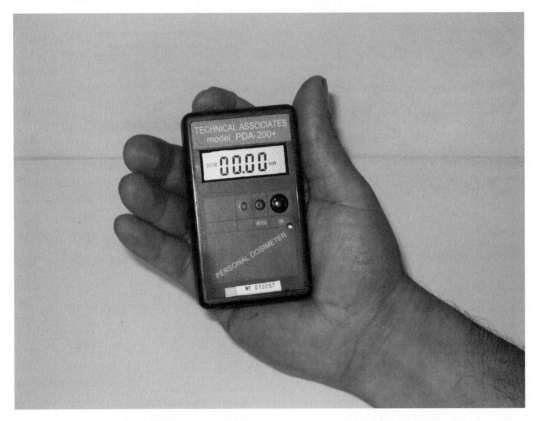

Figure 9-26. Direct-reading electronic dosimeter for personal monitoring. Electronic dosimeters can measure and log beta- and gamma-ray doses from 1 μSv (0.1 mrem) to about 10 Sv (1000 rems) and contain programmable alarms for cumulative dose and for dose rate. (Courtesy of Technical Associates, Canoga Park, CA.)

electronic dosimeters that are more useful for personal dosimetry and dose tracking than either film or TLD (Fig. 9-26). Electronic dosimeters measure and display instantaneous dose rate and integrate over time to obtain, store, and display the cumulative dose. They are also designed to alarm at any desired dose rate or cumulated dose. In the United States of America, the NRC requires all radiographers and their assistants to wear an alarming dosimeter (10 CFR 34). The data are stored in a nonvolatile memory and can be downloaded into a computer for dose-tracking and record-keeping purposes.

Electronic personal dosimeters employ solid-state semiconductors, silicon diodes, to detect beta and gamma radiation over a very wide range of dose rates and doses. With an accuracy of about $\pm10\%$ for ^{137}Cs gammas, electronic personal dosimeters measure dose rates from 1 μSv (0.1 mrem) per hour to 10 mSv (1,000 mrems) per hour and store doses from 1 μSv (0.1 mrem) to 10 Sv (1000 rems). These electronic pocket dosimeters incorporate several detectors, each one responding to radiation that had passed through different filters in order to account for the inherent energy dependence of the detectors. When the outputs of the several detectors are added together, the resulting count rate is approximately proportional to the absorbed dose rate. By this technique, the response of electronic personal dosimeters is approximately energy independent ($\pm25\%$) from 60 keV to 1.5 MeV.

Survey Meters: Ion Current Chambers

Ion current chambers have a response that is proportional to absorbed energy and hence are widely used by health physicists in making dose measurements. Most of these ionization chambers have an air-equivalent wall and therefore measure exposure rather than dose. Exposure, which in the traditional system of units is expressed by the quantity called the *roentgen*, is expressed in SI units by the quantity called the *coulomb per kilogram*, C/kg, or by the *air kerma*, whose units are J kg^{-1} or grays (Gy). The quantitative relationship among these three quantities is

$$1 \text{ R} = 2.58 \times 10^{-4} \frac{\text{C}}{\text{kg}} = 0.0088 \text{ Gy}.$$

For radiation protection purposes, an exposure of 1 R is the equivalent of 1 rem in the traditional system of units, and an exposure of 2.58×10^{-4} C/kg or an air kerma of 0.0088 Gy is the equivalent of 0.01 Sv. Health physics survey meters with air walls may therefore be calibrated to read in units of mR/h, C/kg/h, or μSv/h.

A current ionization chamber consists basically of a gas- or air-filled chamber with two electrodes across which is placed a potential low enough to prevent gas multiplication but high enough to prevent recombination of the ions (Fig. 9-27). The ions that are generated in the chamber are collected and flow through an external circuit. The ion chamber thus acts as a current source of infinite internal resistance. Although, in principle, an ammeter can be placed in the external circuit to measure the ion current, in practice this is not done because the current is very small. Instead, a high-valued load resistor R on the order of 10^9–10^{12} ohms is placed in the circuit and the voltage drop across the load resistor is measured with a sensitive electrometer. Because of the capacitance of the chamber and its associated circuitry C, the voltage across the load resistor varies with time t after closing the circuit, according to the equation

$$V(t) = iR(1 - e^{-t/RC}). \tag{9.9}$$

The product RC is called the *time constant of the detector circuit* and determines the speed with which the detector responds. When t is equal to RC, the exponent in Eq. (9.9) becomes ~1 and the voltage attains 63% of its final value. As t increases beyond several time constants, the instrument reads the final steady-state voltage V_f:

$$V(t) = V_f(1 - e^{-t/RC}). \tag{9.10}$$

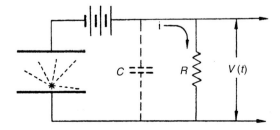

Figure 9-27. Operating principle of a current ionization chamber. The radiation-produced ions are collected from the chamber, thus causing a current i to flow through the external circuit, resulting in a voltage drop $V(t)$ across the high-valued resistor R. C represents all the capacitance associated with the chamber.

The sensitivity of the detector *increases* with increasing resistance of the load resistor. Since the capacitance of the detector and the circuit is fixed, this means that in an instrument with several ranges—which is accomplished by varying the value of R—the more sensitive ranges have longer time constants and hence are slower to respond than the less-sensitive ranges. The time constants for health physics surveying instruments vary up to about 10 s. The magnitude of the time constant is very important when measuring a short pulse of radiation whose duration is of the order of or less than the time constant of the survey instrument, as illustrated in Example 9.5. Laboratory instruments, where fast response is not important, may have much longer time constants.

 EXAMPLE 9.5

A survey meter, whose time constant is 4 seconds reads 10 mR (100 μSv) per hour while measuring the radiation from a dental X-ray exposure of 0.08 second.

(a) What was the actual exposure rate?

(b) What would have been the dose to the dental hygienist if she had been at the point of measurement?

Solution

(a) With Eq. (9.10), we find

$$\dot{D}_f = \frac{\dot{D}_t}{1 - e^{t/RC}} = \frac{10 \; \frac{mR}{h}}{1 - e^{-0.08/4}} = 505 \; \frac{mR}{h} \qquad (5050 \; \frac{\mu \; Sv}{h}).$$

(b)

$$\text{Dose} = \text{Dose rate} \times \text{Exposure time} \qquad \qquad \textbf{(9.11)}$$

$$D = 505 \; \frac{mR}{h} \times \frac{1 \; h}{3600 \; s} \times 0.08 \; s = 0.011 \; \; mR \qquad (1.1 \; \mu \; Sv).$$

Instrument manufacturers often list the response time of an instrument instead of the time constant. The response time is usually the time during which the instrument will reach 90% of its final reading.

When a current ion chamber is exposed to radiation levels of different intensity and the voltage across the chamber is varied, a family of curves, as shown in Figure 9-28, is obtained. The current plateau is called the *saturation current*.

When operated at a voltage that lies on the plateau, all the ions that are produced in the chamber are being collected. The operation of a current ion chamber and the fact that the response is proportional to absorbed energy is shown in the following illustrative example.

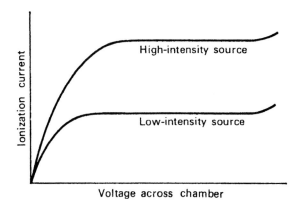

Figure 9-28. Variation of ionization current with voltage across the ionization chamber for different levels of radiation. The plateau represents the saturation current.

EXAMPLE 9.6

A large air-filled ionization chamber has a window whose thickness is 1 mg/cm².

(a) What ionization current will result if 1200 alpha particles from ^{210}Po enter the chamber per minute?

(b) What would be the ionization current if the window thickness were increased to 3 mg/cm²?

Solution

The ionization current within the chamber may be calculated from the following equation:

$$i = \frac{N \dfrac{\alpha}{s} \times \bar{E} \dfrac{eV}{\alpha} \times 1.6 \times 10^{-19} \dfrac{C}{ion}}{w \dfrac{eV}{ion}} \times \frac{1\,A}{C/s}. \tag{9.12}$$

(a) The energy of the alpha particle after it penetrates the window into the chamber is equal to the difference between its initial kinetic energy, 5.3 MeV, and the energy lost in penetrating the window. Assuming the plastic window to be equivalent to tissue in regard to the stopping power, we calculate from Eqs. (5.20) and (5.21) that the range of a 5.3-MeV alpha particle in the plastic of which the window is made is 5.1 mg/cm². After passing through the 1-mg/cm² window, therefore, the alpha particle's remaining kinetic energy is

$$\frac{5.1 - 1}{5.1} \times 5.3 = 4.26\ \text{MeV},$$

and the resulting ion current is, from Eq. (9.12),

$$i = \frac{1.2 \times 10^3 \, \dfrac{\alpha}{\text{min}} \times 4.26 \times 10^6 \, \dfrac{\text{eV}}{\alpha} \times 1.6 \times 10^{-19} \, \dfrac{\text{C}}{\text{ion}}}{60 \, \dfrac{\text{s}}{\text{min}} \times 35 \, \dfrac{\text{eV}}{\text{ion}}} \times \frac{1 \, \text{A}}{\text{C/s}}$$

$$i = 3.9 \times 10^{-13} \, \text{A}.$$

(b) If the window thickness were increased to 3 mg cm^{-2}, the energy of the alpha particle entering into the ionization chamber would be

$$\frac{5.1 - 3}{5.1} \times 5.3 = 2.18 \, \text{MeV},$$

and the ion current would be only 2×10^{-13} A. In both instances alpha particles were entering the ion chamber at the same rate. Therefore, if individual pulses had been counted, the counting rate would have been the same in both cases.

The ionization current, which depends on the volume of the chamber, the air density ρ, and on the exposure rate, is given by

$$i = \frac{V \, \text{cm}^3 \times \rho \, \dfrac{\text{kg}}{\text{cm}^3} \times \dot{X} \, \dfrac{\mu\text{C/kg}}{\text{h}} \times 10^{-6} \, \dfrac{\text{A}}{\mu\text{C/s}}}{3.6 \times 10^3 \, \dfrac{\text{s}}{\text{h}}}. \qquad (9.13)$$

For a 400-cm^3 chamber filled with standard air and an exposure rate of 6.5 μC/kg/h (25 mR/h), the ionization current is found, from Eq. (9.13), to be 9.3×10^{-13} A. To produce a voltage drop of about 1 volt across a resistor requires a resistor of about 10^{11} ohms. If a resistor of this value is used as the load resistor for the most sensitive scale of the instrument, then we need resistors of 10^{10} and 10^9 ohms respectively for full-scale dose-rate measurements in radiation fields 10 and 100 times more intense than that of the most sensitive scale. Ionization-chamber survey meters are relatively energy independent over a wide range of quantum energies, as shown in Figure 9-17.

Certain of the commercially available ionization-chamber survey meters have windows thin enough to admit alpha particles and are fitted with sliding shields that allow the measurement of alpha, beta, and gamma radiation. Other survey meters are available that respond only to betas and gammas or to gammas only. The span of full-scale dose rates in the commonly used ionization-chamber survey meters is from 0 to 0.01 mSv (0–1 mrem) per hour with multipliers of 10, 100, 1000, and 10,000. Good energy response is usual across an energy range of about 30 keV to 1.5 MeV, with an accuracy of about 30% or better.

NEUTRON MEASUREMENTS

Detection Reactions

Neutrons, like gamma rays, are not directly ionizing; they must react with another medium to produce a primary ionizing particle. Because of the strong dependence of neutron reaction rate on the cross section for that particular reaction, we either use different detection media, depending on the energy of the neutrons that we are trying to measure, or we modify the neutron energy distribution so that it will be compatible with the detector. Some of the basic neutron-detection reactions used in health physics instrumentation include the following:

1. $^{10}B(n, \alpha)^7Li$. Boron, which may be enriched in the ^{10}B isotope, is introduced into the counter either as BF_3 gas or as a thin film on the inside surfaces of the detector tube. The intense ionization produced by the alpha particle and by the ^7Li recoil nucleus is counted.

2. Elastic scattering of high-energy neutrons by hydrogen atoms. The scattered protons are the primary ionizing particles, and the ionization they produce is detected and measured.

3. Nuclear fission—fissile material (n, f) fission fragments. The fissile material is deposited as a thin film on the inside surface of a counter tube. Capture of a neutron and splitting of the fissile nucleus results in highly ionizing fission fragments, which can easily be detected. Fission reactions are energy dependent, and several fissile isotopes have a threshold energy below which fission cannot occur.

4. Neutron activation—Many neutron reactions produce radioactive isotopes. The degree of neutron-induced radioactivity of any given substance depends on the total neutron irradiation. By measuring the induced activity and allowing for decay time between exposure and measurement, the integrated neutron exposure can be calculated. Furthermore, since many of these activation reactions have energy thresholds, they can be useful in determining the neutron energy distribution. Tables 9-3 and 9-4 list the materials most commonly used for this purpose. This technique is especially useful in measuring neutron dose at very high dose rates, such as those that would be encountered in a criticality accident. (A criticality accident is an accidental uncontrolled chain reaction in which a very large amount of energy is liberated during a very brief time.) For measuring high neutron fluxes for health physics purposes, a series of threshold detectors of various threshold energies is packaged in a single unit. Exposure to neutrons activates the detectors. Since the induced activity in the threshold detectors depends on the neutron flux whose energy exceeds the threshold energy, the relative counting rates of the threshold detectors after exposure is used as a measure of the spectral distribution of the neutrons, while the absolute activity of the detector is a measure of exposure. A number of different substances may be used as threshold detectors. One type of pocket criticality dosimeter (Fig. 9-29) uses a combination of indium, cadmium-covered indium, sulfur, and cadmium-covered copper. By combining the results of the activity in each of these foils, the total critically neutron spectrum is covered.

The total neutron flux is thus divided into four energy groups, thereby permitting a reasonably accurate means for computing absorbed dose. The threshold detectors

TABLE 9-3. Foil Reactions with Thermal Neutrons

FOIL MATERIAL	TARGET NUCLEUS	TARGET % ABUNDANCE	NUCLEAR REACTION	PRODUCT NUCLEUS	PRODUCT HALF-LIFE	200 m/s ACTIVATION CROSS-SECTION (b)
Ag	^{107}Ag	51.35	n, γ	^{108}Ag	2.3 min	44
Ag	^{109}Ag	48.65	n, γ	^{110}Ag	25 s	110
In	^{115}In	95.77	n, γ	^{116m}In	54 min	145
U (nat.)	^{235}U	0.715	n, f	F.P.	$T^{-1.2}$	582
Dy	^{164}Dy	28.18	n, γ	^{165}Dy	2.32 h	2100
V	^{51}V	99.76	n, γ	$^{52}52 V$	3.77 min	4.5
Mn-Cu	^{55}Mn	80.00	n, γ	^{56}Mn	2.56 h	13.4
Cu	^{63}Cu	69.1	n, γ	^{64}Cu	12.8 h	4.3
Cu	^{65}Cu	30.9	n, γ	^{65}Cu	5.1 min	1.8
Al	^{27}Al	100	n, γ	^{28}Al	2.3 min	0.21
Au	^{197}Au	100	n, γ	^{198}Au	2.7 days	96
Rh	^{103}Rh	100	n, γ	^{104m}Rh	4.4 min	12
Rh	^{103}Rh	100	n, γ	^{104}Rh	44 s	140
Co	^{59}Co	100	n, γ	^{60}Co	5.27 yrs	36.3
NaCl	^{23}Na	100	n, γ	^{24}Na	15 h	0.53
Lu-Al	^{175}Lu	97.5	n, γ	^{176m}Lu	3.7 h	35
B-Al	^{10}B	19.6	n, α	^{7}Li	Stable	4010
Eu-Al	^{151}Eu	47.77	n, γ	^{152}Eu	9.2 h	1400
Pb	^{208}Pb	52.3	n, γ	^{209}Pb	3.2 h	6E−5
Nb	^{93}Nb	100	n, γ	^{94m}Nb	6.6 min	1.0

No adjustment was made for composition of alloys or compounds. This table lists the most useful thermal neutron reactions. (Courtesy of Reactor Experiments, Inc.)

are calibrated by exposing the pack to a known beam of neutrons and then measuring the induced activity. (A thermoluminescent dosimeter may be added to measure the gamma-ray exposure from a criticality accident.)

Neutron Counting with a Proportional Counter

Counting in the proportional region makes it simple to measure neutrons in the presence of gamma radiation. A neutron counter used for this purpose uses BF_3 gas to take advantage of the n, α reaction on ^{10}B:

$$^{10} B(n, \alpha)^7 Li.$$

Boron-10 has a high cross section for this reaction, 4010 barns for thermal neutrons, and consequently makes a very sensitive detecting medium. The alpha particles resulting from this reaction are produced inside the detector. Because of the great difference between the output pulses resulting from the alpha particles and Li ions and those due to gamma rays, it is a simple matter to discriminate electronically against all pulses except those due to the alphas and Li ions when a neutron is captured by ^{10}B.

The sensitivity of a BF_3 neutron detector may be increased by using ^{10}B-enriched BF_3 gas. Naturally occurring boron contains about 19.8% ^{10}B. However, it is possible to concentrate the ^{10}B isotope to the extent that BF_3 gas containing 96% ^{10}B is routinely available from commercial suppliers. The BF_3-filled counter is a sensitive and simple thermal-neutron detector and is widely used by health physicists for measuring thermal-neutron flux. Furthermore, since 680 thermal neutrons/cm^2/s

TABLE 9-4. Threshold Foil Reactions

FOIL MATERIAL	TARGET NUCLEUS	TARGET % ABUNDANCE	NUCLEAR REACTION	PRODUCT NUCLEUS	PRODUCT HALF-LIFE	EFFECTIVE ACTIVATION CROSS-SECTION (b)	EFFECTIVE THRESHOLD ENERGY (MeV)
Ni	58 Ni	67.76	n, p	58 Co	71.3 d	0.42	2.9
Fe	54 Fe	5.84	n, p	54 Mn	314 d	0.61	~3
Fe	56 Fe	91.68	n, p	56 Mn	2.58 h	0.11	7.5
Ti	46 Ti	7.95	n, p	46 Sc	84.1 d	0.23	5.5
S	32 S	95.018	n, p	32 P	14.3d	0.30	2.9
Mg	24 Mg	78.60	n, p	24 Na	15h	0.060	6.3
Al	27 Al	100.0	n, α	24 Na	15 h	0.130	8.7
Zr	90 Zr	51.46	n, 2n	89 Zr	3.3d	1.6	14.0
In, In-Al	115 In	95.77	n, n	115m In	4.5 h	0.2	1.0
NH₄I	127 I	100.0	n, 2n	126 I	13.3d	0.98	11.0
V	51 V	99.76	n, α	48Sc	44 h	0.08×10^{-3}	11.5
Th	232 Th	100.0	n, f	99 Mo	66 h	0.060	1.75
U, depl	238 U	0.415	n, f	99 Mo	66 h	0.55	1.45
U, depl	238 U	0.038	n, f	99 Mo	66 h	0.55	1.45
Si-Al	28 Si	92.27	n, p	28 Al	2.3 min	0.004	6.7

No adjustment was made for composition of alloys or compounds. This table lists the most useful threshold reactions. (Courtesy of Reactor Experiments, Inc.)

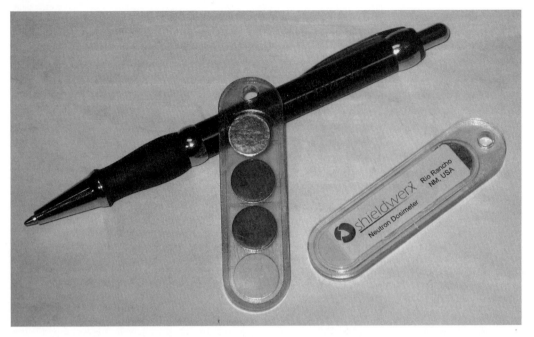

Figure 9-29. Pocket criticality dosimeter for measuring neutron exposure. Inside the dosimeter are four different foils whose induced radioactivity, following exposure to neutrons, depends on the neutron energy and fluence. (Courtesy of Bladewerx, LLC, Rio Rancho, NM.)

for 40 hours corresponds to 100 mrems (1 mSv) per week, it is a simple matter to discriminate electronically against all pulses except those due to the alphas and Li ions when a neutron is captured by ^{10}B.

The capture cross section for the ^{10}B$(n, \alpha)^7$Li reaction, and hence the counting rate of a BF$_3$ detector, depends on the neutron energy. Consider the case of a thermal neutron flux of ϕ neutrons/cm^2/s having a Maxwell–Boltzmann energy distribution and a BF$_3$ counter containing a total of N atoms of ^{10}B. If there is negligible neutron absorption by the counter wall and if the intrinsic counting efficiency is 100%, the counting rate is given by

$$CR = N \int \phi(v)\sigma(v)\,dv, \tag{9.14}$$

where $\phi(v)$ is the flux of neutrons of velocity v and $\sigma(v)$ is the capture cross section for neutrons of velocity v. Substituting $\phi(v) = n(v)v$, where $n(v)$ is the density in neutrons per cm^3 of those neutrons whose velocity is v cm/s; and, from Eq. (5.53), substituting $\sigma(v) = \sigma_0(v_0/v)$ into Eq. (9.14), we have

$$CR = N\sigma_0 v_0 \int n(v)\,dv \tag{9.15}$$

$$CR = N\sigma_0 v_0 n. \tag{9.16}$$

From Eq. (9.16), we see that the counting rate of a BF$_3$ counter is proportional to the total neutron density within the range of energies where the $1/v$ law is valid (up to about 1000 eV). If $\bar{v}$ is the mean neutron velocity (not the velocity corresponding to the mean neutron energy), then

$$\phi = n\bar{v}, \tag{9.17}$$

or $n = \phi/\bar{v}$. Substituting this value for n into Eq. (9.16) and solving for ϕ, we have

$$\phi = \frac{\bar{v}}{v_0} \times \frac{\mathrm{CR}}{N\sigma_0}. \tag{9.18}$$

In the Maxwell–Boltzmann distribution, $\bar{v}/v_0 = 2/\sqrt{\pi} = 1.128$. For thermal neutrons, therefore, the flux is related to the counting rate by

$$\phi = \frac{1.128}{N\sigma_0} \times \mathrm{CR}. \tag{9.19}$$

EXAMPLE 9.7

A thermal neutron counting rate of 600 counts per minute is measured with a BF_3 counter whose inside dimensions are 2 cm (diameter) × 20 cm (length), and is filled with 96% enriched $^{10}BF_3$ to a pressure of 20 cm Hg at a temperature of 27°C. What is the thermal flux? The volume of the counter is $\pi r^2 \times l$, or 62.83 cm³.

Solution

The molar quantity of BF_3 in the counter is

$$m = \frac{PV}{RT} = \frac{\dfrac{20}{76}\,\mathrm{atm} \times 0.06283\,\mathrm{L}}{0.082\dfrac{\mathrm{L\cdot atm}}{\mathrm{mol}} \cdot 300\,\mathrm{K}} = 6.72 \times 10^{-4}\,\mathrm{mol},$$

and the number ^{10}B atoms in the counter is

$$N = 0.96\frac{^{10}\mathrm{B\ atoms}}{\mathrm{molecule}} \times 6.02 \times 10^{23}\frac{\mathrm{molecules}}{\mathrm{mol}} \times 6.72 \times 10^{-4}\,\mathrm{mol}$$

$$= 3.89 \times 10^{20}\ ^{10}\mathrm{B\ atoms}.$$

From Eq. (9.19), we have

$$\phi = \frac{1.128}{3.89 \times 10^{20}\,\mathrm{atoms} \times 4.010 \times 10^{-21}\,\dfrac{\mathrm{cm}^2}{\mathrm{atom}}} \times 10\,\frac{\mathrm{counts}}{\mathrm{s}}$$

$$= 7.2\frac{\mathrm{neutrons}}{\mathrm{cm}^2/\mathrm{s}}.$$

The sensitivity of a radiation detector may be defined as

$$\text{Sensitivity} = \frac{\text{Count Rate}}{\text{Flux}}. \tag{9.20}$$

The sensitivity S of the BF_3 counter in Example 9.4 is

$$S = \frac{CR}{\phi} = \frac{600 \text{ counts/min}}{7.2 \dfrac{\text{neutrons}}{\text{cm}^2/\text{s}}} = 83.3 \frac{\text{counts/min}}{\dfrac{\text{neutrons}}{\text{cm}^2/\text{s}}}$$

Long Counter

One of the earliest fast-neutron counters was the long counter, which consists of a BF_3 counter surrounded by a paraffin moderator. Fast neutrons are sufficiently slowed down by the moderator to allow them to be captured by the ^{10}B. The counting rate of a moderated BF_3 counter in a field of fast neutrons increases with increasing moderator thickness until the paraffin is sufficiently thick to absorb a significant fraction of the thermalized neutrons. Beyond this optimum thickness, the counting rate decreases with further increase in thickness. The exact thickness at which this occurs depends on the energy of the neutrons. A paraffin moderator 2 3/8 in. thick results in an approximately flat response over a neutron-energy span from about 10 keV to better than 1 MeV. The outside of the paraffin may be covered with a thin sheet of cadmium to absorb thermal neutrons while allowing fast neutrons to pass through into the paraffin. The capture gammas due to absorption of thermal neutrons by the cadmium produce very small pulses in the counter, pulses small enough to be rejected by the discriminator. Such a paraffin-surrounded BF_3 counter is called a *long counter* because of its long energy-independent response. In health physics work, it is most useful in the energy range of about 10–500 keV. Measurement of higher energy neutrons with a BF_3 counter requires relatively large amounts of paraffin for slowing down the neutrons, thus making it impractical for many health physics surveying applications. Such a counter, which is reported as having a fairly uniform response from 10 keV to 5 MeV[1] is shown below in Figure 9-30. The counter response is highly directional and is designed to measure neutrons that are incident only on the front face. The layer of paraffin outside the B_2O_3 is a shield designed to remove neutrons that are incident on the sides. The series of eight holes in the front face permit the lower energy neutrons to reach the detector tube after being thermalized. The sensitivity of this counter is about 1 count/s/neutron/cm^2.

Proton Recoil Counter

A proportional counter that responds to recoil protons resulting from the collision of fast neutrons with hydrogen atoms may be used for the detection of neutrons whose energy exceeds 500 keV. (Below this energy, the output pulses from the counter are very weak, and high gain amplification would be required to record them.) Such a counter may be made simply by using a hydrogenous gas, such as methane, in

---

[1] A. O. Hanson and M. L. McKibben. A neutron detector having uniform sensitivity from 10 keV to 5 MeV. *Phys Rev*, 72:673, 1947; and R. A. Nobles, et al. Response of the long counter. *Rev Sci Instrum*, 25:334, 1954,

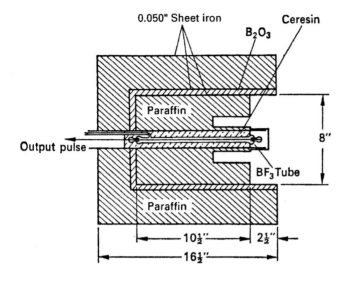

Figure 9-30. Diagram of a long counter, a neutron counter whose response is approximately uniform from about 10 keV to 5 MeV. (Reproduced with permission from Hanson AO, McKibben JL. A neutron detector having uniform sensitivity from 10 kev to 3 Mev. *Phys Rev.* 1947; 72(8):673–677. Copyright © 1947 American physical Society.)

the counter. The counter is enclosed in a thin sheet of cadmium to absorb thermal neutrons in order to prevent pulses due to deuteron recoils following absorption of thermal neutrons by the hydrogen. The hydrogenous material may also be a solid, such as paraffin or polyethylene, incorporated into the wall of the counter. The fast neutrons "knock out" protons from these solids, and the protons dissipate their energy in the counter gas. When used in this way as a source of protons, the hydrogenous substance is called a *proton radiator*.

The sensitivity for fast neutrons of a proton recoil counter is very much less than the sensitivity of a BF_3 counter for thermal neutrons. This is true for two reasons: The cross section of hydrogen for scattering of fast neutrons is very much less than the slow-neutron capture cross section of ^{10}B, and also the energy distribution of the scattered protons includes a large fraction of very low energy protons. For neutron energies up to about 10 MeV, the scattering of neutrons is isotropic. This means that the energy of the scattered proton may vary from zero to the energy of the neutron. The pulses that result from protons to which little energy was imparted during the collision are therefore not counted because of the bias against gamma radiation. Above this threshold, the energy response of the recoil proton proportional counter is determined mainly by the energy dependence of the scattering cross section of hydrogen.

Neutron Dosimetry

The dose equivalent from neutrons depends strongly on the energy of the neutrons, as shown in Table 9-5. We therefore cannot simply convert neutron flux density (fluence) into dose equivalent unless we know the energy spectral distribution of the neutrons. For thermal neutrons, of course, the spectral distribution is known, and a BF_3 counter can be calibrated to read directly in millirads per hour. For higher energy neutrons, neither the moderated BF_3 long counter with its "flat" energy-independent response to fast neutrons nor the simple proton-recoil proportional counter, whose response to fast neutrons depends strongly on the scattering cross section, is suitable for dosimetry.

TABLE 9-5. Values of Neutron Fluence Rates Which, in a Period of 40 Hours, results in a Maximum Dose Equivalent of 1 mSv.

NEUTRON ENERGY (MeV)	NEUTRON FLUENCE RATE (cm²/s)	
	Adapted from NCRP Report No. 38 (NCRP, 1971)[a]	Adapted from Cross and Ing. 1985[a]
2.5E−08	270	280
1E−07	340	—
1E−06	280	280
1E−05	280	280
1E−04	290	290
1E−03	340	280
5E−03	—	310
1E−02	350	300
2E−02	—	250
5E−02	—	110
1E−01	58	40
3E−01	—	20
3.8E−01	—	16
4.4E−01	—	13
5E−01	14	16
6E−01	—	15
8E−01	—	14
9E−01	—	13
1.0	10	9.7
1.20	—	12
2.00	—	11
2.30	—	12
2.50	10	11
3.00	—	11
3.50	—	8.5
4.50	—	9.9
5.00	8.0	9.7
6.25	—	9.2
7.00	8.5	9.0
10.0	8.5	8.0
14.0	6.0	6.8
14.7	—	6.5
20	5.5	
40	5.0	
60	5.5	
100	7.0	
200	6.5	
300	5.5	
400	5.0	

[a]The fluence rates presented here have been obtained from the cited references by dividing the respective reference values for thermal neutrons by 2.5 and the respective values for all the other energies by 2.0. These adjustments have been made to reflect recommendations of the NCRP (1987) to increase the effective quality factors for thermal neutrons and for more energetic neutrons by 2.5 and 2.0 respectively.

Reproduced with permission of the National Council on Radiation Protection and Measurements from *Calibration of Survey Instruments Used in Radiation Protection for the Assessment of Ionizing Radiation Fields and Radioactive Surface Contamination.* Bethesda, MD: National Council on Radiation Protection & Measurement; 1991:92. NCRP Report 112.

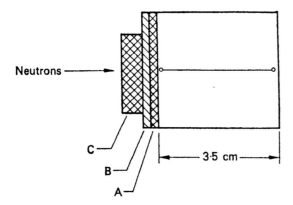

Figure 9-31. Schematic representation of a count-rate fast-neutron dosimeter. A—paraffin (13 mg/cm^2); B—aluminum (29 mg/cm^2); C—paraffin (100 mg/cm^2). Ratio of the paraffin areas, $a_A/a_C = 2.9$. The gas is methane at 30-cm Hg pressure. The counter has a highly directional response, and must be oriented towards the neutron beam, as shown in the diagram. (Reprinted with permission from Hurst GS, Ritchie RH, Wilson HN. A count rate method of measuring fast neutron dose. *Rev Sci Instr.* 1951; 22:981–986. Copyright © 1951 American Institute of Physics.)

Fast Neutrons: Hurst Counter

The proton-recoil proportional counter can be modified to measure fast-neutron dose rate. By using a combination of several different proton radiators and filling gases, as shown schematically in Figure 9-31, the energy distribution of the recoil protons that enter into the gas-filled cavity of a proportional counter is such that the resulting count rate is proportional to the variation of tissue dose with the neutron energy. Hence, the counting rate meter read out from the proportional counter can be calibrated directly in millirads or millisieverts per hour of fast neutrons. Figure 9-32 compares the energy dependence of the dose with the response of the dose–rate dosimeter. Gamma-insensitive fast-neutron dosimeters based on this design principle are commercially available. Because of the design, this instrument is limited to measurement of neutrons in the energy range from 0.2 to 14 MeV. The discriminator settings necessary to obtain the correct dose response rejects all counts due to neutrons whose energy is less than 0.2 MeV. Above 14 MeV, the response of this fast-neutron dosimeter is not proportional to the absorbed dose rate.

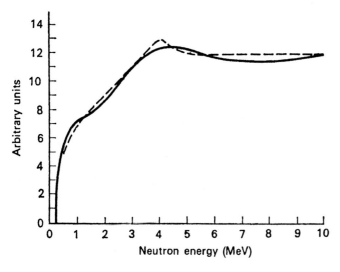

Figure 9-32. Energy response of the Hurst count-rate fast-neutron dosimeter. The solid curve shows the relationship between count rate per unit flux and neutron energy; the broken curve relates the dose rate per unit flux and neutron energy. (Reprinted with permission from Hurst GS, Ritchie RH, Wilson HN. A count rate method of measuring fast neutron dose. *Rev Sci Instr.* 1951; 22:981–986. Copyright © 1951 American Institute of Physics.)

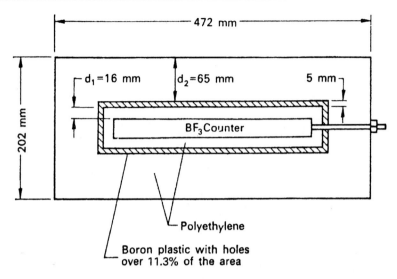

Figure 9-33. Construction of the neutron rem counter. The BF_3 counter embedded in the polyethylene has an outside diameter of 30 mm, a sensitive length of 200 mm, and a total length of 300 mm; it is filled with 94% ^{10}B-enriched BF_3 at a pressure of 600 mm Hg. (Reprinted with permission from Andersson IO, Braun J. A neutron rem counter with uniform sensitivity from 0.025 eV to 10 MeV. In: *Neutron Dosimetry: Proceedings of the Symposium on Neutron Detection, Dosimetry, and Standardization.* Vol 2. Vienna: International Atomic Energy Agency (IAEA); 1963:87–95.)

Thermal and Fast-Neutron Dose-Equivalent Meter

A neutron counter whose count rate is proportional to the dose equivalent across the energy span of 0.025 eV–10 MeV can be made by surrounding a BF_3 proportional counter with two cylindrical layers of polyethylene moderator separated by a boron-loaded plastic (Fig. 9-33). Circular disks of the same materials make up the ends of the cylinders.

In designing the counter, the simplifying assumptions were made that all neutrons entering the counter and making their first collision in the outer polyethylene are absorbed in the boron plastic shield and thus lost for the purpose of detection, while all neutrons making their first collision in the polyethylene inside the boron plastic are considered as having a detection probability k. On the basis of these assumptions, the likelihood of obtaining a pulse from a neutron of energy E that is incident normal to the long axis of the counter is given by

$$P = ke^{-\sum(E)d_2}(1 - e^{-2\sum(E)d_1}), \qquad (9.21)$$

where $\sum(E)$ is the macroscopic total scattering cross section for neutron energy E, and d_1 and d_2 are the thicknesses of the inner and outer polyethylene moderators. Varying d_1 and d_2 changes the energy response. With $d_1 = 16$ mm and $d_2 = 32$ mm, the energy response of the counter very closely approximates, within $\pm15\%$, the curve of rem per neutron per cm^2 versus neutron energy (Fig. 9-34). A commercial survey meter based on this design has a sensitivity of 12 cpm/μSv/h (120 cpm/mrem/h) and a range of 1–1000 μSv (0.1–100 mrems) per hour.

Commercially available neutron dose-equivalent meters (Fig. 9-35) that can measure neutron dose equivalent rates from 1 μSv/h (0.1 mrem/h) to 100 mSv (10,000

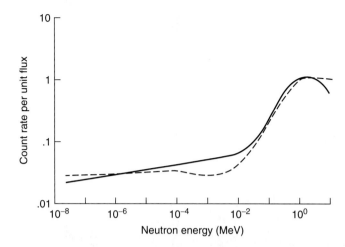

Figure 9-34. Energy response curve (solid line) of a neutron rem counter. The broken line is the dose equivalent per unit flux. Ideally, the response should be 7.6 counts/s/mrem/h. (Reprinted with permission from Andersson IO, Braun J. A neutron rem counter with uniform sensitivity from 0.025 eV to 10 MeV. In: *Neutron Dosimetry: Proceedings of the Symposium on Neutron Detection, Dosimetry, and Standardization.* Vol 2. Vienna: International Atomic Energy Agency (IAEA); 1963:87–95.)

mrems) per hour utilize a thermal-neutron detector surrounded by a spherical or semispherical moderator (remball detector). Either a small (about 4 mm × 4 mm) ^{6}LiI(Eu) scintillating crystal located in the center of the sphere or a ^{10}BF$_3$ counter inserted into the moderator can be used as the neutron detector. However, because the ^{10}BF$_3$ tube is less sensitive to gamma rays than is the scintillation crystal, the ^{10}BF$_3$ counter is the most widely used neutron detector in neutron dose-equivalent meters. However, BF$_3$ tubes are being replaced by tubes filled with ^{3}He. Because of new restrictions on the air transport of BF$_3$, shipping companies are reluctant to ship devices containing BF$_3$ despite the fact that a tube contains only about 0.02 g BF$_3$. The energy response of ^{3}He tubes is the same as that of the BF$_3$ tubes, and the neutron sensitivity of ^{3}He tubes is greater than that of BF$_3$ tubes. Replacement of the BF$_3$ tubes therefore will not lead to any changes in the use of remball detectors.

The response of a spherical neutron dosimeter, when the sphere is 30 cm in diameter, is approximately proportional to the neutron dose-equivalent rate from thermal energies to about 15 MeV. This type of neutron dose-equivalent meter thus may be calibrated with neutrons of any energy within this range. Spheres smaller than 30 cm in diameter are relatively more sensitive to lower energy neutrons. Since the energy response of the instrument depends on the size of the spherical moderator, it is possible to determine the energy distribution in a neutron field by making a series of measurements with different-sized spheres. The spheres used for this method of neutron spectroscopy are commonly called "Bonner spheres"; they range in diameter from 5 to 30 cm.

Superheated Emulsion (Bubble) Dosimeter

A superheated emulsion (bubble) dosimeter (Fig. 9-36) is a sensitive passive neutron dosimeter about the size of a fountain pen, and hence is useful for personal monitoring as well as for area monitoring for stray neutron radiation at a radiotherapy facility using a high-energy particle accelerator. It is completely unresponsive to gamma radiation, and its energy response is such that it approximates the ICRP 60 weighting factors for neutrons, thus allowing calibration and readout directly in microsieverts or in millirems of neutron dose. The bubble detector consists of numerous microscopic droplets of a superheated liquid of a hydrocarbon or halocarbon dispersed in

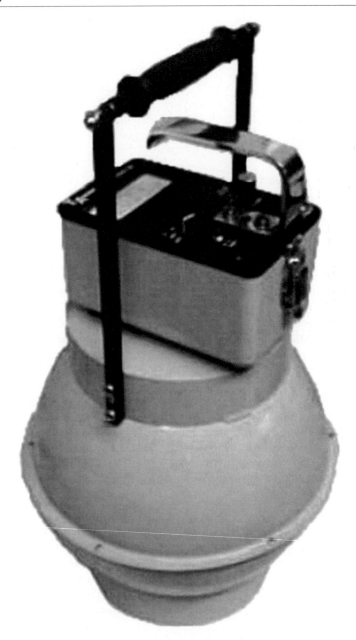

Figure 9-35. Spherical neutron dose-equivalent meter. The sphere is made of polyethelene, 10 inches diameter. The thermalized neutrons are measured with a ^{3}He filled detector. (Courtesy Technical Associates, Canoga Park, CA.)

a gel or an elastic polymer. The potential energy contained in the droplets is released when a droplet is struck by a neutron. This released energy heats the droplet, causing it to vaporize and explode into a visibly and audibly discernible bubble. The resulting bubbles are trapped in the viscous suspending medium, where they can be counted visually. The number of bubbles is directly proportional to the neutron-equivalent dose. Commercially available neutron-bubble dosimeters have a sensitivity of about

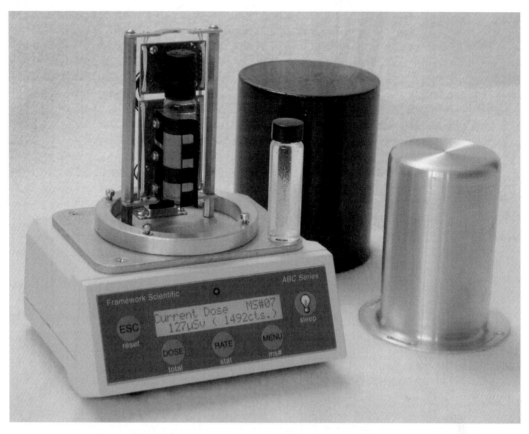

Figure 9-36. Photograph of a superheated emulsion vial and acoustical bubble counter. The lead cylinder in the background is used to extend the response to over 1 GeV. (Courtesy of FrameSci.com.)

10,000 bubbles per mSv (100 bubbles per mrem) and span a range of dose rates from 0.5 to 1000 μSv/h (0.05–100 mrems/h).

CALIBRATION

Radiation survey instruments are used principally to provide a basis for the control of radiation exposure and to evaluate the efficacy of control measures; they also are necessary to demonstrate compliance with radiation safety regulations. It is essential, therefore, that the instruments' readings be sufficiently accurate for these tasks. To this end, survey instruments must be properly calibrated in order that we have confidence in their readings. Calibration is accomplished by exposing the instrument in a radiation field of known intensity, and then adjusting the controls on the instrument to read this intensity. Since the scales of the instrument may not be linear, calibration measurements must be made at several different radiation levels. If the scale is indeed not linear, then a calibration curve of dose rate versus meter reading is drawn for use with the instrument. The radiation characteristics of the source that is used for this calibration should be traceable to an official standards laboratory, such as the NIST (formerly the United States Bureau of Standards). Since a survey instrument can go out of calibration for several different reasons, every survey meter should have a check source attached to it. The meter reading of the check source whenever the instrument is used should be the same as it was at the time the instrument was calibrated. Survey instruments should be recalibrated whenever they fail a check measurement, after any repair, or under any other conditions that may modify their response. As a minimum, all health physics survey instruments should be recalibrated at least once a year.

Gamma Rays

Radium (usually as a radium salt, such as RaBr) in equilibrium with its daughters and sealed into a platinum–iridium capsule was once the most widely used gamma-ray calibration source. The gamma radiation from a radium source is very heterochromatic, and ranges in energy from 0.184 MeV to 2.198 MeV, with a mean energy of 0.7 MeV. The gamma-ray output from a 1-g radium source is 212 μC/kg/h, which is the equivalent of 8.25 mSv (825 mrems) per hour at a distance of 1 m. The distance from the source for any other dose rate may be calculated with the aid of the inverse square law. Because of widespread radium contamination from several accidental ruptures of the platinum capsule due to the pressure of the helium gas that accumulates as alpha radiation is emitted, the use of radium as a calibration source was abandoned. It has been replaced by other sources, such as ^{60}Co and ^{137}Cs. Since these two radionuclides have relatively short half-lives, 5.3 and 30 years, respectively, correction factors—to account for their decreased activity since their original calibration—must be applied when they are used as calibration sources.

In free space, the radiation intensity, or dose rate, from a point source in free space varies inversely with the square of the distance from the point (Eq. [9.22]). This relationship is called the *inverse square law*, and is expressed algebraically as

$$\frac{I_1}{I_2} = \frac{d_2^2}{d_1^2},$$

(9.22)

where I_1 is radiation intensity at distance d_1 and I_2 is radiation intensity at distance d_2.

EXAMPLE 9.8

If the source documentation says that the gamma-ray exposure rate at a distance of 1 m is 0.88 mGy air kerma/h (25.8 μC/kg/h or 100 mR/h) and we wish to calibrate the 0.11 mGy/h (3.2 μC/kg/h or 12.5 mR/h) midpoint on the scale of an instrument that measures 0–0.22 mGy/h air kerma (0–6.4 μC/kg/h or 0–25 mR/h), at what distance from the calibration source should the detector be placed?

Solution

Substituting the values for $I_1 = 0.88$, $I_2 = 0.11$, and $d_1 = 1$ into Eq. (9.22), we have

$$\frac{0.88}{0.11} = \frac{d_2^2}{1^2}$$

$$d_2 = 2.83 \text{ m.}$$

When applied to a point source (for practical purposes, a real source approximates a "point" at distances from the source greater than 10 times the longest linear dimension of the source) the inverse square law is strictly applicable only in a free field, that is, in a field where there is no scattered radiation that can reach the detector. If there is significant scattered radiation, then the fall-off of radiation intensity with distance will be less than that predicted by the inverse square law. Allowance for the scatter can be made in several ways. One method is to measure the radiation at various distances from the calibration source with another calibrated instrument, then plot the radiation level versus distance on log–log paper and calculate the slope of the line. For example, if the slope is found to be –1.8, then instead of an inverse square relationship, we have

$$\frac{I_1}{I_2} = \frac{d_2^{1.8}}{d_1^{1.8}}.$$

Under this condition, d_2, the distance from the source in Example 9.9, would be 3.19 m.

Another method for accounting for scattered radiation is to make two measurements at each calibration distance. One measurement is made with the detector in the radiation beam, and the second reading is made with the direct beam blocked out by a thick piece of lead, whose cross section is that of the detector, placed midway between the detector and the source. The difference between the two readings is due to the scattered radiation, and the appropriate correction can be made. When properly calibrated, a gamma- or X-ray survey meter should measure the radiation within ±10% about 95 times out of 100 measurements.

Beta Particles

Dose–response characteristics of most portable survey instruments for beta particles are strongly energy dependent. As a consequence, survey instruments are used mainly to detect beta radiation rather than to quantify the beta-radiation dose rate. Such instruments are therefore not usually calibrated for beta dose. For those cases where beta calibration is desired, sources of various surface areas are commercially available. These sources, whose calibration is traceable to the NIST, may be calibrated in transformations per minute per square centimeter for use in contamination monitoring or in microsieverts per hour or millirems per hour at the surface and at several distances above the surface. In external dosimetry, we are not concerned with measuring dose from beta particles whose energy is less than 70 keV, because the range of these betas is less than 7 mg/cm^2; therefore, they do not have enough energy to reach the target cells in the skin. Because of the dependence of dose and range of betas on their energy, it is recommended that beta calibration sources be appropriate for the energy of the betas that will be measured with the calibrated instruments. If the instrument will be used for a wide range of beta emitters, then the calibration should be performed with low-, medium-, and high-energy betas. Frequently, an infinitely thick ($\geq$1.1 g/cm^2) source, which gives a surface dose rate of 2.3 mSv/h (230 mrems/h) at a tissue depth of 0.007 cm, is used to calibrate an instrument for beta dosimetry. Table 9-6 lists several different beta sources that are recommended for beta calibration.

Alpha Particles

Portable survey instruments used to measure alpha contamination are usually designed to read in units of counting rate. Calibration sources for these instruments are most often metal disks on which known amounts of an alpha-emitting

TABLE 9-6. Calibration Sources for Beta Particles

RADIONUCLIDE	E$_{max}$(keV)	T$_{1/2}$(yr)	BARE SOURCE DOSE RATE IN AIR^a mGy/h/MBq		
			10 cm	20 cm	30 cm
^{14}C^b	156	5730	0.46		
^{147}Pm^c	225	2.62	0.86	0.053	0.003
^{99}Tc	294	2 $\times 10^5$	1.20	0.16	0.034
^{85}Kr	670	10.8	1.26	0.29	0.13
^{36}Cl	710	3 $\times 10^5$	1.19	0.30	0.13
^{204}Tl	764	3.8	1.21	0.26	0.10
^{90}Sr + ^{90}Y^d	2280	28.6	2.22	0.51	0.21
			(0.78)	(0.19)	(0.086)
Natural or depleted U^e	2290	4 $\times 10^9$	2.3^g		
^{106}Ru + ^{106}Rh ^{f}	3540	1.0	0.82	0.21	0.091

^{a} Dose rates are for point isotropic sources with no source covering other than the air between the source and the dose point unless otherwise noted. The values have been estimated from the data of Cross *et al.*, 1982. Multiply values by 3.7 to obtain mrad/h/μCi. These values are provided as guidance. The particular source fabrication can greatly affect the dose rates that must be evaluated in order to usea a source for calibration.

^{b} If ^{14}C is used as a reference source, it is recommended that another source whose residual maximum beta energy <0.3 MeV also be used as a reference source because most instruments have a very large energy dependence for low energy betas.

^{c}^{147}Pm frequently contains ^{146}Pm (E_{max} = 780 keV).

^{d} The source should be covered with 100 mg/cm^2 (nominal) filtration to remove the ^{90}Sr beta component if the lower energy contribution from the ^{90}Sr is not desired. The dose-rate numbers in the parentheses are for a point source covered with 100 mg/cm^2 of a low atomic number absorber.

^{e} The uranium requires 200 days after separation to achieve greater than 99% equilibrium of short-lived progeny.

^{f} The source should be covered with 10 mg/cm^2 (nominal) filtration to remove the ^{106}Ru beta component. Ten centimeters of air is sufficient for this purpose.

^{g} The recorded dose rate (mGy/h) is the soft tissue dose rare at a tissue depth of 7 mg/cm^2 at the surface of an infinite slab of uranium.

Reproduced with permission of the National Council on Radiation Protection and Measurements from *Calibration of Survey Instruments Used in Radiation Protection for the Assessment of Ionizing Radiation Fields and Radioactive Surface Contamination.* Bethesda, MD: National Council on Radiation Protection & Measurement; 1991:92. NCRP Report 112.

TABLE 9-7. *Calibration Sources for Alpha Particles*

RADIONUCLIDE	ALPHA ENERGY (MeV)	HALF-LIFE
^{235}U	4.37–4.6	7.1×10^8 yr
^{239}Pu	5.11–5.16	24,400 yr
^{210}Po	5.3	138.4 d
^{241}Am	5.44–5.49	433 yr

radioisotope are electroplated. Such sources are listed in Table 9-7 and are readily available through commercial sources or through national standards laboratories.

Neutrons

For fast neutrons, commonly used calibration sources include Po–Be, Ra–Be, and Pu–Be. The approximate neutron yield for each of these sources is given in Table 5-5. The exact output of fast neutrons, in neutrons per second is usually given by the supplier of the source. For intercomparison of sources, the long counter of Hanson and McKibben may be used with an accuracy of ±5%. The neutron flux at a distance d from the source, assuming the source to be a "point," is given by

$$\phi \frac{\text{neutrons}}{\text{cm}^2/\text{s}} = \frac{N \text{ neutrons/s}}{4\pi d^2}. \tag{9.23}$$

All neutron sources supply fast neutrons. For the three α, n sources listed above, the neutron energies span a range from about 1/2 MeV to about 10 MeV, with a mean energy of about 4–5 MeV (Figs. 5-23, 9-37 and 9-38). In using a fast-neutron source for calibration of a dose-equivalent neutron survey meter, attention must be paid to the neutron energy spectrum. For example, let us consider the case of a Pu–Be neutron source (Fig. 9-38) and determine the flux that corresponds to 25 μSv/h (2.5 mrems/h), or to 1 mSv (100 mrems) per 40-hour week. The spectral distribution is given in Table 9-8. From these data, and using the appropriate Q values published in

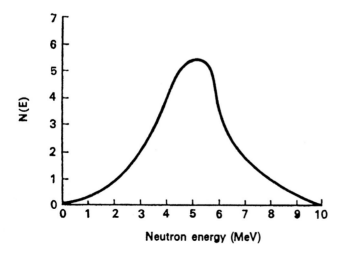

Figure 9-37. Neutron energy spectrum for Ra–Be alpha-neutron source. The neutron spectrum was determined by measuring track lengths in nuclear emulsion. (Source: *Physical Aspects of Irradiation.* Washington, DC: US Government Printing Office; 1964. NBS Handbook 85.)

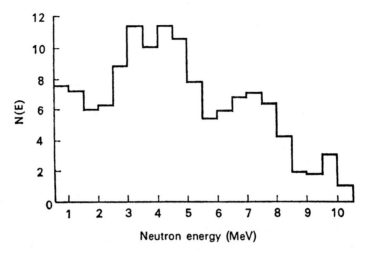

Figure 9-38. Neutron energy spectrum for Pu–Be (α, n). (Reproduced with permission from *Neutron Sources and Their Characteristics*. Ottawa, Canada: Atomic Energy of Canada, Ltd (AECL). Tech Bulletin NS-1.)

TABLE 9-8. Data for Computation of Dose–Equivalent Rate from Pu-Be Neutrons

ENERGY INTERVAL ΔE_i	MEAN ENERGY $\bar{E}_i$	f_i FRACTION OF NEUTRONS IN ΔE_i	FLUX ϕ_i, FOR $\bar{E}_i \times f_i$	FLUX ϕ_i, FOR 25 μSv/h	$\phi_i \times f_i$
0–0.5	0.25	0.038	0.0095	25	0.95
0.5–1	0.75	0.049	0.0368	14.3	0.70
1–1.5	1.25	0.045	0.0563	11.7	0.53
1.5–2	1.75	0.042	0.0735	11.3	0.47
2–2.5	2.25	0.046	0.1035	11.2	0.52
2.5–3	2.75	0.062	0.1705	11	0.68
3–3.5	3.25	0.077	0.2503	9.8	0.75
3.5–4	3.75	0.083	0.3113	9.2	0.76
4–4.5	4.25	0.082	0.3485	8.5	0.70
4.5–5	4.75	0.076	0.3610	9.8	0.74
5–5.5	5.25	0.057	0.2933	9.6	0.55
5.5–6	5.75	0.042	0.2415	9.4	0.39
6–6.5	6.25	0.042	0.2625	9.2	0.39
6.5–7	6.75	0.052	0.3510	9.1	0.47
7–7.5	7.25	0.054	0.3915	9	0.49
7.5–8	7.75	0.051	0.3953	9	0.46
8–8.5	8.25	0.038	0.3135	8.5	0.32
8.5–9	8.75	0.017	0.1488	8.5	0.14
9–9.5	9.25	0.018	0.1665	8	0.14
9.5–10	9.75	0.022	0.2145	8	0.18
10–10.5	10.25	0.007	0.0718	8	0.06
		$\sum = 1.000$	$\sum = 4.5774$		$\sum = 10.39$

10 CFR 20 values for the various neutron energies, expressed as flux that will result in a dose-equivalent of 25 μSv/h (2.5 mrems/h), we calculate that 20 neutrons/cm^2/s corresponds to 25 μSv/h (2.5 mrems/h). If monoenergetic neutrons are required, then one of the γ, n sources listed in Table 5-4 must be used. If thermal neutrons are required for calibration purposes, the fast neutrons emitted from the neutron source must be thermalized. This is easily accomplished by surrounding the source with paraffin. However, it should be emphasized that not all the fast neutrons are thermalized. The beam that emerges from the moderator is heterochromatic, the moderator thus merely extends the lower end of the neutron energy spectrum to thermal energies. If the moderator is too thin, the neutron beam is too rich in fast neutrons; if the moderator is too thick, the ratio of thermal to fast neutrons increases, but the intensity of the neutron beam is decreased. The thickness of paraffin for maximizing the intensity of thermal neutrons from a calibration source is about 4 in. (10 cm). With this thickness, the thermal-neutron flux within a distance of 2 m from the source has been found to be about 40% of the fast-neutron flux that would have been obtained without the paraffin moderator. If a relatively constant ratio of thermal to fast neutrons is required, the paraffin moderator thickness must be increased beyond 4 in. (10 cm).

The exact ratio of thermal to resonance or nonthermal neutrons may be measured by using the neutrons to activate a bare gold foil and a cadmium-covered gold foil. Because of the sharp cadmium absorption cutoff at about 0.4 eV, the induced activity in the cadmium-shielded foil is due only to neutrons whose energy exceeds 0.4 eV, while the activity of the bare foil is due to thermal neutrons as well as to the higher energy neutrons. The cadmium ratio, which is defined by

$$\text{Cd ratio} = \frac{\text{activity of bare foil}}{\text{activity of Cd} - \text{covered foil}} \tag{9.24}$$

is a measure of the purity of a thermal neutron field. The thermal flux may be computed from the gold foil activity measurements with the aid of Eq. (5.73).

EXAMPLE 9.9

A gold foil 2.54 cm (diameter) $\times$ 0.1 mm (thickness) is irradiated, at a temperature of 40°C, in a neutron beam that is thermalized by passing it through 10 cm of paraffin. Another gold foil of the same size is covered with cadmium, and is irradiated in the same beam. After irradiation for 1 hour, both foils are counted in a system whose overall efficiency is 50%. One hour after removal from the beam, the bare foil's count is 6030 cpm and the Cd-covered foil's count is 30 cpm. The activation cross section for the ^{197}Au$(n, \gamma)^{198}$Au reaction is 98.6 b, gold consists only of ^{197}Au, $T_{1/2}$ ^{198}Au = 2.7 days, and density of Au = 19.3 g/cm^3.

(a) What is the ratio of thermal neutrons to resonance neutrons in the beam?

(b) What is the thermal-neutron flux in the beam?

Solution

(a) The ratio of thermal neutrons to resonance neutrons is

$$\frac{\text{therman neutrons}}{\text{resonance neutrons}} = \frac{6030 - 30}{30} = 200 : 1.$$

(b) The thermal neutron flux is calculated with Eq. (5.73):

$$\lambda N = \text{activity} = \phi \sigma n (1 - e^{-\lambda t}) \tag{5.70}$$

The activity, $\lambda N = \dfrac{6000\dfrac{\text{counts}}{\text{min}} \times \dfrac{1\,\text{min}}{60\,\text{s}}}{0.5\,\text{counts/disint}} = 200$ dps.

The number of ^{198}Au target atoms, n, is calculated below:

$$n = \frac{\pi r^2 \times \text{thickness} \times \text{density}}{A\,\text{g/mol}} \times 6.03 \times 10^{23}\,\frac{\text{atoms}}{\text{mol}}$$

$$n = \frac{\pi \times (1.7\,\text{cm})^2 \times 0.01\,\text{cm} \times 19.3\,\dfrac{\text{g}}{\text{cm}^3}}{197\ \text{g/ mol}} \times 6.03 \times 10^{23}\,\frac{\text{atoms}}{\text{mol}}$$

$$= 5.36 \times 10^{21}\,\text{atoms}.$$

The temperature-corrected activation cross section, from Eq. (6.64b) is

$$\sigma = \sigma_0 \times \sqrt{\frac{T_0}{T}} = 98.6\,\text{b} \times 10^{-24}\,\frac{\text{cm}^2}{\text{b}} \times \sqrt{\frac{293}{313}} = 95.4 \times 10^{-24}\text{cm}^2.$$

The ^{198}Au decay rate constant $= \dfrac{0.693}{2.7\,\text{days} \times 24\,\dfrac{\text{h}}{\text{d}}} = 1.07 \times 10^{-2}\text{h}^{-1}.$

When we substitute these values into Eq. (b), and when we add the term for decay between the end of irradiation and the activity measurement, we obtain

$$200\,\frac{\text{dis}}{\text{s}} = \phi\,\frac{n}{\text{cm}^2/\text{s}} \times 95.4 \times 10^{-24}\,\frac{\text{cm}^2}{\text{atom}}$$

$$\times\, 5.36 \times 10^{21}\,\text{atoms} \times (1 - e^{-0.0107/\text{h}\times 1\,\text{h}})(e^{-0.0107/\text{h}\times 1\,\text{h}})$$

$$\phi = \frac{200\ \text{dps}}{95.4 \times 10^{-24}\,\dfrac{\text{cm}^2}{\text{atom}} \times 5.36 \times 10^{21}\,\text{atoms} \times (1 - e^{-0.0107\,\text{h}^{-1}\times 1\text{h}})(e^{-0.0107\,\text{h}^{-1}\times 1\text{h}})}$$

$$\phi = 3.71 \times 10^4\,\frac{\text{neutrons}}{\text{cm}^2/\text{s}}.$$

Flux corresponding to 25 μSv/h (2.5 mrems/h) $= \dfrac{\sum_i \phi_i f_i}{\sum_i f_i} = \dfrac{10.39}{1}$

$= 10.4 \dfrac{\text{neutrons}}{\text{cm}^2/\text{s}}$

Mean neutron energy $= \dfrac{\sum_i \bar{E}_i f_i}{\sum_i f_i} = \dfrac{4.5774}{1} = 4.6$ MeV.

Accuracy

Accuracy is a gauge of how close the measured value is to the actual value. In order for a photon- or neutron-measuring instrument to be acceptably calibrated, we should be 95% certain that the instrument's response to radiation whose energy is the same as that of the calibration source is within ±10% of the true mean calibration value. However, in the field, the accuracy required of health physics instruments depends on how close the actual dose rate is to the prescribed limit. When measurements are made at levels less than 25% of the prescribed limits, a deviation from the true value by a factor of 2 is usually acceptable. Because of the high degree of conservatism built into the ICRP recommendations, an accuracy of ±30% is usually acceptable when the field intensity is close to the prescribed limit. For measurements considerably in excess of the prescribed limits, the deviation of the measured value from the true value should be within 20%, because medical management of overexposed people is strongly influenced by their estimated dose as well as their clinical signs and symptoms. In this discussion, health physics instruments must be sharply distinguished from radiation-measuring instruments used in the calibration of radiation-producing machines in medical radiology. These instruments must have an accuracy of ±3% or better for the radiations for which their use is intended.

COUNTING STATISTICS

The equation for radioactive transformation, Eq. (4.18),

$$A = A_0 e^{-\lambda t}$$

can be derived by statistical reasoning only if we assume that radioactive transformation is a randomly occurring event whose mean rate of occurrence is characteristic of a given radionuclide. The probability of transformation p during a time interval Δt is directly proportional to the length of the time interval:

$$p \propto \Delta t.$$

If λ is the constant of proportionality, then

$$p = \lambda \, \Delta t. \tag{9.25}$$

The probability of surviving the time interval Δt is

$$1 - p = 1 - \lambda \, \Delta t, \tag{9.26}$$

and the probability of surviving the next Δt is also $1 - p$. Therefore, the probability of surviving two successive time periods of Δt each is

$$(1 - p)(1 - p) = (1 - p)^2 = (1 - \lambda \Delta t)^2, \tag{9.27}$$

and the probability of surviving n successive periods of Δt each is

$$(1 - p)^n = (1 - \lambda \Delta t)^n. \tag{9.28}$$

If the n successive intervals of Δt each is the total time t, then

$$t = n \Delta t, \tag{9.29a}$$

or

$$\Delta t = \frac{t}{n}. \tag{9.29b}$$

If Eq. (9.29b) is substituted into Eq. (9.28), we obtain

$$(1 - p)^n = (1 - \lambda \Delta t)^n = (1 - \lambda \frac{t}{n})^n. \tag{9.30}$$

As $\Delta t \to 0$, $n \to \infty$. Furthermore,

$$\lim_{n \to \infty} \left(1 - \frac{\lambda t}{n}\right)^n = e^{-\lambda t}. \tag{9.31}$$

Therefore, $e^{-\lambda t}$ is the probability that a single atom survives for a time t. If A_0 is the initial number of radioactive atoms, then, from Eq. (4.18), the number of atoms that survive for a time t is given as

$$A = A_0 e^{-\lambda t}.$$

Since Eq. (4.18) was derived by assuming that radioactive transformation is a stochastic process whose mean rate of occurrence is characteristic of a given radionuclide, it follows that individual measurements in a series of consecutive counts will differ among themselves and will be randomly distributed around an average value. Because of this fluctuating rate, it is not correct to speak of a *true* rate of transformation (which implies no statistical error in the measurement) but rather of a *true average* rate of transformation. When we make a measurement, we estimate the true average rate from the observed count rate. The *error* of a determination is defined as the difference between the true average rate and the measured rate. We can determine the frequency of occurrence of an error of any given size by applying the laws of probability.

Distributions

Radioactive transformations and other nuclear reactions are randomly occurring events and must therefore be described quantitatively in statistical terms. The sampling distribution of a population of randomly occurring events is called the *binomial distribution* and is given by the expansion of the binomial

$$(p+q)^n = p^n + np^{n-1}q + \frac{n(n-1)}{2!}p^{n-2}q^2 + \frac{n(n-1)(n-2)}{3!}p^{n-3}q^3 + \cdots,$$

(9.32)

where p is the mean probability of the occurrence of an event, q is the mean probability of nonoccurrence of the event, $p + q = 1$, and n is the number of chances of occurrence. The probability of the occurrence of exactly n events is given by the first term of the binomial expansion, the probability of occurrence of $n-1$ events is given by the second term, and so on. Using dice as an example, the likelihood of throwing three ones in three consecutive throws of a die, in which the mean probability of throwing a one is $1/6$, is given by the first term of the expansion, according to Eq. (9.32), of $(1/6 + 5/6)^3$:

$$\left(\frac{1}{6}+\frac{5}{6}\right)^3 = \left(\frac{1}{6}\right)^3 + 3\left(\frac{1}{6}\right)^2\left(\frac{5}{6}\right) + \frac{3\times2}{2!}\left(\frac{1}{6}\right)\left(\frac{5}{6}\right)^2 + \frac{3\times2\times1}{3!}\left(\frac{5}{6}\right)^3$$

$$= \frac{1}{216} + \frac{15}{216} + \frac{75}{216} + \frac{125}{216} = 1$$

The probabilities of 2 ones, 1 one, and no ones are given by the second, third, and fourth terms as $15/216$, $75/216$, and $125/216$, respectively. A plot of these probabilities (Fig. 9-39, curve A), shows the distribution to be very asymmetrical. If we were to make similar calculations for the probability of throwing 6, 5, 4, 3, 2, 1 or

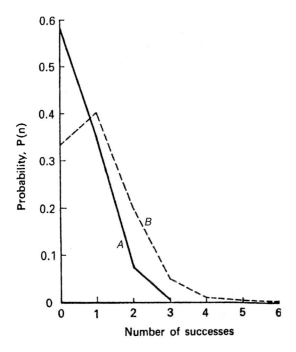

Figure 9-39. Probability of throwing 0, 1, 2, and 3 ones in three throws of a die, curve A; and the probability of throwing 0, 1, 2, 3, 4, 5, and 6 ones in six throws of a die, curve B.

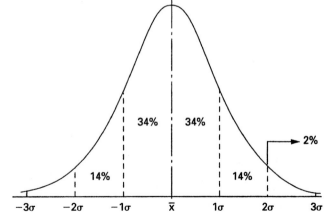

Figure 9-40. Normal curve, showing the percentage of the area between the mean and $\pm 1\sigma$, between 1 and 2σ, and beyond 2σ from the mean. Observed values are plotted along the abscissa (x-axis) and the frequency of these observations are plotted along the ordinate (y-axis).

0 ones in six throws, that is $(1/6 + 5/6)^6$, we would find the distribution given in Figure 9-39, curve B. By comparing curves A and B, we see that the latter curve is closer to symmetry. As *n* increases, the distribution curve becomes increasingly symmetrical around the centerline. For the case where *n* is infinite, we have the familiar bell-shaped *normal curve* (Fig. 9-40). For cases where $n \geq 30$, the binomial sampling distribution curve is, for practical purposes, indistinguishable from a normal curve.

The normal distribution is given by

$$p(n) = \frac{1}{\sigma\sqrt{2\pi}} e^{-(n-\bar{n})^2/2\sigma^2},$$ (9.33)

where

$p(n)$ = probability of finding exactly *n*,
$\bar{n}$ = mean value, and
σ = standard deviation.

Equation (9.33) shows that the normal distribution must be fitted by two parameters: the mean and the standard deviation. The mean is the central tendency, and the standard deviation is a measure of the spread of the data around the mean.

In the practical application of statistical reasoning, the area under the normal curve represents the total population under study. If we measure distances from the mean in units of standard deviations, then an important and useful property of the normal curve is that the fraction of the area under the curve that is contained between any two ordinates at any distance from the mean is fixed, regardless of the numerical values of the mean and the standard deviation. (These fractions are published in tables of areas under the normal curve, which may be found in science and engineering handbooks and in statistics books.) Thus, we find that 34% of the area lies between the mean and 1σ above or below the mean, and about 14% of the area is between 1σ and 2σ, and only about 2% of the total area lies beyond either $+2\sigma$ or -2σ from the mean. Since the curve is symmetrical about the mean, 68% of

TABLE 9-9. Confidence Intervals and Percent of Area Under Normal Curve

CONFIDENCE INTERVAL (%)	NO. OF STANDARD DEVIATIONS
50	0.6745
68	1
90	1.645
95	1.96
96	2
99	2.58

the area lies between $\pm 1\sigma$ and 96% of the area is included between $\pm 2\sigma$. Table 9-9 shows the percentage of the area included between the positive and negative values of several different numbers of standard deviations.

For the case where $p \ll 1$, that is, where the occurrence of an event is highly improbable, the binomial distribution approaches the *Poisson distribution*. Since radioactive decay of a particular atom is a highly unlikely event (in ^{32}P, for example, whose half-life is 14.3 days, the probability of decay of any atom is given by the decay constant as 5.6×10^{-7} s^{-1}), radioactive decay processes are described by Poisson statistics. According to the Poisson distribution, the probability of the occurrence of exactly n events per unit time, if the true average rate is $\bar{n}$, is given by the $(n+1)$ term of the expansion of

$$e^{-\bar{n}} \times e^{\bar{n}} = 1, \tag{9.34}$$

which gives, upon series expansion of $e^{\bar{n}}$:

$$e^{-\bar{n}} \left(1 + \frac{\bar{n}}{1!} + \frac{\bar{n}^2}{2!} + \frac{\bar{n}^3}{3!} + \cdots \right), \tag{9.35}$$

or by the general term for the Poisson distribution

$$p(n) = \frac{(\bar{n})^n \times e^{-\bar{n}}}{n!}. \tag{9.36}$$

For example, if we have 37 Bq (0.001 μCi) of activity, the mean number of transformations per second is 37. The probability of observing exactly 37 transformations in 1 second is calculated from Eq. (9.36) as

$$p(37) = \frac{37^{37} \times e^{-37}}{37!}.$$

Using Sterling's approximation

$$n! = \sqrt{2\pi n} \times \left(\frac{n}{e} \right)^n \tag{9.37}$$

to evaluate 37!, we find $p(37)$ to be equal to 0.066. It thus follows that a wide range of observations around the true mean of 37 would be made in a series of measurements of the 37-Bq source. The width of this range is given by the standard deviation of the distribution of measurements. As in the case of the normal distribution, in a large number of measurements, 68% of all the observations would lie between plus and minus one standard deviation of the mean, 96% between plus and minus two standard deviations, and so on. The normal distribution, given by Eq. (9.33), contains the standard deviation, σ, as one of the parameters. The Poisson distribution (Eq. [9.36]), contains only one parameter, the mean. The standard deviation of the Poisson distribution is equal to the square root of the mean number of observations made during a given measurement interval:

$$\sigma \text{ (Poisson)} = \sqrt{n}. \tag{9.38}$$

The "size" of the sample when we are counting events such as radioactive decay or other nuclear events is the arbitrary length of time over which we are making the measurement. In Eq. (9.38), n is equal to the total number of events that occurred during that time of observation and is thus the average rate for that time interval. Thus, if we observe 10,000 counts during a 10-minute counting interval, the standard deviation of the observation is $\sqrt{10,000} = 100$ counts per 10 minutes. The measurement represents a mean value of 10,000 counts for the 10-minute measurement interval. One of the main virtues of the Poisson distribution is that, for practical purposes, when $n \geq 20$, it is indistinguishable from a normal distribution of the same mean and of standard deviation equal to the square root of the mean. Under these conditions, all statistical tests that are based on a normal distribution, such as the t-test, the chi-square criterion, and the variance ratio test (which is called the F-test) may also be used for Poisson distributions. Although all these tests are applicable to radioactivity measurements, a full discussion of them is beyond the scope of this book. Details and applications of these tests may be found in the Suggested Readings at the end of this chapter.

In the example cited above, where 10,000 counts were recorded during 10 minutes of counting, the mean counting rate, in counts per minute, and the standard deviation of the mean rate is given by

$$r \pm \sigma_r = \frac{n}{t} \pm \frac{\sqrt{n}}{t}. \tag{9.39}$$

Since

$$\sigma_r = \frac{\sqrt{n}}{t} = \sqrt{\frac{n}{t} \times \frac{1}{t}} = \sqrt{r \times \frac{1}{t}},$$

we have

$$r \pm \sigma_r = r \pm \sqrt{\frac{r}{t}}, \tag{9.40}$$

which gives 1000 ± 10 cpm. If the activity had been measured over a 1-minute interval and had given 1000 counts, we would have $1000 \pm \sqrt{1000}$ or 1000 ± 32 cpm.

Precision is a gauge of the reproducibility of a measurement. Thus, we are more likely to observe 1000 cpm during a 10-minute counting time than during a 1-minute counting period. Numerically, precision is given by the *coefficient of variation*, CV, which is defined as the ratio of the standard deviation to the mean:

$$CV = \frac{\sigma}{\text{mean}}, \tag{9.41a}$$

and is often expressed as a percent:

$$\%CV = \frac{\sigma}{\text{mean}} \times 100. \tag{9.41b}$$

Thus, in the case illustrated above, where a mean count rate of 1000 cpm was determined by a 10-minute count and a 1-minute count, the precision of the 10-minute count was ±1% while that of the 1-minute count was ±3.2%.

Standard Deviation of a Sum or a Difference

The square of the standard deviation, σ^2, is called the *variance*. When two quantities, each of which has its own variance, are either added or subtracted, the variance of the sum or difference is equal to the sum of the variance of the two quantities:

$$(A \pm \sigma_A) \pm (B \pm \sigma_B) = (A \pm B) \pm \sigma_{A \pm B}, \tag{9.42}$$

$$\sigma^2_{A \pm B} = \sigma^2_A + \sigma^2_B, \tag{9.43}$$

$$\sigma_{A \pm B} = \sqrt{\sigma^2_A + \sigma^2_B}. \tag{9.44}$$

When making radioactivity measurements, we must usually account for background, and are thus interested in the net counting rate; that is, the difference between the gross counting rate of the sample, which includes background, and the background counting rate. Each of these counting rates has its own standard deviation. The standard deviation of the net counting rate is given as

$$\sigma_n = \sqrt{\sigma^2_g + \sigma^2_b} = \sqrt{\frac{r_g}{t_g} + \frac{r_b}{t_b}}, \tag{9.45}$$

where

σ_g = standard deviation of gross counting rate,
σ_b = standard deviation of background counting rate,
r_g = gross counting rate,
r_b = background counting rate,
t_g = time during which gross count was made, and
t_b = time during which background count was made.

 EXAMPLE 9.10

A 5-minute sample count gave 510 counts, while a 1-hour background measurement yielded 2400 counts. What is the net sample counting rate and the standard deviation of the net counting rate?

Solution

$$r_n = \frac{510 \text{ counts}}{5 \text{ min}} - \frac{2400 \text{ counts}}{60 \text{ min}} = 102 \text{ cpm} - 40 \text{ cpm} = 62 \text{ cpm}$$

$$\sigma_n = \sqrt{\frac{102}{5} + \frac{40}{60}} = 4.6.$$

Therefore,

$$r_n = 62 \pm 4.6 \text{ cpm}.$$

Standard Deviation of a Product or a Quotient

In the case of a product or a quotient of two or more numbers, each with its own standard deviation,

$$\frac{(A \pm \sigma_A) \times / \div (B \pm \sigma_B)}{(C \pm \sigma_C) \times / \div (D \pm \sigma_{D)})} = Y \pm \sigma_Y, \tag{9.46}$$

the coefficient of variation of the answer is given by

$$\frac{\sigma_Y}{Y} = \sqrt{\left(\frac{\sigma_A}{A}\right)^2 + \left(\frac{\sigma_B}{B}\right)^2 + \left(\frac{\sigma_C}{C}\right)^2 + \left(\frac{\sigma_D}{D}\right)^2}. \tag{9.47}$$

 EXAMPLE 9.11

A counting standard whose transformation rate is given as $1000 \pm 30 \text{ min}^{-1}$ is used to determine the efficiency of a counting system. The measured count rate is $200 \pm 10 \text{ min}^{-1}$. What is the efficiency of the counting system and the precision of the measurement?

Solution

The efficiency is

$$\varepsilon = \frac{200 \text{ min}^{-1}}{1000 \text{ min}^{-1}} = 0.2, \text{ or } 20\%,$$

and the standard deviation of the efficiency, from Eq. (9.47), is calculated as

$$\sigma_\varepsilon = 0.2\sqrt{\left(\frac{30}{1000}\right)^2 + \left(\frac{10}{200}\right)^2} = 0.012 = 1.2\%.$$

The statistical error associated with a count ratemeter is a function of the meter's time constant (response time) and is given by

$$\sigma_{CRM} = \sqrt{\frac{\text{count rate}}{2 \times \text{time constant}}}. \tag{9.48}$$

Note that the count rate and the time constant in Eq. (9.48) must be in the same time units.

 ## EXAMPLE 9.12

A survey meter whose time constant is 15 seconds reads 400 cpm. What is the standard deviation of this measurement?

Solution

In this case, the time constant, 15 seconds, corresponds to 0.25 minutes. Therefore, from Eq. (9.48), we find

$$\sigma_{CRM} = \sqrt{\frac{400 \text{ cpm}}{2 \times 0.25 \text{ min.}}} = \pm 28 \text{ cpm.}$$

The standard deviation is a measure of the dispersion of randomly occurring events around a mean. It was pointed out above that if a large number of replicate measurements were made, 68% of the measurements would fall between $\pm 1\sigma$ of the mean. For this reason, we say that 1σ is the 68% confidence interval. Similarly, the 96% confidence interval is $\pm 2\sigma$. If we report data within the limits of 2σ, it means that we are 96% certain that the true value lies within the given interval. Several levels of confidence, together with their corresponding number of standard deviations, are given in Table 9-9. The numerical value of a confidence interval represents the percentage of the area under the normal curve that is included between the corresponding number of standard deviations.

 ## EXAMPLE 9.13

A preliminary measurement made during a short counting time suggested a gross counting rate of 55 cpm. The background counting rate, determined by a 1-hour measurement, is 25 cpm. How long should the sample be counted in order to be 96% certain that the measured net counting rate will be within 10% of the true counting rate?

Solution

The estimated net counting rate is 30 cpm; 10% of this is 3 cpm. Since we want to be at the 96% confidence level, this allowable error of ±3 cpm represents two standard deviations; one standard deviation therefore is 1.5 cpm. Using this value in Eq. (9.45) and substituting the other given values leads to

$$1.5 = \sqrt{\frac{55}{t_g} + \frac{25}{60}}$$

$$t_g = 30.1 \text{ min.}$$

Difference Between Means

In making counting measurements, we are almost always interested in the difference between two counting rates—as, for example, the difference between the sample counting rate and the background counting rate, or the difference between the net counting rates of two samples. If this difference is very great, then we know intuitively that there is a real difference between the two samples. However, if the difference is small, then, because of the fact that radioactive decay is a random process in which we know that 96% of the measurements will lie between the true mean and plus or minus two standard deviations, we cannot decide intuitively whether the observed difference is merely due to errors of random sampling, and that the two measurements are in fact two samples of the same population. To help in our decision, we make use of an objective statistical test based on the *null hypothesis*. The null hypothesis assumes that there is no difference between the two measurements. With this assumption, we calculate the probability that this difference is due to errors of random sampling, and that the two means are samples from the same population. Furthermore, we arbitrarily set a limit to this probability. If the calculated likelihood of randomly finding the measured difference is greater than this limit, then we say that there is no difference between the two counting rates and that the two samples come from the same population. If, on the other hand, the probability of finding the measured difference among samples of the same population is less than the calculated value, then we reject the null hypothesis and say that the difference between the two means is statistically significant; the samples are in fact different. The two arbitrary levels of significance most frequently used in statistical calculations are 1% and 5%. That means, if we choose the 1% level, that if the probability of randomly finding a difference between two samples of the same population as great as that observed in the two sample measurements is greater than 1 in 100, we accept the null hypothesis, and we say that there is no difference between the two samples. If the calculated probability is 1 in 100 or less, then we say that the difference is significant. The significance level is *purely arbitrary* and is set by the experimenter. The experimenter is not bound to the 1% or 5% level; he may, if he wishes, be more liberal and use 10% or any other significance level. However, if he uses a 10% level, he is more likely to accept an apparent difference, which in fact is not real, than he would if he used 5% or 1% criteria. In reading and interpreting experimental data, therefore, it is important to know the probability level that the experimenter used as a criterion for significance.

Determination of the significance of the difference between means is based on the fact that, in a normally distributed population, not only are means of population samples normally distributed about the true means of the population but differences between means are also normally distributed. If we should draw a very large number of duplicate samples from a population, compute the mean for each sample, then subtract the mean of the second sample M_2 from the mean of the first sample M_1 and plot the differences between the means, we will obtain a normal curve about a mean difference of zero. The standard deviation of this distribution of differences between means is called the *standard error of the difference between means.* To estimate the standard error of the difference between means from two samples, we use Eq. (9.45), which can be written in a more general form as

$$\sigma_{\text{diff}} = \sqrt{\sigma_{M_1}^2 + \sigma_{M_2}^2},$$ (9.49)

where σ_M^2 is the square of the standard error of the mean. In counting measurements, the standard error of the mean count rate is given in Eq. (9.40) as

$$\sigma_{\text{r}} = \sqrt{\frac{\text{rate}}{\text{time}}}.$$ (9.50)

The t-test is used to tell us by how many units of the standard error of the difference between means the difference between two measured means differs from zero:

$$t = \frac{|M_1 - M_2|}{\sigma_{\text{diff}}} = \frac{|M_1 - M_2|}{\sqrt{\left(\dfrac{\text{rate}}{\text{time}}\right)_1 + \left(\dfrac{\text{rate}}{\text{time}}\right)_2}}.$$ (9.51)

EXAMPLE 9.14

The background in two adjacent buildings was measured to determine whether the building materials affected the radiation background. In the first building, 1590 counts were recorded during a 30-minute counting time. A 30-minute background count in the second building gave a rate of 50 cpm. At the 95% confidence level, is there a difference between the background levels of the two buildings?

Solution

$$M_1 = \frac{1590 \text{ counts}}{30 \text{ min}} = 53 \text{ cpm}, \quad \text{time}_1 = 30 \text{ min}$$

$$M_2 = 50 \text{ cpm}, \qquad\qquad\qquad \text{time}_2 = 30 \text{ min}$$

$$t = \frac{53 - 50}{\sqrt{\dfrac{53}{30} + \dfrac{50}{30}}} = 1.62.$$

This result shows that the measured difference is 1.62 standard deviations from zero. From a table of areas under a normal curve, we find that 1.62 standard deviations includes 44.74% of the area on each side of the mean, or 89.48% of the area between ± 1.62 standard deviations. We interpret this result as saying that we would expect a difference this great 10 or 11 times out of 100 $(100.00 - 89.48 = 10.52)$ if the two samples came from the same population. Therefore, the difference between the two samples is not statistically significant. To be statistically significant at the 95% confidence level, the difference between the two means would have to be great enough to be observed only 5 times or less out of 100. When we are using the 95% confidence level, there is a 5% chance of incorrectly concluding that there is a difference between the two means when, in fact, the two means are members of the same population, and the observed difference is due to errors of random sampling.

Minimum Detectable Activity

The *minimum detectable activity* (MDA) is important in low-level counting, when the count rate of a sample is almost the same as the count rate of the background, Under these conditions, the background is measured with a blank—that is, with a sample holder, such as a planchet—and everything else that may be counted with the actual sample, except that there is no activity in the blank. The MDA is defined as the smallest quantity of radioactivity that could be distinguished from the blank under specified conditions. The MDA depends on the lower limit of detection and on the counting efficiency of a counting system.

In Example 9.14, we wanted to know whether the two means differed. In determining the MDA, we wish to know whether the sample activity, M_1, is greater than the blank activity, M_2, not merely different from M_2. To answer this question we use a "one-tailed" t test. In the one-tailed test, we resort to the cumulative area under the normal curve. To include 95% of the area under a normal curve, we have 50% from $-\infty$ to the mean, and from the mean to the next 45% of the area is 1.645σ. Therefore, to be significant at the 95% confidence level when the one-tailed test is appropriate, the difference between the means must be $\geq 1.645\sigma$.

To decide whether or not a given sample has activity in it, we arbitrarily choose some count rate greater than that of a zero-activity blank that must be exceeded by the sample. If this decision level L_C is chosen so that it will be exceeded only 5 times out of 100 by a zero-activity blank, then the net count rate of the sample must be greater than that of the blank by 1.645 standard deviations of the net count rate. This decision level considers only an alpha or type 1 error—that is, saying that there is activity in the sample when in fact there is none. Such an error is often called a *false positive*. The 95% confidence level means that we will be wrong, or have false positives 5 times out of 100. A beta, or type 2, error is one where we say that there is no activity when there really is activity. That is, a type 2 error is a *false negative*. It is possible to have a very large type 2 error even if the type 1 error is only 5%. Figure 9-41 illustrates the situation where the sample really contains radioactivity and its mean count rate is equal to the decision level of the background. In this case, the type 2 error can be 50%. The power of a statistical test, which is defined as

$$Power = 1 - \beta, \tag{9.52}$$

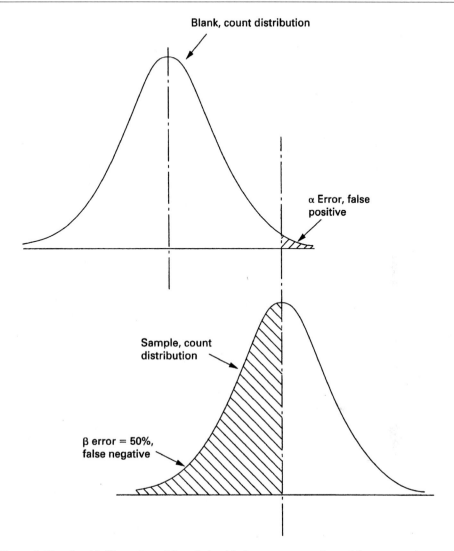

Figure 9-41. Graphic illustration of the relationship between a type 1, or alpha error, and a type 2, or beta error, in low-level counting.

is a measure of the probability of rejecting a false hypothesis when it really is false. Thus, in the case shown in Figure 9-41, although there is only a 5% chance of saying that there is activity when there really is none, there is a 50% chance of saying that there is no activity when there really is activity present in the sample. The power of the statistical test, in this case, is 50%.

The lower limit of detection (LLD) is based on consideration of both the alpha and beta errors (Fig. 9-42). For the case where the alpha and beta errors are both set at 5% and the sample and background counting times are equal, the LLD is given by

$$LLD = (4.66 \times \sigma_b) + 3. \tag{9.53}$$

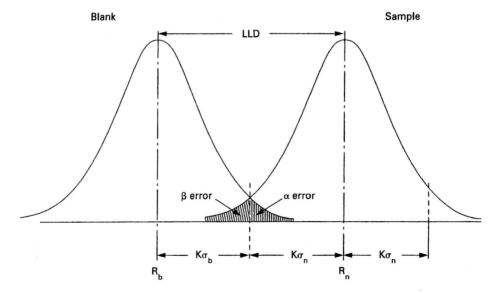

Figure 9-42. Graphic representation of the lower limit of detection based on consideration of both alpha and beta errors. For 95% alpha and beta errors, K = 1.645.

EXAMPLE 9.15

What is the LLD for a 30-minute sample count if a blank gives 45 counts in 30 minutes?

Solution

Substituting $\sqrt{45}$ for σ_b in Eq. (9.53) gives

$$LLD = 4.66 \times \sqrt{45} + 3 = 34.3 \text{ counts}$$

above background, or a gross 30-minute count of $45 + 34.3 = 79$ counts.

The MDA may be defined by the equation

$$MDA = \frac{4.66\sigma_b + 3}{K \times t}, \tag{9.54}$$

where

σ_b = standard deviation of the background;

K = a factor that includes the counter efficiency, the conversion factor for changing transformation rate into Bq if SI units are used, or into pCi if the traditional system of units is used, and chemical yield if chemical extraction is involved in preparation of the sample; and

t = sample counting time and background counting time.

EXAMPLE 9.16

What is the MDA for ^{137}Cs in a water sample when
sample size = 1 L,
sample counting time = 100 minutes,
blank = 169 counts in 100 minutes,
chemical yield = 75%, and
counting efficiency = 25%?

Solution

$$\mathrm{MDA} = \frac{\mathrm{LLD}}{\mathrm{Yield} \times \varepsilon \times 60 \dfrac{\mathrm{tpm}}{\mathrm{Bq}} \times \mathrm{volume} \times t}$$

$$\mathrm{MDA} = \frac{4.66\sqrt{169}+3}{0.75 \times 0.25 \dfrac{\mathrm{cpm}}{\mathrm{tpm}} \times 60 \dfrac{\mathrm{tpm}}{\mathrm{Bq}} \times 1\,\mathrm{L} \times 100\,\mathrm{min}}$$

$$\mathrm{MDA} = 5.65 \times 10^{-2}\ \frac{\mathrm{Bq}}{\mathrm{L}}\left(1.53\ \frac{\mathrm{pCi}}{\mathrm{L}}\right).$$

Equations (9.53) and (9.54) are valid only if the blank and the sample counting times are equal. For the case where this condition is not met, we must use the more general equations:

$$\mathrm{LLD} = 3.29\sqrt{r_b t_g \left(1 + \frac{t_g}{t_b}\right)} + 3 \tag{9.55}$$

$$\mathrm{MDA} = \frac{3.29\sqrt{r_b t_g \left(1 + \frac{t_g}{t_b}\right)} + 3}{K \times t}. \tag{9.56}$$

EXAMPLE 9.17

Strontium-90 is determined by precipitating the ^{90}Sr, then counting the ^{90}Y betas after a suitable ingrowth period. What is the MDA if

^{90}Y counting efficiency = 45%,
blank = 144 counts in 480 minutes,

sample counting time = 100 minutes,
Sr recovery = 80%, and
Y recovery = 96%?

Solution

Substituting the appropriate values into Eq. (9.56), we have

$$\text{MDA} = \frac{3.29\sqrt{\dfrac{144}{480} \times 100\left(1 + \dfrac{100}{480}\right)} + 3}{0.45 \times 0.8 \times 0.96 \times 100} = 0.66\frac{\text{transf}}{\text{min}} = 0.011 \text{ Bq.}$$

Optimization of Counting Time

Optimal use of a given period of time can be made by dividing the time between background counting time and sample counting time in order to minimize the statistical uncertainty of the net counting rate. The standard deviation of the net counting rate is given by Eq. (9.45) as

$$\sigma_n = \sqrt{\sigma_g^2 + \sigma_b^2} = \sqrt{\frac{r_g}{t_g} + \frac{r_b}{t_b}}.$$

Squaring Eq. (9.44) gives

$$\sigma_n^2 = \frac{r_g}{t_g} + \frac{r_b}{t_b}, \tag{9.57}$$

and differentiating Eq. (9.57) with respect to t yields

$$2\sigma_n d\sigma_n = -\frac{r_g}{t_g^2} dt_g - \frac{r_b}{t_b^2} dt_b. \tag{9.58}$$

To minimize t, set $d\sigma_n = 0$

$$0 = \frac{r_g}{t_g^2} dt_g + \frac{r_b}{t_b^2} dt_b, \tag{9.59}$$

which shows that

$$\frac{r_g}{t_g^2} dt_g = -\frac{r_b}{t_b^2} dt_b. \tag{9.60}$$

Since total counting time t is constant

$$t = t_g + t_b, \tag{9.61}$$

and therefore

$$dt_g + dt_b = 0. \tag{9.62}$$

Rearranging Eq. (9.60) and applying Eq. (9.62) yields

$$\frac{r_g/t_g^2}{-r_b/t_b^2} = \frac{dt_b}{dt_g} = \frac{dt_b}{-dt_b} = -1,$$

(9.63)

which leads to the optimum division of the total counting time between sample counting time and background counting time:

$$\frac{t_g}{t - t_g} = \sqrt{\frac{r_g}{r_b}}.$$

(9.64)

EXAMPLE 9.18

A total of 1 hour is available for counting a sample and the background. Preliminary measurements show the background to be about 15 cpm, and the sample count rate to be about 22 cpm. How long should the sample and the background be measured in order to minimize the statistical counting error?

Solution

From Eq. (9.64) we have

$$\frac{t_g}{t - t_g} = \sqrt{\frac{22}{15}}$$

$$t_g = 33 \text{ minutes}$$

$$t_b = 60 - t_g = 27 \text{ minutes}.$$

Weighted Means

Frequently, several different samples are taken from the same batch or universe, and then the value assigned to the universe is the arithmetic mean of the several samples. For example, the mean concentration of activity in a lake or a river is determined from a number of samples taken from the lake or river. This procedure is statistically valid only if all the measurements are made with the same degree of relative precision. If the precision of the measurements differs, we must weight the more-precise measurements more heavily than the less-precise measurements in order to arrive at the best estimate of the true mean. The procedure for weighting the means is illustrated by the following example:

EXAMPLE 9.19

Four samples were taken from a pond for activity determination, and the following counting rates were found, per liter of sample:

95 ± 3
105 ± 10
94 ± 6
118 ± 12.

Calculate the best estimate of weighted mean of the given data.

Solution

The mean and standard deviation of these data are 103 ± 11.2. The standard error of the mean, which is given by

$$\sigma_M = \frac{\sigma}{\sqrt{n-1}},$$ (9.65)

where σ = standard deviation of the distribution and n = number of samples, is found to be ±6.5, and, according to this calculation, the best estimate of the mean counting rate is 103 ± 6.5. However, it should be noted that the precision of the four analytical determinations vary widely, from 3.2% for the first value to 10.2% for the last one. In the calculation above, all the values were given equal consideration in arriving at the mean. Because of the wide variation in precision, the first value should be given greater weight than the last value. This weighting is done in the following manner:

Define a weighting factor

$$w_i = \frac{1}{\sigma_i^2}.$$ (9.66)

The weighted mean is then given by

$$M_w = \frac{\sum_i w_i M_i}{\sum_i w_i},$$ (9.67)

and the standard error of the weighted mean is given by

$$\sigma_{M_w} = \sqrt{\frac{1}{w_1 + w_2 + \cdots + w_n}}.$$ (9.68)

For the data in this example:

$M_i \pm \sigma_i$	σ_i^2	$w_i = 1/\sigma_i^2$	$w_i \times M_i$
95 ± 3	9	0.1111	10.56
105 ± 10	100	0.0100	1.05
94 ± 6	36	0.0278	2.61
118 ± 12	144	0.0070	0.82
		$\sum_i w_i = 0.1559$	$\sum_i w_i M_i = 15.04$

$$M_w = \frac{\sum_i w_i M_i}{\sum_i w_i} = \frac{15.04}{0.156} = 96.5$$

$$\sigma_{M_w} = \sqrt{\frac{1}{w_1 + w_2 + \cdots + w_n}} = \sqrt{\frac{1}{0.156}} = 2.54$$

The best estimate of the true mean, therefore, is 96.5 ± 2.5.

Reliability of a Counting System: Chi-Square

Because of the random nature of radioactive decay, it is highly unlikely that a number of successive counts of the same sample will be exactly the same. Thus, when we count a sample, we cannot be certain that the counting system is operating properly. However, if the counting system is operating properly, successive counts of the same sample will follow a Poisson distribution, and will be distributed around the true mean with a standard deviation whose value is a function of the true mean. To determine the reliability of a counting system, we apply a statistical test, called the *chi-square* test to a series of measurements on the same sample.

Chi-square is a measure of the significance of the difference between an observed distribution and an expected distribution. When applied to determining the statistical reliability of a counting system, it is defined by

$$\chi^2 = \frac{1}{\bar{X}} \sum_{i=1}^{N} (X_i - \bar{X})^{2,} \tag{9.69}$$

Where

X_i = the i th individual measurement,
$\bar{X}$ = mean of all the measurements, and
N = number of measurements.

The numerical value of chi-square depends on the number of measurements that are made. In statistical parlance, we say that the value of chi-square depends on the number of degrees of freedom, df. The df is defined as the number of values in the

TABLE 9-10. Chi-square Confidence Intervals

df	χ^2 (96%)	χ^2 (95%)	χ^2 (90%)	χ^2 (80%)
5	0.75–13.39	0.83–12.83	1.15–11.07	1.61–9.24
6	1.13–15.04	1.24–14.45	1.64–12.59	2.20–10.64
7	1.56–16.63	1.69–16.01	2.17–14.07	2.83–12.02
8	2.03–18.17	2.18–17.53	2.73–15.51	3.49–13.36
9	2.53–19.68	2.70–19.02	3.33–16.92	4.17–14.68
10	3.06–21.16	3.25–20.48	3.94–18.31	4.87–15.99
11	3.61–22.62	3.82–21.92	4.57–19.68	5.58–17.28
12	4.18–24.05	4.40–23.34	5.23–21.03	6.30–18.55
13	4.77–25.47	5.01–24.74	5.89–22.36	7.04–19.81
14	5.36–26.87	5.63–26.12	6.57–23.68	7.79–21.06
15	5.99–28.26	6.26–27.49	7.26–25.00	8.55–22.31
16	6.61–29.63	6.91–28.85	7.96–26.30	9.31–23.54
18	7.90–32.35	8.23–31.53	9.39–28.87	10.86–25.99
20	9.24–35.02	9.59–34.17	10.85–31.41	12.44–28.41

Source: Natrella MG. *Experimental Statistics.* Washington, DC: US Government Printing Office; 1963. NBS Handbook 91.

series of measurements that may be changed without changing the value of the sum. In this case, df $= N - 1$.

For perfect agreement, χ^2 (df) $= 0.5$. This means that there is a 50% chance that we would get a wider distribution of counts, and a 50% chance that we would get a narrower distribution of counts if we were to repeat the series of measurements. From the values of chi-square and df we can determine the probability that the observed departure of the observed distribution of measurements from the expected distribution is due to statistical errors of random sampling or whether the measured distribution differs significantly from the expected distribution, and, therefore, that the counting system is not operating properly. Although the confidence interval used in various laboratories for determining the significance of the chi-square value ranges from 96% to 80%, the counting system usually is considered to be satisfactory when the chi-square value is within the 95% confidence interval, i.e., $0.025 < \chi^2 < 0.975$. Chi-square values for 96%, 95%, and 80% confidence intervals for several different degrees of freedom are given below in Table 9-10.

EXAMPLE 9.20

The following data were obtained in seven replicate 1-minute counts on the same sample. Was the counter operating satisfactorily?

RUN	1	2	3	4	5	6	7	TOTAL
X_i	209	217	248	235	224	223	233	1589
$(X_i - \bar{X})^2$	324	100	441	64	9	16	36	990

Solution

$$\overline{X} = \frac{1589}{7} = 227$$

$$\sum (X_i - \overline{X})^2 = 990$$

$$\chi^2 = \frac{1}{\overline{X}} \sum_{i=1}^{N} (X_i - \overline{X})^2$$

$$\chi^2 = \frac{1}{227} \times 990 = 4.36.$$

Table 9-10 shows that a chi-square value of 4.36 for 6 degrees of freedom lies within the range of all the confidence intervals. The counting apparatus is therefore considered to be operating satisfactorily.

SUMMARY

Humans do not possess any sensory organs for radiation. They must rely solely on instruments to detect and measure radiation and therefore must always have an appropriate, functioning instrument whenever a radiation source is present or is thought to be present. Health physics instruments are designed for specific purposes, such as personnel monitoring or radiation field measurements and surveying. They are also designed to measure either particle flux or radiation dose. The response of an instrument depends on the detector type and wall thickness, type of radiation, and energy of the radiation. Health physics instruments must therefore be calibrated with standardized sources appropriate to the intended use of the instrument.

Radioactive transformation is a randomly occurring process; therefore statistical techniques must be used to distinguish low-level measurements from the omnipresent background and to distinguish between measurements that are relatively close together.

PROBLEMS

9.1. If a counting standard has a mean activity of 400 cpm, what is the probability of

(a) observing exactly 400 counts in 1 minute?

(b) measuring 390–410 counts in 1 minute?

9.2. A sample count was 560 in 10 minutes, while the background count was 390 in 15 minutes.

   (a) What is the standard deviation of the gross and background counting rates?

   (b) What is the standard deviation of the net counting rate?

   (c) What are the 90% and 99% confidence limits for the net counting rate?

9.3. A 10-minute sample count yielded 1000 counts. A 10-minute background measurement gave 250 counts. Assuming negligible radioactive decay of the sample during the counting period, what is the sample's net count rate and its 95% confidence interval?

9.4. A 10-minute sample count was 756, and a 40-minute background count was 600 counts.

   (a) What is the net count rate and its standard deviation?

   (b) What is the precision of the measurement expressed as percent error?

9.5. A background counting rate of 30 cpm was determined by a 60-minute count. A sample that was counted for 5 minutes gave a gross count of 170.

   (a) At the 90% confidence level, is there activity in the sample?

   (b) Is there activity in the sample at the 95% confidence level?

9.6. As a test of the operation of a certain counter, two measurements were made on the same long-lived sample. The first gave 10,210 counts in 10 minutes and the second gave 4995 counts in 5 minutes. Is the counter operating satisfactorily?

9.7. A 1-minute count shows a gross activity of 35 counts. If the background is 1560 counts in 60 minutes, how long must the sample be counted in order to be within ±10% of the true mean activity at the 95% confidence level?

9.8. A sample that had been counted for 15 minutes showed a mean counting rate of 32 cpm. The background, counted for 10 minutes, was 15 cpm.

   (a) What is the net counting rate, at the 95% confidence limit?

   (b) What is the coefficient of variation (relative error at ±1 standard deviation) of the net counting rate?

9.9. A sample has an estimated gross counting rate of 35 cpm (based on a 2-minute count). The background, determined by a 1-hour count, is 10 cpm. How long should the sample be counted if we want to be 95% certain that the net counting rate is within ±5% of the true mean net counting rate?

9.10. (a) The gross 1-minute count on a sample was 100, and a 1-minute background count gave 50 counts. What was the net counting rate and the 90% confidence interval?

   (b) If the sample and background were each counted for 10 minutes and gave counting rates of 100 and 50 cpm respectively, what was the net counting rate and the 95% confidence interval?

9.11. A shielded low-background counter has an average counting rate of 2 cpm. What is the probability that a 1-minute counting period will record

   (a) 2 counts?

   (b) 4 counts?

   (c) 0 counts?

9.12. A sample of river water was taken near the waste-discharge pipe of an isotope laboratory, and another sample was taken upstream of the discharge point. Each sample was counted for 10 minutes and gave 225 and 210 cpm, respectively. At the 99% confidence level, is the downstream water more radioactive than the water upstream?

9.13. A certain counting standard has a true mean counting rate of 50 cpm.

(a) What is the probability of observing exactly 50 counts in one minute?

(b) What is the probability of measuring 43–57 cpm?

(c) What is the probability of finding more than 57 counts in one minute?

9.14. A counting system has a background of 360 counts during a 20-minute counting period. What is the lower limit of detection with this system for counting times of

(a) 2 minutes

(b) 20 minutes

(c) 200 minutes

9.15. To determine possible low-level contamination, smears are counted for 10 minutes at an overall counting efficiency of 10%. The smear is considered positive if its activity exceeds the minimum detectable activity. If the blank gives 400 counts in 10 minutes, what is the minimum detectable activity for this counting system?

9.16. A blank in an alpha counter records 28 counts in 2 hours. Calculate the lower limit of detection for 1-hour and 2-hour sample counts.

9.17. A counting standard was counted for 5 minutes before an experiment and gave a mean count rate of 5965 cpm. After the experiment was over, the standard was counted again and gave 6070 cpm during a 2-minute check. Was the counting system operating as expected?

9.18. An unsealed air-wall ionization chamber whose volume is 275 cm^3 is calibrated at an atmospheric pressure of 760 torr and a temperature of 20°C. A measurement is made at an altitude of 7000 ft (2120 m), where the pressure is 589 torr and the temperature is 25°C. The meter reading was 10 mR/h (0.088 mGy air kerma, 2.58 μC/kg/h). What is the corrected exposure rate?

9.19. A 0.0025-μCi (92.5-Bq) ^{14}C source is placed into an air-filled current ionization chamber whose detection efficiency is 40%. The ionization current produces a 10-mV drop when it flows through a 10^{12}-ohm load resistor. What is the mean energy of the ^{14}C beta particles?

9.20. A survey meter whose time constant is 6 seconds is used to measure the scattered radiation from an X-ray machine. After a 0.2-second exposure time, the meter read 10 mR (2.58 μC/kg, 0.088 mGy air kerma)/h. What was the actual exposure rate?

9.21. What is the gamma threshold energy for a Cerenkov counter whose index of refraction is 1.6?

9.22. An ionization chamber has a window thickness of 2 mg/cm^2. If a 0.01-μCi (370-Bq) ^{210}Po source is located 1 cm in front of the window so that the counting geometry is 25%, calculate the saturation ionization current.

9.23. An air-wall air-filled ionization chamber whose volume is 100 cm^3 gives a saturation current of 10^{-12} A when placed in an X-ray field. If the temperature was 27°C and the atmospheric pressure was 740 mm Hg, what was the radiation exposure rate?

9.24. **(a)** A resistor of what value, to be placed in series with the ion chamber (Problem 9.23), is required to generate a voltage drop of 10 mV?

(b) If the capacitance of the chamber is 250 pF, what is the time constant of detector circuit?

(c) How much time is required before the meter will read 99% of the saturation current?

9.25. A pocket dosimeter has a capacitance of 5 pF and a sensitive volume of 1.5 cm^3. What is the charging voltage if it is to be used in the range 0–200 mR (0–51.5 μC/kg, 0–1.75 mGy air kerma) and if the voltage across the dosimeter should be one-half the charging voltage when the dosimeter reads 200 mR (1.75 mGy air kerma)?

9.26. A Geiger-Müller tube has a capacitance of 25 pF. The time required to collect all the positive ions is 221×10^{-6} seconds. In order to produce sharp output pulses, it is desired to limit the time constant of the detector circuit to 50 μs.

(a) What is the value of the series resistor?

(b) If 10^8 ion pairs are formed per Geiger pulse, what is the upper limit of the output voltage pulse?

9.27. A GM counter has a resolving time of 250 μs. What fraction of the counts is lost due to the counter's dead time if the observed counting rate is 30,000 cpm?

9.28. The fact that the gas multiplication in a proportional counter is very much less than that in a Geiger counter means that a pulse amplifier for use with a proportional counter must have a lower input sensitivity than one used with a Geiger counter. Calculate the input sensitivity for an amplifier to be used with a 2-in. diameter, hemispherical, windowless gas-flow proportional counter whose capacitance is 20 pF and which is operated to give a gas amplification of 5×10^3. Assume that the output pulse is "clipped" to one-half its maximum height.

9.29. What is the sensitivity of a thermal neutron detector whose volume is 50 cm^3 and which is filled with 96% enriched ^{10}BF$_3$ to a total pressure of 70 cm Hg at a temperature of 20°C?

9.30. If the BF$_3$ tube of Problem 9.29 is used as a current ionization chamber, what saturation current would result from a thermal flux of 10^9 neutrons/cm^2/s?

9.31. How long would it take for the sensitivity of the BF$_3$ detector of Problem 9.30 to decrease by 10%?

9.32. What is the sensitivity for 1-MeV and for 10-MeV neutrons (amps per neutron per cm^2/s) of an ion chamber that is filled with CH$_4$ gas to a pressure of 760 mm Hg, if its volume is 500 cm^3?

9.33. A 1000-MBq (27-mCi) ^{60}Co source is lost. At what distance can the lost source be detected with a survey meter whose sensitivity is 0.05 mR/h (0.013 μC/kg/h) above background?

9.34. The thermal-neutron flux from a moderated ^{252}Cf neutron-calibration source is determined by irradiating a gold foil of dimensions 1 cm (diameter) × 0.013 cm (thickness) for a period of 7 days at a distance of 100 cm from the source. The foil was counted immediately after the end of the irradiation period and found to have an activity of 100 Bq (2.7 nCi). What was the thermal flux at the point where the foil was irradiated? The activation cross section for gold is 98.5 b.

9.35. A thermal-neutron counter with dimensions 1 cm (diameter) × 10 cm (length) is filled with BF_3 gas at atmospheric pressure and 20°C. What is the counting rate when the counter is in a thermal-neutron flux ($E_{mp} = 0.025$ eV) of 1000 neutrons/cm^2/s?

9.36. If an irradiated TLD chip is kept at room temperature, the probability that a trapped electron will spontaneously drop to the ground state is 2×10^{-9} s^{-1}. If the TLDs are read at the end of the month, 30 days after distribution, and if an exposure occurred on the day of receipt of the dosimeter, what percent of the original dose information would be lost?

9.37. A thin-walled air ionization chamber whose volume is 0.5 cm^3 collects a charge of 1.65×10^{-9} C when placed into a plastic phantom whose relative mass stopping power is 1.1. When manufactured, the ionization chamber was sealed when the temperature was 25°C and the atmospheric pressure was 770 mm Hg. What was the absorbed dose, in Gy and in rads, at the point of measurement?

9.38. Twelve 1-minute counts on a check source gave the following results:

530   480   520   430   470   450   440   530   540   510   490   500

Using the chi-square criterion at the 96% confidence level, determine whether the counter was operating properly.

9.39. A count-rate frisker whose time constant is 5 seconds reads 500 cpm. What is the 95% confidence interval for this measurement?

9.40. From the following results, which were obtained in a tracer study of the efficiency of a solvent-extraction process, calculate the solvent-extraction efficiency and the 95% confidence interval:

SAMPLE	cpm	COUNTING TIME (min)
Mixture	200	5
Extract	180	5
Background	20	60

9.41. How many total counts are required if we want a 1% counting error at the 95% confidence level?

9.42. A background count of 600 was recorded during a 30-minute counting time. How long should a sample be counted in order to have a 5% precision for the net counting rate, if the gross count rate is about 2000 cpm?

9.43. The radiation background on a 10,000 ft. (3048 m) high mountain is measured with a 1-L capacitor-type air-wall ionization chamber whose capacitance is 50 pF. The chamber was hermetically sealed, at a temperature of 27°C and a pressure of 750 mm Hg. It was charged to 150 V, and was exposed for 30 days. After exposure, the voltage across the chamber had decreased to 100 V. What was the radiation exposure, in mR, over the 30-day period?

9.44. What is the 90% confidence interval of a ratemeter reading of 600 cpm if the meter's time constant is 10 seconds?

9.45. The manufacturer's specifications says that an ion chamber survey meter reaches 90% of its final reading in 4 seconds. Calculate the

(a) time constant, RC, of the meter circuit.

(b) exposure rate if the meter reads 10 mR/h after a 0.2-second X-ray exposure.

SUGGESTED READINGS

Adams, F., and Dams, R. *Applied Gamma-Ray Spectrometry*, 2nd ed. Pergamon Press, Oxford, U.K., 1970.

Attix, F. H. *Introduction to Radiological Physics and Radiation Dosimetry*. Wiley, New York, 1986.

Attix, F. H., Roesch, W. C., and Tochilin, W. C. E., eds. *Radiation Dosimetry, Vol. II. Instrumentation*. Academic Press, New York, 1966.

Birks, J. B. *The Theory and Practice of Scintillation Counting*. Pergamon Press. Oxford, U.K., 1970.

Brodsky, A. Statistical Methods of Data Analysis, in Brodsky, A., ed. *Handbook of Radiation Protection and Measurement, Sec. A, Vol. II. Biological and Mathemetical Information*. CRC Press, Boca Raton, FL, 1982.

Cameron, J. R., Suntharalingham, N., and Kenney, G. N. *Thermoluminescent Dosimetry*. University of Wisconsin Press, Madison, WI, 1968.

Cerenkov, P. A., Frank, I. M., and Tamm, I. E. *Nobel Lectures in Physics*. Elsevier, New York, 1964.

Currie, L. A. Limits for qualitative detection and quantitative determination. *Anal Chem*, **40**:586–593, 1968.

Cross, W. G., Ing, H., Freedman, N. O., Mainville, J. *Tables of Beta Dose Distributions in Water, Air, and Other Media*. Report AECL 7617. Atomic Energy of Canada, Ltd, Chalk River, Ontario, Canada, 1982.

Debertin, K., Helmer, R.G. *Gamma Ray Spectrometry with Semiconductor Detectors*. North Holland Publishing, Amsterdam, 1988.

d'Errico, F. Radiation dosimetry and spectrometry with superheated emulsions. *Nucl Instrum Methods Phys Res, Sec. B*, **184**:229–254, 2001.

d'Errico, F. Status of radiation detection with superheated emulsions, *Radiat Prot Dosimetry*, **120**:475–479, 2006.

Eicholz, C. G., and Posten, J. W. *Principles of Nuclear Radiation Detection*. Ann Arbor Science, Ann Arbor, MI, 1979.

Frame. P.W. A history of radiation detection instrumentation. *Health Phys*, **87**:111–138, 2004.

Gilmore, G., and Hemingway, J. D. *Practical Gamma Ray Spectrometry*. Wiley, New York, 1995.

Golnick, D. A. *Experimental Radiological Health Physics*. Pergamon Press, Oxford, U.K., 1978.

Greening, J. R. *Fundamentals of Radiation Dosimetry*, 2nd ed. Adam Hilger, Ltd., Bristol, U.K., 1985.

Hine, G. J., and Brownell, G. L. *Radiation Dosimetry*. Academic Press, New York, 1956.

International Commission on Radiation Units and Measurements (ICRU), Bethesda, MD. ICRU Publication No.

10b. *Physical Aspects of Irradiation*, 1964.

10f. *Methods of Evaluating Radiological Equipment and Materials*, 1963.

12. *Certification of Standardized Radioactive Sources*, 1968.

20. *Radiation Protection Instrumentation and Its Application*, 1971.

22. *Measurement of Low-Level Radioactivity*, 1972.

26. *Neutron Dosimetry for Biology and Medicine*, 1977.

27. *An International Neutron Dosimetry Intercomparison*, 1978.

28. *Basic Aspects of High Energy Particle Interactions and Radiation Dosimetry*, 1978.

31. *Average Energy Required to Produce an Ion Pair*, 1979.

34. *The Dosimetry of Pulsed Radiation*, 1984.

35. *Radiation Dosimetry: Electron Beams with Energies Between 1 and 50 MeV*, 1984.

36. *Microdosimetry*, 1983.

37. *Stopping Powers for Electrons and Positrons*, 1984.

39. *Determination of Dose Equivalents Resulting from External Radiation Sources*, 1985.

40. *The Quality Factor in Radiation Protection*, 1986.

43. *Determination of Dose Equivalents from External Radiation Sources—Part 2*, 1988.

44. *Tissue Substitutes in Radiation Dosimetry and Measurement*, 1989.

45. *Clinical Neutron Dosimetry—Part 1: Determination of Absorbed Dose in a Patient Treated by External Beams of Fast Neutrons*, 1989.

46. *Photon, Electron, Proton, and Neutron Interaction Data for Body Tissues*, 1992.

46d. *Photon, Electron, Proton, and Neutron Interaction Data for Body Tissues, with Data Disk*, 1992.

47. *Measurement of Dose Equivalents from External Photon and Electron Radiations*, 1992.

50. *Prescribing, Recording, and Reporting Photon Beam Therapy*, 1993.

51. *Quantities and Units in Radiation Protection Dosimetry*, 1993.

52. *Particle Counting in Radioactivity Measurements*, 1994.

53. *Gamma-Ray Spectrometry in the Environment*, 1994.

55. *Secondary Electron Spectra from Charged Particle Interactions*, 1996.

56. *Dosimetry of External Beta Rays for Radiation Protection*, 1997.

57. *Conversion Coefficients for use in Radiological Protection against External Radiation*, 1998.

59. *Clinical Proton Dosimetry, Part I, Beam Production, Beam Delivery, and Measurement of Absorbed Dose*, 1998.

60. *Fundamental Quantities and Units for Ionizing Radiation*, 1998.

62. *Prescribing, Recording, and Reporting Photon Beam Therapy (Supplement to ICRU Report 60)*, 1999.

63. *Nuclear Data for Neutron and Proton Radiotherapy and for Radiation Protection*, 2000.

64. *Dosimetry of High Energy Photon Beams Based on Standards of Absorbed Dose in Water*, 2001.

66. Determination of operational dose equivalent quantities for neutrons. *Jour ICRU,* **1**(3), 2001.

71. Prescribing, recording, and reporting electron beam therapy. *Jour ICRU,* **4**(1), 2004.

72. Dosimetry of beta rays and low energy photons for brachytherapy with sealed sources. *Jour ICRU,* **4**(2), 2004.

Jelly, J. V. *Cerenkov Radiation and Its Applications*. Pergamon Press, London, 1958.

Kleinknecht, K. *Detectors for Particle Radiation*. Cambridge University Press, Cambridge, U.K., 1986.

Knoll, G. F. *Radiation Detection and Measurement*, 3rd ed. Wiley, New York, 2001.

Kocher, D. C. External dosimetry, in Till, J. E., and Meyer, H. R., eds. *Radiological Assessment*. NUREG/CR-3332, U.S. NRC, Washington, DC, 1983.

National Council on Radiation Protection and Measurements (NCRP), Bethesda, MD. (NCRP) Publication No.

23. *Measurement of Neutron Flux and Spectra*, 1960.

25. *Measurement of Absorbed Dose of Neutrons and of Mixtures of Neutrons and Gamma Rays*, 1961.

27. *Stopping Powers for Use with Cavity Chambers*, 1961.

47. *Tritium Measurement Technics*, 1976.

50. *Environmental Radiation Measurements*, 1976.

57. *Instrumentation and Monitoring Methods for Radiation Protection*, 1978.

58. *A Handbook of Radioactivity Measurements Procedures*, 2nd ed., 1985.

69. *Dosimetry of X-Ray and Gamma-Ray Beams for Radiation Therapy in the Energy Range 10keV to 50 MeV*, 1981.

72. *Radiation Protection and Measurement for Low-Voltage Neutron Generators*, 1983.

78. *Evaluation of Occupational and Environmental Exposures to Radon and Radon Daughters in the United States*, 1984.

106. *Limit for Exposure to Hot Particles on the Skin*, 1989.

112. *Calibration of Survey Instruments Used in Radiation Protection for the Assessment of Ionizing Radiation Fields and Radioactive Surface Contamination*, 1991.

122. *Use of Personal Monitors to Estimate Effective Dose to Workers for External Exposure to Low-LET radiation*, 1995.

127. *Operational Radiation Safety Program*, 1998.

144. *Radiation Protection for Particle Accelerator Facilities*, 2003.

Nir-El, Y. Minimum detectable activity in gamma-ray spectrometry—Statistical properties and limits of applicability. *Oper Radiat Saf,* **80**(No. 2): S22–S25, 2001.

Paic, G. *Ionizing Radiation: Protection and Dosimetry*. CRC Press, Boca Raton, FL, 1988.

Poston, J. W., Sr. External dosimetry and personnel monitoring. *Health Phys,* **88**:289–296, 2005.

Price, W. S. *Nuclear Radiation Detection*, 2nd ed. McGraw-Hill, New York, 1965.

Shapiro, J. *Radiation Protection*, 4th ed. Harvard University Press, Cambridge, U.K., 2002.

Sharpe, J. *Nuclear Radiation Detectors*. Methuen, London, 1964.

Siegbahn, K., ed. *Alpha, Beta, and Gamma Ray Spectroscopy, Vol. 1*. North Holland, Amsterdam, 1965.

Snell, A. H., ed. *Nuclear Instruments and Their Uses*. Wiley, New York, 1962.

Tait, W. H. *Radiation Detection*. Butterworths, London, 1980.

Whyte, G. N. *Radiation Dosimetry*. Wiley, New York, 1959.

EXTERNAL RADIATION SAFETY

BASIC PRINCIPLES

Radiation safety practice is a special aspect of the control of environmental health hazards by engineering means. In the industrial environment, the usual procedure is first to try to eliminate the hazard. An example of this is the successive replacement of benzene as a degreasing solvent—first by carbon tetrachloride and later by trichloroethylene. If elimination of the hazard is not feasible, an attempt is made to isolate the hazard. If neither of these techniques is practical, then the hazard can usually be controlled by isolating the worker. The exact manner of application of these general principles to radiation safety practice depends on the individual situation. Radiation safety practice is divided between two principal categories: the safe use of sources of external radiation and prevention of personal contamination resulting from inhaled, ingested, or tactilely transmitted radioactivity.

External radiation originates in X-ray machines and other devices specifically designed to produce radiation; in devices in which production of X-rays is a side effect, as in the case of the electron microscope; and in radioisotopes. If it is not feasible to do away with the radiation source, then exposure of personnel to external radiation must be controlled by concurrent application of one or more of the following three techniques:

1. Minimizing exposure time.
2. Maximizing distance from the radiation source.
3. Shielding the radiation source.

Time

Although many biological effects of radiation are dependent on dose rate, it may be assumed, for purposes of environmental control, that the reciprocity relationship,

$$\text{dose rate} \times \text{exposure time} = \text{total dose},$$

is valid. For total dose that falls within one or two orders of magnitude of the radiation protection guide value, we have no data, neither clinical nor experimental, to contradict this assumption. Thus, if work must be performed in a relatively high radiation field, such as the repair of a cyclotron made radioactive by the absorption of neutrons or manipulation of a radiographic source in a complex casting, then the restriction of exposure time—so that the product of dose rate and exposure time does not exceed the maximum allowable total dose—permits the work to be done in accordance with radiation safety criteria. For example, in the case of a radiographer who must make radiographs 5 days per week while working in a radiation field of 0.25 mSv/h (25 mrems/h), overexposure can be prevented by limiting his daily working time in the radiation field to 48 minutes. His total daily dose would then be only 0.2 mSv (20 mrems). If the volume of work requires a longer exposure, then either another radiographer must be used or the operation must be redesigned in order to decrease the intensity of the radiation field in which the radiographer must work.

Distance

Point Source

Intuitively, it is clear that radiation exposure decreases with increasing distance from a radiation source. When translated into quantitative terms, this fact becomes a powerful tool in radiation safety. We will consider three cases: a point source, a line source, and a surface source.

In the case of a point source, the variation of dose rate with distance is given simply by the inverse square law, Eq. (9.22). Cobalt-60, for example, which emits one photon of 1.17 MeV and one photon of 1.33 MeV per disintegration, has a source strength that is approximated by Eq. (6.17b):

$$\Gamma = 1.2 \times 10^{-7} \sum f_i \times E_i \frac{\text{Sv} \cdot \text{m}^2}{\text{MBq} \cdot \text{h}}.$$

$$= 1.2 \times 10^{-7} (1 \times 1.17 + 1 \times 1.33)$$

$$= 3 \times 10^{-7} \frac{\text{Sv} \cdot \text{m}^2}{\text{MBq} \cdot \text{h}} \left(1.3 \frac{\text{R} \cdot \text{m}^2}{\text{Ci} \cdot \text{h}} \right).$$

For a 3700-MBq (100-mCi) source, the exposure rate at a distance of 1 m is about 1.11×10^{-3} Sv/h (111 mrems/h). If a radiographer were to manipulate this source for 1 hour per day, his maximum dose rate should not exceed 0.2 mSv/h (20 mrems/h) in order to stay within the weekly maximum guide of 1 mSv (100 mrems). This restriction could be attained through the use of a remote handling device whose length, as calculated from the inverse square law, Eq. (9.22), is at least 2.5 m.

If the radiography is to be done at one end of the shop, which is set aside exclusively for this purpose, then either a barricade must be erected outside of which the dose rate does not exceed the maximum allowable weekly rate, or, if this is not possible because of space limitations, a shield must be erected. If the barricade is used, its distance from the source must be such that the dose rate will not exceed

$$\frac{1 \text{ mSv/wk}}{40 \text{ h/wk}} = 0.025 \text{ mSv/h (2.5 mrems/h)}.$$

By the inverse square law, this distance is found to be 2.3 m. Because of the inverse square effect, the dose rate increases rapidly as a person approaches a point source, and it decreases rapidly while the person moves away from the source. At any distance d from a point source of activity A and specific gamma-ray constant Γ, the dose-equivalent rate is given by

$$\dot{H} = \frac{\Gamma \times A}{d^2} \times w_{\mathrm{R}}. \tag{10.1}$$

The total dose to a person approaching a source during the time t is given by

$$H = \int_0^t \dot{H}\, \mathrm{d}t. \tag{10.2}$$

Equation (10.2) can be solved in terms of the velocity of approach v and the closest distance d_0 to which the source is approached. If we let

$$d = d_0 + v \times t, \tag{10.3}$$

then

$$\mathrm{d}d = v\, \mathrm{d}t, \tag{10.4a}$$

$$\mathrm{d}t = \frac{\mathrm{d}d}{v}. \tag{10.4b}$$

If we now substitute Eqs. (10.1) and (10.4b) into Eq. (10.2), we have

$$H = \int_{d_0}^{\infty} \frac{\Gamma \times A \times w_{\mathrm{R}}}{d^2} \times \frac{\mathrm{d}d}{v} = \frac{\Gamma \times A \times w_{\mathrm{R}}}{v} \int_{d_0}^{\infty} \frac{\mathrm{d}d}{d^2}. \tag{10.5}$$

Therefore,

$$H = \frac{\Gamma \times A \times w_{\mathrm{R}}}{v \times d_0}. \tag{10.6}$$

 EXAMPLE 10.1

A 10-Ci (3.7×10^5 MBq) ^{60}Co source failed to be retracted into its shield. The operator walks toward the source at a rate of 1 m/s, and, at a distance of 1 m from the source, he stops, looks at the exposed source for 15 s, realizes that the source is not in the shield, and leaves at a rate of 2 m/s. What is his dose commitment from this exposure?

Solution

His total dose includes the dose during approach to the source, viewing the source, and then leaving. The dose during the approach, from Eq. (10.6), is

$$H(\text{approach}) = \frac{\Gamma \times A \times w_R}{v \times d_0} = \frac{1.3 \, \dfrac{R \cdot m^2}{Ci \cdot h} \times 10 \, Ci \times 1 \, rem/R}{1 \, m \cdot s^{-1} \times 3600 \, s/h \times 1m} = 3.6 \times 10^{-3} \, rem.$$

$$H(\text{viewing}) = \frac{\Gamma \times A \times t \times w_R}{d_0^2} = \frac{1.3 \, \dfrac{R \cdot m^2}{Ci \cdot h} \times 10 \, Ci \times \dfrac{15 \, s}{3600 \, s/h} \times 1 \, rem/R}{(1m)^2}$$

$$= 54.2 \times 10^{-3} \, rem$$

$$H(\text{leaving}) = \frac{\Gamma \times A \times w_R}{v \times d_0} = \frac{1.3 \, \dfrac{R \cdot m^2}{Ci \cdot h} \times 10 \, Ci \times 1 \, rem/R}{2 \, m/s \times 3600 \, s/h \times 1m} = 1.8 \times 10^{-3} \, rem$$

$$\text{Dose commitment} = \sum H = 10^{-3}(3.6 + 54.2 + 1.8) = 60 \times 10^{-3} \, rem$$

$$= 60 \, mrems \, (600 \, \mu Sv).$$

Line Source

In the case of a line source of radiation, such as a pipe carrying contaminated liquid waste, the variation of dose rate with distance is somewhat more complex mathematically than in the case of the point source. If the linear concentration of activity in the line is C_l MBq or curies per unit length of a gamma emitter whose source strength is Γ, then the dose rate at point p (Fig. 10-1), at a distance h from the infinitesimal length dl is given by

$$d\dot{D}_p = \frac{\Gamma \times C_l \times dl}{l^2 + h^2}, \tag{10.7}$$

and for the dose rate due to the activity in the total length of pipe, we have

$$\dot{D}_p = \Gamma \times C_l \int_0^{l_1} \frac{dl}{l^2 + h^2} + \Gamma \times C_l \int_0^{l_2} \frac{dl}{l^2 + h^2}$$

$$\dot{D}_p = \frac{\Gamma \times C_l}{h} \left(\tan^{-1} \frac{l_1}{h} + \tan^{-1} \frac{l_2}{h} \right)$$

$$\dot{D}_p = \frac{\Gamma \times C_l \times \theta}{h}. \tag{10.8}$$

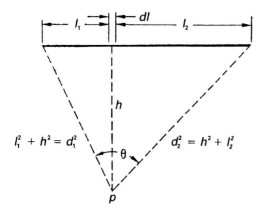

$$l_1^2 + h^2 = d_1^2$$

$$d_2^2 = h^2 + l_2^2$$

Figure 10-1. Geometry for computing gamma-ray dose rate at a finite distance h from a line source of uniform activity C_l per unit length.

EXAMPLE 10.2

Induced ^{24}Na activity in a cooling-water line passes through a small-diameter pipe in an access room 6-m wide. The door to the room is in the center of the 6-m wall, at a distance of 3 m from the pipe, as shown in Figure 10-2. If the linear concentration of activity is 100 MBq/m, what is the

(a) dose-equivalent rate $\dot{H}_1$ in the doorway at point D_1, at a distance of 3 m from the pipe?

(b) dose-equivalent rate $\dot{H}_2$ midway between the pipe and the door, point D_2, at a distance of 1.5 m from the pipe?

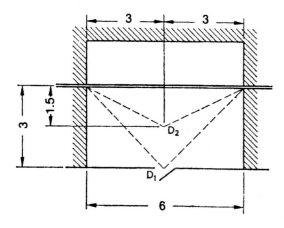

Figure 10-2. Layout of the room described in Example 10.2.

Solution

(a) For ^{24}Na, Γ (air kerma) $= 4.36 \times 10^{-7}$ Sv-m^2/MBq-h (from Table 6-3). The dose-equivalent rate at a distance of 3 m from the pipe is

$$\dot{H}_1 = \frac{2 \times \Gamma \times C_1}{h} \times \tan^{-1} \frac{l}{h}$$

$$= \frac{2 \times 4.36 \times 10^{-7} \, \dfrac{\text{Sv} \cdot \text{m}^2}{\text{MBq} \cdot \text{h}} \times 100 \text{ MBq/m}}{3 \text{ m}} \times \tan^{-1} \frac{3}{3}$$

$$= 2.3 \times 10^{-5} \text{ Sv/h} = 0.023 \text{ mSv/h} \quad (2.3 \text{ mrems/h}).$$

(b) The ratio of the two dose-equivalent rates $\dot{H}_1$ at a distance of 3 m and $\dot{H}_2$ at a distance of 1.5 m is

$$\frac{\dot{H}_1}{\dot{H}_2} = \frac{2\Gamma C_1 / h_1}{2\Gamma C_1 / h_2} \times \frac{\theta_1}{\theta_2}$$

$$\frac{\dot{H}_1}{\dot{H}_2} = \frac{h_2}{h_1} \times \frac{\theta_1}{\theta_2}. \tag{10.9}$$

In this example, $\theta_1 = 2 \tan^{-1} 3/3 = \pi/2$ radians, while $\theta_2 = 2 \tan^{-1} 3/1.5 = 0.7\pi$ radians. Substituting these values into Eq. (10.9) gives

$$\frac{0.023}{\dot{H}_2} = \frac{1.5}{3} \times \frac{\left(\dfrac{\pi}{2}\right)}{0.7\pi}$$

$$\dot{H}_2 = 0.064 \text{ mSv/h} \quad (6.4 \text{ mrems/h}).$$

Area (Plane) Source

Frequently the health physicist may find it necessary to know the quantitative relationship between dose rate and distance from a plane radiation source. If we have a thin source of radius r meters (Fig. 10-3) and a surface concentration C_a MBq/m^2 of a gamma emitter whose source strength is Γ Sv (air kerma) per hour per MBq at 1 m, then, the dose-equivalent rate at a point p, at a distance h along the central axis, is given by

$$\dot{H} = \int_0^r \frac{\Gamma \, \dfrac{\text{Sv} \cdot \text{m}^2}{\text{MBq} \cdot \text{h}} \times C_a \, \dfrac{\text{MBq}}{\text{m}^2} \times 2\pi r \, dr}{r^2 + h^2}$$

$$\dot{H} = \Gamma \times C_a \times \pi \times \ln \frac{r^2 + h^2}{h^2} \text{Sv/h}. \tag{10.10}$$

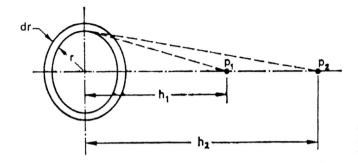

Figure 10-3. Geometry for calculating the variation of dose with distance from a plane source of radiation.

If activity is given in Ci/m^2 and Γ in $R\text{-}m^2/Ci\text{-}h$, and since an exposure of 1 R corresponds to a dose equivalent of 1 rem, the dose-equivalent rate in rems/h can be calculated with Eq. (10.10) by using the traditional units instead of the SI units.

$$\dot{H} = \Gamma \frac{rem \cdot m^2}{Ci \cdot h} \times C_a \frac{Ci}{m^2} \times \pi \times \ln \frac{r^2 + h^2}{h^2} \frac{rem}{h}. \tag{10.11}$$

The ratio of the dose-equivalent rate at a distance h to the dose-equivalent rate at any other distance is given by

$$\frac{\dot{H}_1}{\dot{H}_2} = \frac{\ln\left[\dfrac{(r^2 + h_1^2)}{h_1^2}\right]}{\ln\left[\dfrac{(r^2 + h_2^2)}{h_2^2}\right]}. \tag{10.12}$$

EXAMPLE 10.3

Fifty MBq of $^{24}NaCl$ solution spilled over a circular area 50 cm in diameter. What is the gamma-ray dose-equivalent rate at a height of

(a) 30 cm?

(b) 1 m?

Solution

(a) From Table 6-3, we find the specific gamma-ray emission constant for ^{24}Na to be 4.36×10^{-7} Sv-m^2/MBq-h. The areal concentration $C_a = 50$ MBq/π $(0.25\ m)^2 = 254.65$ MBq/m^2. Substituting the respective values into

Eq. (10.10) yields

$$\dot{H} = 4.36 \times 10^{-7} \frac{\text{Sv} \cdot \text{m}^2}{\text{MBq} \cdot \text{h}} \times 254.65 \frac{\text{Bq}}{\text{m}^2} \times \pi \times \ln\frac{0.25^2 + 0.3^2}{0.3^2}$$

$$\dot{H} = 1.84 \times 10^{-4} \text{ Sv/h}$$

$$= 0.184 \text{ mSv/h} \quad (18.4 \text{ mrems/h}).$$

(b) By substituting the appropriate values into Eq. (10.12), we find

$$\frac{0.184}{\dot{H}_2} = \frac{\ln\left(\dfrac{0.25^2 + 0.3^2}{0.3^2}\right)}{\ln\left(\dfrac{0.25^2 + 1^2}{1^2}\right)}$$

$$\dot{H}_2 = 0.021 \text{ mSv/h} \quad (2.1 \text{ mrems/h}).$$

Volume Source

In an infinitely large volume containing a uniformly distributed radioisotope, the energy emitted per unit volume is equal to the energy absorbed per unit volume. For example, consider the case of a 30-gallon metal drum, 50 cm in diameter and 79 cm high, containing aqueous ^{137}Cs waste at a concentration of 0.1 μCi/cm^3 (3700 MBq/m^3). Cesium-137 emits a 0.661-MeV gamma in 85% of its transformations. Since the attenuation coefficient for 0.661-MeV gammas in water is about 0.089 cm^{-1}, an assumption of an infinite volume is reasonable. The estimated gamma-ray dose rate in the center of the drum is given by

$$\dot{H} = \frac{C \dfrac{\mu\text{Ci}}{\text{cm}^3} \times 3.7 \times 10^4 \dfrac{\text{transf/s}}{\mu\text{Ci}} \times \bar{E} \dfrac{\text{MeV}}{\text{transf}} \times 1.6 \times 10^{-6} \dfrac{\text{erg}}{\text{MeV}} \times 3.6 \times 10^3 \dfrac{\text{s}}{\text{h}}}{\rho \dfrac{\text{g}}{\text{cm}^3} \times 100 \dfrac{\text{ergs/g}}{\text{rad}}} \times 1\frac{\text{rem}}{\text{rad}}$$

$$\dot{H} = \frac{0.1 \dfrac{\mu\text{Ci}}{\text{cm}^3} \times 3.7 \times 10^4 \dfrac{\text{transf/s}}{\mu\text{Ci}} \times 0.85 \times 0.661 \dfrac{\text{MeV}}{\text{transf}} \times 1.6 \times 10^{-6} \dfrac{\text{erg}}{\text{MeV}} \times 3.6 \times 10^3 \dfrac{\text{s}}{\text{h}}}{1 \dfrac{\text{g}}{\text{cm}^3} \times 100 \dfrac{\text{ergs/g}}{\text{rad}}} \times 1 \frac{\text{rem}}{\text{rad}}$$

$$\dot{H} = 0.12 \frac{\text{rem}}{\text{h}} = 120 \frac{\text{mrems}}{\text{h}} \quad \left(1.2 \frac{\text{mSv}}{\text{h}}\right).$$

The dose rate at the surface is 1/2 that in the center of the infinite mass, since the surface is irradiated from one side only, that is, it experiences 2π radiation rather than 4π radiation when it is completely surrounded by radioactivity. The surface gamma-ray dose rate, therefore, is $0.5 \times 120 = 60$ mrems/h (0.6 mSv/h).

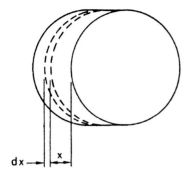

Figure 10-4. Conditions for setting up Eq. (10.13).

The radiation doses rate from a source that is substantially less than infinitely thick, containing a uniformly distributed gamma-emitting isotope, may be estimated from the effective surface activity after allowing for self-absorption within the slab. Consider a large slab of thickness t m (Fig. 10-4), containing C_v MBq/m^3 of uniformly distributed radioactivity. The linear absorption coefficient of the slab material is μ. The activity on the surface due to the radioactivity in the layer dx at a depth of x is

$$d(C_a) = C_v\, d x\, e^{-\mu x}. \tag{10.13}$$

Integrating Eq. (10.13) over the total thickness t yields the effective surface activity:

$$C_a = \int_0^t C_v e^{-\mu x}\, dx = \frac{C_v}{\mu}(1 - e^{-\mu t}). \tag{10.14}$$

Substituting Eq. (10.14) into Eq. (10.10) yields

$$\dot{H} = \pi \Gamma\, \frac{\text{Sv} \cdot \text{m}^2}{\text{MBq} \cdot \text{h}} \times \frac{C_v\, \text{MBq/m}^3}{\mu\, \text{m}^{-1}} (1 - e^{-\mu t}) \times \ln \frac{r^2 + h^2}{h^2}\, \frac{Sv}{h}. \tag{10.15}$$

In traditional units, where activity is in curies and Γ is in units of rems per Ci per hour at 1 m, Eq. (10.15) becomes

$$\dot{H} = \pi \Gamma\, \frac{\text{rem} \cdot \text{m}^2}{\text{Ci} \cdot \text{h}} \times \frac{C_v\, \text{Ci/m}^3}{\mu\, \text{m}^{-1}} \times (1 - e^{-\mu t}) \times \ln \frac{r^2 + h^2}{h^2}\, \frac{\text{rems}}{h}. \tag{10.16}$$

In the illustration above where the surface dose rate of the concrete in the 30-gallon drum was calculated as 60 mrems/h, let us calculate the dose rate on the central axis of the cylinder at a height of 30.5 cm (1 ft.) above the top using Eq. (10.16). The absorption coefficient for 0.661-MeV gammas in water is 0.032 cm^2/g, and the specific gamma-ray constant $\Gamma = 0.33$ R-m^2/Ci-h (7.82×10^{-8} Sv-m^2/MBq-h). Substituting the respective values into Eq. (10.16), we have

$$
\dot{H} = \pi \times 0.33 \, \frac{\mathrm{R \cdot m^2}}{\mathrm{Ci \cdot h}} \times \frac{0.1 \; \mathrm{Ci/m^3}}{3.2 \, \mathrm{m^{-1}}} \times \left(1 - e^{-3.2 \, \mathrm{m^{-1}} \times 0.79 \, \mathrm{m}}\right)
$$

$$
\times \ln \frac{(0.25 \, \mathrm{m})^2 + (0.305 \, \mathrm{m})^2}{(0.305 \, \mathrm{m})^2} \times 1 \, \frac{\mathrm{rem}}{\mathrm{R}}
$$

$$
\dot{H} = 1.5 \times 10^{-2} \; \mathrm{rem/h} = 15.3 \; \mathrm{mrem/h} \; (0.15 \; \mathrm{mSv/h}).
$$

Shielding

In Chapter 5, Eq. (5.27), we saw that, under conditions of good geometry, the attenuation of a beam of gamma radiation is given by

$$
I = I_0 \, e^{-\mu t}.
$$

However, under conditions of poor geometry, that is, for a *broad beam* or for a very thick shield, Eq. (5.27) underestimates the required shield thickness because it assumes that every photon that interacts with the shield will be removed from the beam and thus will not be available for counting by the detector. Under conditions of broad-beam geometry (Fig. 10-5), this assumption is not valid; a significant number of photons may be scattered by the shield into the detector, or photons that had been scattered out of the beam may be scattered back in after a second collision. This effect may be illustrated by Figure 10-6, which shows the broad-beam and narrow-beam attenuation of ^{60}Co gamma rays by concrete. According to Eq. (5.27), about 7 in. of concrete shielding is required to transmit 10% of the incident ^{60}Co radiation, under conditions of good geometry. For a broad beam, on the other hand (Fig. 10-6) shows that this thickness of concrete will transmit about 25% of the radiation incident on it. To transmit only 10% of a broad beam requires about 11 in. of concrete. In designing a shield against a broad beam of radiation, experimentally determined shielding data for the radiation in question should be used whenever they are available. (Broad-beam attenuation curves for radium, ^{60}Co, and ^{137}Cs for concrete, iron, and lead are given in Figures 10-6, 10-7, and 10-8). When such data are not available, a shield thickness for conditions of poor

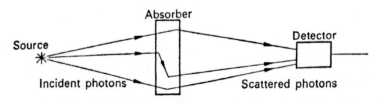

Figure 10-5. Gamma-ray absorption under conditions of *broad-beam* geometry, showing the effect of photons scattered into the detector.

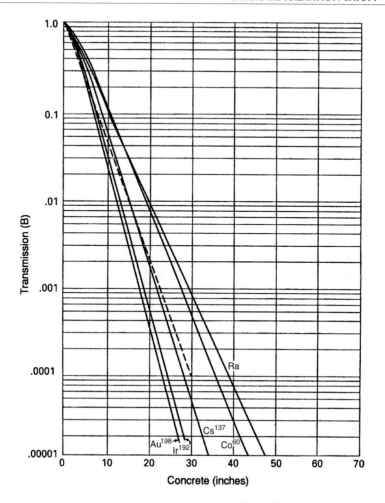

Figure 10-6. Fractional transmission of gamma rays from ^{137}Cs, ^{60}Co, and Ra (in equilibrium with its decay products) through concrete. The solid curves represent transmission of broad beams, and the broken line represents ^{60}Co gamma-ray attenuation under conditions of good geometry. (Reproduced from *Radiological Health Handbook*. Rev ed. Washington, DC: US Government Printing Office; 1970.)

geometry may be estimated by modification of Eq. (5.23) through the use of a *buildup factor B*:

$$I = B \times I_0\, e^{-\mu t}. \tag{10.17}$$

The buildup factor, which is always greater than 1, may be defined as the *ratio of the intensity of the radiation, including both the primary and scattered radiation, at any point in a beam, to the intensity of the primary radiation only at that point.* Buildup factor may apply either to radiation flux or to radiation dose. Buildup factors have been calculated for various gamma-ray energies and for various absorbers.[1] Some of these values are given in Figures 10-9 and 10-10. In these curves, the shield thickness is given

[1]H. Goldstein and J. E. Wilkins. *Calculation of the Penetration of Gamma Rays.* USAEC Report NYO-3075, 1954.

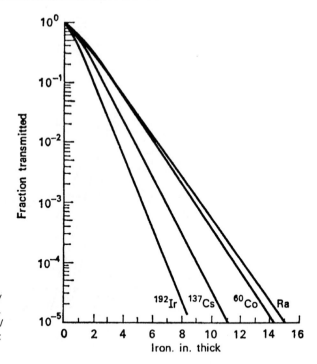

Figure 10-7. Broad-beam attenuation by iron of gamma-rays from ^{192}Ir, ^{137}Cs, ^{60}Co, and radium. (Reproduced from *Radiological Health Handbook.* Rev ed. Washington, DC: US Government Printing Office; 1970.)

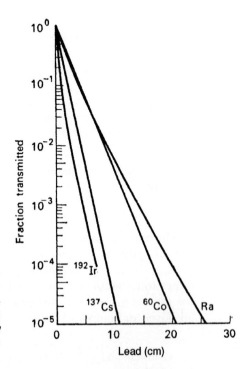

Figure 10-8. Broad-beam attenuation by lead of gamma-rays from ^{192}Ir, ^{137}Cs, ^{60}Co, and radium. (Reproduced from *Protection Against Radiations from Sealed Gamma Sources.* Washington, DC: National Bureau of Standards; 1960. NBS Handbook 73.)

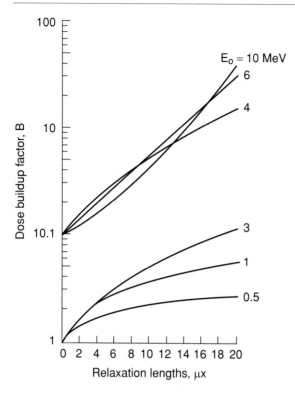

Figure 10-9. Dose buildup factor in lead for a point isotropic gamma-ray source of energy E_0. The 10 in 10.1 on the ordinate applies to the lower curves, while the 1 in 10.1 on the ordinate applies to the upper curves. (Reproduced from *Radiological Health Handbook*. Rev ed. Washington, DC: US Government Printing Office; 1970.)

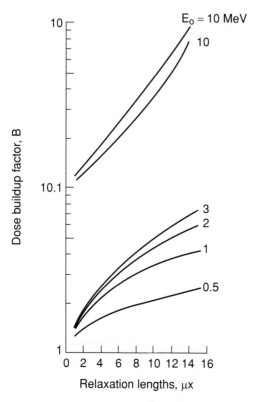

Figure 10-10. Dose buildup factor in lead for a plane monodirectional gamma-ray source of quantum energy E_0. The 10 in 10.1 on the ordinate applies to the lower curves, while the 1 in 10.1 on the ordinate applies to the upper curves. (Reproduced from *Radiological Health Handbook*. Rev ed. Washington, DC: US Government Printing Office; 1970.)

in units of *relaxation lengths*. One relaxation length is that thickness of shield that will attenuate a narrow beam to $1/e$ of its original intensity. One relaxation length, therefore, is numerically equal to the reciprocal of the absorption coefficient. The use of the buildup factor in the calculation of a shield thickness may be illustrated with the following examples:

EXAMPLE 10.4

A 3.7×10^4 MBq (1-Ci) source of ^{137}Cs is to be stored in a spherical lead container when not in use. How thick must the lead be if the air kerma rate at a distance of 1 m from the source is not to exceed 25 μSv/h (2.5 mrems/h)? Assume the source to be sufficiently small to be considered a "point."

Solution

In Table 6-3, we find the specific gamma-ray emission of ^{137}Cs to be 7.82×10^{-8} Sv/h/MBq at 1 m (0.33 R-m^2/Ci-h). The exposure rate at 1 m from the unshielded source, therefore, is

$$\dot{K} = \frac{3.7 \times 10^4 \text{ MBq} \times 7.82 \times 10^{-8} \dfrac{\text{Sv} \cdot \text{m}^2}{\text{MBq} \cdot \text{h}}}{1 \text{ m}^2} = 2.89 \times 10^{-3} \text{ Sv/h}.$$

If there were no buildup, the required thickness of lead would be calculated from Eq. (5.23), using the value for the attenuation coefficient for lead for 0.661-MeV gamma rays from Table 5-2, $\mu = 1.24$ cm^{-1}:

$$I = I_0 \times e^{-\mu t}$$

$$25 = 2890 \times e^{-1.24t}$$

$$t = 3.8 \text{ cm}.$$

This is an underestimate of the required shield thickness, since it does not include the additional thickness to account for buildup.

In Figures 10-9 and 10-10, we see that the buildup factor is a function of the shield thickness. Since the shield thickness is not yet known, Eq. (10.17) has two unknowns, the buildup factor B and the shield thickness t. To determine the proper shield thickness, we estimate a thickness, then substitute this estimated value into Eq. (10.17) to determine whether it will satisfy the dose-rate reduction requirement. The minimum shield thickness can be estimated by assuming narrow-beam attenuation and then increasing the thickness thus calculated by one half value layer (1 HVL) to account for buildup. The HVL of lead for 0.661-MeV gamma rays is

$$\text{HVL} = \frac{\ln 2}{\lambda} = \frac{0.693}{1.24 \text{ cm}^{-1}} = 0.56 \text{ cm}.$$

The estimated shield thickness therefore is 3.84 plus 0.56, or 4.40 cm, which corresponds to $1.24 \times 4.40 = 5.5$ relaxation lengths. From Figure 10-9, we find (by interpolation) the dose-buildup factor for 0.661-MeV gamma rays to be 2.12 for a lead shield of this thickness. Substituting these values for B and t into Eq. (10.17), we have

$$I = 2890 \times 2.12 \times e^{-1.24 \times 4.4}$$

$$= 26 \,\mu\text{Sv/h} \quad (2.6 \,\text{mrems/h}).$$

This calculated reduction in gamma-ray dose rate is just slightly more than the desired value of 2.5 mR/h. The thickness of 4.4, as calculated above, is therefore just about correct. In this example, we found the correct thickness after one attempt in a trial-and-error method. If the calculated reduction in radiation dose rate had not turned out to be so close to the design value with the estimated shield thickness, we would have continued, by trial and error, to estimate thicknesses until the one that results in the desired reduction of dose rate would have been obtained.

EXAMPLE 10.5

Design a spherical, lead storage container that will attenuate the exposure rate from 1 Ci of ^{24}Na to 10 mR/h at a distance of 1 m from the source.

Solution

In each disintegration of a ^{24}Na atom, two gamma rays are emitted in cascade: one of 2.75 MeV and one of 1.37 MeV. The dose rate, at a distance of 1 m, due to each of these photons is, from Eq. (6.18):

$$\Gamma_{2.75} = 0.5 \times 2.75 = 1.38 \,\frac{\text{R} \cdot \text{m}^2}{\text{C} \cdot \text{h}},$$

$$\Gamma_{1.37} = 0.5 \times 1.37 = 0.69 \,\frac{\text{R} \cdot \text{m}^2}{\text{C} \cdot \text{h}}.$$

To reduce the exposure rate from the high-energy photon to 10 mR/h for the condition of good geometry, we use the interpolated value of 0.485 cm^{-1} (Table 5-3) for the attenuation coefficient μ.

$$\frac{I}{I_0} = \frac{10}{1380} = e^{-0.485t}$$

$$t = 10.16 \,\text{cm}.$$

The HVL of lead for 2.75-MeV gammas is 1.43 cm. To account for the 1.37-MeV gamma, let us add one-half an HVL, or 0.72 cm, to the thickness calculated above for the 2.75-MeV gamma. We will then calculate the attenuation of the 2.75-MeV gamma with the new trial thickness, $10.16 + 0.72 = 10.88$ cm.

$$I = 1380 \times e^{-0.485 \times 10.88}$$

$$I = 7.1 \, \text{mR/h.}$$

With this thickness of lead, the 1.37-MeV gamma, whose attenuation coefficient is 0.629 cm^{-1} (Table 5-2) will be attenuated to

$$I = 690 \times e^{-0.629 \times 10.88}$$

$$I = 0.7 \, \text{mR/h,}$$

and the total exposure rate at a distance of 1 m will be the sum of the exposure rates due to the two quantum energies, or 7.8 mR/h.

The calculation above is based on good geometry. Let us now account for buildup in the shield. Considering at this time only the high-energy photon, let us add another half of one HVL to the shield thickness, which gives us 11.6 cm. Since one relaxation length of lead for 2.75-MeV gammas is 2.1 cm, the shield thickness corresponds to 5.5 relaxation lengths. From Figure 10-9, we find the buildup factor to be 3.1. The attenuation of the shield, therefore, according to Eq. (10.17), is

$$I = 1380 \times 3.1 \times e^{-0.485 \times 11.6}$$

$$I = 15.4 \, \text{mR/h.}$$

This exposure rate is too high; the shield thickness must therefore be increased. If we add another HVL to the shield to give us 13 cm, or 6.3 relaxation lengths, and using the corresponding dose buildup factor of 3.4, we find the exposure rate to be 8.5 mR/h for the high-energy photon. For the lower-energy photon, whose relaxation length in lead is 1.6 cm, this shield thickness corresponds to 8.2 relaxation lengths, and the dose buildup factor is 3.6. With these values in Eq. (10.17), the exposure rate due to the 1.37-MeV photons is calculated as 0.7 mR/h. The total exposure rate at a distance of 1 m from the shielded ^{24}Na source is thus 9.2 mR/h. Since this rate may be considered, for most practical purposes, to be equivalent to the design value of 10 mR/h, the required shield thickness is 13 cm. Since the shield may be interposed anywhere between the source and the point where the desired attenuated dose rate is located, and since the volume of lead, for a given wall thickness in a spherical shield, increases rapidly with increasing outer radius according to the expression

$$\text{Volume} = \frac{4}{3}\pi(r_0^3 - r_i^3),$$

the inner radius of the shield is kept as small as possible, consistent with the space requirements set by the physical dimensions of the source. The outside radius then is equal to the sum of the inside radius and the shield thickness.

X-Rays

In Chapter 6 we saw that the roentgen, which had been originally used as a dosimetric quantity, was really a measure of X-ray exposure rather than dose. However, the roentgen continued to be used as a dosimetric quantity because an exposure of 1 R, which deposited 87.8 ergs of energy to a gram of air, deposited 97 ergs of energy to a gram of soft tissue. Since an absorbed dose of 1 rad corresponds to absorption of 100 ergs/g, the absorbed dose from a 1-R exposure is approximately 1 rad. Furthermore, since the radiation weighting factor $w_R = 1$ for X-rays, a 1-rad X-ray dose = 1-rem dose equivalent. Thus, a 1-R exposure leads to an approximate dose equivalent of 1 rem, or, in SI units, to a dose equivalent of 1 cSv (or 10 mSv). However, the roentgen is now an obsolete unit. For X-ray protection purposes, the quantity *air kerma* is often used. This unit is especially useful to express exposure in SI units because exposure measured in air kerma is considered numerically equal to the dose equivalent measured in Sv.

Shielding for protection against X-rays is considered under two categories: source shielding and structural shielding. Source shielding is usually supplied by the manufacturer of the X-ray equipment in the form of a lead shield in which the X-ray tube is housed. The safety standards recommended by the National Council on Radiation Protection (NCRP) specify the following types of protective tube housings for medical X-ray installations (NCRP 102):

1. *Diagnostic type*: It is so built that the leakage-radiation air kerma at a distance of 1 m from the target cannot exceed 1 mGy (100 mrads) in 1 hour when the tube is operated at its maximum continuous rated current and high voltage.
2. *Therapeutic type*:
   a. For X-rays generated at voltages of 5 to 50 kV—The tube housing is built so that the maximum-leakage kerma rate at any point 5 cm from the tube housing does not exceed 1 mGy (100 mrads) in 1 hour when the tube is operated at its maximum rated beam current and high voltage.
   b. For X-rays generated at voltages greater than 50 kV but less than 500 kV—A tube housing built so that the leakage kerma rate at a distance of 1 m from the target does not exceed 1 cGy (1 rad) in 1 hour. Furthermore, the leakage kerma rate at a distance of 5 cm from the tube housing does not exceed 30 cGy/h (30 rads/h).
   c. For X-ray generated at peak voltages of 500 kV or more—A protective source housing built so that (i) the leakage-radiation rate in a region outside of the maximum-sized useful beam but within a 2-m radius circular plane centered on the beam's central axis at the normal treatment distance does not exceed 0.2% of the treated tissue dose rate and (ii) except for this region, the absorbed dose rate at 1 m from the electron path between the source and the target does not exceed 0.5% of the treatment dose rate on the central axis of the beam at the normal treatment distance.

For nonmedical X-rays, a protective tube housing is one that surrounds the X-ray tube itself, or the tube and other parts of the X-ray apparatus (for example, the transformer), and is so constructed that the leakage radiation at a distance of 1 m from the target cannot exceed 1 rem in 1 hour when the tube is operated at any of its specified ratings. Leakage radiation, as used in these specifications for tube housings, means all radiation, except the useful beam coming from the tube housing.

Structural shielding is designed to protect against the useful X-rays, leakage radiation, and scattered radiation. It encloses both the X-ray tube (with its protective tube housing) and the space in which the object being irradiated is located. Structural shielding may vary considerably in form. It may, for example, be either a lead-lined box in the case of an X-ray tube used by a radiobiologist to irradiate small organisms, or it may be the shielding around a room in which a patient is undergoing diagnostic procedures utilizing radiation sources or radiation therapy. In any case, structural shielding is designed to protect people in an occupied area outside an area of high radiation intensity. The structural shielding requirements for a given installation are determined by

1. the maximum kilovoltage at which the X-ray tube is operated,
2. the maximum milliamperes of beam current,
3. the workload (W), which is a measure, in suitable units, of the amount of use of an X-ray machine. For X-ray shielding design, workload is usually expressed in units of milliampere-minutes per week,
4. the use factor (U), which is the fraction of the workload during which the useful beam is pointed in the direction under consideration, and
5. the occupancy factor (T), which is the factor by which the workload should be adjusted to correct for the degree or type of occupancy of the area in question. When adequate occupancy data are not available, the values for T given in Table 10-1 may be used as a guide in planning shielding.

According to the International Commission on Radiological Protection (ICRP) Publication No. 26 (1977)—*General recommendations for protection of radiation workers*—and ICRP 57 (1989)—*Recommendations for protection of workers in medicine and dentistry*—the annual dose limit is 50 mSv (5000 mrems). In ICRP 60 (1990), the

TABLE 10-1. Suggested Occupancy Factors[a]

LOCATION	OCCUPANCY FACTOR (T)
Administrative or clerical offices; laboratories, pharmacies, and other work areas fully occupied by individuals; receptionist areas, attended waiting rooms, children's indoor play areas, adjacent X-ray rooms, film-reading areas, nurse's stations, and X-ray control rooms	1
Rooms used for patient examinations and treatments	1/2
Corridors, patient rooms, employee lounges, staff rest rooms	1/5
Corridor doors[b]	1/8
Public toilets, unattended vending areas, storage rooms, outdoor areas with seating, unattended waiting rooms, patient holding areas	1/20
Outdoor areas with only transient pedestrian or vehicular traffic, unattended parking lots, unattended vehicular drop off areas, attics, stairways, unattended elevators, janitor's closets	1/40

[a]When using a low occupancy factor for a room immediately adjacent to an X-ray room, care *should* be taken to also consider the areas further removed from the X-ray room. These areas may have significantly higher occupancy factors than the adjacent room and may therefore be more important in shielding design despite the larger distances involved.
[b]The occupancy factor for the area just outside a corridor door can often be reasonably assumed to be lower than the occupancy factor for the corridor.
Reproduced with permission of the National Council on Radiation Protection and Measurements from *Structural Shielding Design for Medical X-Ray Imaging Facilities.* Bethesda, MD: National Council on Radiation Protection & Measurement; 2004. NCRP Report 147.

recommended dose limit was changed to 100 mSv (10,000 mrems) over a 5-year period, with a maximum dose in any single year of 50 mSv (5000 mrems). The mean annual dose limit is thus 20 mSv (2000 mrems). These recommendations have been incorporated into the radiation safety regulations of many but not all countries. Since no harmful effects have been observed among workers whose dose was limited to 5000 mrems in one year, radiation safety regulations in the United States continue to be based on an annual occupational dose limit of 5000 mrems (50 mSv) and 100 mrems (1 mSv) in 1 year for the nonoccupationally exposed members of the public. At a uniform rate of exposure over 50 weeks, these maxima correspond to 100 mrems (1 mSv) per week for occupational exposure and to 2 mrems (0.02 mSv) per week for individuals who are not radiation workers.

NCRP 147 Methodology[2]

Recommendations for the design of structural shielding for medical radiation facilities that had been published in NCRP 49 have been updated. The new recommendations for shielding design for medical imaging facilities are found in NCRP 147, and, for therapeutic facilities, the revised recommendations are found in NCRP 151. For X-rays, the updated recommendations specify exposure in units of air kerma, K, rather than in roentgen units, and the minimum distance from a shielded wall to an occupied area is assumed to be 0.3 m. Additionally, the calculational methodology for imaging facilities is based on mathematical models derived from extensive measurements made during a survey made by the American Association of Physicists in Medicine (AAPM) at 14 different medical institutions involving about 2500 patients and 7 types of radiological installations. Shielding design recommendations are made for each of the different types of installations. These include:

- Radiographic installations. These are general-purpose installations that employ X-ray tubes operating at potentials of 50–150 kVp (kV peak). Radiographic installations do not have provisions for fluoroscopy. Three subcategories based on use and orientation of the X-ray tube are described:
  - ○ Rad room (all barriers), used only for secondary barriers,
  - ○ Rad room (chest bucky), and
  - ○ Rad room (floor and other barriers).
- The Rad room (all barriers) is composed of the sum of the other two Rad rooms. These two include beams directed at the floor, or any other directions.
- The walls at which the beam is directed form the primary barriers. For this reason, the Rad room (all barriers) data are used only for the design of secondary barriers.
- Fluoroscopy installations. Since fluoroscopic units also are used for radiographic imaging, two subcategories are considered:
  - ○ Fluoroscopy tube (R & F room). Fluoroscopy is usually done at X-ray potentials of 60–120 kVp. Since the fluoroscopic image receptor is designed

---

[2] This chapter is intended to provide an introduction to NCRP Report No. 147 on *Structural Shielding Design for Medical X-Ray Imaging Facilities*, which contains numerous worked examples and additional information not contained herein. It is recommended that the reader obtain a copy of Report No. 147 from NCRP at http://NCRP publications.org for a more complete treatment of shielding for medical x-ray imaging facilities.

as a primary barrier, all the walls are considered secondary barriers against scattered and leakage radiation.
  ○ Rad Tube (R & F room)
- Chest room, dedicated to chest X-rays only. The image receptor is located at a particular wall, which is the primary protective barrier. All other walls are secondary barriers.
- Mammography room. Mammography is performed at X-ray voltages of 25–35 kVp, and the image receptors of dedicated mammographic units are required to intercept the primary beam. Dedicated mammography installations, therefore, may not require any more shielding than that afforded by the structural materials of the walls of the room.
- Interventional imaging facilities. Two subcategories are considered:
  ○ cardiac angiography
  ○ peripheral angiography

Per patient workload values, which are exposure values for each of these applications that are weighted according to the distribution of operating high voltages for each procedure, are listed in the NCRP report in units of milliamperes-minutes per week (Table 10-2) and are incorporated into the recommended design methodology. The workload for a given facility is defined as the total number of milliamperes-minutes per week that the X-ray tube is in operation. The average workload per patient, which may include multiple exposures due to several different radiological modalities, is called the normalized workload, W_{norm}, and the total workload for a given installation is the product of the normalized workload and the weekly number of patients, N:

$$W = N \times W_{norm}.$$

To decrease the unshielded primary air kerma, $K_P(0)$, at a location at a distance d_P from the X-ray tube, requires a barrier that will transmit the following fraction of the unshielded incident radiation:

$$B_P = \left(\frac{P}{T}\right) \frac{d_P^2}{K_P^1 \times U \times N}, \tag{10.18}$$

TABLE 10-2. Mean per Patient kVp-Weighted Workload, W_{norm}, for Several Medical Imaging Installations

INSTALLATION	W_{norm} (mA-min wk^{-1})	K_P^1 (mGy/ PATIENT)	PATIENTS wk^{-1}
Rad room, all barriers	2.5		110 total for all
Rad room, chest bucky	0.6	2.3	Rad room uses
Rad room floor or other barriers	1.9	5.2	
R & F room, fluoroscopy	13		18
R & F room, radiography	1.5	5.9	23
Chest room	0.22	1.2	210
Mammography room	6.7		47
Cardiac angiography	160		19
Peripheral angiography	64		21

where

P = allowable air kerma rate, either 0.1 mGy/wk for a controlled area or 0.02 mGy/wk for an uncontrolled area,

T = occupancy factor (Table 10-1),

d_P = distance from X-ray tube to point of interest (usually 1 ft., or 0.3 m, from the barrier),

K_P^1 = unshielded primary air kerma per patient at a distance of 1 m,

U = use factor = fraction of the time that the primary beam is directed towards a given primary barrier, and

N = number of patients per week.

Using the kVp weighted values for the workload, and using three empirically determined parameters, mathematical models were fitted to the data obtained for each of the exposure modalities that had been investigated, and broad-beam transmission equations were determined for primary and secondary protective barriers. The thickness of the primary barrier is given by

$$x = \frac{1}{\alpha\gamma}\ln\left[\frac{\left(\dfrac{NTUK_P^1}{Pd_P^2}\right)^\gamma + \dfrac{\beta}{\alpha}}{1 + \dfrac{\beta}{\alpha}}\right],\qquad (10.19)$$

where α, β, and γ are parameters that depend on the barrier material and on the operating potential of the X-ray tube, which is implicit in the imaging modality. NCRP Publication 147 lists the values for these parameters for lead, concrete, gypsum wallboard, steel, plate glass, and wood. Values for lead, concrete, and gypsum wallboard for the several modalities that had been studied are listed in Table 10-3.

For calculating the thickness of a secondary barrier, the following empirical equation is used:

$$x = \frac{1}{\alpha\gamma}\ln\left[\frac{\left(\dfrac{NTK_{\text{sec}}^1}{Pd_{\text{sec}}^2}\right)^\gamma + \dfrac{\beta}{\alpha}}{1 + \dfrac{\beta}{\alpha}}\right].\qquad (10.20)$$

The parameter values for secondary radiation are different from those for primary radiation because of the different X-ray energies of the secondary radiation. Table 10-4 lists some of these values.

Some of the physical factors that determine the shielding requirements for protection from X-ray beams are shown in Figures 10-11, 10-12, and 10-13. A collimated X-ray beam of area F is directed at patient M (or object to be radiographed, in the case of nonmedical radiography) from the shielded X-ray tube. The beam passes through the patient and is attenuated to an acceptable level by the primary protective barrier before irradiating a person in area 1. The leakage radiation from the X-ray tube and the scattered radiations are attenuated to an acceptable level by

TABLE 10-3. Values for the Parameters for Transmission of Broad-Beam Primary X-rays

WORKLOAD DISTRIBUTION[a]	LEAD			CONCRETE[b]			GYPSUM WALLBOARD		
	$\alpha(mm^{-1})$	$\beta(mm^{-1})$	γ	$\alpha(mm^{-1})$	$\beta(mm^{-1})$	γ	$\alpha(mm^{-1})$	$\beta(mm^{-1})$	γ
Rad rooms (all barriers)	2.346	1.590×10^{1}	4.982×10^{-1}	3.626×10^{-2}	1.429×10^{-1}	4.932×10^{-1}	1.420×10^{-2}	5.781×10^{-2}	7.445×10^{-1}
Rad rooms (chest bucky)	2.264	1.308×10^{1}	5.600×10^{-1}	3.552×10^{-2}	1.177×10^{-2}	6.007×10^{-1}	1.278×10^{-2}	4.848×10^{-2}	8.609×10^{-1}
Rad rooms (floor or other barriers)	2.651	1.656×10^{1}	4.585×10^{-1}	3.994×10^{-2}	1.448×10^{-1}	4.231×10^{-1}	1.679×10^{-2}	6.124×10^{-2}	7.356×10^{-1}
Fluoroscopy tube (R&F room)	2.347	1.267×10^{1}	6.149×10^{-1}	3.616×10^{-2}	9.721×10^{-2}	5.186×10^{-1}	1.340×10^{-2}	4.283×10^{-2}	8.796×10^{-1}
Rad tube (R&F room)	2.295	1.300×10^{1}	5.573×10^{-1}	3.549×10^{-2}	1.164×10^{-1}	5.774×10^{-1}	1.300×10^{-2}	4.778×10^{-2}	8.485×10^{-1}
Chest room	2.283	1.074×10^{1}	6.370×10^{-1}	3.622×10^{-2}	1.766×10^{-2}	5.404×10^{-1}	1.286×10^{-2}	3.505×10^{-2}	9.356×10^{-1}
Mammography room	3.060×10^{1}	1.776×10^{2}	3.308×10^{-1}	2.577×10^{-2}	1.765	3.644×10^{-1}	9.148×10^{-2}	7.090×10^{-1}	3.459×10^{-1}
Cardiac angiography	2.389	1.426×10^{1}	5.948×10^{-1}	3.717×10^{-2}	1.087×10^{-1}	4.879×10^{-1}	1.409×10^{-2}	4.814×10^{-2}	8.419×10^{-1}
Peripheral angiography[c]	2.728	1.852×10^{1}	4.614×10^{-1}	4.292×10^{-2}	1.538×10^{-1}	4.236×10^{-1}	1.774×10^{-2}	3.449×10^{-2}	7.158×10^{-1}

[a] The workload distributions are those surveyed by the AAPM.
[b] The fitting parameters for concrete assume standard-density concrete.
[c] The data in this table for peripheral angiography also apply to neuroangiography.
Reproduced with permission of the National Council on Radiation Protection and Measurements from *Structural Shielding Design for Medical X-Ray Imaging Facilities.* Bethesda, MD: National Council on Radiation Protection & Measurement; 2004. NCRP Report 147.

TABLE 10-4. Values for the Parameters for Broad-Beam Secondary Transmission of X-rays[a]

WORKLOAD DISTRIBUTION[b]	LEAD			CONCRETE[c]			GYPSUM WALLBOARD		
	$\alpha\,(mm^{-1})$	$\beta\,(mm^{-1})$	γ	$\alpha\,(mm^{-1})$	$\beta\,(mm^{-1})$	γ	$\alpha\,(mm^{-1})$	$\beta\,(mm^{-1})$	γ
30 kVp	3.879×10^{1}	1.800×10^{2}	3.560×10^{-1}	3.174×10^{-1}	1.725	3.705×10^{-1}	1.198×10^{-1}	7.137×10^{-2}	3.703×10^{-2}
50 kVp	8.801	2.728×10^{1}	2.957×10^{-1}	9.030×10^{-2}	1.712×10^{-1}	2.324×10^{-1}	3.880×10^{-2}	8.730×10^{-2}	5.105×10^{-1}
70 kVp	5.369	2.349×10^{1}	5.883×10^{-1}	5.090×10^{-2}	1.697×10^{-1}	3.849×10^{-1}	2.300×10^{-2}	7.160×10^{-2}	7.300×10^{-1}
100 kVp	2.507	1.533×10^{1}	9.124×10^{-1}	3.950×10^{-2}	8.440×10^{-2}	5.191×10^{-1}	1.470×10^{-2}	4.000×10^{-2}	9.752×10^{-1}
125 kVp	2.233	7.888	7.295×10^{1}	3.510×10^{-2}	6.600×10^{-2}	7.832×10^{-1}	1.200×10^{-2}	2.670×10^{-2}	1.079
150 kVp	1.791	5.478	5.678×10^{-1}	3.240×10^{-2}	7.750×10^{-2}	1.566	1.040×10^{-2}	2.020×10^{-2}	1.135
Rad room (all barriers)	2.298	1.738×10^{1}	6.193×10^{-1}	3.610×10^{-2}	1.433×10^{-1}	5.600×10^{-1}	1.380×10^{-2}	5.700×10^{-2}	7.937×10^{-1}
Rad room (chest bucky)	2.256	1.380×10^{1}	8.837×10^{-1}	3.560×10^{-2}	1.079×10^{-1}	7.705	1.270×10^{-2}	4.450×10^{-2}	1.049
Rad room (floor or other barriers)	2.513	1.734×10^{1}	4.994×10^{-1}	3.920×10^{-2}	1.464×10^{-1}	4.486×10^{-1}	1.640×10^{-2}	6.080×10^{-2}	7.472×10^{-1}
Fluoroscopy tube (R&F room)	2.322	1.291×10^{1}	7.575×10^{-1}	3.630×10^{-2}	9.360×10^{-2}	5.955×10^{-1}	1.330×10^{-2}	4.100×10^{-2}	9.566×10^{-1}
Rad tube (R&F room)	2.272	1.360×10^{1}	7.184×10^{-1}	3.560×10^{-2}	1.114×10^{-1}	6.620×10^{-1}	1.290×10^{-2}	4.570×10^{-2}	9.355×10^{-1}
Chest room	2.288	9.848	1.054	3.640×10^{-2}	6.590×10^{-2}	7.543×10^{-1}	1.300×10^{-2}	2.970×10^{-2}	1.195
Mammography room	2.991×10^{1}	1.884×10^{2}	3.550×10^{-1}	2.539×10^{-2}	1.8411	3.924×10^{-1}	8.830×10^{-2}	7.526×10^{-1}	3.786×10^{-1}
Cardiac angiography	2.354	1.494×10^{1}	7.481×10^{-1}	3.710×10^{-2}	1.067×10^{-1}	5.733×10^{-1}	1.390×10^{-2}	4.640×10^{-2}	9.185×10^{-1}
Peripheral angiography[d]	2.661	1.954×10^{1}	5.094×10^{-1}	4.219×10^{-2}	1.559×10^{-1}	4.472×10^{-1}	1.747×10^{-2}	6.422×10^{-2}	7.299×10^{-1}

[a]The values cf parameters are applicable to barrier thicknesses within the range of Figures 10-17, 10-18, and 10-19.

[b]The 30 kVp and mammography room data are for molybdenum-anode X-ray tubes. All other data are for tungsten-anode.

[c]Standard-density concrete is assumed.

[d]The data for peripheral angiography also apply to neuroangiography.

Reproduced with permission of the National Council on Radiation Protection and Measurements from *Structural Shielding Design for Medical X-Ray Imaging Facilities*. Bethesda. MD: National Council on Radiation Protection & Measurement; 2004. NCRP Report 147.

535

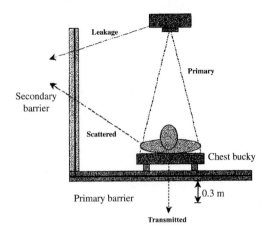

Figure 10-11. Diagram showing primary, scattered, leakage, and transmitted radiation in a radiographic room with a patient standing against the chest bucky. The distance from the shielded wall to an occupied point is assumed to be 0.3 m. (Reproduced with permission of the National Council on Radiation Protection and Measurements from *Structural Shielding Design for Medical X-Ray Imaging Facilities*. Bethesda, MD: National Council on Radiation Protection & Measurement; 2004. NCRP Report 147.)

Figure 10-12. A typical medical imaging room layout. For the indicated tube orientation, the person in area 1 would need to be shielded from the primary beam, with the distance from the X-ray source to the shielded area equal to d_P. The person in area 2 would need to be shielded from scattered and leakage radiations, with the indicated scattering distance d_L. The primary X-ray beam has area F at distance d_F. It is assumed that persons in occupied areas are at a distance of 1 ft. (0.3 m) beyond the barrier walls, 1.7 m above the floor below, and 0.5 m above occupied floor levels in rooms above the imaging room. (Reproduced with permission of the National Council on Radiation Protection and Measurements from *Structural Shielding Design for Medical X-Ray Imaging Facilities*. Bethesda, MD: National Council on Radiation Protection & Measurement; 2004. NCRP Report 147.)

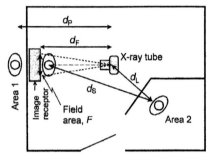

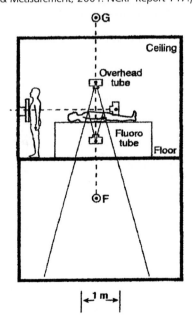

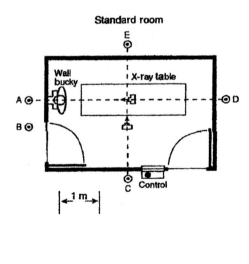

Figure 10-13. Elevation (*Left*) and plan (*Right*) views of a representative radiographic and fluoroscopic room. Points A, B, C, D, and E represent a distance of 0.3 m (1 ft.) from the respective walls. Point F is 1.7 m above the floor below. Point G is 0.5 m above the floor of the room below. (Reproduced with permission of the National Council on Radiation Protection and Measurements from *Structural Shielding Design for Medical X-Ray Imaging Facilities*. Bethesda, MD: National Council on Radiation Protection & Measurement; 2004. NCRP Report 147.)

a secondary protective barrier before reaching points outside the walls where other people may be irradiated.

The application of these equations is illustrated below in Example 10.6.

 # EXAMPLE 10.6

Calculate the thicknesses of

(a) the primary barriers and

(b) secondary barriers

to permit safe operation of a dedicated chest X-ray unit under the following conditions:

- 50 patients per day × 5 days per week = 250 patients per week.
- X-ray beam is always directed to the same wall, therefore, use factor, $U = 1$.
- Chest bucky image receptor area = 1833 cm² at a source-to-image distance = 2 m.
- Adjacent rooms are fully occupied and not controlled.
- Distance to occupied space in room adjacent to primary wall, $d_P = 3$ m.
- Distance from X-ray tube and from patient to occupied space in side room, $d_{sec} = 1.7$ m.
- Image receptor is a wall-mounted cassette holder, equivalent thickness = 0.85 mm Pb.
- Wall consists of two 5/8-in.-thick gypsum wallboards nailed to the opposite sides of 2 in. × 4 in. studs.

Solution

(a) Primary protective barrier
The unshielded primary air kerma from a given procedure, $K_P(0)$, at the closest distance to the protected point, d_P, is given by

$$K_P(0) = \frac{K_P^1 \frac{\text{mGy} \cdot \text{m}^2}{\text{patient}} \times N \frac{\text{patients}}{\text{wk}} \times U}{(d_P \text{ m})^2},$$ **(10.21)**

where U is the use factor, that is, the fraction of the primary-beam workload during which the X-ray beam is directed at the primary barrier. In the case of a dedicated chest room, $U = 1$. The mean unshielded air kerma per patient, K_P^1 at 1 m, is found in Table 10-5 to be 1.2 mGy per patient. Inserting 1.2 mGy

TABLE 10-5. Unshielded Primary and Secondary Air Kerma (mGy per Patient) for the Indicated Workload, W_{norm} (mA-min/wk), normalized to a primary beam distance of 1 m

WORKLOAD DISTRIBUTION	W_{norm}^a	$K_P^{1\,b}$	$K_{sec}^{1\,c}$	$K_{sec}^{1\,d}$
Rad room (chest bucky)	0.6	2.3	5.3×10^{-3}	7.3×10^{-3}
Rad room (floor or other barriers)	1.9	5.2	2.3×10^{-2}	3.3×10^{-2}
Rad tube (R & F room)	1.5	5.9	2.9×10^{-2}	4.0×10^{-2}
Chest room	0.22	1.2	2.7×10^{-3}	3.6×10^{-3}
Cardiac angiography	160	N/A	2.7	3.8

[a]For the indicated clinical installations, W_{norm} is the average workload, mA per patient.
[b]These values for the primary air kerma, mGy per patient, ignore the attenuation available in the radiographic table and image receptor.
[c]Leakage and side scatter.
[d]Leakage and forward/backscatter.
Reproduced with permission of the National Council on Radiation Protection and Measurements from *Structural Shielding Design for Medical X-Ray Imaging Facilities*. Bethesda, MD: National Council on Radiation Protection & Measurement; 2004. NCRP Report 147.

per patient, 250 patients per week, 1 for the use factor, and 3 m for the distance to the nearest point to be protected into Eq. (10.21), we have

$$K_P(0) = \frac{1.2 \dfrac{\text{mGy} \cdot \text{m}^2}{\text{patient}} \times 250 \dfrac{\text{patients}}{\text{wk}} \times 1}{(3\,\text{m})^2} = 33.3 \text{ mGy/wk}.$$

The required transmission factor for the primary barrier is calculated from

$$B_P = \frac{P \text{ mGy/wk}}{K_P(0)}. \tag{10.22}$$

Since the area to be protected is not controlled, the limiting radiation dose there is 0.02 mGy/wk (2 mrems/wk). The required primary transmission factor therefore is

$$B_P = \frac{0.02 \text{ mGy/wk}}{33.3 \text{ mGy/wk}} = 6 \times 10^{-4}.$$

The wall consists of two 5/8-in.-thick gypsum wallboards, or a single wallboard with a total thickness of 28 mm. We will first determine the transmission of the gypsum wallboard to see whether it is sufficient. If not, we will determine the thickness of additional lead sheeting that must be hung on the wall to transmit no more than 6×10^{-4}, or 0.06%, of the incident radiation.

Based on the workloads listed in Table 10-2, broad-beam transmission curves for the primary X-ray spectra and for the secondary (leakage and scattered) radiation generated by each of the imaging applications have been published in NCRP 147 for lead, concrete, gypsum wallboard, steel, plate glass, and wood. The curves for gypsum and concrete are reproduced in Figures 10-14 and 10-15.

Figure 10-14 shows that 28 mm (the two gypsum wallboards, 14 mm each) gypsum wallboard transmits 0.35 (35%) of the "chest room" incident radiation. However, we need a transmission no greater than 6×10^{-4} (0.06%).

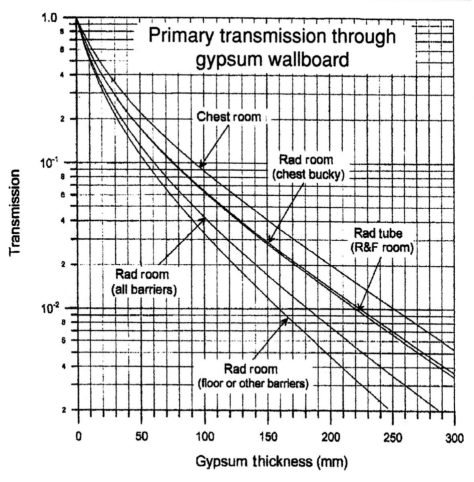

Figure 10-14. Primary broad-beam transmission through gypsum wallboard. A nominal 5/8-in. sheet of "type X" gypsum wallboard has a minimum gypsum thickness of ~14 mm. (Reproduced with permission of the National Council on Radiation Protection and Measurements from *Structural Shielding Design for Medical X-Ray Imaging Facilities*. Bethesda, MD: National Council on Radiation Protection & Measurement; 2004. NCRP Report 147.)

We therefore must add additional shielding. The final transmission (B_{final}) of the barrier is equal to the product of the transmission factor of the shielding already in place ($B_{in\ place}$) and the transmission of the additional shielding (B_{add}):

$$B_{final} = B_{in\ place} \times B_{add} \tag{10.23}$$

$$6 \times 10^{-4} = 3.5 \times 10^{-1} \times B_{add}$$

$$B_{add} = 1.7 \times 10^{-3}.$$

Let us use lead sheet for the additional barrier thickness. In NCRP 147, Figure B.3, we find that 1.62-mm lead transmits 1.7×10^{-3} of the incident radiation.

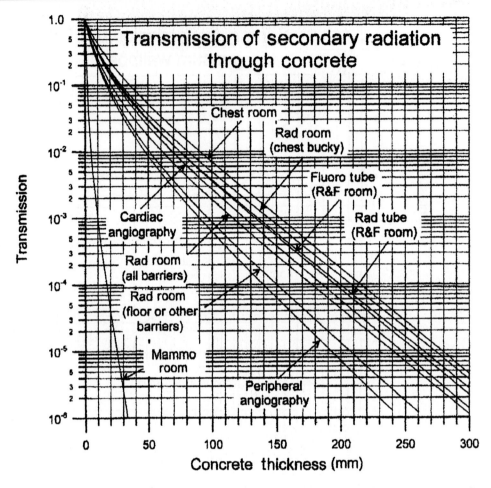

Figure 10-15. Transmission of secondary radiation through standard weight concrete (147 #/ft³, 2.4 g cm⁻³). (Reproduced with permission of the National Council on Radiation Protection and Measurements from *Structural Shielding Design for Medical X-Ray Imaging Facilities.* Bethesda, MD: National Council on Radiation Protection & Measurement; 2004. NCRP Report 147.)

In Table 10-6, we find that commercial lead sheet with a thickness of 5/64 in. (1.98 mm) fits the requirements and, in fact, provides additional reduction in dose below the 0.02 mGy/wk design goal.

(b) Secondary protective barrier

(i) Wall

The room adjacent to the chest room is fully occupied and not controlled. The design maximum air kerma, therefore, is 0.02 mGy/wk. The dimensions of the room are such that the distance to the protected person in the adjacent room, d_{sec} is 2.5 m. From Table 10-5, we find that the total unshielded secondary air kerma (leakage + side scatter) is 2.7×10^{-3} mGy per patient at 1 m. The unshielded air kerma from the secondary radiation at the point of

TABLE 10-6. Commercial Lead Sheets

THICKNESS		NOMINAL WEIGHT	
mm	in.	#/ft²	kg/m²
0.79	1/32	2	10
1.00	5/128	2 1/2	12
1.19	3/64	3	15
1.58	1/16	4	20
1.98	5/64	5	24
2.38	3/32	6	29
3.17	1/8	8	39
4.76	3/16	12	59
6.35	1/4	16	78
8.50	1/3	20	98
10.1	2/5	24	117
12.7	1/2	30	146
16.9	2/3	40	195
25.4	1	60	293

interest is

$$K_{sec}(0) = \frac{K_{sec}^1 \dfrac{mGy \cdot m^2}{patient} \times N \dfrac{patients}{wk}}{(d_{sec}\, m)^2} \qquad (10.24)$$

$$K_{sec}(0) = \frac{2.7 \times 10^{-3} \dfrac{mGy \cdot m^2}{patient} \times 250 \dfrac{patients}{wk}}{(2.5\, m)^2} = 0.11 \frac{mGy}{wk}.$$

The secondary barrier must therefore attenuate the secondary radiation to

$$B_{sec} = \frac{I}{I_0} = \frac{0.02\ mGy/wk}{0.11\ mGy/wk} = 0.18.$$

The present wall consists of two gypsum wallboards whose total gypsum thickness is 28 mm. We will determine the required secondary barrier thickness to transmit 18% of the incident secondary radiation using Eq. (10.20) instead of the graphical method that we used to determine the primary barrier in the first part of this example. The empirically determined values for parameters α, β, and γ, which depend on the barrier material and on the X-ray energy, are found in Table 10-4. From Eq. (10.20), we have

$$x = \frac{1}{\alpha\gamma} \ln \left[\frac{\left(\dfrac{NTK_{sec}^1}{Pd_{sec}^2}\right)^\gamma + \dfrac{\beta}{\alpha}}{1 + \dfrac{\beta}{\alpha}} \right].$$

For gypsum wallboard and for the chest room, $\alpha = 1.3 \times 10^{-2}\ mm^{-1}$, $\beta = 2.97 \times 10^{-2}\ mm^{-1}$, and $\gamma = 1.195$.

For the other variables in Eq. (10.20), we have

$N = 250$ patients per week,

$T =$ occupancy factor $= 1$,

$K_{sec}^1 = 2.7 \times 10^{-3}$ mGy per patient at 1 m (Table 10-5),

$P = 0.02$ mGy/wk, and

$d_{sec} = 2.5$ m.

When we substitute these values into Eq. (10.20) we have

$$x = \frac{1}{0.013 \times 1.195}$$
$$\times \ln \left[\frac{\left(\dfrac{250 \, \dfrac{\text{patients}}{\text{wk}} \times 1 \times 2.7 \times 10^{-3} \, \dfrac{\text{mGy} \cdot \text{m}^2}{\text{patient}}}{0.02 \, \dfrac{\text{mGy}}{\text{wk}} \times (2.5 \text{ m})^2} \right)^{1.195} + \dfrac{0.0297}{0.013}}{1 + \dfrac{0.0297}{0.013}} \right]$$

$x = 70.28$ mm gypsum wallboard.

If we were to use sheets of gypsum as the secondary barrier, we would need a total of

$$\frac{70.28 \text{ mm}}{14 \, \dfrac{\text{mm}}{\text{wallbord}}} = 5 \text{ wallboards.}$$

Since we already have 2 wallboards, we need an additional 3 gypsum wallboards.

Let us calculate the thickness of lead to be added to the existing wall if we wished to use a layer of lead sheet instead of 3 additional layers of wallboard, then the 2 gypsum wallboards provide 2/5, or 40%, of the required barrier thickness. If there were no gypsum, then the required barrier thickness of lead is calculated with Eq. (10.20), by using the α, β, and γ values for lead for secondary radiation in a chest room. In Table 10-4, we find that for lead barriers in a chest room,

$\alpha = 2.288$ mm^{-1},

$\beta = 9.848$ mm^{-1}, and

$\gamma = 1.054$.

The other values for substituting into Eq. (10.20) are the same as for the calculation of the required gypsum wallboard barrier thickness. Substituting these values into Eq. (10.20) gives:

$$x = \frac{1}{2.288 \times 1.054}$$
$$\times \ln \left[\frac{\left(\dfrac{250 \, \dfrac{\text{patients}}{\text{wk}} \times 1 \times 2.7 \times 10^{-3} \, \dfrac{\text{mGy} \cdot \text{m}^2}{\text{patient}}}{0.02 \, \dfrac{\text{mGy}}{\text{wk}} \times (2.5 \, \text{m})^2} \right)^{1.195} + \dfrac{9.848}{2.288}}{1 + \dfrac{9.848}{2.288}} \right]$$

$x = 0.332$ mm lead.

From Table 10-6, we find that the thinnest commercially available lead sheet is 0.79 mm, or 1/32 in. thick. The additional 1/32-in.-thick sheet of lead is much more than adequate to meet the design criteria for radiation safety. The architect may choose either to have a wall that is 5 gypsum wallboards thick, or to hang a 1/32-in.-thick lead sheet on the 2 wallboard thick wall in accordance with ALARA and depending on cost and space considerations, and possible increased workload in the future.

(ii) Floor

We will use Eq. (10.20) to calculate the thickness of a concrete barrier required to attenuate the secondary radiation from the chest room to the design level of 0.02 mGy/wk:

$$x = \frac{1}{\alpha \gamma} \ln \left[\frac{\left(\dfrac{NTK^1_{\sec}}{Pd^2_{\sec}} \right)^{\gamma} + \dfrac{\beta}{\alpha}}{1 + \dfrac{\beta}{\alpha}} \right].$$

In Table 10-5, we see that the total (side scattered + leakage) secondary air kerma at 1 m, $K^1_{\sec}$, is 2.7×10^{-3} mGy/patient, and in Table 10-4, we find the values of α, β, and γ for concrete to be

$\alpha = 0.0364$ mm^{-1},

$\beta = 0.0659$ mm^{-1}, and

$\gamma = 0.7543$.

When we insert the respective values into Eq. (10.20), we have

$$x = \frac{1}{0.0364 \times 0.7543}$$

$$\times \ln \left[\frac{\left(\dfrac{250 \, \dfrac{\text{patients}}{\text{wk}} \times 1 \times 2.7 \times 10^{-3} \, \dfrac{\text{mGy} \cdot \text{m}^2}{\text{patient}}}{0.02 \, \dfrac{\text{mGy}}{\text{wk}} \times (3 \, \text{m})^2} \right)^{0.7543} + \dfrac{0.0659}{0.0364}}{1 + \dfrac{0.0659}{0.0364}} \right]$$

$$= 17 \, \text{mm concrete.}$$

Since the floor is already thicker than the required 17 mm concrete, no additional barrier thickness is necessary.

EXAMPLE 10.7

Calculate the shielding requirement for the wall of a hospital room where cardiac angiography will be performed. Cardiac angiography is an interventional diagnostic procedure for locating and evaluating coronary artery disease. To do this, a catheter, about 2–3-mm diameter, is inserted through a skin puncture into an artery in the groin or in the arm, and then is carefully advanced into the opening of a coronary artery. An iodine solution, which is opaque to X-rays, is injected into the artery, and X-ray images that are taken show the location and severity of blockages in the artery. The catheter is removed after the procedure. The entire procedure is done under fluoroscopy and requires about 25–30 minutes for examining all the coronary arteries. With good technique, the effective radiation dose to the patient for this procedure usually is in the range of 4.6 mSv (460 mrems) to 15.8 mSv (1,580 mrems).

Given the following information, calculate the shielding requirements for one of the walls and for the floor:

- 30 patients per week.
- All adjacent rooms are fully occupied, $T = 1$; and not controlled, $P = 0.02$ mSv (2 mrems) per week.
- Walls are made of hollow concrete blocks whose total wall thickness is 2 in. (5 cm), with 5/8-in.-thick gypsum wallboard on each side.
- Floor and ceiling consist of 4 in. (10 cm) thick concrete.
- Floor-to-floor distance = 3.5 m.

- Distance to protected point on other side of wall is 3 m from X-ray unit isocenter.
- Only secondary radiation is considered in the shielding design, since the image receptor acts as the primary-beam stopper, therefore, $K_{sec}^1 = 3.8$ mGy/patient at 1 meter (from Table 10-5).
- Assume forward or backscatter in calculating the level of the secondary radiation, $K_{sec}^1 = 3.8$ mGy/patient at 1 meter (from Table 10-5).

Solution

To find the unshielded air kerma at the point to be shielded, we insert the respective values into Eq. (10.24):

$$K_{sec}(0) = \frac{K_{sec}^1 \dfrac{mGy \cdot m^2}{patient} \times N \dfrac{patients}{wk}}{(d_{sec}\, m)^2}$$

$$K_{sec}(0) = \frac{3.8 \dfrac{mGy \cdot m^2}{patient} \times 30 \dfrac{patients}{wk}}{(3\, m)^2} = 12.7 \frac{mGy}{wk}.$$

The required maximum transmission of the shielding barrier is

$$B_{sec} = \frac{P}{K_{sec}} = \frac{0.02\ mGy/wk}{12.7\ mGy/wk} = 1.6 \times 10^{-3}.$$

From Figure 10-15, we find that 50 mm (2 inches) concrete attenuates the radiation to 2.5×10^{-2}, and we find in NCRP 147, Figure C.4 that 31.25-mm gypsum wallboard attenuates the radiation from cardiac angiography to 3×10^{-1}. The total attenuation by the existing wall therefore is

$$B_{sec}(existing\,wall) = 2.5 \times 10^{-2} \times 3 \times 10^{-1} = 7.5 \times 10^{-3}.$$

We need a transmission factor of 1.9×10^{-3}. The additional reduction factor is calculated from Eq. (10.22):

$$1.9 \times 10^{-3} = 7.5 \times 10^{-3} \times B_{sec}(additional)$$
$$B_{sec}(additional) = 0.25.$$

If we decide to provide the additional shielding with lead, we find, in NCRP 147, Figure C.2, that 0.14-mm lead will attenuate the cardiac angiography radiation to 0.25. The next largest commercially available lead sheet is 0.79 mm (1/32 inch) thick. If we should wish to provide the additional shielding by adding another sheet of gypsum wallboard, we find from figure in NCRP 147, Figure C.4 that 22 mm, or a single 5/8-in.-thick wallboard, which is 16 mm thick, will reduce the radiation to lower than the design criterion.

Computed Axial Tomography

Computed axial tomography (CAT or CT) is a diagnostic tool that uses X-rays and computers to construct a cross-sectional image of any part of the body. CAT is based on the principle that an image of an object can be constructed from attenuation of numerous X-ray beams that pass through the object from different angles. To accomplish this, CT scanners have a circular ring-shaped gantry (Figure 10-16), an X-ray source, and one or more detectors located diametrically opposite to the X-ray tube. The patient is placed inside the circular gantry, and the gantry rotates at a rate of about 60–120 RPM (1–2 revolutions per second) while the table on which the patient lies is moved horizontally through the gantry. In this mode of operation, the X-ray beam traces a helix, which allows manipulation of the resultant image.

The X-ray beam that is directed at the patient is narrowly collimated along the axis of rotation, resulting in a narrow beam along the axis, on the order of 1–10 mm, and is fan-shaped in the radial direction. As the X-ray tube is rotated, the incident beam is attenuated in a manner dependent on the local tissue composition (greater attenuation for bones, lesser for soft tissues). These attenuation changes are measured by the detectors, and from the relationship between the signals generated by the attenuated beam and their radial distribution, a computer constructs an image representing the cross section of the scanned area. The energy of the X-ray beam (determined by tube potential and filtration) and photon fluence (determined

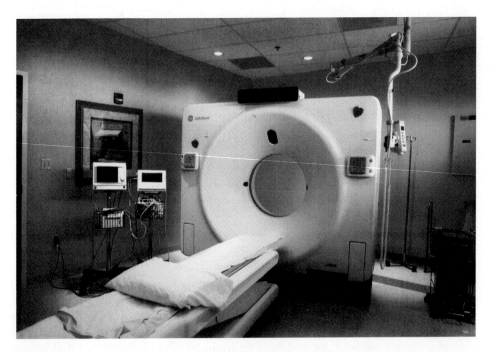

Figure 10-16. Computed axial tomography, CT, scanner. (Reproduced with permission of the National Council on Radiation Protection and Measurements from *Structural Shielding Design for Medical X-Ray Imaging Facilities.* Bethesda, MD: National Council on Radiation Protection & Measurement; 2004. NCRP Report 147.)

by the product of tube current and time) are among the main factors that affect the radiation dose to the patient.

In conventional radiography, radiation dose decreases continuously from the beam's entrance into the body to its exit. In CT, the dose is distributed more uniformly across the scanning plane because the patient is equally irradiated from all directions by the rotating X-ray source. In a CT examination of the head, for instance, the dose is relatively uniform across the field of view. In larger objects such as the chest or abdomen, the dose is equally distributed around the surface of the skin, and decreases by a factor of about two near the center of the object. Dose comparisons, therefore, between CT and conventional radiography in terms of skin dose are not appropriate. Furthermore, the radiation energy delivered by CT is not fully contained within the scanning volume. Scattered radiation, divergence of the radiation beam, and limits to the efficiency of beam collimation all contribute to the radiation dose outside scan volume. In the case of the multiple scans required to image some length of a patient's body, it becomes necessary to consider the radiation dose delivered beyond the boundaries of a single scan.

The principal metric used in CT dosimetry is called the CT dose index, or $CTDI_{100}$. The $CTDI_{100}$ integrates the radiation dose along the axis for the entire scan; it includes radiation scattered into adjacent tissue from slices being scanned, as well as radiation scattered beyond the ends of the scan. The $CTDI_{100}$ is measured with a 100-mm-long ionization chamber and two different phantoms: a 16-cm diameter phantom to represent the head, and a 32-cm diameter phantom to represent the trunk. When designing shielding for rooms where CT scanning will be performed, only secondary radiation is considered, since the primary X-ray beam is attenuated to a very low level and essentially stopped by the detector assembly and by the gantry. The scattered radiation at 1 meter per rotation is given by

$$K_{sec}^{1} = \kappa \frac{L}{p} \times CTDI_{100},$$ **(10.25)**

where $\kappa =$ the X-ray scatter fraction per cm, and has the following experimentally determined values:

$$\kappa_{head} = 9 \times 10^{-5} cm^{-1}$$ **(10.26a)**

$$\kappa_{body} = 3 \times 10^{-4} cm^{-1}$$ **(10.26b)**

$$L = \text{length of the scan, cm}$$

$$p = \text{pitch} = \frac{\text{horizontal movement of the patient / gantry rotation}}{\text{beam width}}.$$

The value of the $CTDI_{100}$ for any specific scanner depends on the X-ray high voltage and on the exposure in mA-seconds (mA-s). Values of the $CTDI_{100}$ vary from one model scanner to another, and are measured and supplied by the manufacturer of the scanner. If we normalize the $CTDI_{100}$ to per mA-s and we call it $_nCTDI_{100}$, then we obtain

$$K_{sec}^1 = \kappa \frac{L}{p} \times {}_nCTDI_{100}. \tag{10.27}$$

EXAMPLE 10.8

Given the following information about a hospital room where a CT scanner will be installed:

- Walls are made of hollow concrete blocks painted on both sides. The effective concrete thickness is 2 in. (50 cm).
- One wall, which has a door, separates the CT room from a corridor ($T = 1/5$), the other side of the opposite wall is an unattended parking lot ($T = 1/40$), and the other two walls connect with fully occupied offices.
- All adjacent areas are not controlled, therefore, $P = 0.02$ mGy/wk.
- The room is in the basement, so there is nothing below; the room above is a fully occupied laboratory. The floor-to-floor distance to the room above is 3 m, and the ceiling consists of a 4-in. (101-mm) thick concrete slab.
- Distance from gantry isocenter to protected point in corridor is 2.5 m, and in adjacent rooms is 3 m; distance from isocenter to floor is 1.5 m.
- Expected maximum workload is 75 body scans of 50-cm average length at 250 mA-s, 140 kVp, and 1.3 pitch; and 25 head scans, mean length of 20 cm, per week at 300 mA-s and 140 kVp, and a pitch of 1.0.
- The $_nCTDI_{100}$ values are listed by the manufacturer as 0.225 mGy per mA-s for the head and 0.140 mGy per mA-s for the body.

Calculate the lead thickness for the door, and any additional thickness of lead, if needed, by the

(a) corridor wall,

(b) wall to the adjacent room, and

(c) ceiling.

Solution

(a) The secondary air kerma at a distance of 1 m from a patient from a head scan and from a body scan is calculated by inserting the values for κ_{head} and κ_{body}

from Eqs. (10.26a) and (10.26b) into Eq. (10.27):

$$K^1_{\text{sec}}(\text{head}) = 9 \times 10^{-5}\text{cm}^{-1} \times \frac{20\,\text{cm}}{1} \times 300\frac{\text{mA} \cdot \text{s}}{\text{patient}} \times 0.225\frac{\text{mGy}}{\text{mA} \cdot \text{s}}$$

$$= 0.122\frac{\text{mGy}}{\text{patient}}$$

$$K^1_{\text{sec}}(\text{body}) = 3 \times 10^{-4}\text{cm}^{-1} \times \frac{50\,\text{cm}}{1.3} \times 250\frac{\text{mA} \cdot \text{s}}{\text{patient}} \times 0.140\frac{\text{mGy}}{\text{mA} \cdot \text{s}}$$

$$= 0.404\frac{\text{mGy}}{\text{patient}}.$$

The unshielded secondary radiation at a distance of 2.5 m is:

$$K_{\text{sec}} = \left(\frac{1\text{m}}{2.5\,\text{m}}\right)^2 \left(25\,\frac{\text{patients}}{\text{wk}} \times 0.122\,\frac{\text{mGy}}{\text{patient}} + 75\,\frac{\text{patients}}{\text{wk}} \times 0.404\,\frac{\text{mGy}}{\text{patient}}\right)$$

$$K_{\text{sec}} = 5.34\,\text{mGy/wk}.$$

For the corridor door and wall, the maximum barrier transmission of the secondary radiation is

$$B_{\text{sec}}(\text{corridor}) = \frac{P}{K_{\text{sec}} \times T} = \frac{0.02\,\text{mGy/wk}}{5.34\,\text{mGy/wk} \times \dfrac{1}{5}} = 1.9 \times 10^{-2}.$$

Door—From Figure 10-17, we find that 0.52-mm lead is required for the door (neglecting the shielding effect of the wooden door). From Table 10-6, we find the next thicker, commercially available lead sheet to be 0.79 mm (1/32 in.) thick, which we will specify for the door.
Corridor wall—The transmission factor for the corridor wall, as calculated above, is 1.9×10^{-2}. The effective thickness of the hollow concrete block wall is 50 mm. Figure 10-18 shows that 50-mm concrete will reduce the secondary CT radiation to 1.3×10^{-1}. Therefore, we need to add more shielding to the wall. The additional transmission factor is calculated with Eq. (10.23):

$$0.13 \times B_{\text{add}} = 0.019$$

$$B_{\text{add}} = 0.15.$$

In Figure 10-17, we see that 0.35-mm lead will attenuate the secondary radiation from a 140 kVp CT scanner to 0.15. To specify a commercially available lead sheet to attach to the corridor wall, we go to Table 10-6, which shows the next thicker, commercially available lead sheet to be 0.79 mm (1/32 in.).

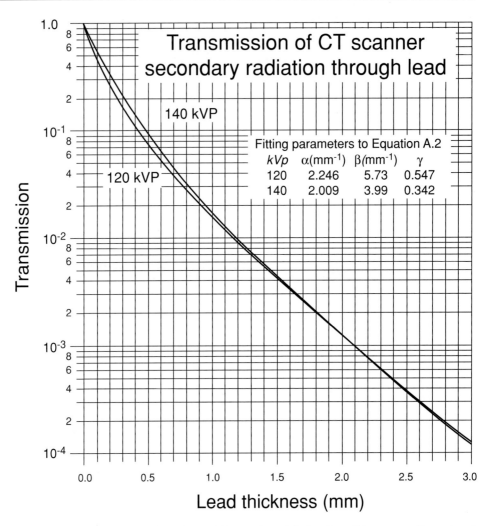

Figure 10-17. Transmission through lead of secondary radiation from CT scanners. (Reproduced with permission of the National Council on Radiation Protection and Measurements from *Structural Shielding Design for Medical X-Ray Imaging Facilities.* Bethesda, MD: National Council on Radiation Protection & Measurement; 2004. NCRP Report 147.)

(b) *Adjacent room*—The unshielded secondary radiation at a distance of 3 m from the isocenter is calculated in the following manner:

$$K_{sec} = \left(\frac{1\,m}{3\,m}\right)^2 \left(25\,\frac{patients}{wk} \times 0.122\,\frac{mGy}{patient} + 75\,\frac{patients}{wk} \times 0.404\,\frac{mGy}{patient}\right)$$

$$K_{sec} = 3.7\ mGy/wk.$$

The barrier transmission to reduce the unshielded radiation to 0.02 mGy/wk is

$$B_{sec}(\text{adjacent room}) = \frac{0.02\,mGy/wk}{3.7\,mGy/wk \times 1} = 5.4 \times 10^{-3}.$$

TABLE 10-7. Primary Barrier Tenth Value Layers (TVLs) for Ordinary Concrete (2.35 g/cm³), Steel (7.87 g/cm³) and Lead (11.35 g/cm³)

ENDPOINT ENERGY	MATERIAL	TVL₁ (cm)	TVLₑ(cm)
4	Concrete	35	30
	Steel	9.9	9.9
	Lead	5.7	5.7
6	Concrete	37	33
	Steel	10	10
	Lead	5.7	5.7
10	Concrete	41	37
	Steel	11	11
	Lead	5.7	5.7
15	Concrete	44	41
	Steel	11	11
	Lead	5.7	5.7
18	Concrete	45	43
	Steel	11	11
	Lead	5.7	5.7
20	Concrete	46	44
	Steel	11	11
	Lead	5.7	5.7
25	Concrete	49	46
	Steel	11	11
	Lead	5.7	5.7
30	Concrete	51	49
	Steel	11	11
	Lead	5.7	5.7
Co-60	Concrete	21	21
	Steel	7.0	7.0
	Lead	4.0	4.0

The first (TVL₁) and equilibrium (TVLₑ) tenth-value layers are used to account for the spectral changes in the radiation as it penetrates the barrier.
Reproduced with permission of the National Council on Radiation Protection and Measurements from *Structural Shielding Design and Evaluation for Megavoltage X-and Gamma-Ray Radiotherapy Facilities*. Bethesda, MD: National Council on Radiation Protection & Measurement; 2005, NCRP Report 151.

Since the concrete block wall attenuates the secondary radiation to 1.3×10^{-1}, we will need additional shielding. The additional transmission factor is calculated with Eq. (10.23):

$$1.3 \times 10^{-1} \times B_{\text{add}} = 5.4 \times 10^{-3}$$

$$B_{\text{add}} = 4.2 \times 10^{-2}.$$

In Figure 10-17. we see that 0.72-mm lead will reduce the radiation level in the adjacent room to the design level of 0.02 mGy/wk. Table 10-7 shows that we specify 0.79-mm (1/32-in.) thick lead sheeting to affix to the wall.

(c) *Ceiling*—The shielding design distance for the floor above is 1.7 m above the floor, which corresponds to 3.2 m above the isocenter. Since the room is fully occupied and not controlled, $P = 0.02$ mGy/wk and the use factor,

$T = 1$. The unshielded secondary radiation at a distance of 3.2 m is

$$K_{sec} = \left(\frac{1\,m}{3.2\,m}\right)^2 \left(25\,\frac{patients}{wk} \times 0.122\,\frac{mGy}{patient} + 75\,\frac{patients}{wk} \times 0.404\,\frac{mGy}{patient}\right)$$

$K_{sec} = 3.26$ mGy/wk.

The maximum barrier (ceiling) transmission is

$$B_{sec}(room\ above) = \frac{0.02\,mGy/wk}{3.26\,mGy/wk \times 1} = 6.1 \times 10^{-3}.$$

From Figure 10-18, we find that 101-mm (4-in.) concrete transmits 0.02 of the incident radiation, and we need to reduce the transmission to 0.0061. Therefore, the additional barrier transmission factor is calculated:

$$0.02 \times B_{add} = 0.0061$$

$$B_{add} = 0.31.$$

According to Figure 10-17, 0.2-mm lead will give the required degree of transmission. The next thicker, commercially available lead sheet (Table 10-7) is 0.76 mm (1/32 in.) thick. This calculation was for the shortest distance from the source of secondary radiation to the point of interest. Further calculations show that a large area in the room above would exceed the radiation safety criterion unless it was shielded. In this case, therefore, it is reasonable to shield the entire area by affixing the lead sheet to the ceiling of the CT room, or covering the floor in the room above with the lead sheet.

Positron Emission Tomography

Positron emission tomography (PET) is a diagnostic technique that is useful in identifying tissues in which there is a high rate of metabolism. PET differs from other radiation-based diagnostic modalities. Whereas other imaging modalities produce an anatomic image of a tissue or organ, PET images sites of metabolic activity. The basic principle here is that the rate of cellular utilization of sugar increases with increased metabolic rate. Fluorodeoxyglucose (FDG) is an analog of glucose, and is metabolized like sugar.

In PET applications, FDG is labeled with the 110-minute positron emitting radioisotope ^{18}F to make 18F-fluorodeoxyglucose (18FDG), and the labeled 18FDG is injected into the patient. After about 45 minutes, the 18FDG will have been absorbed and widely distributed throughout the body. At sites of high metabolic activity, such as in that part of the brain where certain neurologic processes are occurring, or in malignant tumors whose growth requires a relatively high rate of sugar use, there will be a relatively greater concentration of 18FDG and its metabolic products than in other regions of the body. In conditions where there is decreased metabolic

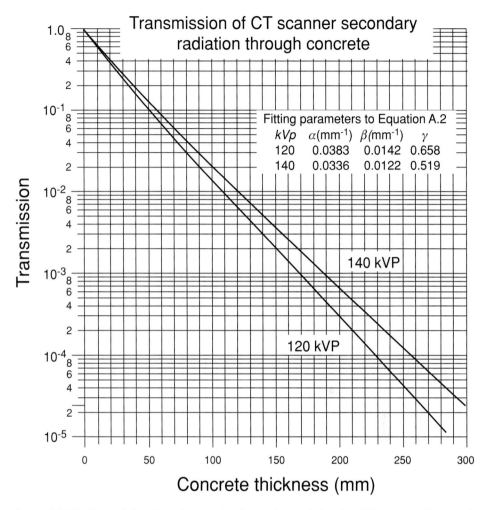

Figure 10-18. Transmission through concrete of secondary radiation from CT scanners. Computed axial tomography (CAT) scanner. (Courtesy of InnerVision Advanced Medical Imaging, Lafayette, IN)

activity, such as occurs in the brains of Alzheimer's disease sufferers and in nonviable heart muscle, the decrease from normal metabolic activity will be seen in a PET scan. This fact is used to distinguish between densities on radiographs that are not malignant, such as fibrotic tissue or scar tissue, whose cells do not metabolize rapidly, and primary or metastatic cancers whose cells do undergo rapid metabolism.

The metabolically hyperactive site is visualized in a PET scan by measuring the intensity of the 0.51-MeV gamma photons that are produced when the positrons from the ^{18}F are annihilated on interaction with the electrons within the metabolically active cells. The annihilation photons travel in a straight line in diametrically opposite directions. The patient is inserted into a circular ring, which is lined with detectors that respond to the annihilation radiation. Each pair of diametrically opposite detectors is connected to a coincidence circuit. Only coincident counts are recorded, since only coincident counts represent the photons from the annihilation of a single positron. Electronic analysis of these coincident pulses allows the construction of an image of the metabolically active sites in that section of the body that is within the detector ring. Since this is not an anatomical image of the site, the PET image can be combined with a CT image, or an MRI image, both of which are anatomical renderings of organs, to visualize the anatomical site of the abnormal metabolic activity.

The short half-life of ^{18}F made it necessary for the early PET centers to produce their own ^{18}F in specially designed cyclotrons. Now, because of the relatively widespread use of PET scanning, regional laboratories have found it feasible to produce the radiofluorine and to distribute it to the users in the region. The 110-minute half-life makes it necessary to produce much more ^{18}F activity than will be administered to a patient.

In shielding for all the other radiation-based diagnostic modalities, we deal with relatively low quantum energies, almost always ≤ 150 kV. In PET scanning, however, we must shield against high-energy gamma radiation, 0.51 MeV, or 510 keV. For this relatively high-energy radiation, the usual wall materials, such as gypsum wallboard, hollow concrete, or cinder blocks provide little shielding. For example, the HVL for 150-kVp X-rays is 0.3 mm-Pb and 22-mm concrete. For 0.51-MeV gammas, the HVLs are 5-mm Pb and 98-mm concrete. Additional lead shielding therefore must always be added to the walls of the PET suite. Also, in most other modalities, we deal with a small radiation source, the X-ray target or the relatively small scattering area where the primary beam strikes the patient, which can reasonably be approximated as a "point" for the purpose of shielding design. In the case of PET, the activity is distributed throughout the body, and we have an extended source whose radiation is partly absorbed by the body tissues.

A typical PET suite (Figure 10-19) consists of an imaging room, a patient dosing room, and a control room. The patient is injected with 10–20 mCi (370–740 MBq) 18FDG, and then is held for 45 minutes while the FDG is distributed within the patient's body. Considering the radioactive decay of the ^{18}F, the activity in the patient when he leaves the dosing room A_{dr} is

$$A_{dr} = A_0\, e^{-\frac{0.693}{110\text{min}} \times 45\,\text{min}} = 0.75\, A_0.$$

The mean activity in the patient while he is in the dosing room is

$$\bar{A}_{dr} = \sqrt{A_0 \times 0.75\,A_0} = 0.87\,A_0.$$

If a patient receives 20 mCi (740 MBq) ^{18}F, then the average activity while he is in the dosing room is $0.87 \times 20 = 17.4$ mCi. About 20% of the injected FDG is excreted via the urine during the first 2 hours after injection. Thus, after 45 minutes, $45/120 \times 20\% = 7.5\%$ will have accumulated in the patient's bladder, and will have been voided before the patient enters the imaging room. This patient, therefore, will void about $0.075 \times 20 = 1.5$ mCi upon leaving the dosing room. His activity when he enters the imaging room will be $0.75 \times 20 - 1.5 = 13.5$ mCi. If 15 minutes transpire between his departure from the dosing room and the start of the scan, and if the scan lasts 45 minutes, then radioactive decay for 60 minutes will decrease the activity to $0.69 \times 13.5 = 9.3$ mCi (344 MBq), and the mean activity while the patient is in the imaging room is

$$\bar{A}_{ir} = \sqrt{13.5 \times 9.5} = 11.3 \text{ mCi} \quad (418\text{MBq}).$$

EXAMPLE 10.9

Calculate the lead equivalent glass for the control room of the PET suite shown in Figure 10-19. Since the radioactivity is an extended source that is distributed throughout the patient's body, and undergoes some degree of self-absorption by the body, calculation of the shielding becomes a complex problem. The source term can be modeled as a sphere for the head, cylinders for the limbs, and a right ellipsoid or

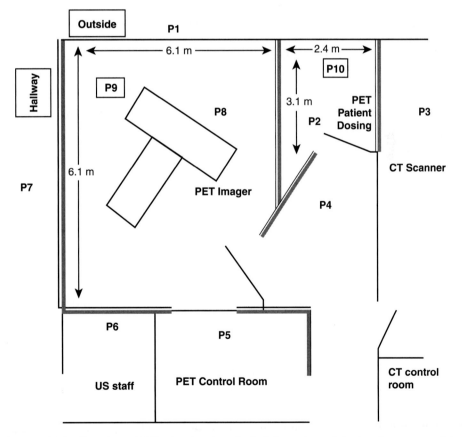

Figure 10-19. Plan view of PET suite showing physical dimensions of the imaging room and the patient dosing room. Also indicated are the dose points, P, of interest. Not drawn to scale. (Reproduced with permission from Methé BM, Shielding design for a PET imaging suite: a case study. *Health Phys.* 2003;84(5 Suppl):S 83–S 88.)

a cylinder for the body, with the distribution of the radionuclide considered either uniform throughout the body or concentrated in certain regions. Calculation of the air kerma rate at the dose point is thus seen to be a very complex problem that is best done with a computer program (such as MicroShield). In this exercise, we will make the simplifying assumption that the source term is a point source, and use the following information as the design basis for determining the required lead thickness:

- 40 patients per week,
- 20 mCi (740 MBq) per patient,
- 45 minutes in dosing room,
- 60 minutes in imaging room,
- occupancy factor of control room $= 1$,
- 4.6 m (15 ft.) from patient on imager to dose point,
- shielding design level $= 0.02$ mGy/wk air kerma for all areas,
- $\Gamma(^{18}\text{F}) = 4.9 \times 10^{-3} \dfrac{\text{mGy} \cdot \text{m}^2}{\text{mCi} \cdot \text{h}}$,
- the source's activity is the mean activity in the patient while he is in the imager, and
- μ(broad beam, Pb, 0.51 MeV) = 1.92 cm^{-1}.

Solution

The unshielded air kerma at 1 m from each patient for an exposure time of t hours is

$$K^1 = \Gamma \ \frac{\text{mGy} \cdot \text{m}^2}{\text{mCi} \cdot \text{h}} \times A \ \frac{\text{mCi}}{\text{patient}} \times t \text{ hours}$$

$$K^1 = 4.9 \times 10^{-3} \ \frac{\text{mGy} \cdot \text{m}^2}{\text{mCi} \cdot \text{h}} \times 11.3 \ \frac{\text{mCi}}{\text{patient}} \times 1 \text{ hour} = 5.5 \times 10^{-2} \frac{\text{mGy} \cdot \text{m}^2}{\text{patient}}.$$

The unshielded air kerma at the dose point in the control room from 40 patients per week is calculated from Eq. (10.21):

$$K(0) = \frac{5.5 \times 10^{-2} \ \dfrac{\text{mGy} \cdot \text{m}^2}{\text{patient}} \times 40 \ \dfrac{\text{patients}}{\text{wk}}}{(4.6 \, \text{m})^2} = 1.04 \times 10^{-1} \ \frac{\text{mGy}}{\text{wk}}.$$

The required transmission for the leaded glass barrier is

$$B = \frac{0.02 \text{ mGy/wk}}{1.04 \times 10^{-1} \text{ mGy/wk}} = 1.93 \times 10^{-1}.$$

The required lead-equivalent leaded glass window is calculated from

$$B = \frac{I}{I_0} = e^{-\mu t}$$

$$t = \frac{\ln B}{-\mu} = \frac{\ln 0.193}{-1.92\,\text{cm}^{-1}} = 0.86\,\text{cm} = 8.6\,\text{mm} = \frac{11}{32}\text{in.}$$

This simplified calculational model was used to illustrate some of the considerations in the design of shielding for a PET facility without either a cyclotron or a CT scanner. A computerized shielding model using a realistic body phantom as the source term, calculated a window thickness of 9.9-mm lead equivalent for exposure conditions similar to those in this simplified illustration.[3]

Radiotherapy Machines[4]

Radiation from radiotherapy machines span a very wide range of energies, from 15 keV Grenz ray X-rays for superficial therapy to 25 MeV accelerators for deep therapy. The basic principles of shielding radiotherapy devices is the same as for diagnostic devices, as is the basic calculational methodology. In all cases, we

1. must know the maximum radiation level to be produced by the device,
2. calculate the unshielded radiation level at the dose point that we wish to protect,
3. calculate the required degree of attenuation, or the maximum transmission, of the shielding barrier, taking into account the use of protected area, and
4. calculate the thickness of the barrier that will give the required degree of attenuation of the radiation.

Although the basic principles are the same for all shielding-design calculations, there are significant difference in the details. Some of these differences include

1. Photoneutrons are produced when high-energy X-rays, $E > 10$ MeV, interact with matter, such as collimaters, shielding, etc. Thus, when discussing shielding of high-energy machines, we have two categories:

    a. ≤ 10MeV, where we do not have neutrons because the threshold energy for photoneutron production is about 8.5 MeV for most materials, and the cross section remains very small until the quantum energy exceeds 10 MeV.
    b. >10 MeV, where we have neutrons that contribute significantly to the radiation dose, and which, therefore, must be shielded.

2. Because of the presence of photoneutrons, safety criteria are expressed in Sv rather than Gy.
3. Specification of the workload—For diagnostic X-ray machines, the workload is specified in milliamp-minutes per week at a given kVp. For therapeutic facilities,

---

[3] Methe, Brian M. *Oper Rad Saf*, S83-S88, May, 2003.
[4] This introduction to radiotherapy machine shielding design is based on NCRP Report 151, *Structural Shielding Design and Evaluation for Megavoltage X- and Gamma Ray Radio Therapy Facilities*. Complete detailed information can be found in NCRP 151.

the workload is specified as the weekly dose at the gantry isocenter, usually at a distance of 1 m from the X-ray source, in Gy per week.

4. An additional safety requirement that the dose-equivalent in any unrestricted area be ≤ 0.02 mSv (2 mrems) in any 1-hour period. This additional requirement is called the *time averaged dose-equivalent rate* (TADR), and is 1-hour dose averaged over a period of 1 week. The weekly TADR, R_W for a dose point behind a primary barrier is given by

$$R_W = \frac{\text{IDR Sv/h} \times W_{\text{pri}} \text{ Gy/wk} \times U_{\text{pri}}}{\dot{D}_O \text{ Gy/h}}, \tag{10.28}$$

where

IDR = instantaneous dose-equivalent rate, Sv/h, measured as the design dose point,

$\dot{D}_O$ = maximum absorbed dose output rate at 1 m, Gy/h,

(A) Section View

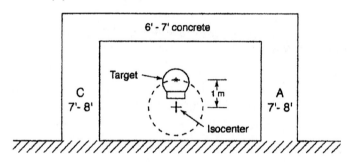

(B) Floor Plan

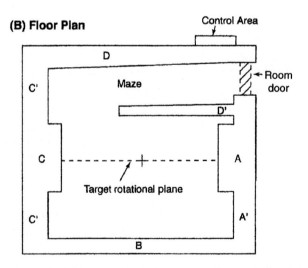

Figure 10-20. Simplified schematic of a typical high-energy treatment room. All barriers are constructed of standard concrete (147 lb ft^{-3}). (Reproduced with permission from McGinley PH. *Shielding Techniques for Radiation Oncology Facilities.* 2nd ed. Madison, WI: Medical Physics Publishing Corp; 2002:Fig 2-1, pg 10.)

W_{pri} = primary barrier weekly workload, Gy/wk, and
U_{pri} = use factor for that dose point.

A generic layout of a typical high-energy treatment room is shown in Figure 10-20.

EXAMPLE 10.10

Calculate the primary concrete barrier thickness for a 6-MV linear accelerator, given the following operational data:

- 40 patients per day, 5 days per week,
- 3.5 Gy per patient,
- 5000 Gy per year for calibration, quality assurance measurements, and maintenance, annual workload, measured at 1 m = 3.5 Gy/patient × 40 patient/d × 5 d/wk × 52 wk/yr + 5000 Gy/yr = 41, 400 Gy/yr, weekly workload, $W = 41,400 \div 52 \approx 800$ Gy/wk,
- $\dot{D}_0 = 10$ Gy/min at 1 m = maximum output from the accelerator,
- $d_{\mathrm{pri}} = 6.3$ m from isocenter to dose point,
- $d_{\mathrm{sca}} = 1$ m = distance from X-ray source to isocenter (scattering point),
- $d_{\mathrm{sec}} = 6.3$ m = distance from scattering point to dose point,
- $d_{\mathrm{L}} = 6.4$ m = leakage distance from X-ray source to dose point,
- maximum field size at isocenter = 40 cm × 40 cm,
- design dose point is in the corridor, occupancy factor $T = 1/5$,
- use factor $U = 0.5$,
- $P = 20 \times 10^{-6}$ Sv/wk   (0.02 mSv/wk) .

Solution

The transmission of the primary barrier is given by

$$B_{\mathrm{pri}} = \frac{P \dfrac{\mathrm{Gy}}{\mathrm{wk}} \times \left(\dfrac{d_{\mathrm{pri}}}{d_1}\right)^2}{W \dfrac{\mathrm{Gy}}{\mathrm{wk}} \times U \times T} \tag{10.29}$$

$$B_{\mathrm{pri}} = \frac{20 \times 10^{-6} \dfrac{\mathrm{Sv}}{\mathrm{wk}} \times \left(\dfrac{6.3\,\mathrm{m}}{1\,\mathrm{m}}\right)^2}{800 \dfrac{\mathrm{Sv}}{\mathrm{wk}} \times 0.5 \times 0.2} = 9.92 \times 10^{-6}.$$

The number of tenth value layers (TVLs) necessary to accomplish this degree of attenuation is calculated from

$$n = \log \frac{1}{B_{\mathrm{pri}}} \tag{10.30}$$

$$n = \log \frac{1}{9.92 \times 10^{-6}} = 5.0.$$

Table 10-7 lists the first TVL, TVL_1, and the equilibrium TVL, TVL_e, for concrete, steel, and lead for various primary-beam quantum energies. The TVL_1 differs from TVL_e in order to account for changes in the spectral distribution of the radiation as it penetrates the shielding barrier. In Table 10-7, we find TVL_1 to be 37-cm concrete, and TVL_e to be 33-cm concrete. The required thickness of concrete is

$$t_{barrier} = TVL_1 + (n-1)TVL_e \tag{10.31}$$

$$t_{barrier} = 37\,cm + (5.0-1) \times 33\,cm = 169\,cm\,(66.5\,in.)$$

Now we must see whether this barrier thickness meets the TADR limit of 20×10^{-6} Sv in 1 week (2 mrems in 1 week). The maximum IDR at the dose point, with the calculated transmission factor of 7.2×10^{-6} is calculated as follows:

$$IDR = \frac{600\,\dfrac{Sv}{h} \times 9.92 \times 10^{-6} \times (1m)^2}{(6.3\,m)^2} = 1.5 \times 10^{-4}\,\frac{Sv}{h}.$$

When we substitute this value into Eq. (10.28), we have

$$R_W = \frac{IDR\,\dfrac{Sv}{h} \times W_{pri}\,\dfrac{Gy}{wk} \times U_{pri}}{\dot{D}_0\,\dfrac{Gy}{h}}$$

$$= \frac{1.5 \times 10^{-4}\,\dfrac{Sv}{h} \times 800\,\dfrac{Gy}{wk} \times 0.5}{600\,\dfrac{Gy}{h}}$$

$$= 100 \times 10^{-6}\,\frac{Sv}{wk} = 100\,\mu\frac{Sv}{wk}.$$

This TADR is five times greater than the required value of 20 μSv/wk. Increasing the thickness of the concrete barrier by 3 HVLs (1 TVL = 3.3 HVL) would decrease the TADR to 12.5 μSv/wk, which is reasonably conservative and would allow for an increased utilization of the facility. If we choose to do this, then the barrier thickness would be

$$t_{barrier} = 165\,cm + 3\,HVL \times \frac{\dfrac{33\,cm}{TVL}}{\dfrac{3.3\,HVL}{TVL}} = 195\,cm.$$

Since the primary barrier is much thicker than the other walls, which shield the secondary (scatter and leakage) radiation, the width of the primary barrier is usually restricted to one that is functionally effective. Good design practice specifies that the width of the primary barrier must be greater by at least 30.5 cm (1 ft.) on each side of the maximum-sized projection of the primary beam on the barrier (Fig. 10-21). That is, its width is 61 cm (2 ft.) greater than the projection of the primary beam at its greatest possible size. The widest possible beam projection occurs when the collimator is rotated by 45°. Since the diagonal of a square is equal to 1.414 $\times$ length of the side, and the length of the projected side is given by

$$\frac{s_1\,cm}{d_1} = \frac{s_2\,cm}{d_2},$$

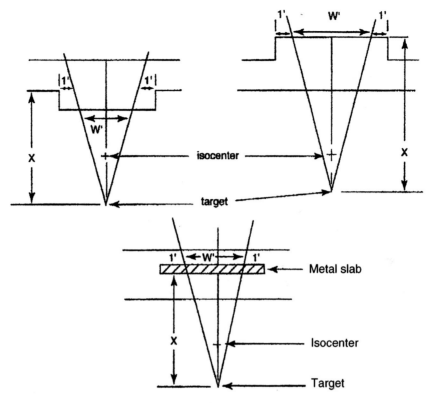

Figure 10-21. Widths of primary barriers. The lower figure shows a metal slab that is embedded in the concrete to provide the additional shielding for the primary beam. (Reproduced with permission from McGinley PH. *Shielding Techniques for Radiation Oncology Facilities.* 2nd ed. Madison, WI: Medical Physics Publishing Corp; 2002:Fig 2-3, pg 27.)

where

s_1 = length of side at distance d_1 from the X-Ray target and

s_2 = length of projected side at a distance of d_2 from the X-Ray target.

The width of the projected beam on the primary barrier wall is

$$w\,(\text{projected beam}) = 1.414 \times s_1 \times \frac{d_2}{d_1}. \tag{10.32}$$

For this example:

$s_1 = 40$ cm,
$d_2 = 7.3$ m $-\,0.3$ m $-\,1.95$ m $= 5.05$ m, and
$d_1 = 1$ m.

The width of the primary barrier, therefore, is

$$w\,(\text{primary barrier}) = 1.414 \times 40\,\text{cm} \times \frac{5.05\,\text{m}}{1\,\text{m}} + 61\,\text{cm} = 347\,\text{cm}.$$

EXAMPLE 10.11

Calculate the secondary concrete barrier thickness for the wall that separates the therapy room in Example 10.10 from a laboratory, given the following additional information:

- $P = 20 \times 10^{-6}$ Sv/wk (0.02 mSv/wk), since the laboratory is not controlled,
- d_{sec}, dose control point, is equidistant from the X-ray target in the accelerator head and the patient scattering position at the isocenter, $d_{sec} = 7.1$ m,
- mean treatment field size, F, = 225 cm^2,
- dose point in the adjacent laboratory is directly opposite the isocenter, and
- T = occupancy factor = 1.

Solution

The origin of most secondary radiation from accelerators whose photon energy ≤10 MeV is radiation scattered by the patient and leakage radiation from the accelerator head. When designing the secondary barrier, only radiation scattered from materials in the primary beam is considered. Scattered radiation intensity depends on the scattering angle, on the energy of the primary beam, and on the scattering area (field size). Table 10-8 lists the intensity ratio, at a scattering angle of 90°, of the scattered-to-incident radiation at a distance of 1 m from the scatterer for a field size (scattering area) of 400 cm^2. On the assumption that the intensity of the scattered radiation varies inversely with the square of the distance from the scatterer and varies directly with the scattering area, the exposure from the scattered radiation, the maximum barrier transmission for radiation scattered by the patient is given in NCRP 147 as

$$B_{ps} = \frac{P}{\alpha\,WT} \times d_{sca}^2 \times d_{sec}^2 \times \frac{400}{F} \tag{10.33}$$

where

P = shielding design goal, usually expressed as Sv or mSv per week,
α = fraction of the absorbed dose in the primary beam that is scattered by the patient through a given angle; in shielding design, scatter through 90° is considered appropriate,

TABLE 10-8. 90° Scatter Fraction (α) at 1 m From a Human-Sized Phantom, Target-to-Phantom Distance of 1 m, and Field Size of 400 cm^2

ACCELERATOR VOLTAGE (MV) →	6	10	18	24
α →	4.26×10^{-4}	3.81×10^{-4}	1.89×10^{-4}	1.74×10^{-4}

Abstracted from *Structural Shielding Design and Evaluation for Megavoltage X- and Gamma-Ray Radiotherapy Facilities.* Bethesda, MD: National Council on Radiation Protection & Measurement; 2005. NCRP Report 151.

W = workload, Gy/wk,

T = occupancy factor, and

F = actual cross-sectional area of the beam at 1 meter, cm^2.

The barrier transmission factor for leakage radiation is given in NCRP 147 as

$$B_L = \frac{1000 \times P \times d_L^2}{W \times T}.$$

The factor of 1000 accounts for the fact that leakage radiation at a distance of 1 m from the target may not exceed 0.1% of the workload.

The scattered radiation barrier transmission is found by substituting the appropriate values into Eq. (10.33). The value of α for 90° scatter is found in Table 10-8.

$$B_{ps} = \frac{P}{\alpha\, WT} \times d_{sca}^2 \times d_{sec}^2 \times \frac{400}{F}$$

$$B_{ps} = \frac{20 \times 10^{-6}\ \dfrac{Sv}{wk}}{4.26 \times 10^{-4} \times 800\ \dfrac{Gy}{wk} \times 1} \times (1\,\mathrm{m})^2 \times (6.3\,\mathrm{m})^2 \times \frac{400\,\mathrm{cm}^2}{225\,\mathrm{cm}^2} = 4.1 \times 10^{-3}.$$

The number of TVLs to attain this degree of attenuation is

$$n = \log\frac{1}{B_{ps}} = \log\frac{1}{4.1 \times 10^{-3}} = 2.4.$$

The required maximum transmission of leakage radiation is calculated by substituting the appropriate values in Eq. (10.33):

$$B_L = \frac{1000 \times P \times d_L^2}{W \times T} = \frac{1000 \times 20 \times 10^{-6}\ \dfrac{Gy}{wk} \times (6.3\,\mathrm{m})^2}{800\ \dfrac{Gy}{wk}} = 9.9 \times 10^{-4}.$$

The number to TVLs required to reach 9.9×10^{-4} is

$$n = \log\frac{1}{B_L} = \log\frac{1}{9.9 \times 10^{-4}} = 3.$$

According to the recommended design practice, when the two calculated barrier thicknesses are close together, as in this case, we add 1 HVL to the thicker barrier. If the two barrier thicknesses differ by a TVL or more, we simply use the thicker barrier. In this example, the barrier thickness for the leakage radiation is not much greater than that for the scattered radiation. We therefore add 1 HVL to the thicker barrier. In Table 10-9, we find TLV$_1$ and the TLV$_e$ for 6-MV X-rays to be 34- and 29-cm concrete respectively. Since 3.3 HVL = 1 TVL, the required barrier thickness is

$$t_{secondary} = 34\,\mathrm{cm} + (3-1) \times 29\,\mathrm{cm} + \frac{29\,\mathrm{cm}}{3.3} = 101\,\mathrm{cm}.$$

TABLE 10-9. Tenth Value Layers (TVLs) of Concrete for Leakage Radiation

ACCELERATOR VOLTAGE (MV)	TVL$_1$ (cm)	TVL$_e$(cm)
4	33	28
6	34	29
10	35	31
15	36	33
18	36	34
20	36	34
25	37	35
30	37	36
^{60}Co	21	21

Reproduced with permission of the National Council on Radiation Protection and Measurements from *Structural Shielding Design and Evaluation for Megavoltage X- and Gamma-Ray Radiotherapy Facilities.* Bethesda, MD: National Council on Radiation Protection & Measurement; 2005. NCRP Report 151.

As shown in the example above, even the secondary barrier is very thick, usually on the order of 1–1.25 m (3–4 ft.) concrete. To shield the entrance doorway into the treatment room would require a massive amount of lead, the exact thickness would depend on the distance of the doorway from the accelerator head. To reduce the shield thickness at the door, megavoltage therapy rooms are designed in the form of a maze (Fig. 10-20). The maze wall is a barrier that reduces the patient-scattered radiation and the leakage radiation at the door to a manageable level. To reach the door, the patient-scattered radiation must again be scattered through a large angle, thereby greatly decreasing the energy of the scattered photons and making it easier to shield the radiation at the door. Details for the design of a maze may be found in NCRP 151.

Neutron Production

Except for the ^{9}Be$(\gamma, n)^8$Be reaction whose gamma threshold energy is 1.666 MeV, all other thresholds for photoneutron production are about 8.5 MeV, and production becomes significant at quantum energies greater than 10 MeV. The neutron energy spectrum is almost independent of the photon energy at these energies, and the average neutron energy is about 1–2 MeV, depending on the exact photodisintegration reaction. The energy spectrum of the neutrons is important to the health physicist because the response of the neutron survey meter may depend on energy of the neutrons. Most neutron-surveying instruments are calibrated with one of the following three sources:

- Pu–Be, whose average neutron energy = 4.2 MeV,
- Am–Be, whose average neutron energy = 4.5 MeV, or
- ^{252}Cf, whose fission neutron spectrum is similar to the spectral distribution of the photoneutrons, and whose average neutron energy, 2.2 MeV, is not far from that of the photoneutrons.

Photoneutron production is important in shielding design for three reasons:

- Neutrons add to the X-ray dose, and must be accounted for in the shield design.
- The neutrons may be absorbed by material in the environment and make the absorbing atoms radioactive, thus leaving radioactivity and a radiation field after the machine is turned off.

- Gamma rays (capture gammas) are almost always produced in the neutron absorption reactions. The average energy of capture gammas in concrete is 3.6 MeV.

Shielding design of high-energy radiotherapy facilities is based on well-known principles of bremsstrahlung production, interaction of photons with matter, neutron production, and neutron interactions, including absorption and activation. However, the application of these principles to the design of a particular facility is a very complex undertaking. Detailed application of these principles may be found in several applied publications, such as NCRP 144, NCRP 147, and NCRP 151. The complexity of shielding design for high-energy radiation therapy facilities makes shielding design an ideal candidate for computerization, and numerous computer codes may be found in the literature.

Airborne Contaminant Production

Interaction of energy by the atmosphere from environmental radiation fields can lead to radiolytic dissociation of oxygen and nitrogen molecules in the air. The resulting disrupted molecules can recombine to form ozone, nitrogen oxide, and nitrogen dioxide. Ozone, whose OSHA permissible exposure level (PEL) is 0.1 parts per million (ppm), and nitrogen dioxide, whose PEL is 5 ppm, are of concern because of their relatively high toxicity. Neutrons can interact with the ^{40}Ar constituent in ordinary air to produce 110-minute half-lived ^{41}Ar, and with atmospheric dusts to produce airborne radioactive particles. According to NCRP 147, ventilation of a normal clinical treatment room at a rate of three air changes per hour is sufficient for health protection.

Beta Shielding

Two factors must be considered in designing a shield against high-intensity radiation—namely, the beta particles and the bremsstrahlung that are generated due to absorption in the source itself and in the shield. Because of these factors, the beta shield consists of a low-atomic-numbered substance (to minimize the production of bremsstrahlung) sufficiently thick to stop all the betas, followed by a high-atomic-numbered material thick enough to attenuate the bremsstrahlung intensity to an acceptable level.

TABLE 10-10. Tenth Value Layers (TVLs) of Concrete for Patient-Scattered Radiation at 90° Scattering Angle

ACCELERATOR VOLTAGE (MV)	TVL (cm)
4	17
6	17
10	18

Reproduced with permission of the National Council on Radiation Protection and Measurements from *Structural Shielding Design and Evaluation for Megavoltage X- and Gamma-Ray Radiotherapy Facilities*. Bethesda, MD: National Council on Radiation Protection & Measurement; 2005. NCRP Report 151.

EXAMPLE 10.12

Fifty milliliters of aqueous solution containing 37×10^4 MBq (10 Ci) carrier-free ^{90}Sr in equilibrium with ^{90}Y is to be stored in a laboratory. The health physicist requires the dose-equivalent rate at a distance of 50 cm from the center of the solution to be no greater than 0.1 mSv (10 mrems) per hour. Design the necessary shielding to meet this requirement.

Solution

The maximum and mean beta energies of ^{90}Sr and ^{90}Y are as follows:

	E_{max}(MeV)	E_{mean} (MeV)
^{90}Sr	0.54	0.19
^{90}Y	2.27	0.93
Sum		1.12

The beta shield must be thick enough to stop the 2.27-MeV ^{90}Y betas. From Figure 5-4, the range of a 2.27-MeV beta is found to be 1.1 g/cm^2. Let us use a bottle made of polyethylene, specific gravity $= 0.95$, as the container for the radioactive solution. The wall thickness of the bottle must be

$$t_{wall} = \frac{1.1 \ \dfrac{g}{cm^2}}{0.95 \ \dfrac{g}{cm^3}} = 1.16 \, cm.$$

The bremsstrahlung is especially important in this case, since ^{90}Sr and ^{90}Y are pure beta emitters, and thus there are no gammas to be shielded. To estimate the bremsstrahlung dose rate at a distance of 50 cm, we first calculate the rate at which energy is carried by the betas:

$$\dot{E}_\beta = 3.7 \times 10^{11} Bq \times 1 \ \frac{tps}{Bq} \times 1.12 \ \frac{MeV}{transf} = 4.14 \times 10^{11} \ \frac{MeV}{s}.$$

Then we calculate the fraction of this beta energy that is converted into bremsstrahlung with the aid of Eq. (5.12):

$$f = 3.5 \times 10^{-4} \times Z_e \times E_{max}.$$

In this case, most of the beta-ray energy will be dissipated in the water. The effective atomic number Z_e for bremsstrahlung production of a mixture or compound is

$$Z_e = \frac{N_1 Z_1^2 + N_2 Z_2^2 + \cdots N_i Z_i^2}{N_1 Z_1 + N_2 Z_2 \cdots N_i Z_i} = \frac{\sum_i N_i Z_i^2}{\sum_i N_i Z_i} \qquad \textbf{(10.34)}$$

where

N_i = number of atoms of the ith element per cm^3 and

Z_i = atomic number of the ith element.

For water, H_2O, density = 1 g/cm^3, formula weight = 18, we have

$$N_H = 1\,\text{cm}^3 \times 1\,\frac{\text{g}}{\text{cm}^3} \times \frac{1\,\text{mol}}{18\,\text{g}} \times 6.03 \times 10^{23}\,\frac{\text{molecules}}{\text{mol}} \times 2\,\frac{\text{atom}}{\text{molecule}}$$

$$N_H = 6.7 \times 10^{22}\ \text{atoms/cm}^3,$$

and

$$N_O = 0.5 \times N_H = 3.35 \times 10^{22}\ \text{atoms/cm}^3.$$

Substituting the numerical values into Eq. (10.34) gives $Z_e = 6.6$, and substituting this value for Z_e into Eq. (5.12a) gives us the fraction of the beta-ray energy that is converted into bremsstrahlung:

$$f = 3.5 \times 10^{-4} \times 6.6 \times 2.27 = 5.24 \times 10^{-3}.$$

If the bremsstrahlung is considered to radiate from a virtual point in the center of the solution, then the exposure dose rate at a distance d meters from this point is given by

$$\dot{D} = \frac{f \times E\,\dfrac{\text{MeV}}{\text{s}} \times 1.6 \times 10^{-13}\,\dfrac{\text{J}}{\text{MeV}} \times \mu\,\text{m}^{-1} \times 3.6 \times 10^3\,\dfrac{\text{s}}{\text{h}}}{1.293\,\dfrac{\text{kg}}{\text{m}^3} \times 4\pi\,d^2 \times 1\,\dfrac{\text{J/kg}}{\text{Gy}} \times 10^{-3}\,\dfrac{\text{Gy}}{\text{mSv}}}, \tag{10.35}$$

where μ is the linear energy absorption coefficient for the quantum energy of the bremsstrahlung. In calculating bremsstrahlung dose rate for radiation safety purposes, we use the quantum energy corresponding to the average beta-ray energy, which in the case of ^{90}Y is 0.93 MeV. Using the value $\mu = 3.7 \times 10^{-3}\ \text{m}^{-1}$ (from Fig. 5-19), we use Eq. (10.35) to calculate the bremsstrahlung exposure dose rate at a distance of 0.5 m from the aqueous solution of ^{90}Sr—^{90}Y to be 1.14 mSv (114 mrads) per hour.

   If we add a lead shield of thickness t cm, then the attenuation of the bremsstrahlung exposure dose rate can be calculated from Eq. (5.27), using a value of μ corresponding to the maximum energy beta particle. From Table 5-3, we find that $\mu = 0.51\ \text{cm}^{-1}$ for 2.27 MeV. Thus, we have

$$I = I_0 e^{-\mu t}$$

$$0.1 = 1.14 \times e^{-0.51 \times t}$$

$$t = 4.8\,\text{cm}.$$

Use of a buildup factor in this case is not explicitly necessary, since it was assumed in the calculation of the shield thickness that all the bremsstrahlung had quantum energy equal to the maximum energy of the beta particles that gave rise to the X-rays. However, this quantum energy is, in fact, the upper limit of the bremsstrahlung energy, and all the bremsstrahlung is much lower in energy than this upper limit. The thickness calculated above, therefore, implicitly accounts for buildup through the use of an attenuation coefficient for the upper-energy limit of the X-rays rather than for their average energy.

Neutrons

Shielding against neutrons is based on slowing down fast neutrons and absorbing thermal neutrons. In Chapter 5, it was seen that attenuation and absorption of neutrons is a complex series of events. Despite the complexity, however, the required shielding around a neutron source can be estimated by the use of removal cross sections. (For neutron energies up to 30 MeV, the removal cross section is about three-quarters of the total cross section.) In designing shielding against neutrons, it must be borne in mind that absorption of neutrons can lead to induced radioactivity and to the production of gamma radiation (capture gammas) when the neutron is absorbed into a nucleus.

 EXAMPLE 10.13

Design a shield for an 18.5×10^4 MBq (5 Ci) Pu–Be neutron source that emits 5×10^6 neutrons/s, such that the dose rate at the outside surface of the shield will not exceed 0.02 mSv/h (20 μSv/h or 2 mrems/h). The mean energy of the neutrons produced in this source is 4 MeV.

Solution

Let us make the shield of water and compute the minimum radius for the case of a spherical shield. Since we know that the capture of a neutron by hydrogen produces a 2.26-MeV gamma ray, let us allow for the gamma-ray dose by designing the shield to give a maximum fast-neutron dose rate of 0.01 mSv/h (1 mrem/h), which corresponds to a fast flux of 3.7 neutrons/cm^2/s (Table 9-5). The total cross section for 4-MeV neutrons for hydrogen and oxygen are 1.9 and 1.7 b, respectively. Since water contains 6.7×10^{22} hydrogen atoms and 3.35×10^{22} oxygen atoms per cm^3, the linear absorption coefficient, Σ, of water is

$$\sum = 1.9 \times 10^{-24} \frac{cm^2}{atom} \times 6.7 \times 10^{22} \frac{atoms}{cm^3} + 1.7 \times 10^{-24} \frac{cm^2}{atom} \times 3.5 \times 10^{22} \frac{atoms}{cm^3}$$

$$\sum = 0.187 \, cm^{-1},$$

which corresponds to an HVL of 3.71 cm. The Pu–Be may be considered as a point source of neutrons, with the neutron flux decreasing with increasing distance as a result of both inverse square dispersion and attenuation by the water. If S is the source strength in neutrons s^{-1}, $T_{1/2}$ is the HVL in cm, n is the number of HVL, and B is the buildup factor, the fast-neutron flux, after passing through a thickness of $nT_{1/2}$ cm, is

$$\phi = \frac{BS}{4\pi\,(nT_{1/2})^2} \times \frac{1}{2^n} = \frac{\text{neutrons}}{\text{cm}^2/\text{s}}. \tag{10.36}$$

For radioactive neutron sources on the order of several curies, the shield thickness is relatively large, and a significant dose buildup due to scattered neutrons results. For a hydrogenous shield at least 20 cm thick, the dose-buildup factor is approximately 5. Using a value of 3.7 neutrons/cm^2/s for ϕ, 3.71 cm for $T_{1/2}$, and 5 for B, Eq. (10.36) may be solved for n to give about 9 HVLs, which corresponds to a thickness of 34 cm of water.

The thermal neutrons that would escape from the surface of a spherical water shield may be estimated with the aid of Eq. (5.65):

$$\phi_{\text{th}} = \frac{S}{4\pi\,RD} \times e^{-R/L}.$$

Since the shield radius calculated above is much greater than the fast diffusion length (which is equal to 5.75 cm), we may assume, for the purpose of this calculation, that essentially all the fast neutrons are thermalized and that the thermal neutrons are diffusing outward from the center. Substituting the appropriate numbers (D and L from Table 5-6 and R = shield radius) into Eq. (5.65), we have

$$\phi_{\text{th}} = \frac{5 \times 10^6 \text{ neutrons} \cdot \text{s}^{-1}}{4\pi \times 34 \text{ cm} \times 0.16 \text{ cm}} \times e^{-34/2.8} = 0.4 \frac{\text{neutrons}}{\text{cm}^2/\text{s}}.$$

This thermal-neutron flux is so small relative to the recommended maximum thermal flux of 270 neutrons/cm^2/s (Table 9-5), that it may, for most practical purposes, be ignored.

Capture of a thermal neutron by a hydrogen atom results in the prompt emission of a 2.26-MeV gamma ray. The water shield, therefore, acts as a distributed source of gamma radiation. Since 3.7 fast neutrons/cm^2/s escape from the surface, the total number of those that escape from a sphere of radius 34 cm is 5.4×10^4 neutrons/s, or approximately 0.96% of the source neutrons. The remaining 99.04% are absorbed in the water, thus giving a mean "specific activity" for 2.26-MeV photons of

$$\frac{4.95 \times 10^6 \text{ neutrons/s}}{\frac{4}{3}\pi\,(34 \text{ cm})^3} = 30 \frac{\text{"Bq"}}{\text{cm}^3} \left(\frac{810\text{"pCi"}}{\text{cm}^3} \right).$$

The dose rate at the surface of a sphere containing a uniformly distributed gamma emitter is, from Eqs. (6.66) and (6.71),

$$\dot{D} = \frac{1}{2} \times C\Gamma \times \frac{4\pi}{\mu}(1 - e^{-\mu r}). \tag{10.37}$$

Using a value 2.7 mSv/h per MBq (10^4 mrems/h per mCi) at 1 cm for Γ, 0.022 cm^{-1} for μ in case of 2.26-MeV photons in water, and 34 cm for the radius gives

$$\dot{D} = \frac{1}{2} \times 30 \times 10^{-6} \frac{\text{Bq}}{\text{cm}^3} \times 2.7 \frac{\text{mSv} \cdot \text{cm}^2}{\text{MBq} \cdot \text{h}} \times \frac{4\pi}{0.022 \, \text{cm}^{-1}} (1 - e^{-0.022 \times 34})$$

$$\dot{D} = 1.2 \times 10^{-2} \, \text{mSv/h} \, (1.2 \, \text{mrems/h}).$$

The dose rate at the surface of the shield due to both neutrons and gamma rays is 22 μSv/h (2.2 mrems/h), which is very close to the desired figure of 20 μSv/h (2 mrems/h). The gamma-ray dose rate could be reduced either by increasing the gamma-ray absorption coefficient of the water shield by dissolving a high-atomic-numbered substance, such as BaCl$_2$, or by reducing the rate of production of the gamma radiation. Of these possible alternatives, the simplest one is the reduction in the production of gamma radiation. This is easily accomplished merely by dissolving a boron compound in the water. Boron captures thermal neutrons with a capture cross section of 755 b, according to the reaction $^{10}\text{B} + ^1 n \rightarrow ^7 \text{Li} + \gamma$ (0.48 MeV). The 0.48-MeV gamma is emitted in 93% of the captures. Either sodium tetraborate (borax), Na$_2$B$_4$O$_7 \cdot 10 \text{H}_2\text{O}$, or boric acid, H$_3BO_3$, both of which are highly soluble in water and very inexpensive, may be considered for this application. If suppression of gamma radiation is the objective, boric acid may be preferred over borax, since the sodium in the borax has a relatively high cross section, 505 mb, for the $^{23}\text{Na}(n, \gamma)^{24}\text{Na}$ reaction. As a consequence of this reaction, a 6.96-MeV capture gamma is emitted and radioactive ^{24}Na, which emits one 1.39-MeV beta, one 1.37-MeV gamma, and one 2.75-MeV gamma per disintegration is produced.

The solubility of boric acid in water at room temperature is 63.2 g/L. The formula weight of H$_3$BO$_3$ is 61.84. The concentration of boron atoms in the saturated solution is

$$C_{\text{boron}} = \frac{63.2 \, \frac{\text{g}}{\text{L}} \times 10^{-3} \, \frac{\text{L}}{\text{mL}} \times 6.02 \times 10^{23} \, \frac{\text{molecules}}{\text{mol}} \times 1 \, \frac{\text{atom B}}{\text{molecule}}}{61.84 \, \frac{\text{g}}{\text{mol}}}$$

$$C_{\text{boron}} = 6.15 \times 10^{20} \, \text{atoms/mL}.$$

If we consider the macroscopic cross sections for thermal-neutron capture of the dissolved boron Σ_B and of the hydrogen Σ_H, we find that

$$\frac{\Sigma_H}{\Sigma_B} = \frac{0.13 \, \text{cm}^{-1}}{0.42 \, \text{cm}^{-1}} = 0.31.$$

The flux of 2.26-MeV hydrogen gamma rays, and consequently the dose rate, will be reduced by this factor to 0.31×0.012 mSv/h $= 3.7 \times 10^{-3}$ mSv/h (0.37 mrem/h). The dose rate due to the ^{10}B capture gammas, which is calculated from Eq. (10.37) using a photon specific activity of $0.69 \times 30 \times 10^{-6}$ "MBq"/cm^3 (5.6×10^{-7} "mCi"/cm^3), an absorption coefficient for 0.48-MeV photons in water of 0.033 cm^{-1}, and a value for Γ of 0.62 mGy-cm^2/MBq-h (2300 mrads-cm^2/mCi-h), is found to be 1.7×10^{-3} mSv/h (0.17 mrem/h). The total dose-equivalent rate at the shield surface, therefore, is

    0.01 mSv/h (1 mrem/h) fast neutrons

$+$ 0.0037 mSv/h (0.037 mrem/h) from hydrogen capture gammas

$+$ 0.0017 mSv/h (0.17 mrem/h) due to boron capture gammas

$=$ 0.015 mSv/h (1.5 mrem/h) if we saturate the water with boric acid.

OPTIMIZATION

According to ICRP recommendations, and recommended maximum dose limits notwithstanding, operations involving exposure to ionizing radiation should be designed so that "any unnecessary exposure should be avoided" and that "all exposures shall be kept as low as reasonably achievable (ALARA), economic and social factors being taken into account." Because the ICRP radiation safety recommendations are based on a zero-threshold dose-response model, and because we do not have infinite resources to commit to radiation safety, the ICRP went on to recommend that this ALARA principle be implemented on the basis of optimization of radiation protection efforts. *Optimization* is the attainment of a balance between the radiation safety benefits obtained from the resources committed to radiation safety and benefits obtained by committing these resources to other avenues. This method of cost–benefit optimization is illustrated in Figure 10-22. This figure shows graphically the cost of the sum of the detrimental effects of radiation, the *detriment*, which are assumed to be directly proportional to the collective dose to the population being protected plus the cost of radiation protection as a function of the collective dose. The amount of radiation protection leading to the minimum in the curve is considered the optimum degree of radiation protection. This ALARA concept has been incorporated into the International Atomic Energy Agency's Basic Safety Standards and into the regulations of the various national regulatory agencies.

Expressed mathematically, the net benefit B of a given procedure is determined by the following equation:

$$B = V - P - X - Y, \tag{10.38}$$

where

    $V =$ gross value of the procedure,

    $P =$ cost of the procedure, exclusive of the cost of protection,

    $X =$ protection cost, and

    $Y =$ detriment cost.

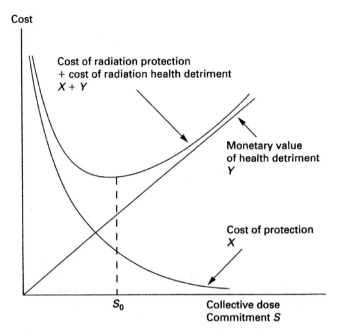

Figure 10-22. Optimization of radiation protection. (Reproduced with permission from *Basic Safety Standards for Radiation Protection*. Vienna, Austria: International Atomic Energy Agency; 1982.)

To optimize protection, $X + Y$ must be minimized. If $\alpha =$ cost per unit radiation detriment and the detriment from a given procedure is S, then the cost of this detriment is

$$Y = \alpha S, \tag{10.39}$$

and the quantity to be minimized is

$$X + Y = X + \alpha S. \tag{10.40}$$

If the costs of protection and detriment are a function of a parameter Z (for example, increased shielding thickness or increased ventilation rate), the minimum in the curve of cost versus dose in Figure 10-26 occurs when

$$\frac{dX}{dZ} + \alpha \frac{dS}{dZ} = 0, \tag{10.41}$$

that is,

$$\frac{dX}{dZ} = -\alpha \frac{dS}{dZ}. \tag{10.42}$$

If we wish to optimize a shield thickness, then the cost of the shield is

$$X = CAt, \tag{10.43}$$

where

C = cost per unit volume of the shield,

A = area of the shield, and

t = thickness of the shield.

The decreased radiation detriment due to the additional shielding, expressed as decreased collective dose, is given by

$$S = \dot{H} e^{-\mu t} \times f \times N \times \tau, \tag{10.44}$$

where

$\dot{H}$ = maximum dose-equivalent rate in the shielded area,

f = ratio of the average to maximum dose rates in the shielded area,

N = number of people in the shielded area,

τ = lifetime of the shielded installation,

μ = effective attenuation coefficient of shielding material, and

t = thickness of the additional shielding.

When we differentiate X and S with respect to the shield thickness t, we get

$$\frac{dX}{dt} = C \times A \tag{10.45}$$

and

$$\frac{dS}{dt} = \dot{H} \times f \times N \times \tau (-\mu) e^{-\mu t}. \tag{10.46}$$

Substituting these two derivatives into Eq. (10.42), we have

$$CA = \alpha \times \dot{H} \times f \times N \times \tau \times \mu e^{-\mu t} \tag{10.47}$$

$$e^{-\mu t} = \frac{CA}{\alpha \times \dot{H} \times f \times N \times \tau \times \mu}. \tag{10.48}$$

Equation (10.48) may be solved for t, the optimum shield thickness:

$$t = \left(\ln \frac{CA}{\alpha \times \dot{H} \times f \times N \times \tau \times \mu} \right) \times \left(\frac{1}{-\mu} \right). \tag{10.49}$$

EXAMPLE 10.14

A concrete shield 1 m thick × 2.5 m high × 4 m wide is designed to reduce the radiation level to 25 μSv (2.5 mrems) per hour at the surface of the shield. If 15 persons work in the shielded area, their average dose rate is 2.5 μSv (0.25 mrem) per hour, and the installation is expected to last 20 years, how much additional shielding, if any, should be added if concrete costs $150 m^{-3} and a person-Sv is worth $1,000,000 ($10,000 per person-rem). The effective μ of the concrete, including the buildup factor at this shield thickness, is 0.17 cm^{-1}.

Solution

If we substitute the respective values into Eq. (10.49), we obtain

$$
t = \ln \left(\frac{\dfrac{\$150}{m^3} \times 10\,m^2}{\dfrac{\$10^6}{(\text{person} \cdot \text{Sv})} \times 25 \times 10^{-6}\,\dfrac{\text{Sv}}{\text{h}} \times 0.1 \times 2000\,\dfrac{\text{h}}{\text{yr}} \times 15\,\text{persons} \times 20\,\text{years} \times \dfrac{17}{m}} \right) \times \left(\dfrac{m}{-17} \right)
$$

$t = 0.57\,\text{m additional concrete thickness.}$

SUMMARY

Protection against external radiation is based on the application of one or more of the following three basic principles:

- *Time*—Minimizing exposure time.
- *Distance*—Maximizing distance from the source.
- *Shielding*—Interposing a shield between the source and the receptor.

The dose rate at any distance from a source may be estimated if we know the activity of the source, the specific gamma-ray constant, and the geometric configuration (i.e., a point, plane, or volume source). Gamma and X-ray shields do not completely stop all the radiation. However, the radiation intensity can be reduced to any desired level by specifying the appropriate shield thickness. Generally, high-atomic-numbered materials, such as lead, are more effective than low-atomic-numbered materials in shielding X-rays or gamma rays.

In the case of beta radiation, on the other hand, low-atomic-numbered shielding material is preferred over high-atomic-numbered shields because bremsstrahlung production increases as the atomic number of the beta shield is increased. In the case of beta shielding, the beta radiation can be completely stopped by making the shield thickness equal to or greater than the range of the betas. In designing a shield for a pure high-energy beta emitter, the bremsstrahlung produced in the shield must be considered in the shielding design.

Neutron shielding is based on slowing down fast neutrons to thermal energies and then absorbing the thermal neutrons. Low-atomic-numbered materials, such as water, and hydrogenous compounds, such as paraffin, are effective slowing-down materials. The thermalized neutrons are most readily absorbed by materials that have a high absorption cross section, such as boron or cadmium. In designing shielding against neutrons, it must be remembered that absorption of neutrons can lead to capture gammas and to induced radioactivity and the consequent production of gamma radiation.

Although radiation protection measures can be designed to reduce radiation dose to levels approaching that of the natural background, expenditure of resources to do this may be wasteful since the benefits that accrue from such low doses are less than the benefits that might result from expenditure of these resources in other avenues. Accordingly, we optimize the degree of radiation protection at the level at which the benefits are equal to the cost of protection.

PROBLEMS

10.1. A Po–Be neutron source emits 10^7 neutrons/s of average energy 4 MeV. The source is to be stored in a paraffin shield of sufficient thickness to reduce the fast flux at the surface to 10 neutrons/cm^2/s. Consider paraffin to be essentially CH$_2$ (for the purpose of this problem) and to have a density of 0.89 g/cm^3.

  (a) What is the minimum thickness of the paraffin shield?

  (b) If the slowing-down length is 6 cm, the thermal diffusion length is 3 cm, and the diffusion coefficient is 0.381 cm, what will be the thermal-neutron leakage flux at the surface of the shield?

  (c) What is the gamma-ray dose rate, due to the hydrogen-capture gammas, at the surface of the paraffin shield?

10.2. An X-ray therapy machine operates at 250 kVp and 20 mA. At a target to skin distance of 100 cm, the dose rate is 0.2 Gy/min. The workload is 100 Gy/wk. The X-ray tube is constrained to point vertically downward. At a distance of 4 m from the target is an uncontrolled waiting room. Calculate the thickness of lead to be added to the wall if the total thickness of the wall (which is made of hollow tile and plaster, density 2.35 g/cm^3) is 2 in. (5 cm).

10.3. A 7.4×10^{13} Bq (2000 Ci) ^{60}Co teletherapy unit is to be installed in an existing concrete room in the basement of a hospital so that the source is 4 m from the north and west walls—which are 30 in. thick. Beyond the north wall is a fully occupied controlled room. Beyond the west wall is a public parking lot. The useful beam is to be directed toward the north wall for a maximum of 5 hours per week during radiation therapy. The beam will be directed at the west wall 1 hour per week. Considering only the radiation from the primary beam, how much additional shielding, if any, is required for each of the walls?

10.4. A radiochemist wants to carry a small vial containing 2×10^9 Bq (~ 50 mCi) ^{60}Co solution from one hood to another. If the estimated carrying time is 3 minutes, what would be the minimum length of the tongs used to carry the vial in order that his dose not exceed 60 μGy (6 mrads) during the operation?

10.5. A viewing window for use with an isotope that emits 1-MeV gamma rays is to be made from a saturated aqueous solution of KI in a rectangular battery jar. What will be the attenuation factor, assuming conditions of good geometry, if the solution thickness is 10 cm and if the glass walls are equivalent in their attenuation property to 1-mm lead? A saturated solution of KI may be made by adding 30-g KI to 21-mL water to give a 30-mL solution at 25°C. Total attenuation cross sections for 1-MeV gamma rays for the elements in the solution are given in the table below:

ELEMENT	ATTENUATION CROSS SECTION (BARNS)
K	4
H	0.2
I	12
O	1.7

10.6. Lead foil, whose specific gravity is 10.4, consists of an alloy containing 87% Pb, 12% Sn, and 1% Cu. If the mass attenuation coefficients for these three elements are 3.50, 1.17, and 0.325 cm^2/g respectively for X-rays whose wavelength is 0.098 Å, and if the specific gravities of the three elements are 11.3, 7.3, and 8.9, respectively:

(a) Calculate the mass and linear attenuation coefficients for lead foil.

(b) What thickness of lead foil would be required to attenuate the intensity of ^{57}Co gamma-rays by a factor of 25?

10.7. A hypodermic syringe that will be used in an experiment in which ^{90}Sr solution will be injected has a glass barrel whose wall is 1.5 mm thick. If the density of the glass is 2.5 g/cm^3, how thick, in millimeters, must we make a Lucite sleeve that will fit around the syringe if no beta particles are to come through the Lucite? The density of the Lucite is 1.2 g/cm^3.

10.8. A room in which a 7.4×10^{13} Bq (2000 Ci) ^{137}Cs source will be exposed has the following layout:

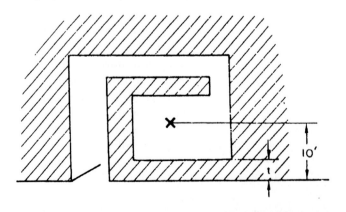

Calculate the thickness t of concrete so that the exposure rate at the outside surface of the wall does not exceed 0.025 mSv (2.5 mrems) per hour.

10.9. What minimum density thickness must a pair of gloves have to protect the hands from ^{32}P radiation?

10.10. When a radium source containing 50-mg Ra encapsulated in 0.5-mm-thick Pt is placed into a Pb storage container, the measured exposure rate at a distance of 1 m from the source is 5.41 μC/kg (21 mR) per hour. If this same container is used for storing ^{137}Cs, how many MBq may be kept in it for a period of 4 hours without exceeding an exposure of 10.3 μC/kg (40 mR) at a distance of 50 cm from the source?

10.11. What is the maximum working time in a mixed radiation field consisting of 6 μC kg^{-1} (23 mR) per hour gamma, 40 μGy (4 mrad) per hour fast neutrons, and 50 μGy (5 mrads) per hour thermal neutrons if a maximum dose equivalent of 3 mSv (300 mrems) has been specified for the job?

10.12. Maintenance work must be done on a piece of equipment that is 2 m from an internally contaminated (with ^{137}Cs) valve. The exposure rate at 30 cm from the valve is 500 R/h (0.13 C/kg/h). If 4 h is the estimated repair time, what thickness of lead shielding is required to limit the dose equivalent of the maintenance men to 1 mSv (100 mrems)?

10.13. Calculate the exposure rate from a 100,000-MBq (2.7-Ci) ^{60}Co "point" source, at a distance of 1.25 m, if the source is shielded with 10-cm Pb.

10.14. A stainless steel bolt came loose from a reactor vessel. It is planned to pick up the bolt with a remotely operated set of tongs and transport it for inspection and study. The bolt had been in a mean thermal-neutron flux of 2×10^{12} neutrons/cm^2/s for a period of 900 days and will be picked up 21 days after reactor shutdown. Calculate the gamma-ray dose rate at a distance of 1 m from the bolt if the bolt weighs 200 g and has the following composition by weight:

Fe	80%
Ni	19%
Mn	0.5%
C	0.5%

10.15. A circular area 1 m in diameter is accidentally contaminated with 10 MBq (270 μCi) ^{131}I. What is the maximum dose-equivalent rate at a distance of 1 m above the contaminated area?

10.16. Design a spherical lead storage container that will attenuate the radiation dose rate from 5×10^{10} Bq (1.35 Ci) ^{24}Na to 100 μGy/h (10 mrads/h) at a distance of 1 m from the source. (The source is physically small enough to be considered a "point.")

10.17. What thickness of standard concrete is needed to reduce the intensity of a collimated beam of 10-MeV X-rays from 10^4 mW/cm^2 to an intensity corresponding to 2.5×10^{-3} cSv/h?

10.18. A Ra–Be neutron source emits about 1.2×10^7 fast neutrons (average energy = 4 MeV) per gram Ra. What fraction of the dose equivalent from an unshielded source is due to the neutrons?

10.19. Transport regulations for shipping a radioactive package specify a maximum surface dose rate equivalent of 2 mSv/h (200 mrems/h) and a maximum of 0.1 mSv/h (10 mrems/h) at 1 m from the surface. If aqueous ^{137}Cs waste is to be mixed with cement for disposal, what is the maximum specific activity of the concrete if it is to be cast in 20-L cylindrical polyethylene containers 30 cm diameter for shipment to the waste burial site?

10.20. A technician's job in a radiopharmaceutical laboratory involves simultaneous handling of 5000 MBq (135 mCi) ^{125}I, 4000 MBq (108 mCi) ^{198}Au, and 2000 MBq (54 mCi) ^{24}Na for 1 hour per day, 5 days per week, for an indefinitely long period of time. Her average dose equivalent during the other 7 hours will be 0.01 mSv (1 mrem). Her body will be 75 cm from the sources while she works with them, and manipulators will be provided so that her hands will not be exposed inside the shield.

  (a) What is the source strength for each of the sources?

  (b) What thickness of lead shielding is required if her weekly dose equivalent is to be within ALARA guidelines, that is, at one-tenth of the maximum permissible dose?

10.21. Design a spherical shield for a 1×10^{11} Bq (2.7 Ci) ^{90}Sr "point" source so that the dose-equivalent rate at the surface will not exceed 2 mSv (200 mrems) per hour. What is the dose-equivalent rate at a distance of 1 m from the shielded source?

10.22. A 10 mCi (370 MBq) ^{60}Co source is to be shielded in order to reduce the dose rate at 30 cm to 2 mrems/h (0.02 mSv/h). How many HVLs of lead are needed? If the HVL for ^{60}Co gammas is 12 mm, how thick must the shield be?

10.23. The air kerma of an X-ray beam is reduced from 10 mGy/h to 1.25 mGy/h by 2-mm lead. Calculate the

  (a) TVL,

  (b) HVL, and

  (c) relationship between the TVL and the HVL.

10.24. If a gamma ray beam is attenuated to 5% of the incident level by 3-mm Pb, what is the thickness of a TVL of lead?

10.25. A technician wears a 1-mm Pb equivalent leaded apron. The HVL for the radiation with which she is working is 0.25-mm Pb. If the unshielded exposure level from the source with which she is working is 25 R/h at 1 cm, what is the shielded dose equivalent rate, mrems/h, at a distance of 1 m from the source?

10.26. What is the maximum working time in a mixed radiation field consisting of 20 mR/h gamma, 4 mrads/h fast neutrons, and 5 mrads/h thermal neutrons, if a maximum dose equivalent of 100 mrems has been specified for the job?

10.27. The exposure rate from an under-the-table fluoroscope operating at 120 kVcp (kV constant potential) is 19 mR/(mA-s) at 1 m from the X-ray target. During fluoroscopy, the X-ray target is 40 cm from the patient, and the tube is operating at 80 kVcp and 5 mA. What is the exposure rate, mR/s at the beam entrance to the patient? Ignore the attenuation of the table.

10.28. **(a)** Dose rates to members of the general public, at a distance of 1 m from large externally contaminated surfaces, are frequently given in units of mrems/yr per μCi/m^2. For occupational exposure, the dose conversion factor is often given as mrems/h per dpm/100 cm^2. Derive the factor for converting each of these units to the corresponding SI units.

(b) The Department of Energy Publication DOE/EH/0070 lists the dose conversion factor for the skin as 58.4 mrem/yr per μCi/m^2 for ^{90}Sr. Calculate the corresponding dose conversion factor as Sv/yr per Bq/m^2.

SUGGESTED READINGS

American Association of Physicists in Medicine. Comprehensive QA for radiation oncology: Report of AAPM Radiation Therapy Committee Task Group 40. *Med Phys*, **21**:581–618, 1994.

American Nuclear Society. *Gamma-ray attenuation coefficients and buildup factors for engineering materials.* ANSI/ANS-6.4.3, American Nuclear Society, La Grange Park, IL, 1991.

Annals of the ICRP, International Commission on Radiological Protection (ICRP). Pergamon Press, Oxford, U.K. ICRP Publication No.

26. *Recommendations of the International Commission on Radiological Protection*, **1**(3), 1977.

34. *Protection of the Patient in Diagnostic Radiology*, **9**(2,3), 1983.

36. *Protection Against Ionizing Radiation in the Teaching of Science*, **10**(1), 1983.

37. *Cost Benefit Analysis in the Optimization of Radiation Protection*, **10**(2,3), 1983.

38. *Radionuclide Transformations: Energy and Intensity of Emissions*, **11–13**, 1983.

42. *A Compilation of the Major Concepts and Quantities in Use by ICRP*, **14**(4), 1984.

44. *Protection of the Patient in Radiotherapy*, **15**(2), 1985.

51. *Data for Use in Protection Against External Radiation*, **17**(2,3), 1988.

52. *Protection of the Patient in Nuclear Medicine*, **17**(4), 1988.

55. *Optimization and Decision Making in Radiological Protection*, **20**(1), 1989.

57. *Radiological Protection of the Worker in Medicine and Dentistry*, **20**(3), 1990.

60. 1990 *Recommendations of the International Commission on Radiological Protection*, **21**(1–3), 1991.

84. *Pregnancy and Medical Radiation*, **30**(1), 2000.

86. *Prevention of Accidents to Patients Undergoing Radiation Therapy*, **30**(3), 2000.

Blatz, H. *Radiation Hygiene Handbook.* McGraw-Hill, New York, 1959.

Blizzard, E. P., and Abbott, L. S. *Reactor Handbook, Vol. III B, Shielding.* Interscience, New York, 1962.

Braestrup, C. B., and Wyckoff, H. O. *Radiation Protection.* Charles C Thomas, Springfield, IL, 1958.

Dresner, L., translator. *Jaeger's Principles of Radiation Protection Engineering.* McGraw-Hill, New York, 1965.

Etherington, H., ed. *Nuclear Engineering Handbook.* McGraw-Hill, New York, 1958.

Faw, R., and Shultis, J. K. *Radiological Assessment.* Prentice-Hall, Englewood Cliffs, NJ, 1993.

Goldstein, H. *Fundamental Aspects of Reactor Shielding.* Addison-Wesley, Reading, MA, 1959.

Health Physics Society. *Health Physics of Radiation-Generating Machines.* Proceedings of the 30th Midyear Topical Meeting. Health Physics Society, McLean, VA, 1997.

International Atomic Energy Agency, Vienna.

Optimization of Radiation Protection. Proceedings of a symposium, 1986.

Design and Implementation of a Radiotherapy Programme: Clinical, Medical Physics, Radiation Protection and Safety Aspects. IAEA-TECDOC-1040, 1998.

Radiological Safety Aspects of the Operation of Neutron Generators. Safety Series No. 42, 1976.

Absorbed Dose Determination in External Beam Radiotherapy. Technical Report Series No. 398, 2000.

Assessment of Occupational Exposure Due to External Sources of Radiation. Safety Standards Series No. RS-G-1.3, 1999.

Radiological Protection for Medical Exposure to Ionizing Radiation. Safety Standards Series No. RS-G-1.5, 2002.

Categorization of Radioactive Sources Safety Guide. Safety Standards Series No. RS-G-1.9, 2005.

Applying Radiation Safety Standards in Diagnostic Radiology and Interventional Procedures Using X-Rays. Safety Reports Series No. 39, 2006.

International Commission on Radiological Protection (ICRP). Pergamon Press, Oxford, U.K. ICRP Publication No.

3. *Report of Committee III on Protection Against X-rays up to Energies of 3 MeV and Beta and Gamma-Rays from Sealed Source,* 1960.

15. *Protection Against Ionizing Radiation from External Sources,* 1970.

16. *Protection of the Patient in X-Ray Diagnosis,* 1970.

21. *Data for Protection Against Ionizing Radiation from External Sources: Supplement to ICRP Publication 15,* 1973.

International Electrotechnical Commission. *Guidelines for Radiotherapy Treatment Rooms Design.* IEC 61859, International Electrotechnical Commission, Geneva, 1997.

International Electrotechnical Commission. *Particular Requirements for the Safety of Electron Accelerators in the Range of 1MeV to 50 MeV.* IEC 60601-2-1, 1998.

Jaeger, R. G., ed. *Engineering Compendium on Radiation Shielding.* Springer-Verlag, Berlin, 1968.

Kalra, M. K., Maher, M. M., Toth, T. L., Hamberg, L. M., Blake, M. A., Shepard, J., and Saini, **S**. Strategies for CT radiation dose optimization. *Radiol,* **230**:619–628, 2004.

Kinsmen, S. *Radiological Health Handbook,* Rev ed. U.S. Dept. of Health, Education, and Welfare, Rockville, MD, 1970.

McGinley, P. H. *Shielding Techniques for Radiation Oncology Facilities.* Medical Physics Publishing, Madison, WI, 1998.

Medich, D. C., and Martel, C. eds. *Medical Health Physics.* Medical Physics Publishing, Madison, WI, 2006.

Methe, B. Shielding design for a PET imaging suite: A case study. *Oper Radiat Saf,* **84**:S83-S88, 2003.

Mutic, S., Low, D. A., Klein, E. E., Dempsey, J. F., and Purdy, J. A. Room shielding for intensity-modulated radiation treatment facilities. *Int J Radiat Oncol Biol Phys,* **50**:239–246, 2001.

National Council on Radiation Protection and Measurements (NCRP), Bethesda, MD. NCRP Report No.

32. *Radiation Protection in Educational Institutions,* 1966.

33. *Medical X-ray and Gamma Ray Protection for Energies Up to 10 MeV: Equipment Design and Use,* 1968.

35. *Dental X-ray Protection,* 1970.

36. *Radiation Protection in Veterinary Medicine,* 1970.

38. *Protection Against Neutron Radiation,* 1971.

39. *Basic Radiation Protection Criteria,* 1971.

48. *Radiation Protection for Medical and Allied Health Personnel,* 1976.

49. *Structural Shielding Design and Evaluation for Medical Use of X-Rays and Gamma Rays of Energies Up to 10 MeV,* 1976.

51. *Radiation Protection Guidelines for 0.1–100 MeV Particle Accelerator Facilities,* 1977.

68. *Radiation Protection in Pediatric Radiology,* 1981.

72. *Radiation Protection and Measurement for Low-Voltage Neutron Generators,* 1983.

85. *Mammography—A User's Guide,* 1986.

99. *Quality Assurance for Diagnostic Imaging,* 1988.

102. *Medical X-Ray, Electron Beam, and Gamma-Ray Protection for Energies up to 50 MeV.* Equipment Design, Performance, and Use, 1989.

105. *Radiation Protection for Medical and Allied Health Personnel,* 1989.

106. *Limit for Exposure to "Hot Particles" on the Skin,* 1989.

107. *Implementation of the Principle of As Low As Reasonably Achievable (ALARA) for Medical and Dental Personnel,* 1990.

116. *Limitation of Exposure to Ionizing Radiation,* 1993.

120. *Dose Control at Nuclear Power Plants,* 1994.

147. *Structural Shielding Design for Medical X-Ray Imaging Facilities,* 2004.

151. *Structural Shielding Design and Evaluation for Megavoltage X- and Gamma Ray Radiotherapy Facilities,* 2005.

OECD. *Optimization in Operational Radiological Protection.* Nuclear Energy Agency, Organization for Economic Co-Operation and Development, Paris, 2005.

Okunade, A. A. Effective dose as a limiting quantity for the evaluation of primary barriers for diagnostic X-ray facilities. *Health Phys,* **89**(Suppl 5): S100–S116, *Operational Radiation Safety,* 2005.

Orn, M. K. *Handbook of Engineering Control Methods for Occupational Radiation Protection.* Prentice Hall, Englewood Cliffs, NJ, 1992.

Paic, G. *Ionizing Radiation: Protection and Dosimetry.* CRC Press, Boca Raton, FL, 1988.

Patterson, W., and Thomas, R. H. *Accelerator Health Physics*. Academic Press, New York, 1973.

Price, B. T., Horton, C. C., and Spinney, K. T. *Radiation Shielding*. Pergamon, New York, 1957.

Profio, E. *Radiation Shielding and Dosimetry*. Wiley, New York, 1979.

Rockwell, T., ed. *Reactor Shielding Design Manual*. McGraw-Hill, New York, 1956.

Schaefer, N. M., ed. *Reactor Shielding for Nuclear Engineers*. TID-25951, U.S. Atomic Energy Commission, Washington, DC, 1973.

Schleien, B. S., Slabeck, L. A., Jr, Kent, B. K. *Handbook of Health Physics and Radiological Health*. Williams and Wilkins, Baltimore, 1998.

Shapiro, J. *Radiation Protection*, 4th ed. Harvard University Press, Cambridge, 2002.

Shultis, J. K., and Faw, R. E. Radiation shielding technology. *Health Phys*, **88**:297–322, 2005.

Stedfore, B., Morgan, H. M., Mayless, W. P. M., eds. *The Design of Radiotherapy Treatment Room Facilities*. Institute of Physics and Engineering in Medicine, York, U.K., 1997.

Turner, J. E. *Atoms, Radiation, and Radiation Protection*. McGraw-Hill, New York, 1986.

Van Pelt, W. R., and Drzyzga, M. Beta radiation shielding with lead and plastic: Effect on bremsstrahlung radiation when switching the shielding order. *Oper Radiat Saf*, **92**(2):S13–S17, 2007.

Zacarias, A., Balog, J., and Mills, M. Radiation shielding design of a new tomography facility. *Health Phys*, **91**:289–295, 2006.

11

INTERNAL RADIATION SAFETY

INTERNAL RADIATION

Internal radiation exposure occurs when radionuclides from environmental contamination enter the body. The consequences of this internal contamination may range from innocuous to very serious, depending on the quantity of the contaminating radionuclide and the dose that it delivers. In many instances, the level of contamination is known only after a lengthy investigation, which may include bioassay measurements. Accordingly, internal radiation safety is concerned mainly with preventing or minimizing the intake of radionuclides into the body and the deposition of radioactivity on the body. This is accomplished by a program designed to keep environmental contamination within acceptable limits and as low as reasonably achievable. This last point, keeping environmental contamination levels as low as reasonably achievable, is especially important in the context of internal radiation safety.

External radiation exposure is due to radiation originating in sources outside the body; there is no physical contact with the radiation source, and exposure ceases when one leaves the radiation area or when the source is removed. Since external radiation may be measured with relative ease and accuracy, the potential or actual hazards may be estimated with a good deal of confidence. In the case of internal contamination, on the other hand, the radiation dose cannot be directly measured; it can only be calculated. As a consequence of the fact that radioactivity is deposited on or within the body, irradiation of the contaminated person continues even after the person leaves the area where the contamination occurred. It must be emphasized, however, that the fact that an internally deposited radioisotope continues to irradiate as long as it is in the body is explicitly considered in calculating the dose from an internally deposited radionuclide or when calculating the annual limits of intake (ALIs) of the various radionuclides. In the context of potential harm, the radiation dose from an internally deposited radionuclide is no different from the same dose absorbed from external radiation. Therefore, it must be emphasized that, *dose for dose, the consequences of internal radiation are the same as those from external radiation; a milligray is a milligray and a millirem is a millirem, regardless of whether it was delivered from an internally deposited radionuclide or from external radiation.*

PRINCIPLES OF CONTROL

Radioactive substances, like other noxious agents, may gain entry into the body through three pathways:

1. Inhalation—by breathing radioactive gases and aerosols.
2. Ingestion—by drinking contaminated water, eating contaminated food, or tactilely transferring radioactivity to the mouth.
3. Absorption—through the intact skin or through wounds.

Basically, therefore, safety measures to counter internal radiation are designed to either block the portals of entry into the body or to interrupt the transmission of radioactivity from the source to the worker. This can be effected either at the source, by enclosing and confining it, or at the worker, through the use of protective clothing and respiratory protective devices. Additionally, work practices and schedules should be designed so as to minimize contamination and exposure to contaminated environments. It should be noted that these control measures are the same as those employed by the industrial hygienist in the protection of workers from the effects of nonradioactive noxious substances. However, the degree of control required for radiological safety almost always greatly exceeds the requirements for chemical safety. This point is made clear by the figures in Table 11-1, which compare the maximum allowable atmospheric concentrations of several nonradioactive noxious substances to the maximum concentrations recommended by the International Commission on Radiological Protection (ICRP) for radioactive forms of the same element.

Control of the Source: Confinement

The simplest type of confinement and enclosure may be accomplished by limiting the handling of radioactive materials to well-defined, separated areas within a laboratory and by the use of subordinate isolating units such as trays. For low-level work, where there is no likelihood of releasing a gas, vapor, or aerosol to the atmosphere in a quantity exceeding 1 ALI, this may be sufficient. If the possibility exists of releasing to the atmosphere—either as gas, vapor, or aerosol—amounts of radioactivity between

TABLE 11-1.   Concentration Limits of Several Substances Based on Chemical and Radiological Toxicity

	CONCENTRATION LIMITS (mg/m^3)	
	Nonradioactive	**Radioactive**
Beryllium	0.002	^7Be 1.7×10^{-8}
Mercury	0.1	^{203}Hg 5×10^{-9}
Lead	0.05	^{210}Pb 1×10^{-9}
Arsenic	0.01	^{74}As 3×10^{-9}
Cadmium	0.1	^{115}Cd 4×10^{-10}
Zinc	5	^{65}Zn 1.2×10^{-8}

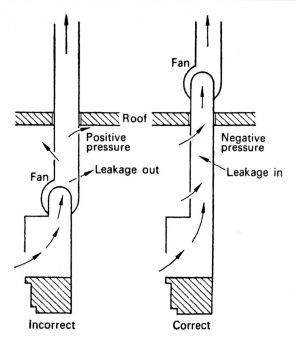

Figure 11-1. *Effect of fan location on direction of leakage in the ductwork. The fan should be close to the discharge end, thereby creating a negative pressure in the ductwork and causing ductwork leakage to be into the duct.*

1 and 10 times the ALI, the usual practice is to use a ventilated hood. The purpose of the ventilated hood is to dilute and to sweep out the released radioactivity with the air that flows through the hood. In order to accomplish this purpose, it thus is essential to have a sufficient amount of air flowing through the hood at all times. Constant airflow velocity may be maintained by using a bypass that opens as the face of the hood is closed. Openings along the bottom of the front-face frame facilitate the flow of air when the face is closed. Figure 11-1 shows a typical radiochemistry fume hood. The face velocity must be great enough to prevent contaminated air from flowing out of the face into the laboratory but not great enough to produce turbulence around the edges, which would allow the contaminated air from the hood to spill out into the laboratory. It has been found that velocities of 125–275 ft/min (0.6–1.4 m/s) are required. To minimize the possibility of contaminating the working environment with the exhaust from the hood, all ductwork must be kept under negative pressure. Any leakage in the ductwork will then be *into* the duct. This is most easily accomplished by locating the exhaust fan at the discharge end of the exhaust line, as shown in Figure 11-1.

For purposes of environmental control and hazard evaluation, aerosols are defined as airborne particles and are classified according to their size and manner of production:

Fumes—Solid particles resulting from a change of state. For example, lead monoxide (PbO) fumes are produced when lead is vaporized, whereupon the molecules are oxidized and then condensed to form solid particles. The particle sizes are less than 0.1 μm.

Dusts—Solid particles resulting from pulverizing large chunks of matter or resuspending previously pulverized matter. Particle sizes range from ~0.1 μm to
30 μm. Particles larger than 30 μm are not considered to be inhalable.

Inertials—Particles that are about 50 μm or greater in size.

Smokes—Products of combustion. Sizes range from submicron to several millimeters.

Mists—Liquid particles of any size.

If a hood is designed to remove only gases and vapors, an air velocity in the
ductwork of about 2000 ft/min (~10 m/s) is sufficient. For fumes, the recommended
duct velocity is 2500 ft/min (12–13 m/s). Since larger particulate matter tends to
settle out, the air transport velocity must be on the order of 3500–4500 ft/min (18–
22 m/s) if particle fallout is to be minimized. If the exhaust from the hood is of such a
nature that it may create a radioactive pollution problem, the effluent from the hood
must be decontaminated by an appropriate air-cleaning device. For this purpose, if
the pollutant is an aerosol, a rough filter followed by a fire-resistant, high-efficiency
filter is commonly employed. As used in this context, a high-efficiency filter is one
that removes at least 99.995% of 0.3-μm-diameter homogeneous particles of dioctylphthalate (DOP). The filter should not offer a resistance greater than 1 in. (25.4
mm) water when air at 70°F (21°C) and 29.9 in. (760 mm) Hg flows through it at its
rated capacity. A manometer or other device should be used to indicate when the
filter is loaded and ready to be changed.

A filter loaded with radioactive dust can easily become a source of contamination
if adequate precautions to prevent the dust from falling off the filter during the
changing operation are not taken. A simple way to minimize dispersal of loose dust
when removing the filter is to spray the filter faces with an aerosol lacquer before
removing the filter, thereby trapping the radioactive dust in the filter. For this purpose, access ports upstream and downstream of the filter should be provided in the
ductwork.

If the nature of an operation involving radioactivity is such that it must be completely enclosed—that is, if the operation is potentially capable of contaminating the
working environment with more than 10 times the recommended maximum body
burden or when the large quantities of air required by a hood are not available—
then a glove box (Fig. 11-2) is used. It should be reemphasized here that, whereas the
main function of a fume hood is to dilute and remove atmospheric contaminants,
the main function of a glove box is to isolate the contaminant from the environment by confining it to the enclosed volume. Accordingly, the airflow through the
glove box may be very small—on the order of 0.01–0.02 m^3/s (25–50 ft^3/min). Air
is usually admitted into the glove box through a high-efficiency fiber-glass filter (to
prevent discharge of radioactive dust into the room in case of an accidental positive
pressure inside the glove box) and is exhausted through a series of fire-resistant,
rough, and high-efficiency filters. Airborne particles small enough to be carried by
this flow of air are thus transferred out of the glove box into the filter; larger particles
fall out inside the glove box and remain there until cleaned out. A negative pressure
of at least 13 mm (0.5 in.) water inside the glove box assures that any air leakage will
be into the box. Despite the negative pressure, however, it may be assumed that a
small fraction, about 10^{-8}, of the activity inside the glove box will leak out during the
course of normal use of the glove box. The laboratory should be prepared to handle

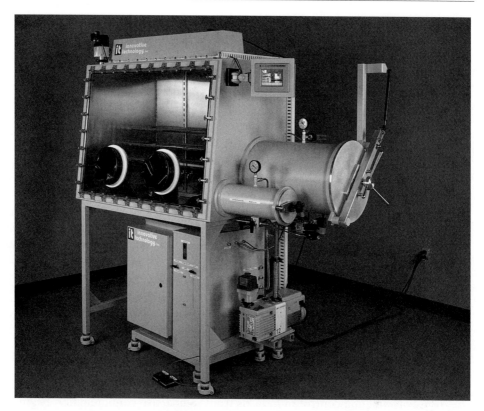

Figure 11-2. Glove box for operations with low-intensity radioactive materials that might accidentally become dispersed into the environment if not handled in an enclosed volume. In use, long rubber gloves fit over the port flanges; material transferred into or out of the glove box through the air lock at the right of the glove box. (Courtesy of Innovative Technology, Inc.)

such contamination, and the health physicist should be prepared to account for this activity in the design and operation of the surveillance program. For maximum safety, transfer of materials and apparatus into or out of the glove box is always done through an air lock. The viewing panel may be heat-resistant safety plate glass. Glove boxes are unshielded when used for handling radioisotopes that do not create high radiation levels. For radioisotopes that do create high levels of radiation, shielding must be added. When handling a high-energy, beta-emitting radioisotope, it may be necessary to use extra-thick gloves.

When we wish to contain substances that have a high degree of toxicity, we must have a highly effective containment. However, no hood provides absolutely perfect containment; some very small fraction of the noxious material that is emitted in the hood will escape to the environment. The effectiveness of a hood is determined by a number of factors, including its physical construction, face velocity, air currents in the laboratory, and so on. Several different methods are used to determine the effectiveness of a hood. All depend on releasing a vapor or a gas in the hood and then measuring the concentration of the test gas in the breathing zone directly in front of the hood. In a commonly used method, a test gas or vapor, such as alcohol or acetone, is released in the hood, and its concentration in the exhaust air is measured. At the same time, a breathing-zone measurement is made. The hood protection factor, HPF, is defined as

$$HPF = \frac{\text{exhaust concentration}}{\text{breathing-zone concentration}}.$$ (11.1)

EXAMPLE 11.1

Acetone is introduced into a chemical fume hood and is found to have a concentration of 1000 ppm in the hood's exhaust. A breathing zone sample taken with a charcoal tube shows a breathing-zone concentration of 1 ppm. Calculate the value of HPF.

Solution

With the aid of Eq. (11.1), we find the HPF to be 1000. Hoods designed for radioisotope use have HPF values on the order of 10,000 or more.

Environmental Control

Environmental control of hazards from radioactive contamination begins with the proper design of the buildings, rooms, or physical facilities in which radioisotopes will be used; it continues with the proper design of the procedures and processes in which radioactivity will be employed. Since a finite probability exists that an accidental breakdown of a mechanical device or a human failure will occur despite the best efforts to prevent such a breakdown, the course of action to be taken in the event of an emergency must be known before the emergency occurs.

In the design of the physical facilities, attention must be paid to the decontaminability of working surfaces, floors, and walls; plumbing and means for monitoring or storing radioactive waste, both liquid and solid; means for incinerating radioactive waste; isotope storage facilities; change rooms and showers; and ventilation and the direction of airflow. Airflow should be directed from office to corridor to area where radioisotopes are handled to exhaust through an air-cleaning system that will assure radiological safety outside the building. Strict control—including monitoring of all persons, materials, and equipment leaving the radiation area—must be maintained over the area where radioisotopes are being used or stored in order to prevent the spread of contamination outside the radiation area. The degree to which each of these control measures is implemented depends, of course, on the types and amounts of isotopes handled and on the consequences of an accidental release of radioactivity to the environment. Radionuclides that are not in use should be stored in a locked cabinet or area to prevent loss of control when the legitimate user is not in the laboratory or in the workplace.

In order to maintain a radiologically safe environment and to prevent internal radiation hazards, good housekeeping and good ventilation must be practiced. In regard to ventilation requirements, several important facts should be emphasized. The first is that fine particles under the influence of gravity do not, for practical purposes, move independently of the air in which they are suspended. Such particles behave effectively as if they were weightless and can be assumed to remain suspended indefinitely in the air. *Control of airborne dust particles, thus, is reduced to a matter of airflow control.*

Control of the Worker: Protective Clothing

Radiation safety philosophy advocates the restriction of radiation exposure to levels as far below the recommended maximums as is reasonably achievable. Since it is extremely difficult to maintain absolute radiological asepsis when working with unsealed sources and the possibility of an accidental spill or release to the environment of radioactivity always exists, it is customary to require radioisotope workers to wear protective clothing in order to prevent contamination of the skin. Workers in nuclear power plants may be simultaneously exposed to multiple hazards, such as heat, noise, electric shock, physical trauma, and chemicals in addition to the radiation environment. They, therefore, may require special protective equipment and clothing, such as heat-resistant garments with built-in cooling systems to prevent heat stress, ear plugs prevent hearing loss, and rubber gloves to prevent electric shock. Clothing worn to prevent skin contamination (anti-C clothing), which may include laboratory coats, coveralls, caps, gloves, and shoes or shoe covers, must be restricted to the contaminated area. Protective clothing is always assumed to be contaminated and therefore must be removed when the worker leaves the contaminated area. To be most effective, the protective clothing should be designed so that the worker can remove it easily and without transferring contamination from the clothing to his or her skin or to the environment. To this end, the worker should be instructed in the proper sequence of removal of the protective clothing before stepping out of the contaminated area into a clean area. Workers should always be monitored before leaving the contaminated area.

Protective clothing, by its very nature, must become contaminated; its main function is to intercept radioactivity that would otherwise contaminate the worker's skin or the clothing worn outside the radioactivity area. The degree of allowable contamination on the protective clothing varies with the type of work that the wearer does. For this reason, the degree of contamination permitted on protective clothing is determined by the individual installation. Table 11-2 lists the guidelines used in nuclear facilities for maximum contamination levels for protective clothing.

TABLE 11-2. Guideline for Protective Clothing Used in Nuclear Facilities[a]

GARMENT	MAXIMUM RADIATION LEVEL, β, γ [b]
Coveralls, lab coats, and hats or hoods	2.5 mrems/h[c]
Gloves and shoe covers	10 mrems/h

[a.] Clothing normally laundered after each use. May be reworn when previously worn in areas less than 10,000 dpm/100 cm^2 removable contamination. (*Note:* dpm = disintegrations per minute)
[b.] If guideline is extended, the clothing should be stored for use in the contaminated area.
[c.] This is an average value over the garment as long as any one spot does not exceed 10 mrems/h.

Laundering contaminated protective equipment is a complex operation. It requires knowledge of the mechanisms of cleaning and of the effects of the cleaning agents on the composition and construction of the protective clothing. For most isotope laboratories, the simplest method for dealing with contaminated protective clothing is to rent the protective clothing from a commercial supplier and to return the contaminated clothing to the supplier. For those installations that do their own laundry, ordinary laundering procedures, using sodium hexa-meta-phosphate or sodium ethylene-diamine-tetra-acetic acid (Na-EDTA) added to the wash water may facilitate the removal of the contaminants. After laundering, the protective clothing should be monitored to ascertain that it has, in fact, been decontaminated to some previously determined limit. If a piece of protective clothing is unusually or very severely contaminated, it may be simpler to dispose of the item as low-level radioactive waste (LLRW) rather than to try to decontaminate it. Unless the wash water meets regulatory requirements for discharge into the sanitary sewer system (such as 10 CFR 20, Appendix B, Table 3), it must be treated as LLRW.

Control of the Worker: Respiratory Protection

When a worker is likely to be exposed to airborne radioactivity, respiratory protection must be considered. According to as low as reasonably achievable (ALARA) requirements, the sum of the internal and external doses must be minimized. Wearing a respirator decreases a worker's efficiency by about 20–25%. Thus, if exposure to airborne radioactivity occurs simultaneously with external radiation exposure, an ALARA-based decision must be made regarding the use of a respiratory protective device, as explained in Chapter 8.

Medical Assessment

It must be strongly emphasized that a worker must be medically approved for respirator use before being allowed to put on a respirator or being fitted for one. Wearing a respirator effectively increases the volume of the upper respiratory tract, thereby decreasing the volume of air that reaches the deep respiratory tract (where gas exchange occurs). To compensate for this decreased air supply, the body's homeostatic mechanisms increase the respiratory rate and the rate of blood flow through the lungs. These rate increases lead to increased demands on the heart muscle. If the worker's cardiovascular and respiratory systems are in good health, then these increased cardiac demands are safely met. On the other hand, if the worker has an impaired cardiovascular system, the heart may not be capable of meeting this increased demand and a heart attack may ensue. For this reason, a worker who may have to wear a respirator on the job *must* be tested and approved for respirator use by a *qualified* physician before he or she is allowed to use a respirator.

Respiratory Protective Devices

The exact type of respiratory protective device that may be required depends on the nature of the airborne contaminant. *Respiratory protective devices may be used only for those hazards for which they are designed.* Half-mask or full-mask facepieces must not leak and must fit properly. Accordingly, the wearer of a respirator must be fit-tested before a respirator is assigned. Respiratory protective devices for radiological protection may be classified into several major categories, as shown in Table 11-3.

TABLE 11-3. Protection Factors for Respirators[a]

DESCRIPTION[c]	MODES[d]	PROTECTION FACTORS[b]		TESTED AND CERTIFIED EQUIPMENT National Institute for Occupational Safety and Health/Mine Safety and Health Administration Tests for Permissibility
		Particles Only	Particles, Gases, and Vapors	
1. Air-purifying Respirators				
Facepiece, half-mask	NP	10		30 CFR Part 11, Subpart K
Facepiece, full	NP	50		
Facepiece, half-mask, full, hood	PP	1000		
2. Atmosphere-supplying respirators				
a. Air-line respirator				
Facepiece, half-mask	CF		1000	30 CFR Part 11, Subpart J
Facepiece, half-mask	D		5	
Facepiece, full	CF		2000	
Facepiece, full	D		5	
Facepiece, full	PD		2000	
Hood	CF		(h)	
Suit	CF		(i)	
b. Self-contained breathing apparatus (SCBA)				
Facepiece, full	D		50	30 CFR Part 11 Subpart H
Facepiece, full	PD		10,000	
Facepiece, full	RD		50	
Facepiece, full	RP		5000	
3. Combination respirators:				
Any combination of air-purifying and atmosphere-supplying respirators	Protection factor for type and mode of operation as listed above			30 CFR Part 11, § 11.63(b)

[a]For use in the selection of respiratory protective devices that are to be used only where the contaminants have been identified and the concentrations (or possible concentrations) are known. (Hoods and suits are excepted.)

[b]The protection factor is a measure of the degree of protection afforded by the respirator, defined as the ratio of the concentration of airborne radioactive materials outside the respiratory protective equipment to that inside the equipment (usually inside the facepiece) under conditions of use. It is applied to the ambient airborne concentration to estimate the concentrations inhaled by the wearer according to the following formula:

$$\text{Concentration inhaled} = \frac{\text{Ambient airborne concentration}}{\text{Protection factor}}$$

[c]Only for shaven faces where nothing interferes with the seal of tight-fitting facepieces against the skin. (Hoods and suits are excepted.)

[d]The mode symbols are defined as follows: CF = continuous flow; D = demand; NP = negative pressure (i.e., negative phase during inhalation); PD = pressure demand (i.e., always positive pressure); RD = demand, recirculating (closed circuit); RP = pressure demand, recirculating (closed circuit).

Source: Abstracted from NRC Regulations: 10 CFR Part 20, Appendix A.

Air-purifying respirators remove the contaminant, either by use of a filter for aerosols or by chemical cartridges that remove gases. Because of the specific action of the chemical agents on the contaminant, different canisters must be used for different gases. For this reason, gas masks are not usually recommended for use against radioactive gases.

Supplied air respiratory protective devices may be used against either or both radioactive gases or radioactive aerosols. In this category of protective devices, we have two subcategories: (1) airline hoods, which utilize uncontaminated air under positive (with respect to the atmosphere) pressure supplied from a remote source, and (2) self-contained breathing apparatus (SCBA), in which breathing air is supplied either from a bottle carried by the user or from a canister containing oxygen-generating chemicals. The advantage of the supplied air device is that the pressure in the breathing zone is higher than atmospheric pressure. As a consequence, leakage is from the inside to outside. When using a supplied air device, it is imperative that the time limitation on the supply air is known. It is also imperative that the breathing air coupling *must be* incompatible with couplings for all other gases or nonrespirable laboratory or plant air, in order to prevent such gases from being inadvertently supplied to the airline respirator. Color coding of couplings and outlets for this purpose is *not sufficient*, because a color-blind person would not recognize the color code.

As shown in Example 8.12, use of a respirator in an area where there is both external radiation and airborne radioactivity may actually increase the worker's total effective dose equivalent (TEDE). In instances of both radiation and airborne radioactivity, the health physicist will recommend, on the basis of TEDE minimization, whether the worker should wear a respiratory protective device. A worker may insist on wearing a respirator, even if this results in an increased TEDE, in the mistaken belief that a rem from internal exposure is more serious than a rem from external exposure.

SURFACE CONTAMINATION LIMITS

Contamination of personnel and/or equipment may occur either from normal operations or as a result of the breakdown of protective measures. An exact quantitative definition of contamination that would be applicable in all situations cannot be given. Generally, contamination means the presence of undesirable radioactivity—undesirable either in the context of health or for technical reasons, such as increased background, interference with tracer studies, etc. In this discussion, only the health aspects of contamination are considered.

Surface contamination falls into two categories, fixed and loose. In the case of fixed contamination, the radioactivity cannot be transmitted to personnel, and the hazard, consequently, is that of external radiation. For fixed contamination, therefore, the degree of acceptable contamination is directly related to the external radiation dose rate. Setting a maximum limit for fixed surface contamination thus becomes a relatively simple matter. The hazard from loose surface contamination arises mainly from the possibility of tactile transmission of the radioactive contaminant to the mouth or to the skin or of resuspending the contaminant and then inhaling it. It follows that the degree of hazard from surface contamination is strongly dependent on the degree to which the contaminant is fixed to the surface.

Dealing with loose surface contamination limits is not as straightforward as dealing with contamination of air and water. In the case of air and water contamination, safety standards can be easily set—at least in theory—on the basis of recommended dose limits. Using these criteria, we can calculate maximum annual intake of a radionuclide that would lead to the recommended dose limit. From the calculated intake limit, we go one step further from the basic radiation safety criteria and compute the maximum concentrations in air and water which, if continuously inhaled or ingested, would result in the ALI. For the case of surface contamination, we go one more step away from the basic criteria; we try to estimate the surface contamination that, if it were to be dispersed into the environment, would result in concentrations that might lead to an excessive body burden. Thus, specification of limits for loose surface contamination is three steps removed from the basic safety requirements.

From the foregoing discussion, it is clear that limits for surface contamination cannot be fixed in the same sense as limits for the concentration of radionuclides in air and water. Nevertheless, it is useful to compute a number that may serve as a guide in the evaluation of the hazard to workers from surface contamination and to assist the health physicist in deciding whether or not to require the use of special protective measures for workers in contaminated areas.

On the basis of per-unit quantity of radioactivity, inhalation is considered the most serious route of exposure. Surface contamination, therefore, is usually limited by the inhalation hazard that may arise from resuspension of the contaminant. The quantitative relationship between the concentration of loose surface contamination and consequent atmospheric concentration above the contaminated surface due to stirring up the surface is called the *resuspension factor*, f_r, and is defined by

$$f_r = \frac{\text{atmospheric concentration Bq/m}^3}{\text{surface concentration Bq/m}^2}. \qquad \textbf{(11.2)}$$

Experimental investigation of the resuspension of loose surface contamination shows that the resuspension factor varies from about 10^{-4} to 10^{-8}, depending on the conditions under which the studies were conducted. A value of 10^{-6} is reasonable for the purpose of estimating the hazard from surface contamination.

 EXAMPLE 11.2

Estimate the maximum surface contamination of "insoluble" strontium 90 (^{90}Sr) dust that may be allowed before taking special safety measures to protect personnel against a contamination hazard.

Solution

The derived atmospheric concentration of ^{90}Sr recommended in ICRP 30 is 60 Bq/m^3 (2×10^{-9} μCi/cm^3). Using a value of 10^{-6} m^{-1} for the resuspension factor in Eq. (11.2), we have

$$10^{-6} \text{m}^{-1} = \frac{60 \text{ Bq/m}^3}{\text{surface concentration}}.$$

Therefore, surface concentration $= 60 \times 10^6$ Bq/m^2 = 60 MBq/m^2 (2×10^{-3} μCi/cm^2).

A figure for loose surface contamination calculated by the method of Example 11.2 is intended only as a guide. In any particular case, the health physicist may, at his or her discretion and depending on the nature of the operation, the degree of ventilation, and other relevant factors, such as the area of contamination and the

TABLE 11-4. Recommended Action Levels for Removable Surface Contamination in Manufacturing Plants

	TYPE OF RADIOACTIVE MATERIAL			
	ALPHA EMITTERS		Beta- or X-ray Emitters (μCi/cm^2)	Low-Risk Beta- or X-Ray Emitters (μCi/cm^2)
TYPE OF SURFACE	High Toxicity (μCi/cm^2)	Lower Toxicity (μCi/cm^2)		
1. Unrestricted areas	10^{-7}	10^{-7}	10^{-6}	10^{-6}
2. Restricted areas	10^{-4}	10^{-3}	10^{-3}	10^{-2}
3. Personal clothing worn outside restricted areas	10^{-7}	10^{-7}	10^{-6}	10^{-6}
4. Protective clothing worn only in restricted areas	10^{-5}	10^{-5}	10^{-4}	10^{-4}

Note on Skin Contamination: Skin contamination should always be kept ALARA. Exposed areas of the body of persons working with unsealed radioactive materials should always be monitored and should be washed when any contamination is detected. It is important, however, that contaminated skin should not be so treated or scrubbed that the chance of intake of radioactivity into the body is increased.

High toxicity alpha emitters include Am-243, Am-241, Np-237, Ac-227, Th-230, Pu-242, Pu-238, Pu-240, Pu-239, Th-228, and Cf-252. Lower toxicity alpha emitters include those having permissible concentrations in air greater than that for Ra-226 (s) in 10 CFR Part 20, Appendix B, Table 1, Column 1. Beta- or X-ray emitter values are applicable for all beta- or X-ray emitters other than those considered low risk. Low-risk nuclides include those whose beta energies are less than 0.2 MeV, whose gamma- or X-ray emission is less than 0.1 R/h at 1 m/Ci, and whose permissible concentration in air in 10 CFR Part 20, Appendix B, Table 1, is greater than $10^{-6}\mu$Ci/mL.

Contamination limits for unrestricted (noncontamination-controlled) areas in this table are considered to be compatible in level of safety with those for release of facilities and equipment for unrestricted use, as given in Regulatory Guide 1.86, "Termination of Operating Licenses for Nuclear Reactors," and in "Guidelines for Decontamination of Facilities and Equipment Prior to Release for Unrestricted Use or Termination of Licenses for Byproduct, Source, or Special Nuclear Material," which is available from the Division of Fuel Cycle and Material Safety, Office of Nuclear Material Safety and Safeguards, U.S. Nuclear Regulatory Commission, Washington, D.C. 20555.

As adapted from Table 1 of Reference 4. Averaging is acceptable over inanimate areas of up to 300 cm^2 or, for floors, walls, and ceiling, 100 cm^2. These limits are allowed only in those restricted areas where appropriate protective clothing is worn.

Reprinted with permission from King S H, Granlund RW. Organization and management of a radiation safety office. In: Miller KL. *Handbook of Management of Radiation Protection Programs.* 2nd ed. Boca Raton, FL: CRC Press; 1992.

TABLE 11-5. Surface Contamination Limits Used by the U.S. Department of Energy

NUCLIDE[a]	REMOVABLE dpm/100 cm^{2b,c}	TOTAL FIXED PLUS REMOVABLE (dpm/100 cm^2)
U-natural, U-235, U-238, and associated decay products	1000 alpha	5000 alpha
Transuranics, Ra-226, Ra-228, Th-230, Th-228, Pa-231, Ac-227, I-125, I-129	20	500
Th-natural, Th-232, Sr-90, Ra-223, Ra-224, U-232, I-126, I-131, I-133	200	1000
Beta–gamma emitters (nuclides with decay modes other than alpha emission or spontaneous fission) except Sr-90 and others noted above. Includes mixed fission products containing Sr-90	1000 beta-gamma	5000 beta-gamma
Tritium organic compounds, surfaces contaminated by HT, HTO, and metal tritide aerosols	1,0000	1,0000

[a]The values in this table apply to radioactive contamination deposited on but not incorporated into the interior of the contaminated item. Where contamination by both alpha- and beta–gamma-emitting nuclides exists, the limits established for the alpha- and beta–gamma-emitting nuclides apply independently.

[b]The amount of removable radioactive material per 100 cm^2 of surface area should be determined by swiping the area with dry filter or soft absorbent paper while applying moderate pressure and then assessing the amount of radioactive material on the swipe with an appropriate instrument of known efficiency. For objects with a surface area less than 100 cm^2, the entire surface should be swiped, and the activity per unit area should be based on the actual surface area. Except for transuranics, Ra-228, Ac-227, Th-228, Th-230, Pa-231 and alpha emitters, it is not necessary to use swiping techniques to measure removable contamination levels if direct scan surveys indicate that the total residual contamination levels are below the values for removable contamination.

[c]The levels may be averaged over 1 m^2 provided the maximum activity in any area of 100 cm^2 is less than three times the values in Table 11-5.

Source: Adapted from *Radiological Control Manual.* Washington, DC: US Department of Energy.

volume of the workroom, generally use more stringent surface-contamination limits for the use of personal protective clothing. On the basis of the ALARA principle, administrative limits for surface contamination are much more restrictive than those calculated using the resuspension factor. Various laboratories and nuclear installations have set their own limits for contamination of surfaces, personnel, equipment, and protective clothing. Tables 11-4 and 11-5 are given to illustrate some of the contamination standards maintained by several large users of radioisotopes.

WASTE MANAGEMENT

Proper collection and management of radioactive waste is an integral part of contamination control and internal (as well as external) radiation protection. In one sense, we cannot "dispose" of radioactive waste. All other types (nonradioactive) of hazardous wastes can be treated, either chemically, physically, or biologically in order to reduce their toxicity. In the case of radioactive wastes, on the other hand, nothing can be done to decrease their radioactivity, and hence their inherent toxic properties. The only means of ultimate disposal is through time—to allow the radioactivity to decay. However, the wastes can be treated and stored in a manner that essentially eliminates their potential threat to the biosphere. Solid and liquid wastes are treated to minimize their volume, and liquid wastes are converted into solids by such means as vitrification, or by incorporating the liquid either into concrete or asphalt, or into an insoluble plastic. The treated solid waste is packaged in containers according to the class of the waste and buried either in shallow engineered trenches in seismologically and hydrologically stable soil that are then covered with soil, or in deep seismologically and hydrologically stable geologic formations.

Radioactive wastes, which include materials of widely differing types and activities, can originate from any industrial, medical, scientific, university, decommissioning, or agricultural activity in which radioisotopes are used or produced. For regulatory purposes, waste is considered to be radioactive if it contains radionuclides at concentrations or activities greater than those specified by a regulatory authority. For example, the U.S. Nuclear Regulatory Commission (U.S. NRC) regulations state that ^{3}H and ^{14}C in animal tissues and in liquid scintillation media in concentrations not greater than 0.05 μCi (1850 Bq) per gram may be disposed of as if it were not radioactive. It must be emphasized that this definition of radioactive waste is for regulatory purposes only. Waste materials whose activity, quantity, or concentration does not exceed this regulatory lower limit are radioactive from a physical point of view. However, because of their low levels of activity, they are not considered to be hazardous.

Waste Classification

For purposes of management and treatment, radioactive wastes may be classified according to their activity level and their half-lives. For example, the International Atomic Energy Agency (IAEA) defines high-level radioactive waste (HLRW) as the waste from reprocessing of spent nuclear fuel or any other waste whose activity is comparable to fuel-reprocessing waste. Furthermore, HLRW is distinguished by its high rate of heat generation. Low- and intermediate-level wastes are defined by the IAEA as wastes whose radionuclide content and thermal power levels are below those of HLRW. In the United States, the classification of radioactive wastes is similar to that of the IAEA. HLRW includes reprocessing wastes from the nuclear weapons program and spent nuclear fuel from commercial nuclear power plants. When it is removed from the nuclear reactor, spent nuclear fuel contains about 1% ^{235}U, about 95% ^{238}U, and about 5% fission products plus transuranic elements, including plutonium isotopes. Although uranium and plutonium are potentially useful, it was decided for sociopolitical reasons not to reprocess spent nuclear reactor fuel in the United States. Accordingly, the Nuclear Waste Policy Act was passed in 1982. This law mandated that HLRW and spent nuclear fuel are to be stored, under conditions that would ensure safety for thousands of years, in a geologic repository. Following the IAEA classification system, all radioactive waste in the United States that is not classified as HLRW is called *low-level radioactive waste* (LLRW). LLRW is further subclassified, in 10 CFR 61, on the basis of the specific radioisotopes, their concentration, and their half lives into class A, class B, and class C, with class A being the lowest level of potential hazard and class C having the highest degree of potential hazard. Class A and class B waste will decay away within 100 years. Wastes whose activity exceeds that of the class C limit are called greater-than-class-C (GTCC) wastes, and are treated like HLRW.

Prior to 1980, LLRW was put into containers, such as steel drums, after reduction in volume to the minimum practical size and, in the case of liquids, it was immobilized in order to minimize leakage. The drums were then placed into shallow trenches and covered with dirt. Six low-level burial sites were in operation in the United States. In the 1970s, three of these sites were closed because of leakage of radioactivity into the groundwater. As a consequence, and to lessen the burden on the remaining burial sites, the U.S. Congress passed the Low-Level Radioactive Waste Policy Act of 1980. This act made each state responsible for the disposal of waste generated within its borders. However, the states were authorized to form compacts for the establishment and operation of regional facilities for the disposal of LLRW generated within the compact states. As of the middle of 2006, the first LLRW burial site under the provisions of this act had yet to be identified. Currently (2007), there are three sites in the United States where LLRW is accepted for burial: Barnwell, South Carolina; Hanford, Washington; and Clive, Utah.

When we deal with waste disposal, we mean that there is no expectation of ever recovering it. However, the waste disposal site is not abandoned but is kept under surveillance and governmental control for an appropriate period of time. The long-term surveillance and stringent attention to long-term safety is in accordance with the IAEA's principle: "Radioactive waste shall be managed in such a way that will not impose undue burdens on future generations." The objective of shallow land burial is to confine the radioactivity and prevent it from reaching the biosphere for a long enough time that the radioactivity does not represent an unacceptable risk. The fitness of a LLRW disposal site is therefore determined mainly by its hydrogeological characteristics as they relate to the prevention of migration of radioactivity outside of the site or the migration of radioactivity into the groundwater. Any activity that does migrate beyond the limits of the site should be of such low level that it will do no harm to humans or the environment.

Because of the wide range of activity in radioactive waste, ranging from very large amounts from the nuclear fuel cycle (Table 11-6) to the very small amounts from scientific laboratories that use tracer quantities of radioisotopes, several basically

TABLE 11-6. Radioactive Wastes from the Fuel Cycle

		APPROXIMATE RADIOACTIVITY LEVEL	
	TYPES OF WASTES AND PRINCIPAL CONSTITUENTS	**Ci/ton U**	**Bq/ton U**
Mining and milling	Gaseous: ^{222}Rn, ^{218}Po, ^{214}Bi, ^{214}Po	10^{-4}–10^{-3}	4×10^6–4×10^7
	Liquid		
	Solid: U, ^{226}Ra, ^{230}Th, ^{210}Pb	0.5–1	2×10^{10}–4×10^{10}
Refining	Liquid: ^{238}U, ^{234}Th, ^{234}Pa, ^{226}Ra	10^{-4} – 10^{-3}	4×10^6–4×10^7
Fuel fabrication	Liquid		
	Solid: U, Pu, Th	10^{-4} – 10^{-3}	4×10^6–4×10^7
Reactor operation	Gaseous: ^{13}N, ^{41}Ar, ^{89}Kr, ^{87}Kr, ^{138}Xe, ^{135}Xe	10–100^a	4×10^{11}–4×10^{12}
	Liquid		
	Solid: ^{58}Co, ^{60}Co, ^{59}Fe, ^{51}Cr, ^{3}H	50–100^a	2×10^{12}–4×10^{12}
Chemical processing	Gaseous: ^{85}Kr, ^{133}Xe, ^{131}I, ^{129}I, ^{3}H	7000^b	26×10^{13}
	Liquid		
	Solid: Fission products, Pu, Am, Cm	$6,6000,000^b$	22×10^{16}

^{a} At time of waste discharge or shipment based on fuel exposure of 20,000 Mwd/ton of U.
^{b}Waste from fuel at 20,000 Mwd/ton, 120 days cooled.

Source: From ORNL Drawing 69–83 R2. Oak Ridge, TN: Oak Ridge National Laboratory; 1969.

different methods are used in the management of radioactive waste. For very large amounts of radioactivity, the general principle is to concentrate and confine the waste, whereas for very small amounts of radioactivity, the waste may be diluted and dispersed. For radionuclides with very short half-lives, the radioactive waste may be stored until the activity is essentially gone. The exact manner of waste management depends on scientific and engineering criteria and on sociopolitical considerations. Included in the first set of criteria are the activity level and half-life of the waste, the physical quantity of the waste, the nonradioactive matrix in which the radioactivity is dispersed, and whether the waste is in solid, liquid, or gaseous form. The second set of criteria includes consideration of the NIMBY ("not in my back yard") syndrome and the degree of public acceptance of scientifically based public policy decisions.

Mixed Waste

Waste that contains "hazardous waste," as defined by the U.S. Environmental Protection Agency (EPA) regulations in 40 CFR 261, subpart D, as well as radioactive waste is called *mixed waste*. Hazardous waste components are those that possess any one or more of the following characteristics:

- ignitability,
- corrosivity,
- reactivity, and
- toxicity.

A mixed waste often encountered by health physicists in research laboratories is scintillation fluid such as benzene, toluene, or xylene containing ≥ 0.05 μCi $(1850$ Bq$)$ of ^{3}H or ^{14}C per gram of liquid. If the activity concentration of an organic liquid scintillation fluid is <0.05 μCi ^{3}H or ^{14}C, it is considered nonradioactive, but still is considered to be a hazardous material on a chemical basis, and must be disposed of accordingly. A simple method of disposal of such "nonradioactive" scintillation fluid is to burn it in an alcohol burner.

High-Level Liquid Wastes

High-level liquid wastes originate mainly as highly acidic solutions from the chemical processing of burned-up fuel, at specific activities of the order of 10^{12} Bq/L (some hundreds of curies per gallon). In the early years of the nuclear industry, these liquids were reduced in volume by evaporation and then stored in underground tanks. The problem of storing high-level liquid waste was complicated by the fact that the rate of heat production due to radioactive transformation is high. If we assume the mean decay energy to be 1 MeV per transformation, then 10^{13} Bq (270 Ci) generates 1 W of power as heat. Provision must therefore be made to remove this decay heat. Storage tanks for HLRW were designed for strength, corrosion resistance, heat removal, and monitoring for leakage. Typical tanks, on the order of 3800 m^3 (10^6 gal), are steel-lined reinforced concrete, with an outer steel shell to serve as a backup in case of a leak and an integrated monitoring system for leak detection (Fig. 11-3).

Although storage in tanks was considered practical for short-term containment, it proved not to be adequate for long-term retention, on the order of many

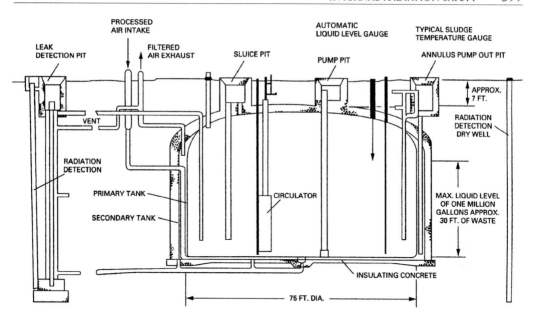

Figure 11-3. Tank for storing high-level liquid radioactive waste. (Reproduced from Roecker JH. *Radioactive Waste Management at Hanford*, 4th rev. Hanford, WA: US Department of Energy; 1979.)

centuries. The potential hazards from high-level nuclear waste are twofold. The greatest threat is from indiscriminate release of the fission product waste to the biosphere. If this were to happen, successive bioconcentration of radionuclides by plants and animals in the food web could lead to unacceptably high levels of radioactivity in our food supply, which, in turn, could lead to an unacceptably high internal dose. The second threat, of smaller magnitude than the first, is the external radiation from the radioactive waste. After extensive research directed toward new treatment methods that would remove these threats, it was found that the internal exposure pathway can be blocked by immobilizing the radioactivity in such a manner as to make it unavailable to the biosphere. This is accomplished by the process of vitrification, whereby the radioactive atoms are chemically incorporated into the chemical structure of glass beads, and become part of the glass itself. When this happens, the only way that the radionuclides can get into the biosphere is by dissolution of the glass, which would require time periods measured in geological terms rather than in historical time units. Thus, even if the glass were to escape from its containment into the environment, the radioactivity would remain locked in the glass and would not be available for uptake by flora or fauna. If an animal were to swallow one of these glass beads, the bead would pass through its gastrointestinal (GI) tract and be eliminated. Of course, the GI tract would be irradiated during passage of the bead, but the animal would not absorb any radioactivity from the bead and irradiation of the GI tract would cease when the bead passes out of it. Experience with thorium and obsidian, a naturally occurring volcanic glass, in the Morro do Ferro (Mountain of Iron) in Brazil proves that glass is stable over geologic time periods. Having thus assured that the HLRW will not enter into the biosphere, the second task is to isolate the radioactive beads so that they do not irradiate people or other living creatures. This can be accomplished by putting the glass beads into a suitable container, and then isolating the container deep underground, in a geologically acceptable formation such as a salt dome, or in the deep tunnels that were used for underground nuclear bomb tests, and thus are already radioactive and useless for most other purposes. By these methods, which effectively cut off exposure pathways, inherently toxic HLRW can be rendered nonhazardous.

Intermediate- and Low-Level Liquid Wastes

In the past, a common method for the disposal of intermediate- and low-level waste was to discharge it into the sea. The tremendous volume of the ocean seemed to make it an ideal medium for the "dilute-and-disperse" technique for the disposal of low- and intermediate-level waste. Furthermore, since seawater already contains a significant amount of radioactivity, mostly in the form of ^{40}K (it is estimated that the total radioactivity content of the oceans is on the order of 2×10^{22} Bq, or about 500,000 MCi), the addition of relatively small quantities of activity in the form of low- and intermediate-level waste would seem to add very little to the total activity of the ocean. However, because of uncertainties regarding the diverse physical, chemical, and biological processes that govern the distribution of radioisotopes in the sea and the possible transmission of these radioisotopes through the food chain to humans, it is very difficult to specify quantitatively the amounts of radioactivity that may be discharged from any point into the sea. Although undersea investigation of former disposal sites have found no deleterious effects, by an international agreement reached in 1993, the disposal of radioactive wastes into the ocean ceased in 1994.

Disposal of low- and intermediate-level wastes directly into the ground had been practiced where the hydrogeologic factors, the ion-exchange properties of the soil, and the population density were favorable. This method of disposal was called the "delay-and-decay" method, because the slow movement of the radioactivity through the ground affords the radionuclides sufficient time to decay to insignificant levels. Characteristics favorable to ground disposal include a deep water table, good ion-exchange properties of the soil in order to extract and retain relatively large fractions of radionuclides from the liquid waste as it percolates through the ground, few bodies of surface water in order to maximize the time of underground flow, a large volume of groundwater flow to maximize dilution if the radioactivity should reach the water table, and a very low population density in the area around the ground-disposal site. In the practice of ground disposal, a wood-lined pit, called a "crib," of appropriate capacity was built into the ground and was filled with gravel. The liquid waste was pumped into the crib, from which it slowly percolated down into the ground. Because of uncertainties in hydrogeologic processes and the fear of serious contamination of the groundwater, direct disposal into the ground was halted.

Chemical processes for the decontamination of low- and intermediate-level liquid wastes include the standard methods of waste-water treatment and ion-exchange methods. Hydroxide flocs, which are produced by adding alum or ferric salts to the liquid wastes and then increasing the pH until aluminum or ferric hydroxide is precipitated, are useful for removing cations other than those of the alkaline earths and alkali metals. This treatment is especially effective for removing alpha emitters; it is not very effective for removing ^{90}Sr. Removal of about 95% of ^{90}Sr may be effected with a calcium phosphate floc under highly basic conditions (pH $\sim$ 11.5). Radiostrontium can also be effectively removed by lime-soda softening of the water. The degree of removal of ^{90}Sr is proportional to the degree of softening, since $^{90}SrCO_3$ is precipitated with $CaCO_3$. Under certain conditions, liquid wastes may be decontaminated by ion-exchange methods. However, since nonradioactive ions are also adsorbed on the ion exchanger, the effectiveness of this method depends on the relative concentrations of radioactive and nonradioactive ions. Better than 99% reduction in radioactivity can be achieved under optimum conditions.

Water may also be decontaminated by biological means. However, biological removal of radionuclides is less effective than chemical treatment. Its main use, consequently, is for those cases where organic matter must be destroyed, as in sewage treatment or where high concentrations of organic complexing agents make ordinary chemical treatment difficult.

For nonvolatile radioactivity, evaporation is an effective means for decontaminating water. However, evaporation is very energy intensive, since the heat of vaporization of water is 544 cal/g (2.28×10^6 J/kg). Because evaporation requires removal of the solvent or the suspending medium, and since this component of the liquid waste usually accounts for more than 95% of the total pretreated volume, evaporation is a relatively expensive method for the treatment of liquid waste. Evaporation is usually reserved for those cases where a very high degree of decontamination is required. By means of evaporation, decontamination factors on the order of 10^4-10^6 may be obtained at vapor mass velocities ranging from about 20 to 3000 kg/m^2/h. The separated radioactivity, now in a relatively small volume, is processed further for disposal.

After separating the bulk of the radioactivity from the suspending liquid, the decontaminated water may be discharged into the storm sewer if it meets the regulatory requirements for such discharge. Very low level wastes, such as those produced in a laboratory handling trace amounts of radioactivity, may also be candidates for discharge into the sewer. Such discharges cannot be done indiscriminately but are subject to strict regulatory control. One reasonable policy that may be adopted for discharge into the public sewer system is that the quantity released in a day, when diluted by the average daily quantity of flow into the sewer from the institution, must not exceed the regulatory limits, such as those published by the NRC in 10 CFR 20, Appendix B, Table 3.

The NRC and EPA have established three layers of radiation protection limits to prevent potential health threats to the public from exposure to radioactive liquid discharges (effluents) from nuclear power plant operations.

- *Layer 1: 3 mrems/yr ALARA objective—Appendix I to 10 CFR Part 50*
  The NRC requires that nuclear plant operators must keep radiation doses from gas and liquid effluents ALARA to people offsite. For liquid effluent releases, such as diluted tritium, the ALARA annual offsite dose objective is 3 mrems effective dose to the whole body and 10 mrems to any organ of a maximally exposed individual who lives in close proximity to the plant boundary.
- *Layer 2: 25 mrems/yr standard—10 CFR 20.1301(e)*
  In 1979, EPA developed a radiation dose standard of 25 mrems to the whole body, 75 mrems to the thyroid, and 25 mrems to any other organ of an individual member of the public. The NRC incorporated these EPA standards into its

regulations in 1981, and all nuclear power plants must now meet these requirements. These standards are specific to facilities that are involved in generating nuclear power (commonly called the "uranium fuel cycle"), including where nuclear fuel is milled, manufactured, and used in nuclear power reactors.

- *Layer 3: 100 mrems/yr limit—10 CFR 20.1301(a)(1)*
  The NRC's final layer of protection of public health and safety is a dose limit of 100 mrems/yr to individual members of the public. This limit applies to everyone, including academic, university, industrial, and medical facilities that use radioactive material.

Although discharge of liquid wastes at concentrations within the legally prescribed limits is allowable, it is not societally acceptable. A convenient way to immobilize the radioactivity in low-level liquid waste is to convert the liquid into concrete and then properly package it and dispose of it in a LLRW repository. This may be accomplished by using the aqueous waste as the water with which the cement is mixed to make the concrete. The radioactive concrete is then poured into a suitable container, such as a 1- or 5-gal can or a larger steel drum if necessary, and sealed. If the waste is to be transported elsewhere for burial, it must be packaged and marked according to transport regulations, and the radiation dose rate must not exceed 2 mGy (200 mrems) per hour on the surface or 0.1 mGy (10 mrems) per hour at 1 m from the surface.

Airborne Wastes

Airborne radioactivity may be either gaseous or particulate. Gases may arise from neutron activation of cooling air in a reactor and from gaseous fission products as well as from radiochemical reactions in which a gaseous product is produced. Particles may be due to a large variety of processes, ranging from condensate droplets formed during the treatment of high-level liquid wastes to dusts from incinerators in which inflammable solids are burned. Hazards from airborne wastes are best controlled at the source of the waste by limiting the production of airborne wastes. If airborne wastes are produced, the air must be sufficiently decontaminated so that it may be safely diluted and discharged into the atmosphere. If the levels of the airborne radioactivity are sufficiently low, the waste may be diluted to concentrations within the regulatory limits and dispersed into the environment without further treatment.

Gases are usually difficult to remove. For small quantities of iodine and the noble gases, adsorption on a bed of activated charcoal that is located in the negative pressure side of the exhaust duct may be used. Most of the radioactive gaseous wastes of the atomic energy industry are very short-lived. Accordingly, these gases may be compressed and stored in tanks until they decay. Some of the methods used against radioactive gases are summarized in Table 11-7. In many instances, the most expedient method for dealing with radioactive gas is to dilute it with ambient atmospheric air discharge it to the atmosphere from a high stack in accordance with the appropriate regulatory limits, and to utilize atmospheric dispersion to further dilute the radioactivity to still lower levels when the effluent reaches ground level.

Particulate matter may be removed from gases by a variety of different devices, listed in Table 11-8, whose operating principles may be based on gravitational, inertial, electrostatic, thermal, or sonic forces; on physicochemical effects; or on filtration

TABLE 11-7. Treatment Methods for Radioactive Gas

TREATMENT	GAS	EFFICIENCY (%)	VELOCITY (fpm)	PRESSURE DROP (Inches of Water)	COMMENTS
Detention chamber	Noble gases	100	0	0	Use to hold up relatively small volumes
Spray tower	Halogens, HF	70–99	50	0.1–1.0	Precleaning or final cleaning for iodine removal
Packed tower	Radioiodine	95–99	50–200	1–10	Heated Berl saddles coated with silver nitrate
Adsorbent beds	Iodine and noble gases	99.95	168	2.8	Activated charcoal or molecular sieves: may be used to decay xenon. May be refrigerated
Limestone beds	Halogens, HF	94–99.9	30	1–3	Experimental only. Some hood applications
Liquifaction column	Noble gases	99.9	—	—	Used to recover small amounts
Stripping column		90–95	—	—	Pilot studies only
Refrigerated carbon catalyst and carbon pellets	Xenon, Krypton	99.9	—	—	Liquid nitrogen used for refrigerant. Gases recovered by desorption

Reproduced with permission from Silverman L. Economic aspects of air and gas cleaning for nuclear energy processes. In: *Disposal of Radioactive Wastes*. Vol 1. Vienna, Austria: International Atomic Energy Agency (IAEA); 1960:147.

TABLE 11-8. Basic Characteristics of Air-Cleaning Equipment

TYPE OF EQUIPMENT	PARTICLE SIZE RANGE, MASS MEDIAN (μm)	EFFICIENCY FOR SIZE IN COLUMN 2 (%)	VELOCITY (fpm)	PRESSURE LOSS, (inches of Water)	CURRENT APPLICATION IN U.S. ATOMIC ENERGY PROGRAMS
Simple settling chambers	>50	60–80	25–75	0.2–0.5	Rarely used except for chips and recovery operations
Cyclones, large diameter	>5	40–85	2000–3500 (entry)	0.5–2.5	Precleaners in mining, ore handling and machining operations
Cyclones, small diameter	>5	40–95	2500–3500 (entry)	2–4.5	Same as above
Mechanical centrifugal collectors	>5	20–85	2500–4000	—	Same as large cyclone application
Baffle chambers	>5	10–40	1000–1500	0.5–1.0	Incorporated in chip traps for metal turning
Spray washers	>5	20–40	200–500	0.1–0.2	Rarely used, occasionally as cooling for hot gases
Wet filters	Gases and 0.1–25 μm mists	90–99	100	1–5	Used in laboratory hoods and chemical separation operations
Packed towers	Gases and soluble particles >5	90	200–500	1–10	Gas absorption and precleaning for acid mists
Cyclone scrubber	>5	40–85	2000–3500 (entry)	1–5	Pyrophoric materials in machining and casting operations, mining, and ore handling. Roughing for incinerators
Inertial scrubbers, power-driven	8–10	90–95	—	3 to 5 HP/1000 cfm	Pyrophoric materials in machining and casting operations, mining and ore handling
Venturi scrubber	>1	99 for H_2SO_4 mist. SiO_2, oil smoke, etc. 60–70	12,000 24,000 at throat	6–30	Incorporated in air-cleaning train of incinerators
Viscous air conditioning filters	10–25	70–85	300–500	0.03–0.15	General ventilation air
Dry spun-glass filters	5	85–90	30–35	0.1–0.3	General ventilation air. Precleaning from chemical and metallurgical hoods
Packed beds of graded glass fibers 1–20 μm 40 in. deep	<1	99.90–99.99	20	10–30	Dissolver off-gas cleaning
High-efficiency cellulose-asbestos filters	<1	99.95–99.98	5 through media 250 at face	1.0–2.0	Final cleaning for hoods, glove boxes, reactor air and incinerators
All-glass web filters	<1	99.95–99.99	5 through media 250 at face	1.0–2.0	Same as above
Conventional fabric filters	>1	90–99.9	3–5	5–7	Dust and fumes in feed materials production
Reverse-jet fabric	>1	90–99.9	15–50	2–5	Same as above
Single-stage electrostatic precipitator	<1	90–99	200–400	0.25–0.75	Final clean-up for chemical and metallurgical hoods. Uranium machining
Two-stage electrostatic precipitator	<1–5	85–99	200–400	0.25–0.50	Not widely used for decontamination

Reproduced with permission from Silverman L. Economic aspects of air and gas cleaning for nuclear energy processes. In: *Disposal of Radioactive Wastes*. Vol 1. Vienna, Austria: International Atomic Energy Agency (IAEA); 1960:139–179.

or barrier effects. The collection efficiencies of the different devices vary over a wide range. In considering an air-cleaning device for radioactive dusts, it should be borne in mind that the collection efficiency given by the manufacturer of air-cleaning devices for nonradioactive dusts is usually based on mass collection. Since the mass of a particle is proportional to the cube of its diameter, a single 10-μm particle is equivalent to a thousand 1-μm particles. Reference to Table 11-1 shows that the maximum allowable concentration of nonradioactive particles is on the order of a million times or more greater than the allowable concentration for radioactive particles. Air-cleaning devices that are designed to remove much mass from the air, and are thus designated as high-efficiency collectors, may nevertheless be inadequate for respirable radioactive dusts. When this is the case, the final air-cleaning device is usually a high-efficiency filter that is designed for radioactive dusts. The performance of some high-efficiency filters is given in Table 11-9.

The extremely rigorous filtration requirements for radioactive dusts makes it desirable to specify the performance of a filter in a more meaningful way than "collection efficiency." Rather than designate the effectiveness of filters by filtration efficiency, in which there appears to be only a small difference between 99.99% and 99.995% (the former passes twice as many particles as the latter, 10 per 100,000 vs. 5 per 100,000), we often used the *decontamination factor* as the figure of merit for a filter. The decontamination factor, df, for a filter whose efficiency is E percent is defined as

$$ \mathrm{df} = \frac{100}{100 - E}. \tag{11.3} $$

The filter whose efficiency is 99.99% and thus passes 10 particles per 100,000 has a decontamination factor of 10,000, while the filter of 99.995% efficiency, which passes 5 particles per 100,000, has a decontamination factor of 20,000.

After filtration, the remaining radioactive particles are discharged into the atmosphere for dispersion of the nonfilterable low levels of activity. If the particles are small, (i.e., <1 μm), the particulate terminal settling velocity is very low and the particles may be considered as part of the gas in regard to their diffusion into the atmosphere and transport with the gases that issue forth from the exhaust stack.

Meteorological Considerations

When a contaminant is discharged from a chimney, it is assumed that the contaminant will be carried downwind while, at the same time, it diffuses laterally and vertically. The two main consequences of this dispersion in the atmosphere are dilution of the contaminant and its eventual return to the breathing zone at ground level. Of particular interest in evaluating the safety of discharge into the air is the relationships between the rate of discharge and the ground-level concentrations—both in the breathing zone and on the ground (as fallout)—of the discharged radioactivity. The ground-level distribution of the discharged radioactivity depends on a number of factors, including atmospheric stability, wind velocity, type of terrain, the nature of the boundary layer of air (the air layer immediately over the ground for a distance of several hundred feet), and the height of the chimney. It is thus very difficult

TABLE 11-9. Performance of High-Efficiency Filters (At Normal Air Temperatures and Standard-Density Air)

MEDIUM	TEST AEROSOL Name	Size in Microns (homogeneous except[a])	AIR VELOCITY fpm	cm/s	RESISTANCE, (Inches of Water)	EFFICIENCY (%)	METHOD	REMARKS
CC-6 Cellulose-asbestos paper	Methylene blue	—	4	2	0.8	99.9871	Discoloration	
	Dioctyl-phthalate (DOP)	0.3	5	2.5	0.67	99.85	Penetrometer	
	Atmospheric dust	0.5[a]	5	2.5	0.67	99.9+	Count	Note excessive velocity causes greater generation of fine size
	Duralumin	0.18	500	250	100	97.7	Count	Reduced velocity improves performance
	Duralumin	0.18	2	1	0.28	99.7	Count	Size for maximum penetration
	Potassium permanganate (KMnO$_4$)	0.02	20	10	2.7	93.0	Count	
AEC No. 1 Cellulose-asbestos	DOP	0.3	5	2.6	0.7	99.78	Penetrometer	
	Duralumin	0.18	2	1	0.28	92.9	Count	
	Duralumin	0.58	40	20	5.6	99.6	Count	
	Atmospheric dust		5	2.5	0.7	99.98	Count	Size for maximum penetration
	KMnO$_4$	0.01 0.02	4	2	0.56	91.0	Count	
All-glass superfine fibers—Hurlbut	DOP	0.3	5	2.5	1.05	99.999	Penetrometer	
	Atmospheric dust	0.5[a]	5	2.5	1.05	99.9+	Count	Size for maximum penetration
MSA1106B	KMnO$_4$	0.015	20	10	4.4	93.0	Count	Size for maximum penetration 69 in. deep: graded size from $2\frac{1}{4}$ – 50 mesh. Will not withstand high moisture conditions
Sand	Cell ventilation gases	1	3–5	1.5–2.5	4.5–5.5	99.5–99.8	Radioactivity	
Composite glass wool	Process off-gases	1	20	10	4.0	99.0	Gravimetric	Composition given in reference
	Methylene blue	0.6 MMD	20	10	4.0	99.99	Gravimetric	Same
Compressed glass fibers	Atmospheric dust	0.5	5.25	2.6	0.69	99.997	Count	0.02 in. thick 50% 1.3 μ and 50% 3.0 μ fibers
Resin wool	Atmospheric dust	0.5	14	7	0.3	99.6	Discoloration	These filters are known to decrease in performance when exposed to ionizing radiation
Glass	Uranium oxide	0.12	2.3–7.8	1.2–3.9	0.30–1.23	95.5–99.5	Gravimetric	Special glass formulation developed by A.D. Little. Aluminum separators and furnace cement seals

[a]Heterogeneous distribution.

Reproduced with permission from Silverman L. Economic aspects of air and gas cleaning for nuclear energy processes. In: *Disposal of Radioactive Wastes*. Vol 1. Vienna, Austria: International Atomic Energy Agency (IAEA); 1960:139–179.

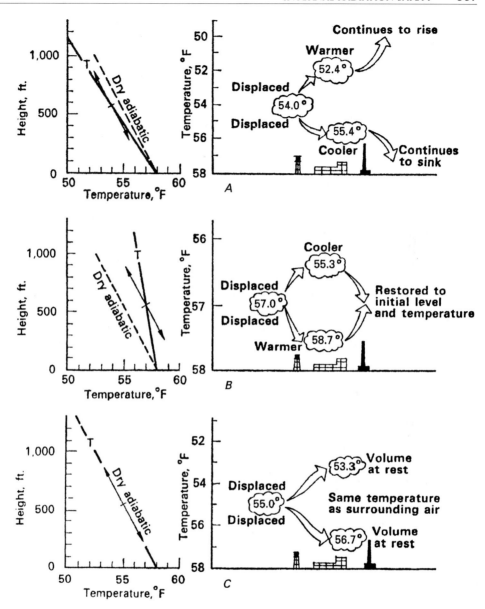

Figure 11-4. Effect of atmospheric temperature gradient—or lapse rate—on a displaced volume of air. (**A**) Unstable lapse rate. (**B**). Stable lapse rate. (**C**). Neutral lapse rate. (Reproduced from *Meteorology and Atomic Energy*. Washington, DC: US Atomic Energy Commission; 1955.)

to predict precisely the pattern of ground-level distribution, although reasonable estimates may be made from one of several different sets of atmospheric diffusion equations.

Atmospheric stability depends on the temperature gradient of the air (Fig. 11-4). Meteorologists refer to the temperature gradient of the atmosphere as the *lapse rate*. A parcel of air that is rising expands as a result of the decreasing atmospheric pressure. If no heat is gained or lost by this parcel of air, the expansion will be adiabatic, and the temperature of the air parcel will drop. For dry air, this adiabatic cooling results in a temperature decrease of 1°C per 100 m (5.4°F per 1000 ft) of ascent; for average moist air, the lapse rate is 0.65°C per 100 m (3.5°F per 1000 ft). If the temperature gradient of the atmosphere is less than adiabatic but still negative, we have a *stable lapse rate*. In this case, a rising parcel of air cools faster than the surrounding atmosphere. It, therefore, is denser than the air in which it is immersed and tends to sink. A sinking parcel of air is warmer than the surrounding air and thus is less dense, which results in a tendency to rise. A stable lapse rate, therefore, tends to restrict the width of the plume in the vertical direction, thereby decreasing the dilution effect of the atmosphere.

If the lapse rate is positive—that is, if the air temperature increases with increasing height—then the superstable condition known as an *inversion* occurs (since the temperature gradient is "inverted"). The rising effluent from the chimney becomes much denser than the surrounding air as it cools adiabatically and thus sinks. The overall effect of an inversion is to trap the effluent from the chimney and to prevent its ascent to higher altitudes.

A *superadiabatic lapse rate*, one in which the rate of decrease of temperature with increasing height is greater than 1°C per 100 m (5.4°F per 1000 ft), produces an unstable condition that helps to promote vertical dispersion of the contaminated effluent from the chimney. Under the conditions of such an unstable lapse rate, a rising parcel of air does not cool fast enough, because of its adiabatic expansion, and therefore it remains warmer and less dense than the surrounding air and thus continues to rise. By the same reasoning, a falling parcel of air continues to fall.

Dispersion of Gas from a Continuous Source

Although we often speak of atmospheric diffusion, the fact is that very little atmospheric dispersion of gases is due to diffusion. The effects of turbulence are usually so great that molecular diffusion is completely masked. For this reason, estimates of the dispersion of gases in the atmosphere are based on mathematical models that consider the meteorological state of the atmosphere rather than on classical diffusion theory. One of the more commonly used models for estimating the ground-level concentration of a gaseous effluent from a point source, such as a chimney, is the Gaussian plume, straight-line trajectory model (Fig. 11-5). In this model, the contaminant is assumed to be normally distributed around the central axis of the plume in both the vertical and the horizontal directions; it is also assumed that atmospheric stability and wind speed determine the atmospheric dispersion characteristics of the contaminant in the downwind direction. This model is described by the Pasquill–Gifford equation:

$$\chi(x, y) = \frac{Q}{\pi \sigma_y \sigma_z \mu} \exp\left[-\frac{1}{2}\left(\frac{y^2}{\sigma_y^2} + \frac{H^2}{\sigma_z^2}\right)\right], \tag{11.4}$$

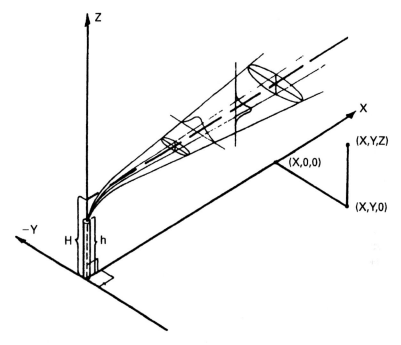

Figure 11-5. Gaussian plume dispersion model for a continuous point source.

where

$\chi(x,y) = $ ground level concentration in Bq (or Ci) per cubic meter at point (x, y),
$x = $ downwind distance on plume center line, meters,
$y = $ crosswind distance, meters,
$Q = $ emission rate, Bq (or Ci) per second,
$\sigma_y \sigma_z = $ horizontal and vertical standard deviations of contaminant concentration in the plume, meters,
$\mu = $ mean wind speed at level of plume center line, meters per second, and
$H = $ effective chimney height, meters.

If the effluent gas has a significant exit velocity or if it is at a high temperature, it will rise to a level higher than the chimney. The *effective chimney height, H,* therefore, is the sum of the actual chimney height plus a factor that accounts for the exit velocity and the temperature of the effluent gas:

$$H = h + d \left(\frac{v}{\mu}\right)^{1.4} \left(1 + \frac{\Delta T}{T}\right), \tag{11.5a}$$

where

$h = $ actual chimney height, meters,
$d = $ chimney outlet diameter, meters,
$y = $ exit velocity of gas, meters per second,
$\mu = $ mean wind speed, meters per second, at top of chimney,
$\Delta T = $ difference between ambient and effluent gas temperatures, and
$T = $ absolute temperature of effluent gas.

Wind velocity, both speed and direction, changes with increasing height. At the ground surface–air interface, the air speed is zero due to friction. As the height above the surface increases, the frictional effect decreases and the wind speed increases. Because the earth is rotating, the frictional effect on the surface "drags" the boundary layer of air with it. With increasing height, the decreasing frictional effect results in less "dragging" of the air, and the wind direction changes. In the Northern Hemisphere, the change with respect to the surface direction is clockwise, and in the Southern Hemisphere, the change is in the counterclockwise direction. ("Ground" level wind speeds are measured at a height of 10 m above ground.) For winds speeds ≥ 6 m/s (13 mph), the directional change is very small; for low wind speeds, the directional changes increase significantly with decreasing wind speed. Changes in wind speed depend on the atmospheric stability and on the surface of the terrain. Air motion is due to atmospheric pressure differences, due to the Coriolis force because of the earth's rotation, and due to frictional forces. When all these forces are balanced, the resulting wind is called the *gradient* wind. The wind speed μ at a height h may be estimated with the following relationship, where μ_{10} is the "ground" level wind speed at a height of 10 m above the ground:

$$\frac{\mu}{\mu_{10}} = \left(\frac{h \text{ m}}{10 \text{ m}} \right)^{\alpha}, \tag{11.5b}$$

where α is a function of the atmospheric stability:

STABILITY	α
Very unstable	0.02
Neutral	0.14
Very stable	0.5

For example, if the ground level wind speed is 6 m/s in a neutral atmosphere, the wind speed at a height of 60 m is:

$$\mu\,(60) = 6 \text{ m/s} \left(\frac{60}{10} \right)^{0.14} = 7.7 \text{ m/s}.$$

Although SI units are shown in Eqs. (11.4) and (11.5), any consistent set of units may be used. The maximum ground-level concentration occurs on the plume center line, at the downwind distance where

$$\sigma_z = \frac{H}{\sqrt{2}}. \tag{11.6}$$

The spread of the plume at any downwind distance is determined by the atmospheric stability, wind speed, and the downwind distance. For purposes of calculating ground-level concentrations with the use of Eq. (11.4), Pasquill proposed the stability categories listed in Table 11-10. For each of the stability categories, the values of the standard deviations in the horizontal and vertical planes through the plume center line, σ_y and σ_z, as a function of downwind distance, are given in Figures 11-6 and 11-7.

TABLE 11-10. Pasquill's Categories of Atmospheric Stability

A: Extremely unstable conditions   D: Neutral conditions[a]
B: Moderately unstable conditions   E: Slightly stable conditions
C: Slightly unstable conditions   F: Moderately stable conditions

SURFACE WIND SPEED (m/s)	DAYTIME INSOLATION			THIN OVERCAST or ≥ 4/8 CLOUDINESS[b]	≤ 3/8 CLOUDINESS
	Strong	Moderate	Slight		
<2	A	A–B	B		
2	A–B	B	C	E	F
4	B	B–C	C	D	E
6	C	C–D	D	D	D
>6	C	D	D	D	D

[a]Applicable to heavy overcast, day or night.
[b]The degree of cloudiness is defined as that fraction of the sky above the local apparent horizon which is covered by clouds.
(Manual of Surface Observations [WBAN], Circular N [7th ed.], paragraph 1210, U.S. Government Printing Office, Washington, July 1960.) Reproduced from Hilsmeier WF, Gifford FA jr. *Graphs for Estimating Atmospheric Dispertion.* Oak Ridge, TN: Oak Ridge National Laboratory; 1962. Report ORO-545.

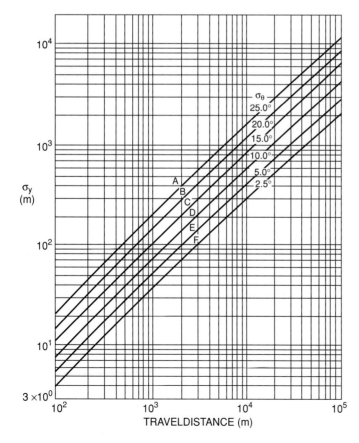

Figure 11-6. Horizontal diffusion standard deviation, σ_y, versus downwind distance from a point source for Pasquill's atmospheric stabilities. (Reproduced from Slade DH. *Meteorology and Atomic Energy.* Washington, DC: US Atomic Energy Commission, Technical Information Division; 1968.)

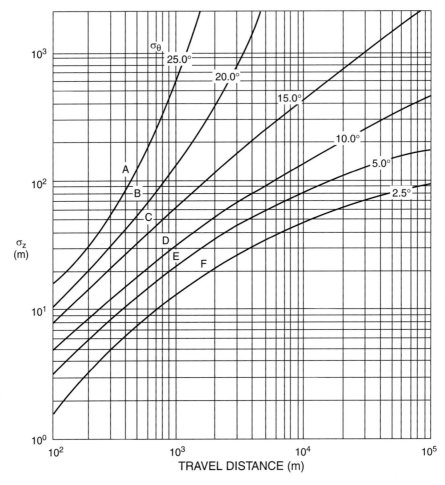

Figure 11-7. Vertical diffusion standard deviation, σ_z, versus downwind distance from a continuously emitting point source for Pasquill's atmospheric stability categories. (Reproduced from Slade DH. *Meteorology and Atomic Energy*. Washington, DC: US Atomic Energy Commission, Technical Information Division; 1968.)

The many uncertainties implicit in Eq. (11.4), such as type of terrain, fluctuations in meteorological conditions, etc., lead to a degree of imprecision in the calculated ground-level concentrations. The standard deviation of the calculated concentration is thought to be about a factor of 3. That is, 68 times out of 100, the true concentration can be expected to lie between $x/3$ and $3x$, while 96 times out of 100, the true concentration can be expected to lie between $x/6$ and $6x$.

EXAMPLE 11.3

The ^{41}Ar effluent from an air-cooled reactor is 40 MBq/s (1.08 mCi/s) on a clear night, through a chimney 75 m high, when the wind speed at the chimney height is 4 m/s and the air temperature is 17°C. The temperature of the effluent gas is 87°C, the effluent velocity is 10 m/s, and the diameter of the chimney orifice is 2 m.

(a) Calculate the effective chimney height.

(b) Calculate the ground-level concentration at 500, 1000, 2000, 4000, and 8000 m downwind on the plume center line.

(c) How far downwind is the maximum ground-level concentration?

(d) What is the ground-level concentration 50 m crosswind from the point of maximum concentration?

Solution

(a) The effective height of the chimney is calculated by substituting the appropriate values into Eq. (11.5a):

$$H = 75 + 2 \left(\frac{10}{4} \right)^{1.4} \left(1 + \frac{87 - 17}{273 + 87} \right) = 83.6 \text{ m}.$$

(b) For the given atmospheric conditions, the Pasquill stability category is found from Table 11-10 to be category E. If we substitute the respective values into Eq. (11.5), including the values of σ_y (Fig. 11-6) and σ_z (Fig. 11-7) for $\chi = 500$ m, we have

$$\chi (500, \ 0) = \frac{40 \times 10^6 \text{ Bq/s}}{\pi \times 29 \text{ m} \ \times 14 \text{ m} \ \times 4 \text{ m/s}} \exp \left[-\frac{1}{2} \left(\frac{83.6 \text{ m}}{14 \text{ m}} \right)^2 \right]$$

$$= 1.4 \times 10^{-4} \text{ Bq/m}^3 \quad (3.8 \times 10^{-15} \ \mu\text{Ci/cm}^3).$$

Similar calculations for the other distances yield

X (m)	σ_y (m)	σ_z (m)	Bq/m³	μCi/cm³
500	29	14	1.4×10^{-4}	3.8×10^{-15}
1000	50	23	3.7	1.0×10^{-10}
2000	100	37	67	1.8×10^{-9}
4000	190	54	94	2.5×10^{-9}
8000	340	78	68	1.8×10^{-9}

(c) Equation (11.6) tells us that the maximum ground-level concentration occurs where the vertical standard deviation is

$$\sigma_z = \frac{83.4 \text{ m}}{\sqrt{2}} = 59 \text{ m}.$$

From Figure 11-7, we find this distance to be 4500 m downwind from the source.

(d) Using Eq. (11.4) and the values for σ_y and σ_z at 4500 m, we have

$$\chi(500, 0) = \frac{40 \times 10^6 \text{ Bq/s}}{\pi \times 205 \text{ m} \times 60 \text{ m} \times 4 \text{ m/s}} \exp\left\{-\frac{1}{2}\left[\left(\frac{50}{205}\right)^2 + \left(\frac{83.6}{60}\right)^2\right]\right\}$$

$$= 95.2 \text{ Bq/m}^3 \quad (2.6 \times 10^{-9} \ \mu\text{Ci/cm}^3).$$

In this calculation, no allowance was made for the fact that ^{41}Ar has a half-life of 110 minutes and thus will undergo a significant decrease in activity during the transit times required for travel of the effluent to the point in question. Generally, if this travel time is significant relative to the half-life of the radioisotope, the emission rate, Q in Eq (11.4), is multiplied by the decay factor $e^{-\lambda t}$, where t is the transit time to the point in question.

Particles

Equation (11.4), which gives the ground-level concentration of a gas that is continuously emitted from a point source, is based on total reflection of the gas by the ground. If the pollutant in the plume were retained on the ground, however, as would be true in the case of particles, then the ground-level concentration would be only one-half of the value given by Eq. (11.4):

$$\chi(x, y) = \frac{Q}{2\pi\sigma_y\sigma_z\mu} \exp\left[-\frac{1}{2}\left(\frac{y^2}{\sigma_y^2} + \frac{H^2}{\sigma_z^2}\right)\right]. \tag{11.7}$$

Furthermore, if a chimney emits particles, then the depletion of the radioactivity in the plume due to gravitational settling, impaction on surfaces protruding from the ground, and precipitation scavenging must be considered in estimating downwind concentrations. Gravitational settling is important for large particles, about 15 μm or larger; impaction and wet deposition are important mechanisms of plume depletion mainly for small particles. Generally, because of the great number of factors that determine depletion of particles, such as particle-size distribution, wetability, solubility, humidity, etc., we can only at best estimate depletion of particles from a plume. The effect of gravitational settling is to tilt the axis of the plume downward through an angle $\theta = \tan^{-1} v_t/\mu$ from the horizontal, where v_t is the terminal settling velocity and μ is the mean wind speed. The effective height of the plume centerline line H' at any downwind distance x becomes

$$H' = H - x \tan\theta \tag{11.8}$$

or

$$H' = H - \frac{xv_t}{\mu}. \tag{11.9}$$

Equation (11.7) may be modified to estimate the concentration of particles at or near ground level by substituting H', from Eq. (11.9), for H in Eq. (11.7):

$$\chi(x, y) = \frac{Q}{2\pi \sigma_y \sigma_z \mu} \exp\left[-\frac{1}{2}\left(\frac{y^2}{\sigma_y^2} + \frac{\left(H - \frac{xv_t}{\mu}\right)^2}{\sigma_z^2}\right)\right]. \tag{11.10}$$

The rate of ground deposition, w, of particles at point (x, y) is found by multiplying the ground-level concentration (Eq. [11.10]) by the deposition velocity v_g of the particulate matter:

$$w \frac{\mathrm{Bq/m^2}}{\mathrm{s}} = \chi \frac{\mathrm{Bq}}{\mathrm{m^3}} \times v_g \frac{\mathrm{m}}{\mathrm{s}}. \tag{11.11}$$

Deposition velocity is determined mainly by micrometeorological conditions near the surface and thus cannot be calculated with any reasonable degree of accuracy. Experimentally determined values range from about 0.1 cm/s to several centimeters per second; an average deposition velocity of about 0.01 m/s is commonly used as a default value.

Solid Wastes

Except for "delay and decay" for short-lived radionuclides, not very much can be done to solid waste to reduce its radioactivity. The main treatment is volume reduction. For noncombustible materials, this can be done by filling a steel drum with the solid waste, covering the drum, and then compressing the drum and its contents into a solid mass with a powerful press. This compressed mass of radioactive waste can then be properly packaged and shipped to a LLRW repository for disposal. Combustible waste can be burned. Incineration may either concentrate the activity by burning away the substrate in which the activity—if nonvolatile—is held, or it may disperse the activity with the effluent from the chimney if the activity is volatile or if the contaminated waste is transformed physically into fly ash. Generally, the chimney effluent passes through an air-cleaning device, such as an electrostatic precipitator, before being discharged to the atmosphere. In the instances where the radioactivity is concentrated in the bottom ash or removed from the effluent stream by the electrostatic precipitator, we have a case of volume reduction. The ashes still must be collected and packaged for disposal. (The collection of ashes from an incinerator in which radioactive waste had been burned should be done under the supervision of a health physicist. Appropriate respiratory protective equipment should be available if necessary.) If the activity goes up the stack to be diluted and dispersed in the atmosphere, the rate of incineration of the radioactive waste should be controlled in order to limit the activity discharged from the stack to acceptable levels.

 EXAMPLE 11.4

Dead rats that had been injected with a ^{14}C-tagged compound are to be burned in an incinerator. The carbon is expected to go up the stack as CO_2, but some of it may also be discharged as carbon particles. About 125 kg of dry, nonradioactive waste are burned per 8-hour day in this incinerator. How much activity may be incinerated if the concentration at the top of the chimney is not to exceed the 10 CFR 20 effluent limit of 3×10^{-7} μCi/mL $(11.1$ kBq/m$^3)$?

Solution

At least 3.5 kg of air per kilogram waste must be supplied to the incinerator. Since 1 m^3 of air weighs 1.2 kg at 22°C and standard atmospheric pressure, the amount of air used during the day is

$$125 \frac{\text{kg waste}}{\text{day}} \times \frac{3.5 \dfrac{\text{kg air}}{\text{kg waste}}}{1.2 \dfrac{\text{kg air}}{\text{m}^3}} = 365 \frac{\text{m}^3}{\text{d}}.$$

To attain a maximum concentration of 3×10^{-7} μCi/mL $(11.1$ kBq/m$^3)$, we may not incinerate more than

$$3 \times 10^{-7} \frac{\mu\text{Ci}}{\text{mL}} \times 10^6 \frac{\text{mL}}{\text{m}^3} \times 365 \frac{\text{m}^3}{\text{d}} = 110 \frac{\mu\text{Ci}}{\text{d}} \left(4.1 \frac{\text{MBq}}{\text{d}}\right).$$

Furthermore, since National Bureau of Standards Handbook 53 recommends a maximum specific activity of 4 μCi (148 kBq) per gram of carbon for particles discharged from a chimney, we shall adhere to this limit. If the incinerated waste is assumed to be 25% carbon by weight, then the amount of C incinerated is

$$\frac{125 \text{ kg waste}}{\text{day}} \times \frac{0.25 \text{ kg C}}{\text{kg waste}} = 31.3 \frac{\text{kg C}}{\text{day}}.$$

The mean specific activity, therefore, if 110 μCi (4.1 MBq) is incinerated per day is

$$\frac{110 \ \mu\text{Ci/d}}{31.3 \dfrac{\text{kg C}}{\text{day}} \times 1000 \dfrac{\text{g C}}{\text{kg C}}} = 3.5 \times 10^{-3} \frac{\mu\text{Ci}}{\text{g C}} \quad \left(130 \frac{\text{Bq}}{\text{g C}}\right),$$

which is very much less than the recommended maximum specific activity.

Let us now consider the rat. It consists of 18% carbon by weight. The maximum activity A_m, in a rat weighing W grams that could be incinerated if there were no isotopic dilution of the carbon is

$$A_m \frac{\mu\text{Ci}}{\text{rat}} = 4 \frac{\mu\text{Ci}}{\text{g C}} \times 0.18 \frac{\text{g C}}{\text{g}} \times W \frac{\text{g}}{\text{rat}}.$$

For a 300-g rat, this corresponds to 216 μCi (8 MBq) per rat. However, because of the very large isotopic dilution of the carbon by the carbon in other wastes, we may allow the daily maximum incinerated activity of 110 μCi (4.1 MBq) to be distributed over any number of rats.

In certain other instances, the radioactivity could be converted into a gas and then discharged to the atmosphere. An illustration of how this may be accomplished within limits prescribed by radiation safety regulations is shown below.

EXAMPLE 11.5

Three hundred and seventy MBq (10 mCi) ^{14}C waste, in the form of 1 g $BaCO_3$, will be disposed of by interacting the $BaCO_3$ with HCl to change the chemical form of the carbon to $^{14}CO_2$ and then discharging the radioactive gas to the atmosphere. The chemical manipulations will be carried out in a fume hood whose face opening is 2 m wide and 0.8 m high and whose face velocity is 0.5 m/s (100 f/min). The $^{14}CO_2$ will be vented to the atmosphere through an exhaust stack from the hood. The chemical conversion from the carbonate to the gas will be accomplished by the addition of 1 N HCl. What is the maximum rate at which acid may be added to the $BaCO_3$ if the maximum effluent concentration of 11.1 kBq/m^3 (3×10^{-7} μCi/cm^3) is not to be exceeded at the discharge end of the exhaust stack?

Solution

The conversion of the carbonate to CO_2 proceeds according to the reaction

$$BaCO_3 + 2HCl \rightarrow BaCl_2 + CO_2 + H_2O.$$

Since the formula weight of $BaCO_3$ is 197.4 (the additional weight due to the ^{14}C is very small, and may be neglected), 1 g $BaCO_3$ is

$$\frac{1 \text{ g}}{197.4 \text{ g/mol}} = 0.00506 \text{ mol}.$$

To convert all the $BaCO_3$ to CO_2, $2 \times 0.00506 = 0.01012$ mol HCl is needed. Since 1 N HCl contains 1 mol acid per liter, the required amount of acid will be contained in 0.01012 L, or 10.12 mL HCl. According to the chemical equation, 1 mol $BaCO_3$ reacts with 2 mol acid to yield 1 mol CO_2. Therefore, if the reaction goes to completion, 0.00506 mol $^{14}CO_2$ will be produced. The gas will occupy a volume, under standard conditions of temperature and pressure, of

$$5.06 \times 10^{-3} \text{ mol} \times 22.4 \text{ L/mol} = 0.113 \text{ L}.$$

The specific activity of the $^{14}CO_2$ produced in this reaction is

$$\frac{10 \text{ mCi} \times 10^3 \frac{\mu \text{ Ci}}{\text{mCi}}}{0.113 \text{ L}} \times 10^{-3} \frac{\text{L}}{\text{mL}} = 88.1 \frac{\mu\text{Ci}}{\text{mL}} \left(3.3 \times 10^{12} \frac{\text{Bq}}{\text{m}^3} \right).$$

According to 10 CFR 20, the maximum permissible effluent concentration for airborne $^{14}CO_2$ is $3 \times 10^{-7} \mu$Ci/mL (11.1×10^3 Bq/m^3). The minimum volume of air in which the generated $^{14}CO_2$ must be mixed in order to meet the required concentration at the point of emission is

$$\frac{10 \text{ mCi} \times 10^3 \frac{\mu\text{Ci}}{\text{mCi}}}{V \text{ mL}} = \frac{3 \times 10^{-7} \mu\text{Ci}}{1 \text{ mL}}$$

$V = 3.33 \times 10^{10} \text{ mL} = 3.33 \times 10^4 \text{ m}^3.$

The volume of air that flows out of the discharge stock is

$$Q = \text{ face area} \times \text{velocity}$$

$$= 2 \text{ m} \times 0.8 \text{ m} \times 30 \frac{\text{m}}{\text{min}} = 48 \frac{\text{m}^3}{\text{min}} \quad (1700 \text{ cfm}).$$

If the conversion of the $BaCO_3$ to CO_2 proceeds at a uniform rate of speed, it must take at least

$$\frac{3.33 \times 10^4 \text{ m}^3}{48 \frac{\text{m}^3}{\text{min}}} = 694 \text{ min}.$$

The 1 N HCl, therefore, must flow into the gas generator at a rate not exceeding

$$\frac{10.12 \text{ mL}}{694 \text{ min}} = 1.46 \times 10^{-2} \frac{\text{mL}}{\text{min}},$$

or about 68.6 min/mL.

ASSESSMENT OF HAZARD

A realistic assessment of hazard based on the dose from an internally deposited radioisotope requires more consideration than merely comparing an environmental concentration to legally prescribed limits. The derived air concentrations (DAC) are not maximum permissible concentrations. They are administrative quantities that are used in radiation protection practice for controlling exposure and for dose tracking as a means of demonstrating compliance with the prescribed dose limit. Nominally, 1 DAC-hour of exposure to an airborne contaminant corresponds to a committed effective dose equivalent of 0.025 mSv (2.5 mrems). However, the ALIs and their corresponding DACs, with few exceptions, are based on generalized properties of classes of compounds, such as oxides, sulfides, etc., rather than on the metabolic characteristics of specific chemical compounds. This fact, together with the successive rounding of the numbers to one significant figure in the calculational steps leading to the ALIs and DACs, may result in large discrepancies between the dose determined from the actual metabolic behavior and the nominal dose based on the administrative equivalence of 1 DAC-hour to 0.025 mSv (2.5 mrems). If the ALI and DAC are calculated from a physiologically based biokinetic model for a specific compound, as is the case for CO and CO_2, then we might expect reasonably close agreement between the nominal dose based on DAC-hours and the calculated dose.

In this regard, the ICRP says that in cases where there are specific data showing that the behavior of any specific material differs significantly from that of the dosimetric model used, then changes should be made in the application of the model to make the model compatible with the specific data.

EXAMPLE 11.6

^{14}CO will be produced in a pilot study in which excess H_2SO_4 will react with H-^{14}CO-ONa, whose specific activity is 47.5 MBq (1.28 mCi) per mmol, to produce ^{14}CO. The OSHA permissible exposure level (PEL) for CO gas, based on its chemical toxicity, is 35 ppm for occupational exposure. The DAC for occupational exposure to ^{14}CO is listed in 10 CFR 20, Appendix B, Table 1, as 7×10^{-4} μCi/mL (26 MBq/m^3).

(a) Will the industrial hygiene control that limits CO to 35 ppm be sufficient to meet the regulatory requirements for radiological safety?

(b) The industrial hygienist, believing that control of the ^{14}CO according to the chemical PEL is sufficient for the radiological hazard, allows a chemical engineer to be exposed to 35 ppm of the ^{14}CO for a period of 2 hours. What is the chemical engineer's dose commitment as a result of his exposure?

Solution

(a) The molar concentration of CO in the atmosphere corresponding to 35 ppm is

$$35 \text{ ppm} = \frac{35 \text{ mol CO}}{10^6 \text{ mol atmosphere}} = 3.5 \times 10^{-5} \frac{\text{mol CO}}{\text{mol atmosphere}}.$$

Since there is one carbon atom per molecule of sodium formate and also only one carbon atom per CO molecule, the specific activity of the tagged ^{14}CO will also be 47.5 MBq (1.28 mCi) per mmol. The radioactivity concentration corresponding to 35 ppm is therefore

$$\frac{3.5 \times 10^{-5} \dfrac{\text{mol CO}}{\text{mol atm}} \times 47.5 \times 10^9 \dfrac{\text{Bq}}{\text{mol CO}}}{22.4 \times 10^{-3} \dfrac{\text{m}^3}{\text{mol atm}}}$$
$$= 7.4 \times 10^7 \text{ Bq/m}^3 \quad (2 \times 10^{-3} \ \mu\text{Ci/mL}).$$

Use of industrial hygiene criteria would, in this case, lead to an atmospheric concentration of ^{14}CO that is

$$\frac{2 \times 10^{-3} \ \mu\text{Ci/mL}}{7 \times 10^{-4} \ \mu\text{Ci/mL}} = 2.9$$

times the DAC limit for continuous exposure.

(b) In order to calculate the absorbed dose, certain facts must be known about the physiological behavior of CO. When CO is inhaled, it diffuses across the capillary bed in the lungs and dissolved in the blood. It is then absorbed by the erythrocytes and combines with the hemoglobin to form carboxyhemoglobin. Since carboxyhemoglobin is incapable of transporting oxygen, the inhalation of CO leads to cellular anoxia, which in turn may lead to unconsciousness or death—depending on the amount of CO that is absorbed into the blood. The maximum amount of an inhaled gas that can be absorbed, which is called the saturation value, depends on the partial pressure (P) of the gas in the atmosphere. The saturation value for CO, S_∞, as percent hemoglobin tied up as carboxyhemoglobin, is given by

$$S_\infty = \frac{210 \times P_{CO}}{(210 \times P_{CO}) + P_{O_2}} \times 100, \tag{11.12}$$

where P_{CO} is the percent CO in the air, and P_{O_2} is the percent oxygen in the alveolar air (P_{O_2} is usually equal to 15). One hundred percent saturation corresponds to 20 mL CO per 100 mL blood. Rate of absorption, in most cases, follows first-order kinetics; that is, the fractional approach to saturation per unit time remains constant. Thus, if 1% of the saturation value is absorbed in 1 minute after a person begins inhaling the gas, 1% of the remaining 99% will be absorbed during the second minute, then 1% of the 98.01% left, and so on. Since saturation is approached asymptotically, we usually refer to the *saturation half time* to designate the rate of absorption of an inhaled gas. The numerical value for the saturation half time is independent of the atmospheric concentration of the gas (except for very high concentrations). For CO, the saturation half time is about 47 minutes. The absorption of CO is analogous to the buildup of a radioactive daughter as it approaches secular equilibrium and is described by a similar equation:

$$S = S_\infty \left(1 - e^{-\frac{0.693}{T} \times t_i}\right), \tag{11.13}$$

where S_∞ is the saturation value corresponding to a particular atmospheric concentration of the CO; S is the percent of the hemoglobin bound with CO; T is the saturation half time; and t_i is the inhalation time.

For an atmospheric concentration of 35 ppm (35×10^{-6} parts CO per part air), which corresponds to $35 \times 10^{-4}\%$, or 0.0035%, the hemoglobin saturation value is calculated from Eq. (11.12) to be

$$S_\infty = \frac{210 \times 0.0035}{(210 \times 0.0035) + 15} \times 100 = 4.7\%.$$

After the 2-hour exposure, the percentage of the worker's hemoglobin that is bound with CO is calculated from Eq. (11.13) to be

$$S = 4.7 \times \left(1 - e^{-\frac{0.693}{47 \text{ min}} \times 120 \text{ min}}\right) = 3.9\%.$$

The blood volume of the reference man is 7.7% of his weight, or 5.4 L for a 70-kg man; it therefore can hold 1/5 of 5.4 L, or 1080 mL CO or oxygen. Since 3.9% of this capacity is tied up with CO, the quantity of CO in the man's body is

$$0.039 \times 1080 \text{ mL} = 42 \text{ mL } {}^{14}CO \text{ at STP} \quad (0°C \text{ and } 760 \text{ mm Hg}).$$

Since the specific activity of the ^{14}CO is 47.5×10^6 Bq (1.28 mCi) per mmol, the body burden following 2 hours of inhalation is

$$\frac{42 \text{ mL}}{22.4 \text{ mL/mmol}} \times 47.5 \times 10^6 \frac{\text{Bq}}{\text{mmol}} = 8.9 \times 10^7 \text{ Bq} \quad (2.4 \text{ mCi}) .$$

Assuming the blood, and hence the ^{14}C, to be uniformly distributed throughout the body of a 70-kg man, the dose rate due to this body burden of ^{14}C is calculated from Eq. (6.47):

$$\dot{D} = \frac{8.9 \times 10^7 \text{ Bq} \times 1 \frac{\text{tps}}{\text{Bq}} \times 5 \times 10^{-2} \frac{\text{MeV}}{\text{transf}} \times 1.6 \times 10^{-13} \frac{\text{J}}{\text{MeV}} \times 3.6 \times 10^3 \frac{\text{s}}{\text{h}}}{70 \text{ kg} \times 1 \frac{\text{J/kg}}{\text{Gy}}}$$

$$= 3.7 \times 10^{-5} \text{ Gy/h} \quad (3.7 \text{ mrads/h}) .$$

If inhalation had continued until the hemoglobin saturation value were attained, the body burden would have reached

$$\frac{4.7}{3.9} \times 8.9 \times 10^7 = 1.1 \times 10^8 \text{ Bq},$$

and the dose rate would have proportionately increased to $\dot{D}_\infty$, the maximum possible value under the conditions of exposure, to 4.5×10^{-5} Gy/h (4.5 mrads/h). In this case, the body burden, and hence the dose rate, varied with time, as shown in Figure 11-8. The instantaneous dose rate during the period of inhalation (period I in Fig. 11-8) is given by

$$\dot{D} = \dot{D}_\infty \left(1 - e^{-kt_i}\right), \tag{11.14}$$

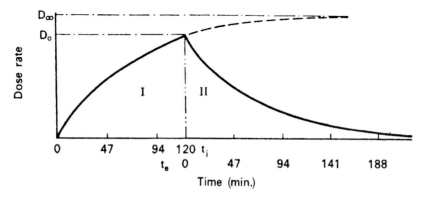

Figure 11-8. Variation of dose rate with time after start of ^{14}CO inhalation. Region I under the curve represents the period of inhalation, and region II represents the period of exhalation. $\dot{D}_0$ is the dose rate at the end of the inhalation period, and $\dot{D}_\infty$ is the dose rate due to the saturation amount of radioactive CO.

where k is the carboxyhemoglobin dissociation rate constant, $0.693/T$, and t_i is the inhalation time. The total dose during the period of inhalation is

$$D_i = \dot{D}_\infty \int_0^{t_i} \left(1 - e^{-kt_i}\right) dt, \qquad (11.15)$$

which, when integrated, yields

$$D = \dot{D}_\infty \left[t_i + \frac{1}{k}\left(e^{-kt_i} - 1\right)\right]. \qquad (11.16)$$

If we substitute the previously calculated values into Eq. (11.16) in order to calculate the absorbed dose during the 2-hour inhalation period, we have

$$D = 4.5 \times 10^{-5} \frac{\text{Gy}}{\text{h}} \left[2\,\text{h} + \frac{1}{0.885\,\text{h}^{-1}}\left(e^{-0.885\,\text{h}^{-1} \times 2\,\text{h}} - 1\right)\right]$$

$$D = 4.8 \times 10^{-5} \text{ Gy} \quad (4.8 \text{ mrads}).$$

The dose absorbed during the time period t_e, when the CO leaves the blood (area II in Fig. 11-8), is given by Eq. (6.58) as

$$D = \frac{D_0}{\lambda_E}.$$

When 3.7×10^{-5} Gy/h is substituted into Eq. (6.58) for the initial dose rate for the exhalation period in Figure 11-8, the dose during the CO elimination period is calculated as follows:

$$D = \frac{3.7 \times 10^{-5} \dfrac{\text{Gy}}{\text{h}}}{0.885\,\text{h}^{-1}} = 4.2 \times 10^{-5} \text{ Gy} \quad (4.2 \text{ mrads}).$$

The dose commitment due to the 2-hour-long inhalation of the ^{14}CO is the sum of the doses during inhalation and elimination, which is equal to 7.9×10^{-5} Gy (7.9 mrads). Since the dose equivalent is numerically equal to the dose for beta radiation, the committed dose equivalent (CEDE) from this exposure is 0.079 mSv or 7.9 mrems. The nominal CEDE from a 2-hour exposure at 2.9 DACs at 0.025 mSv per DAC-hour (2.5 mrems per DAC-hour) is

$$\text{CEDE} = 2\,\text{h} \times 2.9\,\text{DAC} \times 0.025\,\frac{\text{mSv}}{\text{DAC-h}} = 0.15 \text{ mSv} \quad (15 \text{ mrems}).$$

This example shows that if available, biologically based biokinetic information rather than the assumption that 1 DAC-hour is equivalent to 2.5 mrems (0.025 mSv) should be used to estimate the dose from the intake of a radionuclide.

Maximum Credible Accident

The concept of a maximum credible accident is useful in advance planning for the purpose of minimizing radiation dose in the event of an accident or for designing safety limitations into an experiment. Consider the following example.

EXAMPLE 11.7

An engineer wishes to use tritiated water in an experimental study of a closed pressurized system. The system's capacity is 3-L water, which will be kept at a temperature of 150°C (302°F). The experiment will be done in a ventilated laboratory whose dimensions are 3 m × 3 m × 3 m. The maximum credible accident is one in which the system will rupture, and the entire 3 L of tritiated water will be sprayed into the room as steam. The laboratory ventilation rate is 7 m³/min (250 cfm). The laboratory has its own exhaust line and stack, so there is no possibility of spreading the tritium, in the event of an accident, to other laboratories in the building.

What is the maximum amount of tritium, as tritiated water, ^{3}HOH, that may be in the system, assuming a maximum credible accident, if the engineer is not to inhale more tritium than that which would deliver a dose of 30 mGy (3 rads) over a period of 13 weeks. In the event of such an accident, it is estimated that the engineer might remain in the laboratory for as long as 2 minutes.

For tritium:

(a) the critical organ is the total body, weight = 70 kg;

(b) the biological half-time is 12 days;

(c) the radiological half-life is 12.3 years;
   (i)   the effective half-life, from Eq. (6.54), is 12 days;
   (ii)   the effective elimination rate, from Eq. (6.52), is 0.0578 per day;

(d) pure beta emitter, average beta energy = 0.006 MeV; and

(e) all the inhaled tritium is assumed to be absorbed.

Solution

The initial dose rate, $\dot{D}_0$, that will result in a total dose of 30 mGy (3000 mrads) over a period of 13 weeks (91 days) is calculated from Eq. (6.57):

$$30 \text{ mGy} = \frac{\dot{D}_0}{0.0578 \text{ d}^{-1}} \left(1 - e^{-0.0578 \text{ d}^{-1} \times 91 \text{ d}}\right)$$

$$\dot{D}_0 = 1.74 \text{ mGy/d} \quad (174 \text{ mrads/d}) .$$

The body burden, q Bq, that will deliver this initial dose rate is calculated from Eq. (6.47), and is found to be

$$1.74 \times 10^{-3} \text{ Gy/d}$$

$$= \frac{q \text{ Bq} \times 1 \, \dfrac{\text{tps}}{\text{Bq}} \times 6 \times 10^{-3} \, \dfrac{\text{MeV}}{\text{transf}} \times 1.6 \times 10^{-13} \, \dfrac{\text{J}}{\text{MeV}} \times 8.64 \times 10^{4} \, \dfrac{\text{s}}{\text{d}}}{70 \text{ kg} \times 1 \, \dfrac{\text{J/kg}}{\text{Gy}}}$$

$$q = 1.47 \times 10^{9} \text{ Bq} \quad (39.7 \text{ mCi}) .$$

If the entire 3 L of water were vaporized, the density of the steam would be

$$\rho \text{ (steam)} = \frac{3 \text{ kg}}{1000 \text{ m}^3} = 0.003 \text{ kg/m}^3.$$

For the density of water vapor to be this high, the temperature must be 56°C (132°F). This is an unreasonably high ambient temperature. If we assume an ambient temperature of 38°C (100°F), then the saturated water vapor density is 1.275×10^{-3} kg/m^3, and the amount of water in the air is

$$\frac{1.275}{3.00} \times 3 \text{ kg} = 1.275 \text{ kg}.$$

The tritium activity in this amount of water must be restricted to that quantity that would lead to an inhalation of no more than 1.47×10^9 Bq (39.7 mCi) during 2 minutes of breathing air saturated with the tritiated water vapor at a temperature as high as 38°C.

Assume that the worker's breathing rate is 20 respirations per minute and that the tidal volume is 0.5 L. If there were no ventilation and the concentration of the tritium had remained constant, the atmospheric concentration C Bq/L that would lead to the maximum acceptable body burden is

$$C \text{ Bq/L} \times \text{respiration rate, L/min} \times \text{exposure time, min} = q \text{ Bq}.$$

However, the atmospheric concentration does not remain constant; the ventilation system changes the air of the laboratory at a turnover rate k of

$$k = \frac{7 \text{ m}^3/\text{min}}{3 \text{ m} \times 3 \text{ m} \times 3 \text{ m}} = 0.26 \text{ min}^{-1}.$$

The atmospheric concentration of tritium in the laboratory C at any time t after release, assuming instantaneous release and uniform concentration C_0, is given by

$$C = C_0 e^{-k \text{ min}^{-1} \times t \text{ min}}, \tag{11.17}$$

where k is the turnover rate of the air. The total amount of inhaled tritium, during any exposure at a mean respiration rate of RR, is

$$q = \text{RR} \times C_0 \int_0^t e^{-kt} \, dt, \tag{11.18}$$

which yields, upon integration,

$$q = \text{RR} \times \frac{C_0}{k} \left(1 - e^{-kt}\right). \tag{11.19}$$

In the case under consideration, the respiration rate is 0.5 L per inspiration $\times$ 20 inspirations per minute = 10 L min^{-1}. Substituting into Eq. (11.19) to solve for C_0, we have

$$1.47 \times 10^9 \text{ Bq} = 10 \; \frac{\text{L}}{\text{min}} \times \frac{C_0 \text{ Bq/L}}{0.26 \text{ min}^{-1}} \left(1 - e^{-0.26 \text{ min}^{-1} \times 2 \text{ min}}\right)$$

$$C_0 = 9.43 \times 10^7 \text{Bq/L} \quad (2.55 \text{ mCi/L}).$$

Since the room volume is 27 m^3, or 27,000 L, and since only 1.275 kg of the 3 kg of water will be in the vapor state, the maximum amount of tritium that may be contained in the tritiated water is

$$\frac{3}{1.275} \times 9.43 \times 10^7 \frac{\text{Bq}}{\text{L vapor}} \times 2.7 \times 10^4 \text{ L vapor} = 6.0 \times 10^{12} \text{ Bq} \quad (162 \text{ Ci}).$$

According to these calculations the use of no more than 6.0×10^{12} Bq (162 Ci) tritium in the 3 L of tritiated water would ensure against overexposure in the event of the maximum credible accident. If this is not enough activity for the purpose of the experiment, then additional precautions, such as enclosure of the process or increased ventilation, would have to be employed.

Radon

Radon gas is a naturally occurring radioactive gas that occurs in the uranium (4n+2 series) and the thorium (4n series). Since both these series are ubiquitous, radon gas is produced, to a lesser or greater degree in all soils, depending on the concentration of uranium or thorium. The gas diffuses out of the ground and into the air. Because of the relatively slow diffusion rate and the short half-lives of the two Rn isotopes, most of the radon that is exhaled from the ground originates in the top 30 cm (1 foot) of soil. Radon exhalation from the soil is on the order of several picocuries per square meter per second, the exact rate depends on the concentration of the uranium and thorium series precursors in the soil. The concrete foundation or slab on which a building rests acts as a barrier against the radon. However, radon gas can gain entry into the building by diffusing through the concrete or through cracks that may occur in the concrete. Entry rates through such concrete barriers are usually less than one-half the exhalation rate from the soil. Once in the house, air exchange by general ventilation and radioactive decay will lead to a radon and radon daughter concentration that depends on the rate of radon influx into the house, on the ventilation rate, and on the radon concentration in the outside air with which the house is ventilated. In the United States, the average outdoor Rn concentration is 0.4 pCi/L (15 Bq/m^3) and the mean indoor concentration is 1.5 pCi/L (54 Bq/m^3).

In general ventilation, the concentration C to which the airborne contaminant is reduced is determined by the rate of generation G of the contaminant and the ventilation rate Q. The rate of change of the quantity of contaminant in the air is simply the difference between the rate of generation and the rate of removal of the contaminant. If we have a workplace whose volume is V, the rate of change of the quantity of airborne radioactivity is as follows:

Activity change = generated activity − ventilated activity − decayed activity

$$V \, dC = [G - (C \times Q) - (\lambda \times V \times C)] \, dt \tag{11.20}$$

$$V \, dC = [G - C(Q + \lambda V)] \, dt. \tag{11.21}$$

Separating the variables gives

$$\int_{C_0}^{C} \frac{dC}{G - C(Q + \lambda V)} = \int_{0}^{t} \frac{1}{V} dt \tag{11.22}$$

and integrating Eq. (11.22) gives

$$C(t) = \frac{G}{Q + \lambda V} \left[1 - e^{-\left(\frac{Q + \lambda V}{V}\right)t} \right] + C_0 e^{-\left(\frac{Q + \lambda V}{V}\right)t}. \tag{11.23}$$

As $t \to \infty$, $\exp\left[-\left(\dfrac{Q + \lambda V}{V}\right)t\right] \to 0$, and Eq. (11.23) approaches the steady-state concentration of the contaminant:

$$C(\text{steady state}) = \frac{G}{Q + \lambda V}. \tag{11.24}$$

If λV is much less than Q, then Eq. (11.24) reduces to

$$C(\text{steady state}) = \frac{G}{Q}. \tag{11.25}$$

The effective rate of generation of the contaminant is increased if the ventilating air also contains the contaminant. The rate of introduction of the contaminant in the ventilating air (outdoor radon in this case) into the ventilated space is the product of the concentration in the ventilating air, C_V, and the ventilation rate, Q. Thus, the steady state concentration becomes

$$C(\text{steady state}) = \frac{G + (C_V \times Q)}{Q}. \tag{11.26}$$

EXAMPLE 11.8

A single storied house is built on a concrete slab 6.1 m (20 ft.) × 12.2 m (40 ft.). The floor to ceiling distance is 2.5 m (8 ft.). Influx of Rn is 3 pCi/m²/s (0.111 Bq/m²/s), and the air in the house is exchanged twice per hour. The mean Rn concentration in the outside air is 0.4 pCi/L (15 Bq/m³).

(a) Calculate the steady state concentration of the indoor Rn.

(b) Assuming that the Rn–Rn daughter equilibrium ratio is 0.5, calculate the working level (WL) Rn-daughter concentration.

(c) Using an occupancy factor of 0.7, what is the resident's annual exposure, working level months (WLMs)?

Solution

(a) The generation rate of radon by diffusion through the concrete is

$$G = 3 \frac{\text{pCi/m}^2}{\text{s}} \times 6.1 \text{ m} \times 12.2 \text{ m} \times 3600 \frac{\text{s}}{\text{h}} = 8.04 \times 10^5 \frac{\text{pCi}}{\text{h}}.$$

The ventilation rate is:

$$Q = \frac{6.1 \text{ m} \times 12.2 \text{ m} \times 2.5 \text{ m}}{0.5 \text{ hour}} = 372 \frac{\text{m}^3}{\text{h}}.$$

Substituting these values into Eq. (11.26) gives

$$C \text{ (steady state)} = \frac{8.04 \times 10^5 \frac{\text{pCi}}{\text{h}} + (0.4 \frac{\text{pCi}}{\text{L}} \times 372 \frac{\text{m}^3}{\text{h}} \times 1000 \frac{\text{L}}{\text{m}^3})}{372 \frac{\text{m}^3}{\text{h}} \times 1000 \frac{\text{L}}{\text{m}^3}}$$

$$= 2.6 \frac{\text{pCi}}{\text{L}}.$$

(b) The WL was defined in Chapter 7 as the activity of 100 pCi ^{222}Rn in equilibrium with its short-lived progeny. In this case, we have

$$WL = \frac{2.6 \frac{\text{pCi}}{\text{L}}}{100 \text{ pCi/L}} \times 0.5 = 0.013.$$

(c) A WLM was defined in Chapter 7 as exposure for 170 hours, which corresponds to one working month, to a concentration of 1 WL. Therefore, the annual exposure to a resident of this house is

$$WLM \text{ (annual)} = 0.013 \text{ WL} \times 0.7 \times \frac{365 \frac{\text{d}}{\text{yr}} \times 24 \frac{\text{h}}{\text{d}}}{170 \frac{\text{h}}{\text{WLM}}} = 0.47 \frac{\text{WLM}}{\text{yr}}.$$

OPTIMIZATION

Control of airborne contaminants in the workplace is exercised through two different ventilation strategies. One of these, local exhaust ventilation, uses hoods to capture the contaminant at the source, before it escapes to the environment. The second strategy is by general ventilation, which is designed to dilute the airborne contaminant that escapes into the environment to an acceptable level.

EXAMPLE 11.9

An amount of 0.005 μCi/min (185 Bq/min) ^{131}I escapes into the workplace from an enclosed processing unit in a radiopharmaceutical manufacturing laboratory whose dimensions are 10 m × 5 m × 4 m. At what rate should the laboratory be ventilated so that the steady state concentration will not exceed the DAC for ^{131}I, 2 × 10^{-8} μCi/mL (740 Bq/m^3)?

Solution

Substituting into Eq. (11.25) gives us

$$C = \frac{G}{Q}$$

$$2 \times 10^{-8} \, \frac{\mu\text{Ci}}{\text{mL}} = \frac{0.005 \, \dfrac{\mu\text{Ci}}{\text{min}}}{Q \, \text{m}^3 \times 10^6 \, \dfrac{\text{mL}}{\text{m}^3}}$$

$$Q = 0.25 \, \frac{\text{m}^3}{\text{min}} \quad (8.83 \text{ cfm}) \, .$$

Although this ventilation rate will maintain the ^{131}I concentration at the DAC level, it is not necessarily in accord with ALARA. The optimum ventilation rate is that at which the sum of the cost of ventilation plus the cost of the radiation detriment is minimized. For the case of ventilation, the detriment S is given by

$$S = N f T F C = N f T F \frac{G}{Q}, \tag{11.27}$$

where

N = number of workers,
f = fraction "on" time,
T = installation lifetime,
F = dose conversion factor,
C = steady state concentration,
G = activity generation rate, and
Q = ventilation rate.

If α is the cost per unit detriment, then the cost of the detriment Y is

$$Y = \alpha S = \alpha N f T F \frac{G}{Q}. \tag{11.28}$$

The cost of the ventilation x is

$$x = a b f T Q + x_i, \tag{11.29}$$

where

a = cost per unit electricity,

b = units electricity used to move a unit volume of air in the ventilation system, and

x_i = installation cost of the ventilation system.

The total cost U is

$$U = x + y \tag{11.30}$$

$$U = abfTQ + x_i + \alpha NfTF\frac{G}{Q}. \tag{11.31}$$

The optimum ventilation rate Q_0 is the value of Q when U is minimized by setting $dU/dQ = 0$:

$$\frac{dU}{dQ} = abfT - \alpha NfTFG \times \frac{1}{Q^2} = 0, \tag{11.32}$$

$$Q_0 = \sqrt{\frac{\alpha NFG}{ab}}. \tag{11.33}$$

If Q_L is the ventilation rate needed to meet a design criterion, such as the DAC, then the multiplying factor for increasing the ventilation rate needed to achieve the optimum rate is

$$r = \frac{Q_0}{Q_L}. \tag{11.34}$$

But

$$Q_L = \frac{G}{C} = \frac{G}{DAC}. \tag{11.35}$$

Substituting Eqs. (11.33) and (11.35) into Eq. (11.34), we get

$$r = \frac{\sqrt{\dfrac{\alpha NFG}{ab}}}{\dfrac{G}{DAC}} = \frac{\sqrt{\dfrac{\alpha NF}{ab}}}{\sqrt{G}} \times \frac{\sqrt{G}}{\sqrt{G}} \times DAC \tag{11.36}$$

$$r = \sqrt{\frac{\alpha NF}{abG}} \times DAC. \tag{11.37}$$

EXAMPLE 11.10

For the radiopharmaceutical laboratory in Example 11.9, determine the optimum ventilation rate if

$\alpha = \$1000$ per person-rem ($\$100,000$ per person-Sv),

$N = 10$ workers,

$F = 2.7 \times 10^3$ rems/yr per $\mu\text{Ci/m}^3$ (7.3×10^{-4} Sv/yr per Bq/m^3)

$a = \$0.06$ per kW-h,

$b = 1.5 \times 10^{-3}$ kW-h/m^3,

$G = 2.3 \times 10^3 \, \mu\text{Ci/yr}$ (8.5×10^7 Bq/yr), and

DAC $= 2 \times 10^{-8} \, \mu\text{Ci/mL} = 0.02 \, \mu\text{C/m}^3$ (700 Bq/m^3).

Solution

Substituting these values into Eq. (11.37) yields

$$r = \sqrt{\frac{1000 \times 10 \times 2700}{0.06 \times 0.0015 \times 2300}} \times 0.02 = 228.$$

This means that the ventilation rate needed to sustain the airborne concentration at the DAC level should be increased from 0.25 m^3/min by a factor of 228 to $228 \times 0.25 = 57$ m^3/min (2000 cfm).

SUMMARY

Control of internal radiation is based on preventing contamination of the worker through ingestion, inhalation, or absorption either across intact skin or through wounds by radioactive isotopes. This strategy is implemented by blocking the exposure pathways by one or more of several technics: isolating or enclosing the source; control of the environment through good housekeeping, contamination control, ventilation, and waste management; and enclosing the worker in protective clothing and respiratory protective devices. The optimum level for the application of these techniques is determined by minimizing the combined cost of the radiation detriment plus the cost of control.

Although nothing short of allowing natural decay can be done to reduce the radioactivity, and hence the inherent toxic properties, of radioactive wastes, they can be treated to render them essentially nonhazardous. One of the main objectives of waste treatment is to prevent the entrance of radioactive nuclides into the biosphere, where even small amounts might be accumulated by certain plants or animals to potentially toxic concentrations. One treatment method that greatly reduces the potential hazard is immobilization in a highly stable matrix, such as vitrification of high-level liquid waste by incorporating it into glass, or by adsorbing the radionuclides onto clay and then firing the clay at a high temperature, thereby locking the radionuclides into the clay. Both these treatment methods prevent the radionuclides from entering into the biosphere. Other stable matrices include concrete, asphalt, and plastics. Treatment methods include volume reduction of liquid wastes by evaporation and physical compaction of solid wastes, and then packaging and burial in a designated burial site. Low-level liquid wastes may be diluted to concentrations within regulatory requirements, and then released to the environment (although this treatment modality may not be societally acceptable). The exact manner of treatment and disposition is determined by public opinion and by technical and engineering considerations.

PROBLEMS

11.1. A health physicist finds that a radiochemist was inhaling $Ba^{35}SO_4$ particles that were leaking out of a faulty glove box. The radiochemist had been inhaling the dust, whose mean radioactivity concentration was 3.3 MBq/m³ (9×10^{-5} $\mu Ci/cm^3$), for a period of 2 hours. Using the ICRP three compartment lung model, calculate the absorbed dose to the lung during the 13-week period and during the 1-year period immediately following inhalation.

11.2. A tank, of volume 100 L, contained ^{85}Kr gas at a pressure of 10.0 kg/cm². The specific activity of the krypton is 20 Ci/g. The tank is in an unventilated storage room, at a temperature of 27°C, whose dimensions are 3 m × 3 m × 2 m. As a result of a very small leak, the gas leaked out until the pressure in the tank was 9.9 kg/cm². A man unknowingly then spent 1 hour in the storage room. Assume the half-saturation time for krypton solution in the body fluids to be 3 minutes. Henry's law constant for Kr in water at body temperature is 2.13×10^7. Calculate (a) the immersion dose, (b) the internal dose due to the inhaled krypton. The partition ratio of Kr in water to Kr in fat is 1:10.

11.3. If the man in problem 2 turned on a small ventilation fan of capacity 100 ft³/min as he entered the room, calculate his immersion and inhalation doses.

11.4. An accidental discharge of ^{89}Sr into a reservoir resulted in a contamination level of 37 Bq (10^{-3} μCi) per mL of water.

(a) Using the basic radiological health criterion of the ICRP, would this water be acceptable for drinking purposes for the general public if the turnover half-time of the water in the reservoir is 30 days?

(b) If the water were ingested continuously; what maximum body burden would be reached?

(c) How long after the start of ingestion would this maximum occur?

(d) What would be the absorbed dose during the first 13 weeks of ingestion?

(e) What would be the absorbed dose during the first year?

(f) What would be the absorbed dose during 50 years following the start of ingestion?

11.5. Nickel carbonyl $Ni(CO)_4$ has a maximum permissible atmospheric concentration of 1 part per billion (ppb) based on its chemical toxicity. A chemist is going to use this compound tagged with ^{63}Ni. The specific activity of the nickel is 2.5×10^8 Bq/g (6.75 mCi/g). The industrial hygienist is planning to limit the atmospheric concentration of $Ni(CO)_4$ in the laboratory to 0.5 ppb. Will this restriction meet the requirement for the radioactivity DAC of 3×10^{-3} $\mu Ci/mL$?

11.6. Chlorine-36-tagged chloroform, $CHCl_3$, whose specific activity is 100 $\mu Ci/mol$, is to be used under such conditions that 100 mg/h may be lost by evaporation.

The experiment is to be done in a laboratory of dimensions 15 ft × 10 ft × 8 ft. The laboratory is ventilated at a rate of 100 ft^3/min.

(a) Do any special measures have to be taken in order to control the atmospheric concentration of the ^{36}Cl to 10% of its DAC (DAC = 1 × 10^{-6} μCi/cm^3)?

(b) To what concentration of chloroform, in parts per million, does the radiological DAC correspond for this compound? Compare this concentration to the chemical PEL for chloroform.

11.7. For the purpose of estimating hazards from toxic vapors or gases of high molecular weight, it is sometimes incorrectly assumed that settling of the vapor is determined by the specific gravity of the pure vapor, which is defined as

$$\frac{\text{Molecular weight of the pure vapor}}{\text{``Molecular weight'' of air}}$$

instead of the *correct* specific gravity given by

$$\frac{\text{``Molecular weight'' of air and vapor mixture}}{\text{``Molecular weight'' of air}}.$$

(a) If the vapor pressure of benzene (benzol), C_6H_6, is 160 mm Hg at 20°C, calculate the correct specific gravity of a saturated air mixture of benzene vapors and compare it to the specific gravity of the pure vapor.

(b) If the chemical PEL for benzene is 10 ppm by volume, calculate the specific gravity of an air–benzene mixture of this concentration.

(c) What is the maximum specific activity of ^{14}C-tagged benzene in order that one-half the radiological DAC for ^{14}C (DAC = 1 × 10^{-6} μCi/cm^3) not be exceeded by a benzene concentration of 10 ppm?

11.8. Iodine-131 is to be continuously released to the environment through a chimney whose effective height is 100 m and whose discharge rate is 100 m^3/min. The average wind speed is 2 m/s and the lapse rate is stable.

(a) At what maximum rate may the radioiodine be discharged if the maximum downwind ground level concentration is not to exceed 10% of the 10 CFR 20 DAC of 2 × 10^{-8} μCi/cm^3 (700 Bq/m^3).

(b) How far from the chimney will this maximum occur?

11.9. Inhalation exposure is often described as the product of atmospheric concentration and time, as in units of Bq-s/m^3. Using the ICRP assumptions that 23% of inhaled iodine is deposited in the thyroid, and that the thyroid weighs 20 g, calculate the dose to the thyroid due to an acute exposure of 1 Bq-s/m^3 of

(a) ^{131}I.

(b) ^{133}I.

(c) Assuming that the other 77% of the inhaled iodine is absorbed into the blood and is bound to the protein, calculate the total body doses due to the protein-bound iodine.

(d) What is the effective dose from each isotope?

11.10. Disposal of animal carcasses in a biomedical research institution is by incineration. If the incinerator consumes air at the rate of 34 kg/min, how much ^{131}I activity may be incinerated per 40-hour week, assuming that all the radioiodine in the animal carcasses will be volatilized, if the 10 CFR 20 limit of $2 \times 10^{-10} \, \mu\text{Ci/mL}$ in the chimney's effluent is not to be exceeded?

11.11. A graphite-moderated reactor is cooled by passing air at the rate of 680,000 kg/h through the core. The mean temperature in the core is 300°C, and the thermal-neutron flux is 5×10^{13} neutrons/cm^2/s.

    (a) If the air spends an average of 10 seconds in the reactor core, what is the rate of production of ^{41}Ar?

    (b) If the chimney through which the air is discharged is 100 m high and has an orifice diameter of 2 m and the temperature of the effluent air is 170°C, while the ambient temperature is 30°C on a sunny day and if the mean wind velocity is 2 m/s, at what distance from the chimney will the ground-level concentration of ^{41}Ar be a maximum? What will be the value of this maximum concentration (in Bq/m^3)? How does this figure compare to the 10 CFR 20 DAC for ^{41}Ar?

11.12. About 10^{13} Bq (270 Ci) of biomedical ^{14}C waste is generated per year in the United States. If this waste continues to be generated at the same rate:

    (a) What will be the resultant steady-state quantity of ^{14}C waste?

    (b) How long will it take until 99% of the steady-state inventory is reached?

11.13. Analysis of albacore in the Pacific Ocean for ^{137}Cs from nuclear bomb fallout found the mean concentration to be 2.74 Bq/kg (7.4 pCi/kg) wet weight during the period 1965–1971. Calculate the committed dose equivalent due to the consumption of 1 kg albacore per week for 1 year.

11.14. Krypton gas, tagged with ^{85}Kr to a specific activity of 1.3×10^{11} Bq/mol, (3.5 Ci/mol), will be transferred from a tank into another vessel at a rate of 0.1 cm^3/min (at 25°C and 760 torr) through plastic tubing. There is a remote possibility that the tubing connection will break, and the gas will escape into the laboratory. If the laboratory dimensions are 3 m × 4 m × 3 m, what must be the minimum ventilation rate if the steady-state concentration is not to exceed 1/10 of the 10 CFR 20 limit of $1 \times 10^{-5} \, \mu\text{Ci/cm}^3$ (3.7×10^5 Bq/m^3)?

11.15. A 1000-MW (electrical) coal fired power plant burns 6.5 metric tons coal per minute. The ash residue is 10%, of which 90% is bottom ash and 10% is fly ash. The electrostatic precipitator used to collect the fly ash is 98% efficient on a mass basis. The ash contains the following radionuclides, whose inhalation dose conversion factors (DCFs) are listed:

ACTIVITY	CONCENTRATION (pCi/g)	DCF (Sv/Bq)
Uranium	3	3.2E−5
Th-232	9	4.4E−4
Ra-228	3	1.3E−6
Ra-226	3	2.3E−6

A team of 8 workers spend 8 hours repairing a broken water main at a point 500 m directly downwind from the chimney. The effective chimney height is 60 m, the sky is overcast all day, and the ground level wind speed is 2 m/s.

    (a) Calculate the emission rate, pCi/s and Bq/s, for each of the radioisotopes.

(b) Calculate the ground-level concentration of each of the radioisotopes, in pCi/m^3 and Bq/m^3.

(c) If each worker inhaled 10 m³ while on the job, what was the CEDE from the 8-hour inhalation exposure?

11.16. A package of laboratory waste contains ^{140}Ba, $T_{1/2} = 13$ days, and ^{131}I, $T_{1/2} = 8$ days. Ten per cent of the total activity is due to the radiobarium, and 90% of the total activity is due to the radioiodine. What percent of the total activity will the ^{140}Ba contribute 32 days later?

11.17. A 200-L tank contains krypton at a pressure of 1335 psi (9312 kPa) at 70°F (21.1°C). The gas is labelled with ^{85}Kr to a specific activity of 2 Ci per gram Kr. The krypton is leaking out of the tank at a rate of 1 mL (at STP) per minute. The tank is in a storage room 3 m × 3 m × 2 m high, and the air in the room is exchanged 4 times per hour. What is the steady-state concentration in the room, in $\mu Ci/cm^3$ and Bq/m^3?

11.18. A 2-hour air sample at 60 L/min, with a filter efficiency of ~100%, showed 10,000 dpm of ^{90}Sr. The inhalation ALI for class Y ^{90}Sr is 0.1 MBq (4 μCi).

(a) What is the worker's exposure, DAC-hours, if he wore a half-face respirator during the entire 2 hours?

(b) What was the worker's CEDE, in μSv and in mrems, from this exposure?

11.19. Iodine 125 waste, whose half-life is 60 days, is to be disposed of by allowing it to decay away. How long must it be allowed to decay before its activity is reduced by 99.99%?

11.20. To meet regulatory requirements, the activity in a 20-L carboy containing tritiated water must be recorded on the shipping label. A 0.5-mL aliquot is taken, and counted in a liquid scintillation counter whose counting efficiency is 42%. The net counting rate is 13,686 cpm. Calculate the best estimate of the tritium activity in the aqueous waste, in units of μCi and Bq.

SUGGESTED READINGS

American Conference of Governmental Industrial Hygienists. *Industrial Ventilation; A Manual of Recommended Practice*, 25th ed. ACGIH Committee on Industrial Ventilation, Lansing, MI, 2004.

AIChE. *Design Guide for a Radioisotope Laboratory*. American Institute of Chemical Engineers, New York, 1964.

Ayers, J. A., ed. *Decontamination of Nuclear Reactors and Equipment*. Ronald Press, New York, 1970.

Brenk, H. D., Fairobent, J. E., and M, E. H., Jr. Transport of radionuclides in the atmosphere, in Till, J. E. and Meyer, H. R., eds. *Radiological Assessment*. NUREG/CR-3332, U.S. Nuclear Regulatory Commission, Washington, DC, 1983.

Burchsted, C. A., Kahn, J. E., and Fuller, A. B. *Nuclear Air Cleaning Handbook*. ERDA 76-21, NSTIS, Springfield, VA, 1976.

Clayton, G. D., and Clayton, F. E., eds. *Patty's Industrial Hygiene and Toxicology, Vol. I, General Principles*, 4th ed. Wiley Interscience, New York, 1991.

Codell, R. B., and Duguid, J. D. Transport of radionuclides in groundwater, in Till, J. E., and Meyer, H. R., eds. *Radiological Assessment*. NUREG/CR-3332, U.S. Nuclear Regulatory Commission, Washington, DC, 1983.

Cohen, B. L. *The Nuclear Energy Option.* Plenum Press, New York, 1990.

Dennis, R., ed. *Handbook on Aerosols.* TID-26608, NTIS, Springfield, VA, 1976.

Drinker, P. and Hatch, T. *Industrial Dust.* McGraw-Hill, New York, 1954.

Dunlap, R. E., Kraft, M. E., and Rosa, E. A. *Public Reactions to Nuclear Waste.* Duke University Press, Durham, NC, 1993.

Eicholz, G. G. *Environmental Aspects of Nuclear Power.* Ann Arbor Science Publishers, Ann Arbor, MI, 1976.

Eisenbud, M., and Gesell, T. *Environmental Radioactivity: From Natural, Industrial, and Military Sources,* 4th ed. Academic Press, New York, 1997.

Faw, R. E., and Shultis, J. K. *Radiological Assessment.* Prentice-Hall, Englewood Cliffs, NJ, 1993.

Fiber, G. J., Heffter, J. L., and Klement, A. W. Meteorological dispersion of released radioactivity, in Klement, A. W., ed. *Handbook of Environmental Radiation.* CRC Press, Boca Raton, FL, 1982.

Garrick, J. Contemporary issues in risk-informed decision making on the disposition of radioactive wastes. *Health Phys,* **91**:430–448, 2006.

Green, H. L., and Lane, W. R. *Particulate Clouds: Dusts, Smokes, and Mists.* Van Nostrand, Princeton, NJ, 1964.

Hawkins, M. B. The design of laboratories for the safe handling of radioisotopes, in Coleman, H.S., ed. *Laboratory Design.* Reinhold Publishing Co., New York, 1951.

International Atomic Energy Agency (IAEA), Vienna.

Generic Intervention Levels for Protecting the Public in the Event of a Nuclear Accident or Radiological Emergency, 1993.

Handling of Tritium Bearing Wastes, 1981.

Radioactive Waste Management Glossary, 1993.

Separation, Storage, and Disposal of Krypton-85, 1980.

Safety Reports Series No.

21. *Optimization of Radiation Protection in the Control of Occupational Exposure,* 2002.

27. *Monitoring and Surveillance of Residues from the Mining and Milling of Uranium and Thorium,* 2002.

33. *Radiation Protection against Radon in Workplaces other than Mines,* 2003.

34. *Radiation Protection and the Management of Radioactive Waste in the Oil and Gas Industries,* 2003.

35. *Surveillance and Monitoring of Near Surface Disposal Facilities for Radioactive Waste,* 2004.

Safety Series No.

22. *Respirators and Protective Clothing,* 1967.

29. *Application of Meteorology to Safety at Nuclear Plants,* 1968.

30. *Manual on Safety Aspects of the Design and Equipment of Hot Laboratories,* 1981.

45. *Principles for Establishing Limits for the Release of Radioactive Materials into the Environment,* 1978.

39. *Safe Handling of Plutonium,* 1974.

48. *Manual on Decontamination of Surfaces,* 1979.

50. *Atmospheric Dispersion in Nuclear Power Plant Siting,* 1980.

77. *Principles for Limiting Releases of Radioactive Effluents into the Environment,* 1986.

104. *Extension of the Principles of Radiation Protection to Sources of Potential Exposure,* 1990.

115. *Basic Safety Standards for Protection against Ionizing Radiation and for the Safety of Nuclear Sources,* 1996.

Radiation Safety Standards Series No.:

NS-G-3.4. *Meteorological Events in Site Evaluation for Nuclear Power Plants,* 2003.

NS-G-1.13. *Radiation Protection Aspects in the Design of Nuclear Power Plants,* 2005.

RS-G-1.1. *Occupational Radiation Protection,* 1999.

RS-G-1.2. *Assessment of Occupational Exposure Due to Intakes of Radionuclides,* 1999.

RS-G-1.5. *Radiological Protection for Medical Exposure to Ionizing Radiation,* 2004.

RS-G-1.6. *Occupational Radiation Protection in the Mining and Processing of Raw Materials Safety Guide,* 2004.

RS-G-1.8. *Environmental and Source Monitoring for Purposes of Radiation Protection,* 2005.

RS-G-1.9. *Categorization of Radioactive Sources Safety Guide,* 2005.

TS-G-1.2. *Planning and Preparing for Emergency Response to Traffic Accidents Involving Radioactive Material,* 2002.

TS-R-1. *Regulations for the Safe Transport of Radioactive Materials,* 2005.

WS-R-1. *Near Surface Disposal of Radioactive Waste Safety Requirements,* 1999.

WS-R-2. *Predisposal Management of Radioactive Waste, Including Decommissioning Requirements,* 2000.

WS-G-1.2. *Management of Radioactive Waste from the Mining and Milling of Ore,* 2002.

WS-G-2.3. *Regulatory Control of Radioactive Discharges to the Environment*, 2000.

WS-G-2.5. *Predisposal Management of Low and Intermediate Level Radioactive Waste*, 2003.

WS-G-2.6. *Predisposal Management of High Level Radioactive Waste Safety*, 2003.

Symposium Series

a. The Oklo Phenomenon, 1975.

b. Underground Disposal, 1980.

c. Optimization of Radiation Protection, 1986.

d. Environmental Impact of Radioactive Releases, 1995.

e. Radioactive Waste Management—Turning Options into Solutions, 2000.

International Commission on Radiological Protection (ICRP), Pergamon Press, Oxford, U.K.

The Assessment of Internal Contamination Resulting from Recurrent or Prolonged Uptakes. ICRP Publication 10, 1971.

Limits for Intakes of Radionuclides by Workers (8-volume set with index), 1989.

International Commission on Radiological Protection (ICRP). *Annals of the ICRP*, Pergamon Press, Oxford, U.K.

Report No.

25. *Handling and Disposal of Radioactive Materials in Hospitals*, **1**(2), 1977.

29. *Radionuclide Release into the Environment—Assessment of Doses to Man*, **2**(2), 1979.

37. *Cost Benefit Analysis in the Optimization of Radiation Protection*, **10**(2,3), 1983.

38. *Radionuclide Transformations: Energy and Intensity of Emissions*, **11–13**, 1983.

46. *Radiation Protection Principles for the Disposal of Solid Radioactive Waste*, **15**(4), 1986.

47. *Radiation Protection of Workers in Mines*, **16**(1), 1986.

52. *Protection of the Patient in Nuclear Medicine*, **17**(4), 1988.

54. *Individual Monitoring for Intakes of Radionuclides by Workers: Design and Interpretation*, **19**(1–3), 1988.

55. *Optimization and Decision Making in Radiological Protection*, **20**(1), 1989.

56. *Age-Dependent Doses to Members of the Public from Intake of Radionuclides, Part 1*, **20**(2), 1990.

57. *Radiological Protection of the Worker in Medicine and Dentistry*, **20**(3), 1990.

60. *1990 Recommendations of the International Commission on Radiological Protection*, **21**(1–3), 1991.

61. *Annual Limits on Intake of Radionuclides by Workers Based on the 1990 Recommendations*, **21**(4), 1991.

62. *Principles for Intervention for Protection of the Public in a Radiological Emergency*, **22**(4), 1993.

65. *Protection Against Radon-222 at Home and at Work*, 1994.

66. *Human Respiratory Tract Model for Radiological Protection*, **24**(1–3), 1994.

77. *Radiological Protection Policy for the Disposal of Radioactive Waste*, **27**(Supplement), 1998.

78. *Individual Monitoring for Internal Exposure of Workers; Replacement of ICRP Publication 54*, **27**(3,4), 1997.

81. *Radiation Protection Recommendations as Applied to the Disposal of Long-Lived Solid Radioactive Waste*, **28**(4), 1998.

88. *Doses to the Embryo and Fetus from Intakes of Radionuclides by the Mother*, **31**(1–3), 2001.

95. *Doses to Infants from Ingestion of Radionuclides in Mothers' Milk*, **34**(3,4), 2004.

Supporting Guidance 3. *Guide for the Practical Application of the ICRP Human Respiratory Tract Model*, **32**(1,2), 2002.

Jirka, G. H., Findikakis, A. N., Onishi, Y., and Ryan, P. J. Transport of radionuclides in surface waters, in Till, J. E., Meyer, H. R., eds. *Radiological Assessment*. NUREG/CR-3332, U.S. Nuclear Regulatory Commission, Washington, DC, 1983.

Kaye, G. I., Methe, B. M., and Weber, P. B. Low-level waste management in an academic medical center, in Eicholz, G. G., Shonka, J. J., eds. *Hospital Health Physics*. Research Enterprises, Richland, WA, 1993.

Leggett, R. W., and Eckerman, K. F. *Dosimetric Significance of the ICRP's Updated Guidance and Models, 1989–2003, and Implications for U.S. Federal Guidance*, ORNL/TM-2003/207, U.S. Dept of Energy, Washington, DC, 2003.

Lewis, E. E. *Nuclear Power Reactor Safety*. Wiley Interscience, New York, 1977.

Miller, K. L. *Handbook of Management of Radiation Protection Programs*, 2nd ed., CRC Press, Boca Raton, FL, 1992.

More, J. A., and Kearfott, K. J. A simple radon chamber for educational use. *Oper Radiat Saf*, **89**:S78–S84, 2005.

National Bureau of Standards. *Recommendations for the Disposal of Carbon-14 Waste*. NBS Handbook 53, U.S. Govt. Printing Office, Washington, DC, 1953.

National Council on Radiation Protection and Measurement (NCRP). Bethesda, MD.

Report No.

44. *Krypton-85 in the Atmosphere—Accumulation, Biological Significance, and Control Technology,* 1975.

55. *Protection of the Thyroid Gland in the Event of the Release of Radioiodine,* 1977.

60. *Physical, Chemical, and Biological Properties of Radiocerium Relevant to Radiation Protection Guidelines,* 1978.

62. *Tritium in the Environment,* 1979.

65. *Management of Persons Accidentally Contaminated with Radionuclides,* 1979.

75. *Iodine-129: Evaluation of Releases from Nuclear Power Generation,* 1983.

76. *Radiological Assessment: Predicting the Transport, Bioaccumulation, and Uptake by Man of Radionuclides Released to the Environment,* 1984.

88. *Radiation Alarms and Access Control Systems,* 1986.

105. *Radiation Protection for Medical and Allied Health Personnel,* 1989.

116. *Limitation of Exposure to Ionizing Radiation,* 1993.

118. *Radiation Protection for the Mineral Extraction Industry,* 1993.

120. *Dose Control at Nuclear Power Plants* 1994.

139. *Risk-Based Classification of Radioactive and Hazardous Chemical Wastes,* 2002.

141. *Managing Potentially Radioactive Scrap Metal,* 2002.

Plog, B. A., and Quinlan, P. eds. *Fundamentals of Industrial Hygiene,* 5th ed. National Safety Council, Chicago, IL, 2002.

Pritchard, J. A. *A Guide to Industrial Respiratory Protection.* LA-6671-M, NSTIS, Springfield, VA, 1976.

Ryan, M. T., Skrable, K. W., French, C. S., and Potter, C. S., A simple method for assessing exposure to internal emitters. *Oper Radiat Saf,* **88:**S51–S54, 2001.

Sagan, L. A., ed. *Human and Ecologic Effects of Nuclear Power Plants.* Charles C. Thomas, Springfield, IL, 1974.

Shapiro, J. *Radiation Protection,* 4th ed. Harvard University Press, Cambridge, MA, 2002.

Slade, D. H., ed. *Meteorology and Atomic Energy.* TID-24190, NSTIS, Springfield, VA, 1968.

Smith, M., ed. *Recommended Guide for the Prediction of Dispersion of Airborne Effluents.* American Society of Mechanical Engineers, New York, 1968.

Smith, T., and Beresford, N. A., ed. *Chernobyl—Catastrophe and Consequences,* Springer, Secaucus, NJ, 2005.

Steck, D. J., Field, R. W., and Lynch, C. F. Exposure to atmospheric radon, *Environ Health Perspect,* **107**(2), 1999.

Turner, J. E. *Atoms, Radiation, and Radiation Protection,* 2nd ed. McGraw-Hill, New York, 1995.

United Nations Scientific Committee in the Effects of Atomic Radiation (UNSCEAR). United Nations, New York.

Sources and Effects of Ionizing Radiation. A Report to the General Assembly, 2000.

Management of Toxic Chemicals and Hazardous and Radioactive Waste, 2001.

United States Department of Energy (USDOE). *Radiological Control Manual,* DOE/EH-0256T, Washington, DC, 1992.

Wentz, C. A. *Hazardous Waste Management,* 2nd ed. McGraw-Hill, New York, 1995.

Wrixon, A. D., Linsley, G. S., Binns, K. C., and White, D. F. *Derived Limits for Surface Contamination.* NRPB-DL2, National Radiological Protection Board, Harwell, U.K., 1979.

12

CRITICALITY

CRITICALITY HAZARD

Of all the potential radiation hazards with which the health physicist deals, that of an accidental criticality is among the most serious. Criticality may be defined as the attainment of physical conditions such that a fissile material will sustain a chain reaction. During this chain reaction, the nuclei of the fissile material (material whose atoms can be made to fission) splits, thereby liberating tremendous amounts of energy in the form of radiation and producing large quantities of radioactive fission products. In a nuclear reactor, criticality is attained under conditions that are very rigorously controlled in regard to safety and power level. If criticality is accidentally attained outside a reactor during the processing or handling of nuclear fuel, the consequences to personnel and equipment are very grave. The utmost in care and controls, both technical and administrative, must be exercised in the handling, use, or transport of fissile materials if death or serious injury or property damage due to a criticality accident is to be avoided. Generally, such efforts to prevent criticality accidents are called *criticality control* or *nuclear safety*.

NUCLEAR FISSION

The liquid drop model pictures the nucleus as a sphere inside which the nucleons are in constant random motion. As a consequence of this motion, the sphere may become distorted, and, under certain conditions, may become highly deformed and split into several parts: two smaller nuclei, which are called fission fragments, and several neutrons.

For fission to be possible, the following mass–energy relationship must hold:

$$E_f = (M - m_1 - m_2 - m_n)c^2, \tag{12.1}$$

where E_f is the energy released during fission, M is the mass of the fissioned nucleus, m_1 and m_2 are the masses of the fission fragments, and m_n is the mass of the neutrons. This condition can be met only by those isotopes whose atomic number and atomic mass number are such that $Z^2/A \geq 15$. However, although many isotopes at the

TABLE 12-1. Spontaneous Fission Rates

ISOTOPE	FISSIONS/g/s
^{232}Th	4.1×10^{-5}
^{233}U	$<1.9 \times 10^{-4}$
^{234}U	3.5×10^{-3}
^{235}U	3.1×10^{-4}
^{236}U	2.8×10^{-3}
^{238}U	7.0×10^{-3}

upper end of the periodic table meet this requirement, spontaneous nuclear fission is an extremely unlikely event. Table 12-1 lists the spontaneous fission rates for several isotopes that are theoretically fissionable. Although the likelihood of spontaneous fission is almost infinitesimally small, spontaneous fission nevertheless is extremely important in criticality control, since it can, under the proper conditions, initiate an *accidental criticality*, or an uncontrolled nuclear chain reaction. For an isotope where $Z^2/A \geq 49$, the nucleus is unstable toward fission, and the isotope would undergo instantaneous spontaneous fission if it should be produced. All the naturally occurring fissionable isotopes are highly stable against spontaneous fission.

Fissionable isotopes require a certain amount of activation energy in order to cause them to fission. This is due to a potential barrier that must be exceeded before the nucleus splits. For example, let us consider the case where a nucleus of atomic number Z splits into two equal fission fragments of atomic number $Z/2$ and nuclear radius r. In order to part into two distinct fragments as a result of coulombic repulsion, these two fission fragments must be separated by a minimum distance of $2r$. At this separation, the potential energy in the system is at its maximum value of

$$E_m = \frac{\left(Ze/2^2\right)}{2r},$$

and decreases as the distance between the fission fragments increases. At distances less than $2r$, nuclear forces become operative, and the potential energy in the system again decreases, as shown in Figure 12-1. In order for fission to occur, E_f must be equal to or greater than E_m. Thus, if sufficient energy is added to the system to exceed the height of the potential barrier, the fission can be initiated. From Figure 12-1, it can be seen that an isotope whose nuclear potential well is represented by the dotted line requires less activation energy than one whose nuclear potential well is described by the solid line. This difference in activation energy explains why some isotopes, such as ^{235}U and ^{239}Pu are more easily fissionable than others, such as ^{238}U and ^{240}Pu.

Activation energy for nuclear fission may be obtained from the binding energy released when a neutron is absorbed by a fissile nucleus. It was pointed out in Chapter 4 that even–even nuclei are most stable; that is, they have more binding energy per nucleon than isotopes with an odd number of nucleons. Because of this, the addition of a neutron to a nucleus containing an odd number of nucleons, thus producing a nucleus with an even number of nucleons, releases more energy than the addition

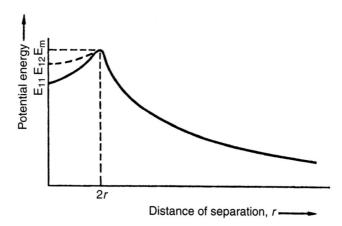

Figure 12-1. Potential energy in a system of two equal fission fragments each of atomic number $Z/2$ and radius r.

of a neutron to a nucleus containing an even number of nucleons. Nuclei with odd numbers of nucleons are consequently more easily fissioned than those with an even number of nucleons. For example, ^{235}U, which fissions after capturing a thermal neutron, is first transformed into an even–even nucleus by the captured thermal neutron and then undergoes nuclear fission:

$$^{235}_{92}\text{U} + ^{1}_{0}\text{n} \rightarrow ^{236}_{92}\text{U}^* \rightarrow \text{fission},$$

whereas ^{238}U, which can also capture a thermal neutron, is transformed into an even–odd nucleus and rids itself of its excitation energy by emitting a gamma ray:

$$^{238}_{92}\text{U} + ^{1}_{0}\text{n} \rightarrow ^{239}_{92}\text{U} + \gamma.$$

The reason for the two different modes of deexcitation of the compound nucleus, nuclear fission and gamma emission, is shown in the following calculation, in which the energy of binding a neutron to ^{235}U and to ^{238}U is calculated. From Eq. (3.19), the nuclear mass for ^{235}U is calculated, then the mass of a neutron is added. We once more use Eq. (3.19), this time to calculate the mass of ^{236}U, then find the binding energy by subtracting the ^{236}U mass from the sum of the masses of ^{235}U and a neutron. This procedure gives

mass of ^{235}U	=	235.04392
mass of neutron	=	1.00867
sum of masses	=	236.05259
minus mass ^{236}U	=	236.04556
mass defect	=	0.00703 amu (atomic mass units)
energy equivalent	=	0.00703 amu × 931 MeV/amu = 6.54 MeV.

In a similar manner, the binding energy of a neutron captured by a ^{238}U nucleus is calculated as 4.80 MeV. Thus, we see that more energy, in the amount of 1.75 MeV, is liberated when a ^{235}U nucleus binds a thermal neutron than when ^{238}U binds such a neutron. In the case of ^{235}U, this additional energy is sufficient to cause fission. Uranium-238 can also be made to fission. This occurs if the ^{238}U nucleus captures a fast neutron. The kinetic energy of the neutron plus the binding energy is sufficient to cause nuclear fission. Experimentally, it has been found that a neutron must have at least 1.1 MeV of kinetic energy in order to induce fission in ^{238}U. Although ^{238}U can undergo "fast fission," the probability of such a reaction is very low in comparison to the probability of thermal fission in ^{235}U. The cross section for fast fission of ^{238}U is 0.29 b, while for thermal fission of ^{235}U, the cross section is 588 b. This great difference in fission cross section is one of the chief reasons for the popularity of ^{235}U-fueled thermal-neutron reactors.

When an atom fissions, it splits into two fission fragments plus several neutrons (the mean number of neutrons per fission of ^{235}U is 2.5) plus gamma rays—according to the conservation equation

$$^{235}_{92}U + ^{1}_{0}n \rightarrow ^{236}_{92}U^* \rightarrow ^{A_1}_{Z_1}F + ^{A_2}_{Z_2}F + \nu ^{1}_{0}n + Q \qquad (12.2)$$

The value of Q in Eq. (12.2), which may be calculated from the mass balance for any particular pair of fission fragments, is about 200 MeV. An approximate distribution of this energy is as follows:

Fission fragments, kinetic energy	167 MeV
Neutron kinetic energy	6
Fission gamma rays	6
Radioactive decay	
Beta particles	5
Gamma rays	5
Neutrinos	11
Total	200 Mev per fission

Most of this energy is dissipated as heat within the critical assembly. In a power reactor, this heat energy is converted into electrical energy. Using a mean value of 190 MeV heat energy per fission, the rate of fission to generate one watt of power is calculated as follows:

$$1\,W = X\,\frac{\text{fission}}{s} \times 190\,\frac{MeV}{\text{fission}} \times 1.6 \times 10^{-13}\,\frac{J}{MeV} \times 1\,\frac{W}{J/s}$$

$$X = 3.3 \times 10^{10}\,\frac{\text{fission}/s}{W}.$$

The amount of ^{235}U burned up to produce 1 MW-day of heat energy is

$$\frac{3.3 \times 10^{10}\,\dfrac{\text{fission}}{W \cdot s} \times 10^6 \dfrac{W}{MW} \times 8.64 \times 10^4\,\dfrac{s}{d}}{\dfrac{6.02 \times 10^{23}\,\text{atoms/mol}}{235\,\text{g/mol}}} = 1.1\,\frac{g}{MW \cdot d}.$$

Fission Products

The atomic numbers of the fission fragments range from 30 (^{72}Zn) to 64 (^{158}Gd). All fission fragments are radioactive, and decay, usually in chains of several members in length, to form *fission products*. Two such chains of fission products that are of special interest to health physicists are

$$^{90}_{36}\text{Kr} (\beta, 33\text{s}) \rightarrow {}^{90}_{37}\text{Rb} (\beta, 2.74 \text{ min}) \rightarrow {}^{90}_{38}\text{Sr} (\beta, 28 \text{ yr}) \rightarrow {}^{90}_{39}\text{Y} (\beta, 64.2 \text{ h})$$

$$\rightarrow {}^{90}_{40}\text{Zr (stable)}$$

and

$$^{137}_{53}\text{I} (\beta, 22 \text{ s}) \rightarrow {}^{137}_{54}\text{Xe} (\beta, 3.9 \text{ min}) \rightarrow {}^{137}_{55}\text{Cs} (\beta, 30 \text{ yr}) \rightarrow {}^{137}_{56}\text{Ba (stable)} .$$

The fission yield for the various fission products are shown in Figure 12-2. After production, each species of fission product decays according to its unique disintegration rate. The total activity at any time after production, therefore, is the sum of the exponential decay curves for each fission product. However, the collective activity, between about 10 seconds and 1000 hours after fission, can be mathematically described by a power function, since the total activity decreases as (time)$^{-1.2}$. The quantity of radioactivity at time ΔT days after fission is given by

$$A = 3.81 \times 10^{-6} \Delta T^{-1.2} \frac{\text{Bq}}{\text{fission}}, \tag{12.3a}$$

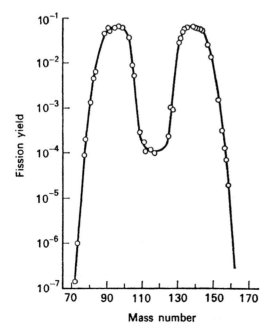

Figure 12-2. Fission product yield from thermal fission of ^{235}U.

or

$$A = 1.03 \times 10^{-16} \Delta T^{-1.2} \frac{\text{Ci}}{\text{fission}},$$ (12.3b)

where T is the time in days after fission.

EXAMPLE 12.1

A certain criticality accident was due to the accumulation, in a 225-gal tank, of 3-kg ^{239}Pu dissolved in an organic solvent (tributylphosphate). When a stirrer began to operate, changes in the density and geometry of the system caused it to become critical, and, in a single burst of about 10 milliseconds, about 10^{17} nuclei fissioned.

(a) How much energy, in kilowatt-hours, was released?

(b) What was the mean power level during criticality?

(c) What was the fission product inventory 1 minute, 1 hour, and 1 day after the accident?

Solution

(a) $E = 10^{17} \text{fiss} \times 190 \dfrac{\text{MeV}}{\text{fiss}} \times 1.6 \times 10^{-13} \dfrac{\text{J}}{\text{MeV}} \times 1 \dfrac{\text{W} \cdot \text{s}}{\text{J}} \times \dfrac{1 \, \text{kW} \cdot \text{h}}{3.6 \times 10^{6} \, \text{W} \cdot \text{s}}$

$E = 0.845 \, \text{kW} \cdot \text{h}.$

(b) $\dfrac{0.845 \, \text{kW} \cdot \text{h} \times 3.6 \times 10^{3} \dfrac{\text{s}}{\text{h}}}{10 \times 10^{-3} \text{s}} = 3.04 \times 10^{5} \, \text{kW} = 304 \, \text{MW}.$

(c) From Eq. (12.3), we find the activity at 1 minute ($1/1440 = 6.95 \times 10^{-4}$ days) to be

$$A = 3.81 \times 10^{-6} \times \left(6.95 \times 10^{-4} \, \text{day}\right)^{-1.2} \frac{\text{Bq}}{\text{fission}} \times 10^{17} \, \text{fissions}$$

$$= 2.35 \times 10^{15} \, \text{Bq},$$

or

$$6.34 \times 10^{4} \, \text{Ci};$$

after 1 hour, the activity is related to the 1-minute activity by

$$\frac{A_1}{A_2} = \frac{(T_1)^{-1.2}}{(T_2)^{-1.2}},$$

$$A_2 = A_1 \left(\frac{T_1}{T_2}\right)^{1.2}$$ (12.4)

$$A_2 = 2.35 \times 10^{15} \text{ Bq} \times \left(\frac{1 \text{ min}}{60 \text{ min}}\right)^{1.2} = 1.73 \times 10^{13} \text{ Bq} \quad (467 \text{ Ci});$$

and after 1 day, we have left

$$A_2 = 2.35 \times 10^{15} \text{ Bq} \times \left(\frac{1 \text{ min}}{1440 \text{ min}}\right)^{1.2} = 3.81 \times 10^{11} \text{ Bq} \quad (10.3 \text{ Ci})$$

CRITICALITY

Criticality is attained when at least one of the several neutrons that are emitted in a fission process causes a second nucleus to fission. However, although a chain reaction may occur whenever fissionable material is irradiated with neutrons, not all systems of fissionable material can go critical. If more neutrons are lost by escape from the system or by nonfission absorption in impurities or "poisons" than are produced in fission, then the chain reaction is not self-sustaining and dies out. In this case, the assembly of fissionable material is called *subcritical*. If we have a sustained chain reaction, and if the rate of fission neutron production exceeds the rate of loss, the assembly is called *supercritical*. When exactly one neutron per fission is available for initiating another fission, the system is called *critical*.

Multiplication Factor: The Four-Factor Formula

The measure of criticality in a given system is expressed by the effective multiplication factor, k_{eff}, which is defined as

$$k_{\text{eff}} = \frac{N_{f+1}}{N_f}, \tag{12.5}$$

where N_{f+1} is the number of neutrons produced in the $(f + 1)$th generation by the number of neutrons N_f of the previous generation. Neutrons of a given generation remain in that generation until they either cause fission or are lost through nonfission process. When k_{eff} is less than 1.0000, the system is subcritical; when k_{eff} exceeds 1.0000, the system is supercritical, and when k_{eff} is exactly equal to 1.0000, the system is critical.

Criticality, or the value of k_{eff}, depends on the supply of neutrons of proper energy to initiate fission and on the availability of fissile atoms. The numerical value of k_{eff}, in turn, depends on two conditions: the composition and the physical arrangement of the fissile assembly and the size of the fissile assembly. Neutrons are lost from the assembly by several nonfission processes, including leakage from the fissile assembly. If the assembly is infinitely large, then no neutrons are lost through leakage, and the multiplication factor is known as the infinite multiplication factor, k_∞. The relationship between k_{eff} and k_∞ is

$$k_{\text{eff}} = L \times k_\infty, \tag{12.6}$$

where L is the nonleakage probability.

The value of k_∞ is determined by four factors whose mutual interrelationship can be demonstrated by following a group of n fission neutrons through a life cycle. If η (eta) is the mean number of neutrons emitted per *absorption in uranium*, then capture of n thermal neutrons will result in $n \times \eta$ fission neutrons. The mean number of neutrons ν (nu) emitted per fission depends on the fuel. For ^{235}U, $\nu = 2.5$; and for ^{239}Pu, $\nu = 3.0$. However, since both ^{235}U and ^{239}Pu also absorb thermal neutrons without fissioning, not every absorption leads to fission, and hence the mean number of fission neutrons per absorption by the fissile material (the fuel) must be less than ν. For pure ^{235}U, $\eta = 2.1$, while for any other degree of enrichment, $\eta < 2.1$ because of nonfission absorption by ^{238}U. The exact value of η depends on the degree of enrichment of the uranium.

EXAMPLE 12.2

Calculate the value of value of η for natural uranium.

Solution

To calculate η for natural uranium

$$\eta = \frac{\Sigma_f}{\Sigma_a} \times \nu = \frac{N_5 \sigma_{f5}}{N_5 \sigma_{a5} + N_8 \sigma_{a8}} \times \nu = \frac{\sigma_{f5}}{\sigma_{a5} + (N_8/N_5)\,\sigma_{a8}} \times \nu, \qquad \textbf{(12.7)}$$

where

Σ_f = macroscopic fission cross section,
Σ_a = macroscopic absorption cross section,
N_5 = ^{235}U atoms per cm^3,
N_8 = ^{238}U atoms per cm^3,
σ_{f5} = fission cross section for ^{235}U = 549 b,
σ_{a5} = absorption cross section for ^{235}U = 650 b,
σ_{a8} = absorption cross section for ^{238}U = 2.8 b, and
ν = average number of neutrons per fission of ^{235}U = 2.5.

For natural uranium,

$$\frac{N_8}{N_5} = 139,$$

and

$$\eta = \frac{549}{650 + (139 \times 2.8)} \times 2.5 = 1.32.$$

Uranium-238 has a small cross section (0.29 b) for fission by fast neutrons. Before becoming thermalized, therefore, some of the fast neutrons will be captured by ^{238}U and will cause "fast fission." If we define the *fast fission factor* ε as

$$\varepsilon = \frac{\text{total number of fission neutrons}}{\text{number of thermal fission neutrons}}, \tag{12.8}$$

then the capture of n thermal neutrons in the fuel will produce $n\eta\varepsilon$ fission neutrons. The value for ε depends on the ratio of moderator to fuel, on the ratio of inelastic scattering cross section to fission cross section, and on the geometrical relationship between uranium and moderator. The maximum value of ε is 1.29 in the case of unmoderated pure uranium metal. In the case of a homogeneous fuel assembly, such as a solution of fuel, ε is very close to 1.

While the fast neutrons are being slowed down, they may be captured by ^{238}U without producing fission; resonances for such capture occur between 200 eV and 5 eV. The probability that a neutron will escape this resonance capture is called the *resonance escape probability* or p and is defined as the fraction of the fast, fission-produced neutrons that finally become thermalized. The value of p depends on the ratio of moderator to fuel. For a very high ratio, p approaches 1, whereas for a very low ratio, p is very small. For pure unmoderated natural uranium, p is 0, which means that natural uranium cannot become critical under any conditions if it is not moderated. The resonance escape probability is given by

$$p = \exp - \left[\frac{N_8}{\xi \Sigma_S} \int (\sigma_a)_{\text{eff}} \frac{\mathrm{d}E}{E} \right], \tag{12.9}$$

where

N_8 = number of ^{238}U atoms per cm^3,
ξ = average logarithmic energy decrement, as defined by Eq. (5.57),
Σ_S = macroscopic scattering cross section for the moderator-uranium mixture, and
$(\sigma_a)_{\text{eff}}$ = effective absorption cross section for the moderator-uranium mixture.

Experimentally, it has been found that for a homogeneous mixture of uranium in a moderator the effective resonance integral can be approximated by

$$\int (\sigma_a)_{\text{eff}} \frac{\mathrm{d}E}{E} = 3.9 \left(\frac{\Sigma_S}{N_8} \right)^{0.415} \text{b.} \tag{12.10}$$

for cases where $\Sigma_S/N_8 = 1000$ b. When Σ_s/N_8 increases beyond 1000 b, the value of the effective resonance integral increases to a limit of 240 b. Some values for the integral are given in Table 12-2.

For a heterogeneous assembly consisting of natural uranium fuel rods,

$$\int (\sigma_a)_{\text{eff}} \frac{\mathrm{d}E}{E} = 9.5 + 24.7 \frac{S}{M} \text{b,} \tag{12.11}$$

where

S = surface area of the uranium in cm^2 and
M = weight of the uranium in grams.

TABLE 12-2. Effective Resonance Integral for Several Values of $\sum_s / N_8$

$\sum_s / N_0$ (barns)	$\int (\sigma_a)_{\text{eff}} \frac{dE}{E}$ (barns)
8.2	9.3
50	20
100	26
300	42
500	51
1000	69
2000	90
3000	101
10,000	125
∞	240

From the original n thermal neutrons, we thus have $n\eta\varepsilon p$ thermal neutrons. Not all of these thermal neutrons produce fission; some are absorbed by nonfuel atoms and some are absorbed by ^{235}U without producing fission. (Only 84% of the thermal neutrons absorbed by ^{235}U cause fission.) The fraction of the total number of thermalized neutrons absorbed by the fuel (including all the uranium) is called the *thermal utilization factor*, f. The total number of new neutrons thus produced by the original n thermal neutrons is $n\eta\varepsilon pf$. From the definition of k in Eq. (12.5), we obtain the *four-factor formula* for criticality in the infinitely large system:

$$k_\infty = \frac{N_{f+1}}{N_f} = \frac{n\eta\varepsilon pf}{n} = \eta\varepsilon pf. \tag{12.12}$$

One of the four factors, η, depends only on the fuel. The other factors, ε, p, and f, depend on the composition and physical arrangement of the fuel: ε varies from a maximum of 1.29 for unmoderated uranium to almost 1 for a homogeneous dispersion of fuel in a moderator; p is on the order of 0.8 to almost 1 (for pure ^{235}U fuel, $p = 1$; for high degrees of enrichment, $p \approx 1$). The thermal utilization factor can be calculated from its definition:

$$f = \frac{\Sigma_{aU}}{\Sigma_{aU} + \Sigma_{aM} + \Sigma_{ap}} = \frac{\sigma_{a5} N_5 + \sigma_{a8} N_{a8}}{\sigma_{a5} N_5 + \sigma_{aM} N_M + (\Sigma \sigma_{ai} N_i)_p}, \tag{12.13}$$

where

Σ_{aU} = macroscopic absorption cross section of uranium,
Σ_{aM} = macroscopic absorption cross section of the moderator,
Σ_{ap} = macroscopic absorption cross section of other substances in the fuel assembly
Σ_{ai} = absorption cross section of the ith element in the "other substances,"
N_i = atoms/cm^3 of the ith element in the other substances,
σ_{a5} = absorption cross section of ^{235}U = 650 b,
σ_{a8} = absorption cross section of ^{238}U = 2.8 b,
N_5 = atoms/cm^3 of ^{235}U, and
N_8 = atoms/cm^3 of ^{238}U.

EXAMPLE 12.3

Calculate f for a solution of 925 g uranium as uranyl sulfate, UO_2SO_4, in 14-L water. The uranium is enriched to 93%.

Solution

The problem may be solved by application of Eq. (12.13). However, it can be slightly simplified since, in a homogeneous mixture, the number of atoms per cm^3 is directly proportional to the molar concentration of the various substances. Therefore, Eq. (12.13) can be rewritten as

$$f = \frac{\sigma_{a5}\, M_5 + \sigma_{a8}\, M_8}{\sigma_{a5}\, M_5 + \sigma_{a8}\, M_8 + \sigma_{aH_2O+}\, M_{H_2O} + \sigma_{aO_2SO_4}\, M_{O_2SO_4}}, \qquad (12.14)$$

where M represents the number of moles of the respective substances in the solution. In 925 g of 93% enriched uranium, we have

$$\frac{0.93 \dfrac{g\ ^{235}U}{g\ U} \times 925\ g\ U}{235 \dfrac{g\ ^{235}U}{mol}} = 3.66\ mol\ ^{235}U,$$

and

$$\frac{0.07 \dfrac{g\ ^{238}U}{g\ U} \times 925\ g\ U}{238 \dfrac{g\ ^{238}U}{mol\ ^{238}U}} = 0.27\ mol\ ^{238}U.$$

For a total of 3.93 moles uranium as UO_2SO_4.

From a table of absorption cross sections, we find that

$\sigma_{aH} = 0.332$ b	$\sigma_{a5} = 650$ b
$\sigma_{aO} = 0.0002$ b	$\sigma_{a8} = 2.8$ b
$\sigma_{aS} = 0.49$ b	

This leads to the following:

MATERIAL	σ_a, BARNS	MOLES	$\sigma_a \times$ MOLES
Uranium-235	650	3.66	2379.00
Uranium-238	2.8	0.27	0.76
Water	0.664	778	516.59
O_2SO_4	0.491	3.93	1.93

Substituting the values from the table above into Eq. (12.14), we have

$$f = \frac{2379 + 0.76}{2379 + 0.76 + 516.59 + 1.93} = 0.82.$$

Note that in this case we used absorption cross sections for 2200 m s^{-1} neutrons, which leads to a conservative result when making criticality calculations for nuclear safety.

The effective multiplication constant is useful for estimating the minimum concentration of a fissile material in a solution of moderator that could become critical.

EXAMPLE 12.4

Estimate the minimum concentration of 93% enriched uranyl sulfate, UO_2SO_4, in water in order that the solution form a critical mass.

Solution

The minimum concentration will occur when the size (or volume) of the solution is infinitely large. In that case, in order to attain criticality,

$$k_{eff} = \eta \varepsilon p f = 1.$$

The value for η is calculated from Eq. (12.7), using the molar ratio of 0.27 : 3.66 from the table in example 12.3 for $^{238}N/^{235}N$:

$$\eta = \frac{549}{650 + \dfrac{0.27}{3.66} \times 2.8} \times 2.5 = 2.11.$$

To calculate f using Eq. (12.14), let us arrange the data as shown in the following table, letting M represent the number of moles of UO_2SO_4 that is to be added to 1 mol of water, to give the minimum concentration that will result in $k_\infty = 1$. In Example 12.3, we calculated an atomic ratio of $^{235}U : U$ to be 3.66 : 3.93. Using this value gives the following:

MATERIAL	σ_a, BARNS	MOLES	σ_a × MOLES
Uranium-235	650	$\dfrac{3.66}{3.93} M$	605 M
Uranium-238	2.8	$\dfrac{0.27}{3.93} M$	0.192 M
Water	0.664	1	0.664
O_2SO_4	0.491	M	0.491M

From the definition of f, Eq. (12.14), we have

$$f = \frac{605\,M + 0.192\,M}{605\,M + 0.192\,M + 0.664 + 0.491\,M} = \frac{605.2\,M}{605.7\,M + 0.664}.$$

Making the very reasonable assumption that ε and p are both equal to 1, the four-factor formula, Eq. (12.12), becomes

$$k_\infty = \eta \varepsilon p f = 1$$

$$1 = 2.11 \times 1 \times 1 \times \frac{605.2\,M}{605.7\,M + 0.664}$$

$$M = 9.85 \times 10^{-4} \frac{\text{mol U}}{\text{mol water}},$$

and, since the molecular weight of the 93%-enriched uranium is $0.93 \times 235 + 0.07 \times 238 = 235.2$, we need

$$235.2 \frac{\text{g U}}{\text{molU}} \times 9.85 \times 10^{-4} \frac{\text{mol U}}{\text{mol water}} = 0.232 \frac{\text{g U}}{\text{mol water}}.$$

Since 1 mole water $= 18$ g ≈ 18 mL, 0.232 g U/mol water corresponds to

$$\frac{0.232 \text{ g U}}{18 \text{ mL water}} \times \frac{1000 \text{ mL}}{\text{L}} = 12.9 \frac{\text{g U}}{\text{L water}}$$

or

$$\frac{363.2 \text{ g UO}_2\text{SO}_4}{235.2 \text{ g U}} \times 12.9 \frac{\text{g U}}{\text{L water}} = \frac{20 \text{ g UO}_2\text{SO}_4}{\text{L water}}.$$

Since the above calculation was based on an infinitely large volume, a concentration less than 12.9 g per L 93%-enriched uranium as UO_2SO_4 can never go critical.

NUCLEAR REACTOR

In a nuclear reactor, these various factors are combined to produce a controlled, sustained chain reaction. The core of a nuclear reactor consists of fuel (^{235}U or ^{239}Pu), a moderator to thermalize the neutrons, a coolant to remove the heat, and control rods to control the chain reaction. In the case of a uranium-fueled reactor, the uranium is usually enriched in the ^{235}U isotope, since natural uranium contains only about 0.7% ^{235}U. Generally, the greater the degree of enrichment, the smaller the size of the reactor. The control rod is made of a metal—such as cadmium, hafnium, or boron steel—that has a very high thermal-neutron capture cross section. When the control rod is fully inserted into the reactor core, the multiplication constant is less than 1 because of the loss of neutrons to the absorber. As the control rod is withdrawn, neutrons that would have been captured by the control rod are now free to initiate a fission reaction. At a certain point of withdrawal, the multiplication factor becomes exactly equal to 1 and the reactor is critical. Should the control rod be kept at that point, there would be no further increase in the power level of the reactor. To increase the power level of the reactor, the rod is withdrawn, so that the multiplication factor k is greater than 1. The power level then increases, and when the desired power level is attained, the control rod is *reinserted* until k is decreased to exactly 1.000000. The reactor then continues to operate at that power level. To decrease the power level, the control rod is inserted into the core, causing k to become less than 1.00000 and the rate of nuclear fission to decrease. When the desired new power level is attained, the control rod is withdrawn to make k exactly equal to 1.0000 once more, and the reactor continues to operate at the reduced power level.

Reactivity and Reactor Control

The increase in the multiplication factor above 1 is called excess reactivity and is defined by

$$\Delta k = k - 1. \tag{12.15}$$

For every n neutrons in one generation, the next generation has $n\Delta k$ additional neutrons. If the lifetime of a neutron generation is l seconds, the time rate of change of neutrons is

$$\frac{dn}{dt} = \frac{n\Delta k}{l}, \tag{12.16}$$

which yields, when integrated from n_0 to n,

$$\frac{n}{n_0} = e^{\left(\frac{\Delta k}{l}\right)t}. \tag{12.17}$$

If we define the *reactor period* T as the time during which the neutrons (and consequently the power level) would increase by a factor of e (an e-fold increase), then, in Eq. (12.17),

$$\frac{\Delta k}{l} = \frac{1}{T},$$

and the reactor period, or e-folding time, is

$$T = \frac{1}{\Delta k}. \tag{12.18}$$

In pure ^{235}U, the mean lifetime, from the birth of a neutron until its absorption, is about 0.001 second. Consider the case where the excess reactivity is 0.1%; that is, $\Delta k = 0.001$. The reactor period is

$$T = \frac{0.001}{0.001} = 1 \text{ second},$$

and the power level would increase by a factor of e, or 2.718 each second. If Δk were increased to 0.5%, then

$$T = \frac{0.001}{0.005} = 0.2 \text{ second},$$

TABLE 12-3.   Delayed Neutrons from the Fission of ^{235}U

GROUP i	YIELD, percent n_i	MEAN GENERATION TIME, seconds T_i	YIELD x MEAN TIME $n_i \times T_i$
1	0.0267	0.33	0.009
2	0.0737	0.88	0.065
3	0.2526	3.31	0.836
4	0.1255	8.97	1.125
5	0.1401	32.78	4.592
6	0.0211	80.39	1.688
	$\sum n_i = 0.6397$		$\sum n_i T_i = 8.315$

and the power level increase in 1 second would be

$$\frac{n}{n_0} = e^{\frac{t}{T}} = e^{\frac{1}{0.2}} = 150 \, \text{fold}.$$

Such rapid increases in the power level as calculated in the example above would make it extremely difficult, if not impossible, to control a reactor. Fortunately, the calculation above is not applicable to a real reactor because, although the mean lifetime of a single neutron from birth until absorption is about 0.001 second, the mean lifetime of a whole generation of a large number of neutrons is much greater than 0.001 second. This increased mean generation time is due to the fact that 0.6407% of fission neutrons are delayed, that is, they are emitted for as long as 80.39 seconds after fission. Six distinct groups of *delayed neutrons* are observed, each group having its own mean delay time. Table 12-3 lists these groups, together with their mean delay (or generation) time.

The mean generation time for all the fission neutrons of a given generation is

$$\bar{T} = \frac{\sum\limits_{i=0}^{6} n_i T_i}{\sum\limits_{i=0}^{6} n_i} = \frac{8.315 + (100.0000 - 0.6397) \times 10^{-3}}{100} = 0.084 \, \text{second}.$$

The group $i = 0$ is the group of *prompt neutrons*, whose yield is 99.359% and whose mean generation time is 0.001 second.

If Δk, is equal to or greater than 0.006407, the reactor is said to be in the *prompt critical* condition, since the chain reaction can be sustained by the prompt neutrons alone. If Δk is less than 0.006407, the reactor is in the *delayed critical* condition, because the delayed neutrons are essential to sustaining the chain reaction. In the delayed critical condition, the reactor period is sufficiently long to allow the power level to be easily controlled.

EXAMPLE 12.5

Compute the reactor period and the increase in power level in 1 second for the case where the mean neutron generation time is 0.084 second for excess reactivity of 0.1% and 0.5%.

For $\Delta k = 0.001$,

$$T = \frac{l}{\Delta k} = \frac{0.084}{0.001} = 84 \, \text{seconds}$$

and

$$\frac{n}{n_0} = e^{\frac{t}{T}} = e^{\frac{1}{84}} = 1.012.$$

For $\Delta k = 0.005$

$$T = \frac{l}{\Delta k} = \frac{0.084}{0.005} = 16.8 \, \text{seconds}$$

and

$$\frac{n}{n_0} = e^{\frac{t}{T}} = e^{\frac{1}{16.8}} = 1.06.$$

Excess reactivity is measured in units of *dollars* and *cents* ($1 = 100¢) and in *inhours* (inverse hours). One dollar's worth of reactivity is that amount of excess reactivity that will cause the reactor to go prompt critical. One inhour is that amount of excess reactivity that results in a reactor period of 1 hour. Two inhours of reactivity give a reactor period of 1/2 hour, etc.

Fission Product Inventory

As a reactor continues to operate, fission products are produced at a rate proportional to the power level; the activity per fission is given by Eq. (12.3). If a nuclear reactor operates at a power level of P watts for a time dt, then the fission product activity at a time T days after shutdown is

$$dA = 3.81 \times 10^{-6} T^{-1.2} \frac{\text{Bq}}{\text{fission}} \times (3.3 \times 10^{10} \times 8.64 \times 10^4) \frac{\text{fission/d}}{\text{W}} \qquad \textbf{(12.19)}$$

$$\times \, PW \times dt \, \text{days}$$

or, combining the numerical constants,

$$dA = 1.09 \times 10^{10} PT^{-1.2} dt. \qquad \textbf{(12.20)}$$

Now referring to Figure 12-3,

if t = reactor operating time, days,
  T = cooling time after reactor shut down, days, and
  τ = total time = $t + T$,

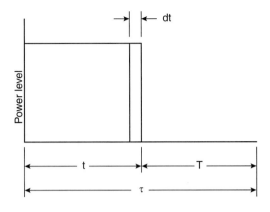

Figure 12-3. Curve showing relationship between reactor operating time at a constant power level and the postoperation cooling time used in the derivation of Eq. (12.23).

then $T = \tau - t$, and Eq. (12.20) may be written as

$$dA = 1.09 \times 10^{10} P(\tau - t)^{-1.2} dt \tag{12.21}$$

$$A = 1.09 \times 10^{10} P \int_0^t (\tau - t)^{-1.2}\, dt \tag{12.22}$$

$$A = 5.45 \times 10^{10} P\left[(\tau - t)^{-0.2} - \tau^{-0.2}\right] \text{Bq}, \tag{12.23a}$$

or, if activity is expressed in Ci,

$$A = 1.46\, P\left[(\tau - t)^{-0.2} - \tau^{-0.2}\right] \text{Ci}. \tag{12.23b}$$

EXAMPLE 12.6

A power reactor operates at a thermal power level of 500 MW for 200 days. It is then shut down for refueling. What is the fission product inventory

(a) 1 day after shutdown?

(b) 10 days after shutdown?

Solution

Substituting 5×10^8 W and the appropriate time periods into Eq. (12.23b), we get

(a) $A = 1.46 \times 5 \times 10^8 [(201 - 200)^{-0.2} - (201)^{-0.2}]$
$= 1.46 \times 5 \times 10^8 [1 - 0.346] = 4.8 \times 10^8$ Ci $(1.8 \times 10^{19}$ Bq).

(b) $A = 1.46 \times 5 \times 10^8 [(210 - 200)^{-0.2} - (210)^{-0.2}]$
$= 1.46 \times 5 \times 10^8 [0.631 - 0.343] = 2.1 \times 10^8$ Ci $(7.8 \times 10^{18}$ Bq).

Tables 12-4 and 12-5 list the fission product activity resulting from operation at a power level of 1MW; Figure 12-4 graphically illustrates the fission product activity–time relationship.

TABLE 12-4.   Production of Important Fission Products in a Reactor

FISSION PRODUCT	ACTIVITY (CURIES)[a] AFTER SELECTED PERIODS OF CONTINUOUS OPERATION OF A REACTOR AT A POWER LEVEL OF OF 1000 kW		
	100 Days	1 Year	5 Years
Kr-85	53	191	818
Rb-86	0.25	0.26	0.26
Sr-89	28,200	38,200	38,500
Sr-90	402	1430	6700
Y-90[b]	402	1430	6700
Y-91	34,800	48,900	49,500
Zr-95	32,900	49,200	50,300
Nb-95(35 H)[b]	446	687	704
Nb-95(35 D)[b]	20,900	48,200	50,500
Ru-103	25,100	30,900	31,000
Rh-103[b]	25,100	30,900	31,000
Ru-106	753	2180	4220
Rh-106[b]	753	2180	4220
Ag-111	151	151	151
Cd-115	4.8	5.9	5.9
Sn-117	83	84	84
Sn-119	<24	<24	<100
Sn-123	4	9	10
Sn-125	100	101	101
Sb-125[b]	12	43	139
Te-125[b]	5	34	136
Sb-127	787	787	787
Te-127(90 D)[b]	146	260	277
Te-127(9.3 H)[b]	808	922	939
Te-129(32 D)	1410	1590	1590
Te-129(70 M)[b]	1410	1590	1590
I-131	25,200	25,200	25,200
Xe-131[b]	250	252	252
I-132	36,900	36,900	36,900
I-132[b]	36,900	36,900	36,900
Xe-133	55,300	55,300	55,300
Cs-136	52	52	52
Cs-137	300	1080	5170
Ba-137[b]	285	1030	4910
Ba-140	51,500	51,700	51,700
La-140[b]	51,300	51,700	51,700
Ce-141	43,000	47,800	47,800
Pr-143	45,000	45,300	45,300
Ce-144	9860	26,700	44,000
Pr-144[b]	9860	26,700	44,000
Nd-147	21,800	21,800	21,800
Pm-147[b]	1290	4900	16,000
Sm-151	9	37	175
Eu-155	23	74	207
Eu-156	108	109	109
Total	563,691	693,573	767,547

[a]Calculated using fission product yields.
[b]Daughter product.

Reproduced from *Radiological Health Handbook.* Rev ed. Washington, DC: US Dept Health Education & Welfare; 1970.

TABLE 12-5. Activity of Fission Products in Curies at Specified Times (T) after Removal from a Reactor That Has Operated 1000 kW for 1 Year

FISSION PRODUCT	$T = 0$[a]	$T = 100$ DAYS	$T = 1$ YEAR	$T = 5$ YEARS
Kr-85	191	187	177	132
Rb-86	0.26	—	—	—
Sr-89	38,200	10,300	321	—
Sr-90	1430	1420	1380	1200
Y-90[b]	1430	1420	1380	1200
Y-91	48,900	14,500	577	—
Zr-95	49,200	17,000	1000	—
Nb-95(90 H)[b]	687	152	15	—
Nb-95(35 D)[b]	48,200	28,700	2140	—
Ru-103	30,900	5920	74	—
Rh-103[b]	30,900	5920	74	—
Ru-106	2180	1800	1090	68
Rh-106[b]	2180	1800	1090	68
Ag-111	151	—	—	—
Cd-115	5.9	1.2	—	—
Sn-117	84	0.7	—	—
Sn-119	<64	<48	<23	<0.4
Sn-123	9	5	1	—
Sn-125	101	0.1	—	—
Sb-125[b]	43	41	34	12
Te-125[b]	34	39	36	13
Sb-127	787	—	—	—
Te-127(90 D)[b]	260	123	16	—
Te-127(9.3 H)[b]	922	124	16	—
Te-129(32 D)	1590	182	0.6	—
Te-129(70 M)[b]	1590	182	0.6	—
I-131	25,200	4	—	—
Xe-131[b]	252	1.5	—	—
Te-132	36,900	—	—	—
I-132[b]	36,900	—	—	—
Xe-133	55,300	—	—	—
Cs-136	52	0.3	—	—
Cs-137	1080	1070	1060	970
Ba-137[b]	1030	1020	1010	920
Ba-140	51,700	230	—	—
La-140[b]	51,700	265	—	—
Ce-141	47,800	4740	10	—
Pr-143	45,300	288	—	—
Ce-144	26,700	20,800	10,700	268
Pr-144[b]	26,700	20,800	10,700	268
Nd-147	21,800	40	—	—
Pm-147[b]	4900	4800	3950	1360
Sm-151	37	37	36.6	35
Eu-155	74	67	52	13
Eu-156	109	1.2	—	—
Eu-156	109	—	—	—
Total	693,573	144,130	36,964	6527

[a]Calculated using fission product yields.
[b]Daughter product.

Reproduced from *Radiological Health Handbook.* Rev ed. Washington, DC: US Dept Health Education & Welfare; 1970.

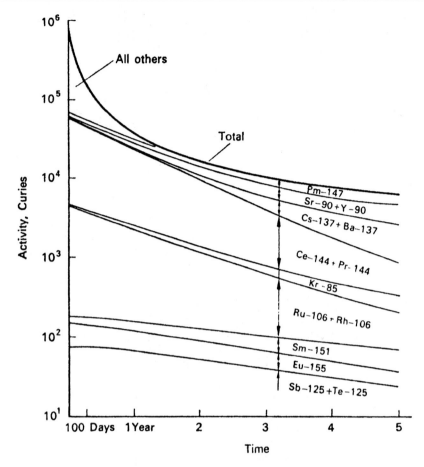

Figure 12-4. Activity–time relationship of certain fission products after removal from a reactor that had been operating at a power level of 1 MW for 1 year. (Reproduced from *Radiological Health Handbook.* Rev ed. Washington, DC: US Dept Health Education & Welfare; 1970.)

CRITICALITY CONTROL

The occurrence of an accidental criticality depends on the following factors:

1. Quantity of fissile material.
2. Geometry of the fissile assembly.
3. Presence or absence of a moderator.
4. Presence or absence of a neutron reflector.
5. Presence or absence of a strong neutron absorber (poison).
6. Concentration of fissile material, if the fissile material is in solution.
7. Interaction between two or more assemblies or arrays of fissile materials, each one of which is subcritical by itself. Consideration of this possibility is important in the transport and storage of fissile materials.

TABLE 12-6.   Minimum Critical Mass or size of 93.5% Enriched ^{235}U

CONDITION	CRITICAL MASS OR SIZE OF ^{235}U
Aqueous solution containing not more than 11.94 g ^{235}U/L	∞
Bare sphere of metallic uranium	48.6 kg
Water-reflected sphere of metallic uranium	22.8 kg
Unreflected sphere containing an aqueous solution of 75 g^{235}U/L	1.44 kg
Water-reflected sphere containing an aqueous solution of 75 g ^{235}U/L	0.83 kg
Infinitely long unreflected cylinder containing an aqueous solution of 75 g^{235}U/L	<8.7-in. diameter
Infinitely low water-reflected cylinder containing an aqueous solution of 75 g ^{235}U/L	<6.3-in. diameter

The influence of some of these factors is shown in Table 12-6, which lists the minimum critical mass of size of 93.5% enriched ^{235}U for several different conditions.

Generally, nuclear safety can be assured by limiting at least one of the factors that determine criticality in such a manner that it becomes physically impossible to initiate a sustained chain reaction. The basic control methods for assuring nuclear safety include the following:

1. *Mass control*—Limiting the mass of fissile material to less than the critical mass under any conceivable condition.
2. *Geometry control*—Having a geometric configuration that is "always safe"; that is, it can never become critical because the surface-to-volume ratio is such that excessive neutron leakage makes it impossible to attain a multiplication factor as great as 1.
3. *Concentration control*: The size of a critical mass depends strongly on the ratio of fissile atoms to moderating atoms. Thus, if this ratio is kept sufficiently small, that is, if the solution of fissile material is sufficiently dilute, absorption of neutrons by the hydrogen atoms makes a sustained chain reaction impossible. The degree of enrichment of ^{235}U is especially important in concentration control. In this connection it should be pointed out that a homogeneous mixture or a solution of natural uranium in water can never become critical, regardless of the concentration. For an aqueous mixture or solution of uranium, the ^{235}U must be enriched to about 1% before it can be made to attain criticality.

Nuclear safety by one of these three basic methods of control can be maintained by restricting any one of the control parameters to the maximum values listed in Table 12-7. It should be emphasized that the values listed in the table are independent of each other; that is, restriction of any one of the parameters to the value listed in the table allows other restrictions to be relaxed. It is considered good practice, however, to design processes and equipment in such a way that at least two highly unlikely independent events occur simultaneously before a criticality accident can occur. In this connection, it should be pointed out that it is considered better practice to rely primarily on safety designed into the equipment rather than on safety designed into a process. Thus, for example, a process may be designed to meet the concentration or enrichment criteria of Table 12-7. However, it would not be too difficult to cause

TABLE 12-7. Values of Basic Nuclear Safety Parameters[a]

| ISOTOPE | PARAMETER | VALUE | | | | MINIMUM SAFETY FACTOR |
| | | MODERATED | | UNMODERATED | | |
		Recommended Maximum	Minimum Critical	Recommended Maximum	Minimum Critical	
^{235}U	Mass	350 g	820 g	10.0 kg	22.8 kg	2.3
	Diameter of infinite cylinder	5.0 in.	5.4 in.	2.7 in.	3.1 in.	1.1
	Thickness of infinite slab	1.4 in.	1.7 in.	0.5 in.	0.6 in.	1.2
	Volume of solution	4.8 L	6.3 L	—	—	1.33
	Concentration (aqueous)	10.8 g/L	12.1 g/L	—	—	1.12
	Enrichment of ^{235}U	0.95	1.0	—	—	
^{233}U	Mass	250 g	590 g	3.2 kg	7.5 kg	2.3
	Diameter of infinite cylinder	3.7 in.	4.4 in.	1.7 in.	1.9 in.	1.1
	Thickness of infinite slab	0.8 in.	1.2 in.	0.2 in.	0.3 in.	1.2
	Volume of solution	2.3 L	3.3 L	—	—	1.33
	Concentration (aqueous)	10.0 g/L	11.2 g/L	—	—	1.12
^{239}Pu	Mass	220 g	510 g	2.6 kg	5.6 kg	2.3
	Diameter of infinite cylinder	4.2 in.	4.9 in.	1.4 in.	1.7 in.	1.1
	Thickness of infinite slab	0.9 in.	1.3 in.	0.18 in.	0.24 in.	1.2
	Volume of solution	3.4 L	3.5 L	—	—	1.33
	Concentration (aqueous)	6.9 g/L	7.8 g/L	—	—	1.12

[a]Moderation by H_2O is assumed; and all values, moderated and unmoderated, assume water reflection.

Reproduced from *Nuclear Safety Guide*. Washington, DC: US Atomic Energy Commission; 1961. AEC Report TID 7016, Rev-1.

a criticality inadvertently by using the wrong material. On the other hand, if the equipment were designed according to "always safe" geometry, such as limiting the diameter of a pipe or the capacity of a vessel, then an accidental criticality could not possibly occur under any conceivable operating condition.

When fissile material is being either stored or transported, it is especially important to prevent an interaction between two subcritical units. This is accomplished by packaging the fissile materials (in subcritical quantities) in containers of such design that the fissile materials are properly spaced. Such containers consist of two parts: a unit container in which the fissile material is placed, and a spacing container, whose function is to ensure the physical separation of the unit containers. One common type of shipping and storage container, which is called a "birdcage," is a weldment consisting of a steel pipe with end-caps (the unit container) in the center of a large angle-iron frame (the spacing container). A variation of this type of container may be made by welding the unit container coaxially, using appropriate spacers, in a 55-gal steel drum. The drum, in this case, is the spacing container. The spacing containers should be of such size that the closest distance (surface to surface) between unit containers cannot be less than 8 in. (204 mm). With this much distance between the unit containers, criticality due to interaction between two or more units is impossible even if the containers are immersed in water. No criticality restrictions on transportation or storage are necessary for

1. Uranium enriched to 0.95% or less as a homogeneous aqueous mixture.
2. Uranium metal enriched to 5% or less provided that there is no hydrogenous material within the container.
3. Aqueous solutions of ^{235}U at concentrations that do not exceed 10.8 g/L of ^{233}U at concentrations that do not exceed 10.0 g ^{233}U/L or of ^{239}Pu at concentrations that do not exceed 6.9 g/L.

SUMMARY

Criticality is a chain reaction in fissile materials (which include isotopes of thorium, uranium, and plutonium) in which the splitting, or fission, of a fissile nucleus leads to the fission of at least one more fissile nucleus. Nuclear fission leads to the release of very large amounts of energy in the form of heat and gamma radiation and to the production of radioactive fission products. Under controlled conditions, as in a nuclear reactor, this released energy is safely put to useful purposes. An accidental criticality, on the other hand, can lead to grave consequences for people and equipment. Accordingly, the handling, use, transport, or storage of fissile material must be done under very strictly controlled conditions.

Criticality occurs when at least one of the several neutrons that are emitted when a fissile nucleus is split causes a second nucleus to split. Criticality is determined by four different factors, including the number of fission neutrons produced per neutron absorbed in uranium, the fraction of those that initiate fast fission (fast-fission factor), the fraction of those that reach thermal energy (resonance escape probability), and the fraction of the thermalized neutrons absorbed by the fuel (thermal-utilization factor). The numerical values for each of these four factors depend on the quantity, composition, and physical arrangement of fissile and nonfissile materials. By controlling one or more of these factors to a level where criticality is physically impossible, we can prevent accidental criticalities.

 PROBLEMS

12.1. Cooling water circulates through a water boiler reactor core at a rate of 4 L/min through a coiled stainless steel tube of 6.4 mm inside diameter and 213 cm in length. The concentration of Na and Cl in the water is 5 atoms each per million molecules H_2O. What is the concentration of induced Na and Cl radioactivity in the cooling water after a single passage through the reactor core if the mean thermal flux is 10^{11} neutrons/cm^2/s and the mean core temperature is 80°C?

12.2. If the cooling water in problem 1 circulates through a heat-exchange reservoir containing 400-L water (including the water in the pipes between the core and the reservoir), what will be the concentration of induced activity in the reservoir after 7 days of operation of the reactor?

12.3. If the tank of problem 2 is spherical, what will be the surface dose rate due to the induced radioactivity one week after the start of operation?

12.4. A research reactor, after going critical for the first time, operates at a power level of 100 W for 4 hours. How much fission product activity does the reactor contain at the following times after shutdown of the reactor?

   (a) 1 hour,

   (b) 8 hour,

   (c) 7 days, and

   (d) 30 days.

12.5. A research reactor, after going critical for the first time, operates at a power level of 100 W for 4 hours. How many curies of fission product activity does that core contain?

12.6. An accidental criticality occurred in an aqueous solution in a half-filled mixing tank 25 cm (diameter) × 100 cm (height). The energy released during the burst was estimated at 1800 J. Assuming that, on the average, each disintegration of a fission product is accompanied by a 1-MeV gamma ray, estimate the gamma-ray dose rate at the surface of the tank (which maintained its integrity during the criticality) and at a distance of 25 ft from the tank at 1 minute, 1 hour, 1 day, and 1 week after the criticality accident.

12.7. A slab of pure natural uranium metal weighing 1 kg is irradiated in a thermal flux of 10^{12} neutrons/cm^2/s for 24 days at a temperature of 150°F. If the fission yield for ^{131}I is 2.8%, how many millicuries of ^{131}I will be extracted 5 days after the end of the irradiation?

12.8. What is the uranium concentration of uranyl sulfate UO_2SO_4 aqueous solution that can go critical if the uranium is enriched to (a) 10% and (b) 90%?

12.9. Calculate η for ^{239}Pu, given that the fission cross section is 664 b and the nonfission absorption cross section is 361 b.

12.10. The blood plasma from a worker who was overexposed during a criticality accident had a ^{24}Na specific activity of 37 Bq (0.001 μCi) per mL 15 hours after the accident. The accidental excursion lasted 10 milliseconds. All the Na in nature is ^{23}Na. The thermal neutron activation cross section for 2200 m/s neutrons is 0.53 b. What was the absorbed dose due to (a) the ^{14}N$(n, p)^{14}$C reaction and (b) the autointegral gamma-ray dose due to the n, γ reaction on hydrogen?

12.11. **(a)** For the case where $k = 1.0025$ and the initial number of neutrons is 1000, how many neutrons will be present after 10 generations?

(b) After how many generations will the neutron flux be doubled?

12.12. At 20 minutes after a criticality accident the dose rate in a laboratory from the fission products was 15 Gy/h (1500 rad/h). If the laboratory ventilation system was shut down at the time of the criticality, how long would it take before a person could enter the laboratory if his dose equivalent during a projected 15-minute exposure time is not to exceed 50 mGy (5 rads)?

12.13. A transient burst of 1×10^{15} fissions in an unshielded accumulation of fissile materials causes a total dose equivalent of 0.25 Sv (25 rems) at a distance of 2 m. If the neutron-to-gamma dose-equivalent ratio is $9 : 1$, what were the absorbed doses from the gammas and from the neutrons?

12.14. The composition, by weight percent, of a concrete mix used in reactor shielding consists of oxygen, 52.17%; Si, 34.0%; Ca, 4.4%; Al, 3.5%; Na, 1.6%; Fe, 1.5%; K, 1.3%; and H, 1.0%. The density of the concrete is 2.35 g/cm^3.

(a) Find and tabulate the thermal (2200 m/s) absorption cross section for each element.

(b) Calculate the linear absorption coefficient (macroscopic cross section) of the concrete.

12.15. The ^{131}I fission yield is 2.77%. What is the ^{131}I activity in the core of a power reactor that had been operating at a power level of 3000 MW (t) for

(a) 8 days,

(b) 30 days,

(c) 60 days, and

(d) 180 days?

12.16. Tritium is produced in a nuclear reactor in *ternary fission,* in which one ^{3}H nucleus is produced in every 10^4 fissions. What is the tritium activity in a reactor core that had been operating at a mean power level of 3000 MW(t) for 2 years?

SUGGESTED READINGS

Ayers, J. A., ed. *Decontamination of Nuclear Reactors and Equipment.* Ronald Press, New York, 1970.

Clark, H. K. *Handbook of Nuclear Safety.* Report No. DP-J32, TID-4500, Office of Technical Services, Washington, DC, 1961.

Etherington, H., ed. *Nuclear Engineering Handbook.* McGraw Hill, New York, 1958.

Farmer, F. R., ed. *Nuclear Reactor Safety.* Academic Press, New York, 1977.

Foster, A. R., and Wright, R. L., Jr. *Basic Nuclear Engineering,* 4th ed. Allyn and Bacon, Boston, MA, 1983.

Glasstone, S., and Edmund, M. C. *The Elements of Nuclear Reactor Theory.* D. Van Nostrand, Princeton, NJ, 1952.

Glasstone, S, and Sesonske, A. *Nuclear Reactor Engineering,* 4th ed. Chapman and Hall, New York, 1994.

Health Physics Society. *Selected Topics on Reactor Health Physics.* Proc. of the Health Physics Society, 1981 Summer School, Health Physics Society, McLean, VA, 1981.

Health Physics Society. *Power Reactor Health Physics.* Proc. 21st Mid-Year Topical Meeting, Health Physics Society, McLean, VA, 1987.

Heinrichs, D. P., and Koponen, B. L. *Technical Information Resources for Criticality Safety.* UCRL-JC-128203, Lawrence Livermore National Laboratory, CA, 1997.

Henry, H. F. *Guide to Shipment of ^{235}U Enriched Uranium Materials.* TID-7019, Office of Technical Services, Washington, DC, 1959.

International Atomic Energy Agency (IAEA), Vienna.

Criticality Control of Fissile Materials, 1966.

Surveillance of Items Important to Safety in Nuclear Power Plants. Safety Series No. 50-G-08 (Rev. 1), 1990.

The International Chernobyl Project. Technical Report by an International Advisory Committee, 1991.

INES: The International Nuclear Event Scale, 1990.

Provision of Operational Radiation Protection Services at Nuclear Power Plants. Safety Series No. 103, 1990.

Safety of New and Existing Research Reactor Facilities in Relation to External Events. Safety Report Series No. 41, 2005.

Chernobyl Forum: 2003–2005. *Chernobyl's Legacy: Health, Environmental, and Socio-Economic Impacts,* 2006.

Engineering Safety Aspects of the Protection f Nuclear Power Plants against Sabotage. Nuclear Security Series No. 4, 2007.

Safety Standards Series No.

SF-1. *Fundamental Safety Principles,* 2006.

NS-G-1.2. *Safety Assessment and Verification for Nuclear Power Plants,* 2002.

NS-G-1.13. *Radiation Protection Aspects of Design for Nuclear Power Plants,* 2005.

NS-G-2.4. *The Operating Organization for Nuclear Power Plants,* 2002.

NS-G-2.7. *Radiation Protection and Radioactive Waste Management in the Operation Nuclear Power plants,* 2002.

NS-R-1. *Safety of Nuclear Power Plants: Design,* 2005.

NS-R-2. *Safety of Nuclear Power Plants: Operation,* 2000.

INSAG Series No.

1. *Summary Report on the Post-Accident Review Meeting on the Chernobyl Accident,* 1986.

2. *Radionuclide Source Terms from Severe Accidents to Nuclear Power Plants with Light Water Reactors,* 1987.

3. *Basic Safety Principles for Nuclear Power Plants,* 1988.

4. *Safety Culture,* 1991.

5. *The Safety of Nuclear Power,* 1992.

6. *Probabilistic Safety Assessment,* 1992.

7. *The Chernobyl Accident: Updating INSAG 1,* 1993.

8. *The Common Basis for Judging the Safety of Nuclear Power Plants Built to Earlier Standards,* 1995.

9. *Potential Exposures in Nuclear Safety,* 1995.

10. *Defence in Depth in Nuclear Safety,* 1996.

11. *The Safe Management of Sources of Radiation,* 1999.

12. *Basic Safety Principles for Nuclear Power Plants,* 1999.

13. *Management of Operational Safety in Nuclear Power Plants,* 1999.

14. *Safe Management of the Operating Lifetimes of Nuclear power Reactors,* 1999.

15. *Key Practical Issues in Strengthening Safety Culture,* 2002.

16. *Maintaining Knowledge, Training, and Infrastructure for Research and Development in Nuclear Safety,* 2003.

18. *Managing Change in the Nuclear Industry: The Effects on Safety,* 2003.

20. *Stakeholder Involvement in Nuclear Issues,* 2006.

21. *Strengthening the Global Nuclear Safety Regime,* 2006.

International Commission on Radiological Protection (ICRP). *Annals of the ICRP.* Pergamon Press, Oxford. U.K.

Publication No.

29. *Radionuclide Release into the Environment Assessment of Doses to Man,* **2**(2), 1979.

63. *Principles for Intervention for Protection of the Public in a Radiological Emergency,* **22**(4), 1993.

Kemeny, J. G. *The Accident at TMI.* Pergamon Press, New York, 1979.

Knief, R. A. *Nuclear Criticality Safety, Theory and Practice.* American Nuclear Society, La Grange Park, IL, 1944.

Lamarsh, J. R. *Introduction to Nuclear Engineering,* 2nd ed. Addison-Wesley, Reading, MA, 1983.

LeClerk, J. *The Nuclear Age.* Sodel, Paris, 1986.

Lewis, E. E. *Nuclear Power Reactor Safety.* Wiley Interscience, New York, 1977.

McCullough, C. R. *Safety Aspects of Nuclear Reactors.* D. Van Nostrand, Princeton, NJ, 1952.

Miller, K. L., ed. *CRC Handbook of Radiation Protection Programs,* 2nd ed. CRC Press, Boca Raton, FL, 1992.

National Council on Radiation Protection and Measurements (NCRP). National Council on Radiation Protection, Bethesda, MD.

NCRP Report No.

120. *Dose Control at Nuclear Power Plants,* 1994.

121. *Principles and Application of Collective Dose in Radiation Protection,* 1995.

122. *Use of Personnel Monitors to Estimate Effective Dose Equivalent and Effective Dose to Workers for External Exposure to Low LET Radiation,* 1995.

123. *Screening Models for Releases of Radionuclides to Atmosphere, Surface Water, and Ground,* 1996.

130. *Biological Effects and Exposure Limits for "Hot Particles,"* 1999.

139. *Risk-Based Classification of Radioactive and Hazardous Chemical Wastes,* 2002.

NEA/OECD. *Chernobyl, Ten Years On, Radiological and Health Impact.* OECD, Paris, 1996.

Okrent, D. *Nuclear Reactor Safety.* University of Wisconsin Press, Madison, WI, 1981.

Organization for Economic Cooperation and Development. *Criticality Control.* OECD, Karlsruhe, Germany, 1961.

Pendlebury, E. D., Woodcock, E. R., Thomas, A. F., et al. *Lectures on Criticality.* UKAEA Report AHSB(S) R4, H.M. Stationery Office, London, U.K., 1961.

Prince, R. J., and Bradely, S. E. Light water reactor health physics. *Health Phys,* **87:**469–474, 2004.

Rhodes, R. *The Making of the Atomic Bomb.* Simon & Schuster, New York, 1988.

Rhodes, R., and Beller, D. The need for nuclear power. *Foreign Aff,* **79:**30–44, 2000.

Rogovin, M., and Frampton, G. T. Jr. *Three Mile Island: A Report to the Commissioners and to the Public.* National Technical Information Services, Springfield, VA, 1980.

Rust, J. H., and Weaver, L. E. eds. *Nuclear Power Safety.* Pergamon Press, New York, 1976.

Schleien, B. S., Slabeck, L. A. Jr, and Kent, B. K. *Handbook of Health Physics and Radiological Health.* Williams and Wilkins, Baltimore, MD, 1998.

Thomas, A. F., and Abbey, F. *Calculational Methods for Interacting Arrays of Fissile Materials.* Pergamon Press, Oxford, U.K., 1977.

United Nations Scientific Committee on the Effects of Atomic Radiation. Exposures and effects of the Chernobyl accident, Appendix J in *Sources and Effects of Ionizing Radiation, A Report to the General Assembly.* United Nations, New York, 2000.

U.S. Nuclear Regulatory Commission, Washington, DC.

Nuclear Safety Guide. TID-7016, Revision 2, NUREG/CR-0095 and ORNL/NUREG/CSD-6, 1978.

Reactor Safety Study (Rasmussen Report). WASH-1400, U.S.NRC, 1975.

Report on the Accident at the Chernobyl Nuclear Power Station. NUREG 1250, 1987.

Vargo, G.J., ed. *The Chernobyl Accident: A Comprehensive Risk Assessment,* Battelle Press, Columbus, OH, 2000.

EVALUATION OF RADIATION SAFETY MEASURES

The effectiveness of safety measures against radiation hazards is evaluated by a surveillance program that includes the observation of both people and their environments. Such a surveillance program may employ one or more of a variety of techniques, depending on the nature of the hazard and the consequences of a breakdown in the system of controls. These techniques may include preemployment and periodic physical examinations, estimation of internally deposited radioactivity by bioassay and total-body counting, personnel monitoring, radiation and contamination surveys, and continuous environmental monitoring.

MEDICAL SURVEILLANCE

The great degree of overexposure required before clinical signs or symptoms of overexposure appear precludes the use of medical surveillance of radiation workers as a routine monitoring device. Nevertheless, medical supervision may play an important role in protecting radiation workers against possible radiation damage. Among the main tasks of medical supervision is the proper placement of radiation workers according to their medical histories, physical condition, and history of previous radiation exposure. Dermatitis, cataracts, and blood dyscrasias, including leukemia, are effects associated with radiation exposure. A preemployment physical examination, therefore, should be given if the nature of the work, including consideration of possible accidental overexposures, warrants it. Special attention is paid to physical conditions including fitness for use of respirators that may lead to, or be suggestive of, susceptibility to any of these effects. Possible indirect effects from working with radioisotopes are also considered by the examining physician. For example, sensitivity or allergy may contraindicate work that requires the wearing of rubber gloves or that may require washing the hands or body with strong detergents or harsh chemicals in order to decontaminate the skin. In addition to the preemployment examination, the radiation worker may be routinely examined at periodic intervals to ascertain that he or she continues to be free of signs that would contraindicate further occupational exposure to radiation. The physician is thus instrumental in preventing damage or injury that could otherwise arise, either directly or indirectly, as a consequence of working with radioisotopes or exposure to radiation. Medical supervision of radiation workers may also be necessary to evaluate overexposure, to treat radiation injuries, and to decontaminate personnel. These activities of the physician are, of course, in addition to the provision of routine health services that are not connected to radiation hazards. It should be pointed out that medical surveillance of workers is not unique to the field of radiation health. All good occupational health programs include preemployment examinations, consideration of medical findings in job placement, and continuing medical surveillance to help maximize the protection of workers against the harmful effects of toxic substances.

ESTIMATION OF INTERNALLY DEPOSITED RADIOACTIVITY

One of the techniques for estimating the intake of radioactivity or the radiation dose from that intake in order to demonstrate compliance with regulatory requirements for limiting the total effective dose equivalent (TEDE) is by a program of routine bioassay. Since the likelihood of intake is related to the level of environmental contamination, routine bioassay programs are designed to verify the efficacy of environmental contamination controls. In routine bioassay, the worker's body burden of radioactivity is determined periodically on a fixed frequency. The results are then compared to an arbitrarily established reference level that is not expected to be reached if there is no breakdown in contamination control measures. The method and frequency of routine bioassay monitoring is determined by the radiation characteristics and metabolic kinetics of the radionuclides of interest as well as by the sensitivity of the monitoring methods, the acceptable degree of uncertainty of the implied dose, and the ease and convenience of the method.

In addition to routine bioassay, special bioassay determinations are made in cases of suspected or known accidental exposures by inhalation, ingestion, or through wounds. When used as a monitoring technique, an administrative level, called an *investigation level*, is set. An investigation level is an estimated intake or committed dose that is higher than expected and above which the result is considered sufficiently significant to warrant further investigation.

Bioassay programs rely on two general techniques. One of these techniques is called in vivo bioassay; it is the direct determination of internal radionuclides by whole-body counting and is useful only for gamma-emitting radionuclides or beta emitters that give rise to suitable bremsstrahlung. The other technique is called in vitro bioassay, and involves the analysis of body fluids, exhaled air, or excreta for the purpose of estimating the intake.

In Vitro Bioassay

The underlying rationale for in vitro bioassay is that a quantitative relationship exists among inhalation or ingestion of a radionuclide, the resulting body burden, and the rate at which the radionuclide is eliminated. From measurements of activity in the urine or feces, therefore, we should be able to infer the body burden, and from the body burden, we can estimate the resulting dose. Unfortunately, the kinetics of metabolism of most substances in any particular individual is influenced by a large number of factors; as a consequence, there is a great deal of uncertainty about the exact quantitative relationships among elimination rates, body burden, and radiation dose. In most instances, therefore, bioassay data give only a very approximate estimate of the intake and dose. Although both urine and feces are available for bioassay measurements in case of an accidental inhalation or ingestion of a large amount of radioactivity, routine bioassay monitoring is usually done with urine samples, because of the ease of sample collection and also for esthetic reasons.

Readily soluble radionuclides may be grouped into three categories according to their metabolic pathways and distribution within the body: (1) those that are uniformly distributed throughout the body, such as ^3H in tritiated water or radiosodium ions; (2) those that concentrate mainly either in specific organs, such as iodine in the thyroid gland or mercury in the kidney; and (3) those that are deposited in the skeleton. Bioassays are most reliable in the case of the first category, the widely distributed radionuclides. In this case, the radioactivity in the body decreases exponentially at a rate given by the effective elimination constant λ_E and the body burden $A(t)$ at any time t after an intake $A(0)$ given by

$$A(t) = A(0)e^{-\lambda_E t}. \tag{13.1}$$

If a constant fraction of the isotope f_U is eliminated in the urine, then the activity in the urine $U(t)$ at time t after ingestion is given by

$$U(t) = f_U \frac{dA(t)}{dt} \tag{13.2}$$

and

$$U(t) = f_U A(0) \lambda_E e^{\lambda_E t}. \tag{13.3}$$

The principles of internal exposure evaluation may be illustrated with an example using tritium as tritiated water. Tritiated water taken in by a reference person either by inhalation, ingestion, or through the intact skin is completely absorbed and instantaneously and uniformly distributed throughout the body fluids in the soft tissues. In this case, the tritium concentration in the urine is the same as that in the body fluids and, hence, serves as a measure of the ^3H body burden.

The reference adult male body contains 42 L of water. Three liters of water are turned over per day through the ordinary excretion pathways (Table 13-1). The daily turnover rate of body water λ_B in the reference adult male is

$$\lambda_B = \frac{3 \frac{L}{d}}{42\ L} = 0.071 \text{ per day},$$

which corresponds to a biological half-time T_B of 9.7 days. Of the 3 L of water lost per day, 1.4 L, or 47%, is excreted in the urine. Studies on humans found that the retention of ^3H following an intake of tritiated water is described mathematically

TABLE 13-1. Water Balance for Reference People

	ADULT MAN		ADULT WOMAN		CHILD (10-YEARS-OLD)	
	Gains (mL/d)	Losses (mL/d)	Gains (mL/d)	Losses (mL/d)	Gains (mL/d)	Losses (mL/d)
Milk	300	1400 in urine	200	1000 in urine	450	1000 in urine
Tap water	150	100 in feces	100	90 in feces	200	70 in feces
Other	1500	850 insensible loss	1100	600 insensible loss	750	580 insensible loss
	—		—		—	
Total fluid intake	1950		1400		1400	
In food	700	650 in sweat	450	420 in sweat	400	350 in sweat
By oxidation of food	350		250		200	
	—	—	—	—	—	—
Totals	3000	3000	2100	2100	2000	2000

(International Commission on Radiological Protection [ICRP] 30 and 54) by a three-component intake retention function (IRF):

$$R(t) = Ae^{-0.693t/T_1} + Be^{-0.693t/T_2} + Ce^{-0.693t/T_3}, \qquad (13.4)$$

where T_1 ranges from 6 to 18 days, T_2 from 21 to 34 days, and T_3 from 250 to 550 days. The last two components represent tritium in organic compounds and together contribute no more than 10% of the absorbed dose. For this reason, we assume that the retention of ^{3}H taken in as tritiated water is adequately described by a single-component exponential equation with a half-time of 10 days. If the activity of the intake is $A(0)$, then the activity retained after a time t days following the intake is

$$R(t) = A(0) e^{-0.693t/10} = A(0) e^{-0.069t}, \qquad (13.5)$$

and the intake retention fraction, IRF, is

$$\text{IRF}(t) = \frac{R(t)}{A(0)} = e^{-0.069t}. \qquad (13.6)$$

Since the specific activity of the urine is the same as the specific activity of the tritiated water in the body, and since the water volume of the reference adult is 42,000 mL, then the expected specific activity C_U of the urine at time t days after a single intake is

$$C_U(t) = \frac{A_0}{42,000\,\text{mL}} \times e^{-0.069t}. \qquad (13.7)$$

EXAMPLE 13.1

After a maintenance mechanic at a heavy-water reactor finished a certain repair job, it was realized that the working environment had been contaminated with tritiated water vapor of unknown atmospheric concentration. To estimate the mechanic's dose, a urine assaying program was started and 24-hour urine samples were collected and analyzed by liquid scintillation counting. To increase the elimination of tritium from his body, the mechanic greatly increased his water consumption. The following data were obtained:

Day	1	2	3	4	5	6	7
kBq/mL	3.00	2.70	2.43	2.20	2.00	1.80	1.65

(a) What was the mechanic's intake of tritium?

(b) What was the dose commitment from this intake?

Solution

(a) If the tritium turnover rate were in fact 0.069 per day, then Eq. (13.7) could be used to estimate the initial body burden. Thus, after day 1, when the specific activity of the urine was 3.00 kBq/mL, we can estimate the intake $A(0)$ as follows:

$$3.00 \, \frac{kBq}{mL} = \frac{A(0) \, kBq}{42,000 \, mL} \times e^{-0.069 \, day^{-1} \times 1 \, day}$$

$$A(0) = 1.35 \times 10^5 \, kBq \quad (3.65 \times 10^3 \, \mu Ci).$$

(b) The inhalation annual limit of intake (ALI) for tritiated water is 3×10^9 Bq $(8 \times 10^4 \mu Ci)$. Since our estimated intake, 1.35×10^8 Bq, is much less than the ALI, we would not expect any medical consequences from this exposure. If we use the dose conversion factor from ICRP 78, which is 1.8×10^{-11} Sv/Bq $(6.3 \times 10^{-2}$ mrems/$\mu Ci)$, the estimated effective dose equivalent based on the single measurement is

$$1.8 \times 10^{-11} \, \frac{Sv}{Bq} \times 1.35 \times 10^8 \, Bq = 2.4 \times 10^{-3} \, Sv \quad (240 \, mrems).$$

However, we have reason to believe that the tritium turnover rate in Eq. (13.6) is not valid in this case, since the mechanic consumed a large amount of water in order to induce diuresis and thus hasten the elimination of the tritium. This hyperhydration probably resulted in an increase in the water turnover rate, which means that the exponent in Eq. (13.6) is too small for this particular case. To find the actual value for the tritium turnover rate, we can plot the excretion data on semilog paper (Fig. 13-1). The slope of the excretion curve is the value of the daily ^{3}H clearance rate. In this case, the clearance half-time is found to be 6 days, which corresponds to a clearance rate of 0.116 per day. Using this measured value of 0.116 per day in Eq. (13.1), we find that the initial concentration of tritium in the urine is 3.4 kBq/mL. The dose commitment is calculated with Eq. (6.58):

$$D = \frac{\dot{D}_0}{\lambda_E},$$

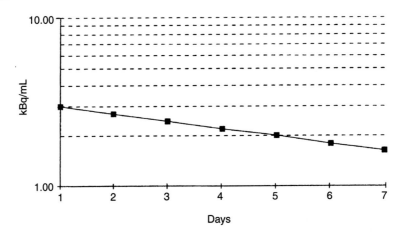

Figure 13-1. Concentration of tritium in urine for the case illustrated in Example 13.1.

where $\dot{D}_0$, the initial dose rate, is the dose rate due to the initial body burden

$$3400 \frac{\text{Bq}}{\text{mL}} \times 42,000 \text{ mL} = 1.4 \times 10^8 \text{ Bq} \quad (3.9 \times 10^3 \ \mu\text{Ci}).$$

The initial dose rate is calculated with Eq. (6.47):

$$\dot{D}_0 = \frac{1.4 \times 10^8 \text{ Bq} \times 1 \frac{\text{tps}}{\text{Bq}} \times 5.7 \times 10^{-3} \frac{\text{MeV}}{\text{transf}} \times 1.6 \times 10^{-13} \frac{\text{J}}{\text{MeV}} \times 8.64 \times 10^4 \frac{\text{s}}{\text{d}}}{(70-7)\text{kg} \times 1\frac{\text{J/kg}}{\text{Gy}}}$$

$$\dot{D}_0 = 1.75 \times 10^{-4} \frac{\text{Gy}}{\text{d}} \quad \left(1.75 \times 10^{-2} \frac{\text{rad}}{\text{d}}\right),$$

and the committed effective dose equivalent (CEDE) is

$$\text{CEDE} = \frac{1.75 \times 10^{-4} \frac{\text{Gy}}{\text{day}} \times 1 \frac{\text{Sv}}{\text{Gy}}}{0.116 \text{ day}^{-1}}$$

$$= 1.51 \times 10^{-3} \text{ Sv} \quad (151 \text{ mrems}).$$

The calculated dose commitment based on urinalyses over a 7-day period differs from that estimated from just a single urine sample. The difference in this case is due to the fact that the mechanic's tritium clearance rate differed significantly from the clearance rate on which the ICRP model is based. In case of a real or suspected overexposure, it is recommended that as many real data as are available be used to estimate intake or to calculate the dose from the estimated intake. Generally, if an accidental intake estimate that is based on ICRP IRFs shows the intake to have been much less than the ALI, no further attempts at increased accuracy are necessary. However, if the estimated intake is significant relative to the ALI, then additional data should be obtained in order to determine the intake and the resultant dose as accurately as possible. Such additional data may include further bioassay data from sequential sampling, as in the example above, breathing-zone atmospheric concentrations from air sampling, and whole-body counting if applicable.

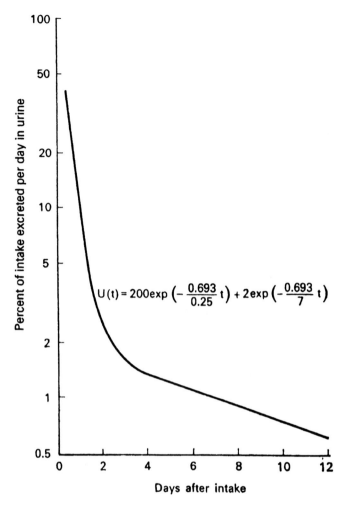

$$U(t) = 200 \exp\left(-\frac{0.693}{0.25}\,t\right) + 2\exp\left(-\frac{0.693}{7}\,t\right)$$

Figure 13-2. Urinary excretion curve of ^{35}S after a single intake of soluble, inorganic sulfate. The general shape of the curve is typical for a readily soluble compound that concentrates in a single organ. (Reproduced with permission from Jackson S, Dolphin GW. Report AHSB (RP) R 51. UK: Atomic Energy Authority (UK AEA); 1965.)

For the second category, those radionuclides that concentrate in one or more organs, there is a greater degree of uncertainty in the intakes and doses estimated from bioassay monitoring than in the case of the widely distributed radionuclides. These radionuclides are absorbed, after ingestion or inhalation, into the body fluids and the blood plasma. From these fluids, they pass into the organs in which they concentrate; a dynamic equilibrium eventually results between the concentration of the nuclide in the organ and that in the body fluids. While the isotope is equilibrating between the body fluids and the organ of concentration, it is also being filtered by the kidney into the urine. This leads to a clearance curve (Fig. 13-2) that is the sum of at least two exponential components. The first component, which falls steeply, represents the clearance of the isotope from the body fluids, while the second component represents the clearance of the isotope from the organ of concentration. The slope and magnitude of the first component may be influenced by a number of factors, such as the amount of the nonradioactive form of the same element that was inhaled or ingested, the amount of water intake, the physiologic state of the kidney, etc., which makes it extremely difficult to relate the intake of the radionuclide to the urinary excretion data during the first few days after a single intake. The component that represents the clearance from the organ of concentration is much less influenced by these factors. An approximate estimate, therefore, of the radionuclide in the organ of concentration following a single exposure can often be made from the urinary excretion after sufficient data become available to establish the second component of the curve.

The third category, which comprises the elements absorbed into the bone, is a special case of the category of isotopes concentrated in an organ or tissue. Bone seekers differ from other radionuclides mainly in the elimination of the isotope. Whereas clearance half-times for non–bone seekers are measured in days or weeks, retention times for the bone seekers are measured in years. Furthermore, the clearance rate from the skeleton is not constant but decreases with increasing time. This is due to the fact that the skeleton is not a single "compartment" but rather a number of different compartments, each of which has its own clearance rate. Over a long period of time, the IRF, which is the sum of all the exponentials representing these different compartments, can be approximated by a power function of the form

$$R(t) = At^{-n}, \tag{13.8}$$

where

$R(t)$ = fractional retention t days after intake,
A = normalized fraction of the intake retained at the end of 1 day, and
n = an empirical constant.

For the case of ^{226}Ra, for example, $A = 0.54$, and $n = 0.52$.

Later studies on radium retention were able to resolve the bone into five compartments, and the following retention equation, which gives the activity retained per unit activity uptake at time t days after the uptake, was fitted to the observational data (ICRP 54):

$$R(t) = 0.54e^{-1.73t} + 0.29e^{-0.139t} + 0.11e^{-0.116t} + 0.04e^{-9.9\times10^{-4}t} + 0.02e^{-1.39\times10^{-4}t}. \tag{13.9}$$

The corresponding urinary excretion curve, expressed as the fraction of the uptake activity per 24-hour urine sample at time t days after the uptake, is

$$f_U = 0.047e^{-1.73t} + 0.002e^{-0.139t} + 6.6\times10^{-5}e^{-0.116t} + 2\times10^{-6}e^{-9.9\times10^{-4}t}$$
$$+1.4\times10^{-7}e^{-1.39\times10^{-4}t} \tag{13.10}$$

The body burden of radium may also be inferred from measurements of radon concentration in the breath. Radium transforms directly into radon; some of the radon dissolves in the body fluids and in the adipose tissue, and the balance is exhaled. Although the fractional retention of radon in the body varies for a short time after deposition of the radium, the mean exhalation is given as 70%. The exhaled radon activity, A_e, is related to the body burden q by the equation

$$A_e \text{ Bq/min} = 0.7 \times q \text{ Bq} \times \lambda \text{ min}^{-1}, \tag{13.11}$$

where λ, the decay constant for radium, is 8.1×10^{-10} min^{-1}. The concentration of radon in the breath, C_B for a volumetric respiration rate of V L/min is given by

$$C_B \frac{\text{Bq}}{\text{L}} = \frac{A_e \text{ Bq/min}}{V \text{ L/min}}. \tag{13.12}$$

Under resting conditions, the respiration rate is about 20 per minute and the tidal volume is about 0.5 L; the ventilation rate V, therefore, is about 10 L/min. For analysis, radon from a measured volume of exhaled breath is adsorbed on activated charcoal. It is then desorbed and transferred into an ionization chamber or scintillation cell for counting.

For strontium, another bone seeker, the biological retention function, after uptake of a unit of Sr, is given (ICRP 54) by the sum of three exponentials, with biological half-times of 3 days, 44 days, and 4000 days (11 years):

$$R(t) = 0.73e^{-\frac{0.693}{3} \times t} + 0.1e^{-\frac{0.693}{44} \times t} + 0.17e^{-\frac{0.693}{4000} \times t}, \tag{13.13}$$

and the urinary excretion function, f_U, expressed as the fraction of the uptake strontium excreted in a 24-hour urine sample t days after the uptake, is

$$f_U(t) = 0.13e^{-\frac{0.693}{3} \times t} + 0.001e^{-\frac{0.693}{44} \times t} + 2.4 \times 10^{-5}e^{-\frac{0.693}{4000} \times t}. \tag{13.14}$$

EXAMPLE 13.2

A chemist in a radiopharmaceutical laboratory was exposed to an ^{89}Sr aerosol during an accidental release of ^{89}SrCl$_2$ particles. To estimate his intake of ^{89}Sr and the resultant dose, 24-hour urine samples were collected and analyzed for ^{89}Sr with the following results. Estimate his intake and the dose commitment.

Day	1	2	3	9	14
kBq	100	78	65	14.9	5.1

Solution

The urinary excretion function, Eq. (13.14), describes the biological excretion only and does not consider radioactive decay. In the case of ^{89}Sr, the radioactive half-life is only 51 days. Therefore, the exponents in Eq. (13.14) must be modified by using the effective half-times for each of the three components. For the first component, the effective half-time is calculated from Eq. (6.54) as follows:

$$T_E = \frac{T_R \times T_B}{T_R + T_B} = \frac{51 \times 3}{51 + 3} = 2.83 \text{ days},$$

and the corresponding effective elimination constant, from Eq. (6.52), is

$$\lambda_E = \frac{0.693}{T_E} = \frac{0.693}{2.83 \text{ days}} = 0.245 \text{ per day}.$$

Similarly, we calculate λ_E (44 days) = 0.0294 d^{-1} and λ_E (4000 days) = 0.0138 d^{-1}. The urinary excretion function for ^{89}Sr, which gives us the number of becquerels excreted per day in the urine per becquerel uptake, therefore, is

$$f_U\left(^{89}\text{Sr}\right) = 0.13e^{-0.245t} + 0.0013e^{-0.029t} + 2.4 \times 10^{-5} \times e^{-0.0138t}. \tag{13.15}$$

If we solve the equation for $t = 1$ day after uptake, we find that $f_U = 0.103$. The estimated uptake, therefore, is calculated from

$$f_U(t) = \frac{A_U(t), \text{ activity in urine at time } t}{\text{uptake}} \qquad (13.16)$$

$$\text{Uptake} = \frac{A_U(1)}{f_U(1)} = \frac{100 \text{ kBq}}{0.103} = 971 \text{ kBq}.$$

When similar calculations are made for the other four urine samples, we get

DAY	$f_u(t)$	$A_u(t)$	UPTAKE (kBq)
1	0.103	100	971
2	0.081	78	963
3	0.0635	65	1024
9	0.0154	14.9	968
14	0.0051	5.1	1000

Our best estimate of the uptake is the average of the five individual estimates, or 985 kBq.

To go from the uptake to the intake, we must consider the fraction of the inhaled activity that was deposited in the lungs and then the fraction of the deposited activity that was transferred to the blood. Table 8-7 tells us that when 1-μm AMAD (activity median aerodynamic diameter) particles (the default size) are inhaled or "taken in," 63% of the intake is deposited in the lungs. Table 8-8 shows that the fraction of the lung burden that is transferred to the blood for class D particles is $0.48 + (0.15 f_1)$, where f_1 is the fraction of the element absorbed into the blood from the gastrointestinal tract. For Sr, $f_1 = 0.3$; therefore, the estimated intake I is

$$985 \text{ kBq} = 0.63 \left[0.48 + (0.15 \times 0.3) \right] \times I$$

$$I = 2.98 \times 10^3 \text{ kBq} = 2.98 \times 10^6 \text{ Bq} \quad (80 \, \mu\text{Ci}).$$

The inhalation ALI is listed in ICRP 30 as 3×10^7 Bq, and in 10 Code of Federal Regulations (CFR) 20 as 800 μCi. For dose-tracking purposes, in order to demonstrate compliance with U.S. Nuclear Regulatory Commission (NRC) regulations, the assigned committed effective dose equivalent (CEDE) from this accidental exposure is calculated:

$$\text{CEDE} = \frac{80 \, \mu\text{Ci}}{800 \dfrac{\mu\text{Ci}}{\text{ALI}}} \times \frac{5000 \text{ mrems}}{\text{ALI}} = 500 \text{ mrems} \quad (5 \text{ mSv}).$$

If we use the inhalation dose coefficient listed in IAEA Safety Series No. 115-1 for 5-μm, solubility-type-F particles, we have

$$3 \times 10^6 \text{ Bq} \times 1.4 \times 10^{-9} \frac{\text{Sv}}{\text{Bq}} = 4.2 \times 10^{-3} \text{ Sv} \quad (420 \text{ mrems}).$$

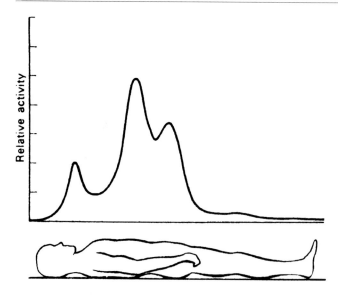

Figure 13-3. Whole-body scan, with a crystal gamma-ray detector, 2 hours after ingestion of Tc. (Reproduced with permission from Beasley TM, Palmer HE, Nelp WB. Distribution and excretion of technetium in humans. *Health Phys.* 1966; 12(10): 1425–1435.)

Using the principles described above, together with data from physiologically based biokinetic models applied to the reference man, tables of IRFs and urinary and fecal elimination fractions for most radionuclides that were ingested or inhaled were calculated and together with the calculational methodology for their application, are published in Lessard (1987)[1] and in ICRP 78.

In Vivo Bioassay

In vivo bioassay may range from simply measuring the radiation from the thyroid gland under standardized conditions with a simple detector such as the Geiger counter probe, with a scintillation detector from a health physics surveying instrument, or with a highly sophisticated, heavily shielded, low-background whole-body counter. The simple determination may be used in routine "go–no go" monitoring to determine whether a previously established reference level has been reached, while measurements with the sophisticated system are useful to learn how much and what kind of activity is in the body. A whole-body count directly measures the radiation emitted from the internally deposited radionuclides. This information is used to determine the nature and location of the radionuclide and to quantitatively estimate the amount in the body, as shown in Figure 13-3. Generally, gamma emitters whose quantum energy exceeds about 30–50 keV can be determined using in vivo techniques. When in vivo methods are used to determine internal emitters, the in vivo data are customarily used as the data of record for demonstrating compliance with radiation safety regulations.

[1]Lessard, E. T. et al. *Interpretation of Bioassay Measurements.* NUREG/CR-4884, BNL-NUREG-52063, U.S. Nuclear Regulatory Commission, Washington, DC, 1987.

EXAMPLE 13.3

In a routine annual whole-body count in a laboratory where there is known to be airborne radioactivity, a worker was found to have 5.4×10^{-3} μCi (200 Bq) ^{137}Cs, 4.1×10^{-3} μCi (152 Bq) ^{60}Co, and 1.4×10^{-3} μCi (52 Bq) ^{54}Mn. Since we do not know exactly when the intakes occurred, we assume the radionuclides to have been inhaled immediately after the previous whole-body count 1 year ago. The 365-day IRFs and the ALIs for the inhaled radioisotopes are given in the following table:

ISOTOPE	BODY BURDEN (μCi)	IRF	ALI (μCi)
^{137}Cs	5.4×10^{-3}	5.93×10^{-2}	2×10^{2}
^{60}Co	4.1×10^{-3}	1.30×10^{-2}	2×10^{2}
^{54}Mn	1.4×10^{-3}	2.79×10^{-4}	8×10^{2}

Calculate

(a) the estimated intake.

(b) the assigned dose from these intakes.

Solution

(a) The estimated intake is calculated from the following equation:

$$I = \frac{\text{Body burden } (t)}{\text{IRF } (t)}.$$

$$^{137}\text{Cs} = \frac{5.4 \times 10^{-3} \mu\text{Ci}}{5.93 \times 10^{-2}} = 9.11 \times 10^{-2} \mu\text{Ci}.$$

$$^{60}\text{Co} = \frac{4.1 \times 10^{-3} \mu\text{Ci}}{1.3 \times 10^{-2}} = 3.15 \times 10^{-1} \mu\text{Ci}.$$

$$^{54}\text{Mn} = \frac{1.4 \times 10^{-3} \mu\text{Ci}}{2.79 \times 10^{-4}} = 5.02 \, \mu\text{Ci}.$$

(b) The assigned dose from these intakes is

$$\text{CEDE} = 5000 \text{ mrems/ALI} \times \sum_{i=1} \frac{I_i \, \mu\text{Ci}}{\text{ALI}_i \, \mu\text{Ci/ALI}}$$

$$= 5000 \left(\frac{0.0911}{200} + \frac{0.315}{200} + \frac{5.02}{800} \right) = 42 \text{ mrems} \quad (0.42 \text{ mSv}).$$

EXAMPLE 13.4

A maintenance worker in a nuclear power plant was accidentally exposed to an aerosol consisting of ^{60}Co (1-μm AMAD, class W), and ^{54}Mn (1-μm AMAD, class D). Follow-up dosimetry included whole-body counting, and urine and feces analyses. However, the data from the urine and feces were found to be useless. Using the following sequential postexposure measured body burdens of the two isotopes, infer the intake and calculate the dose assigned to the accidental exposure. (Data adapted from Lessard, 1987.[2])

DAYS POST INTAKE	MEASURED BODY BURDEN (Bq)		TOTAL BODY IRF	
	^{60}Co	^{54}Mn	^{60}Co	^{54}Mn
1	3.4×10^4	3×10^3	5.66×10^{-1}	5.77×10^{-1}
2	3.7×10^4	2.6×10^3	4.23×10^{-1}	4.96×10^{-1}
8	2.2×10^3	1.8×10^3	1.71×10^{-1}	3.39×10^{-1}
41	1.9×10^3	8.3×10^2	1.08×10^{-1}	1.57×10^{-1}

Solution

If there had been only one measurement of the body burdens, then our best estimate of the intake would have been determined by dividing the measured body burden by the appropriate IRF. However, since we have four measurements made at successive times after exposure, we must consider statistical variability and possible differences among the variances (recall that the variance is the square of the standard deviation) of the several measurements. Since the variance of a radioactivity measurement is the number of counts, the measurement with the greatest number of counts will have the greatest effect on the best estimate of the intake. To account for this variability, the best estimate of the intake is given by

$$I = \frac{\sum_i (\text{IRF})_i}{\sum_i \dfrac{(\text{IRF})_i^2}{A_i}}, \tag{13.17}$$

where

A_i = the ith measurement of the body burden and
$(\text{IRF})_i$ = IRF associated with the ith measurement.

[2]Lessard, E. T. et al. *Interpretation of Bioassay Measurements.* NUREG/CR-4884, BNL-NUREG-52063, U.S. Nuclear Regulatory Commission, Washington, DC, 1987.

When we substitute the respective values for ^{60}Co and ^{54}Mn into Eq. (13.17), we have

$$I\left(^{60}\text{Co}\right) = \frac{0.566 + 0.423 + 0.171 + 0.108}{\dfrac{(0.566)^2}{3.4 \times 10^4} + \dfrac{(0.423)^2}{3.7 \times 10^4} + \dfrac{(0.171)^2}{2.2 \times 10^3} + \dfrac{(0.108)^2}{1.9 \times 10^3}} = 3.8 \times 10^4 \text{ Bq} \quad (1\ \mu\text{Ci}),$$

$$I\left(^{54}\text{Mn}\right) = \frac{0.577 + 0.496 + 0.339 + 0.157}{\dfrac{(0.577)^2}{3.0 \times 10^3} + \dfrac{(0.496)^2}{2.6 \times 10^3} + \dfrac{(0.339)^2}{1.8 \times 10^3} + \dfrac{(0.157)^2}{8.3 \times 10^2}}$$

$$= 5.2 \times 10^3 \text{ Bq} \quad (0.14\ \mu\text{Ci}).$$

The 10 CFR 20 lists the ALI for class W ^{60}Co particles as 200 μC, and for the class D ^{54}Mn particles the ALI is 900 μCi. The assigned dose from these intakes, therefore, is

$$CEDE = 5000 \frac{\text{mrems}}{\text{ALI}} \times \sum_{i=1} \frac{I_i\ \mu\text{Ci}}{ALI_i \dfrac{\mu\text{Ci}}{\text{ALI}}} = 5000 \left(\frac{1}{200} + \frac{0.14}{900} \right)$$

$$= 26 \text{ mrems} \quad (0.26 \text{ mSv}).$$

INDIVIDUAL MONITORING

Personal monitoring for external radiation is the continuous measurement of an individual's exposure dose by means of one or more types of suitable instruments, such as pocket ionization chambers, film badges, electronic dosimeters, and thermoluminescent dosimeters (Chapter 9), which are carried by the individual at all times. The choice of personal monitoring instrument must be compatible with the type and energy of the radiation being measured. For example, a worker who is exposed only to ^{3}H, ^{14}C, or ^{35}S would wear no personal monitoring instrument, since these isotopes emit only beta particles of such low energy that they are not recorded by any of the commercially available personal monitoring devices. In vitro bioassay procedures would be indicated if personal monitoring were necessary.

Workers who may be exposed to radioactive aerosols may wear a personal air sampler. This usually consists of a cassette that holds a 37-mm-diameter membrane filter through which air is drawn at a rate of 2–5 L per min by a battery-operated pump. The cassette is clipped to the worker's garment near his nose or mouth, and thus produces a breathing-zone sample; the pump, which has an integral air-measuring device, such as a rotameter, is worn on the worker's belt. After exposure, the filter is removed from the cassette, and the activity on its surface is measured in the counting laboratory. Such an open-faced filter collects particles of all sizes. In order to better evaluate the hazard from an aerosol, we often resort to size-selective collectors to collect a sample of "respirable dust." The most commonly used size-selective collector is the cyclone sampler, which is designed to capture particles with ≤ 4-μm AMAD. In this collector, the airstream is forced to travel in a circular path, and particles greater than a given size will be removed from the airstream by centrifugal force. A membrane filter upstream of the cyclone captures the particles that were not removed by the centrifugal force. Since the centrifugal force is a function of the particle speed, the airflow rate of the sampling system must be carefully regulated.

The main purpose of personal monitoring is to obtain information on the exposure of an individual. In addition to this main purpose, personal monitoring is also used to observe trends or changes (in time) in the working habits of a single individual or of a department and thus to measure the effectiveness of a radiation control program. Whereas the distribution of personal-monitoring data might all appear to lie within a normal range when viewed as individual readings, statistical analysis of the grouped data may reveal small but significant differences among different control measures or different operating procedures or work habits that might otherwise have escaped the attention of the radiation safety officer.

RADIATION AND CONTAMINATION SURVEYS

A *survey* is a systematic set of measurements made by a health physicist in order to determine one or more of the following:

1. an unknown radiation source,
2. dose rate,
3. surface contamination, and
4. atmospheric contamination.

In order to make these determinations, the health physics surveyor must choose the appropriate instruments and must use them properly.

Choosing a Health Physics Instrument

The choice of a surveying instrument for a specific application depends on a number of factors. Some general requirements include portability, mechanical ruggedness, ease of use and reading, ease of servicing, ease of decontamination, and reliability. In addition to these general requirements, health physics survey instruments must be calibrated for the radiation that they are designed to measure, and they must have certain other characteristics.

1. *Ability to respond to the radiation being measured.* This point can be clarified with a practical example: a commonly used side window beta–gamma probe has a window thickness of 30 mg/cm^2. This probe would be worse than useless if one wished to survey for low-energy beta radiation, such as ^{14}C or ^{35}S, or for an alpha contaminant such as ^{210}Po. Each of these radioisotopes emits only radiation whose range is less than 30 mg/cm^2—radiation not sufficiently penetrating to pass through the window of the probe. Incorrect use of this probe, therefore, may falsely indicate safe conditions when, in fact, there may be severe contamination. Similarly, incorrect inferences may be drawn if a neutron monitor is used to measure gamma radiation or if an instrument designed to measure gamma rays is used for neutrons. Another serious source of error may arise if we use particle-counting instrument to measure the radiation level from a pulsed source, such

as an accelerator. Consider a machine whose pulse repetition rate is 120 s^{-1}, and the pulse width is 5 μseconds. If we use a particle-counting instrument whose resolving time is greater than the pulse width but less than the time between pulses, the instrument will merely record the pulse repetition rate, 120 cps in this case. It is essential that radiation survey instruments be used only for the radiations they are designed to measure.

2. *Sensitivity.* The instrument must be sufficiently sensitive to measure radiation at the desired level. Thus, an instrument to be used in a search for a lost radium needle should be more sensitive than a survey meter used to measure the radiation levels inside the shielding of an accelerator. In the latter case, where the radiation levels may reach hundreds of milligrays per hour (thousands of millirads per hour), an ionization chamber whose sensitivity is about 0.01 mGy/h (1 mrad/h), is suitable. In searching for the lost radium needle, on the other hand, a sensitivity of 0.01 mGy/h (1 mrad/h) would greatly limit the area that could be covered in the search; a Geiger counter survey meter that has a sensitivity of about 0.5 μGy/h (0.05 mrad/h) is much more useful. For example, if a 1-mg radium needle were lost, the distance within which it could be detected with the ionization chamber is about 90 cm, while the Geiger counter will respond to the lost radium at a distance of 400 cm. In this case, the Geiger counter can thus cover a search area about 20 times greater than the ionization chamber. Too great a sensitivity, on the other hand, may be equally undesirable. The range of radiation levels over which the instrument is to be used should be matched by the range of radiation levels for which the instrument is designed. Sensitivity is determined mainly by the value of the input resistor across the detector, R in Figures 9-1 and 9-27. The sensitivity of the detector is directly proportional to the size of the input resistance.

3. *Response time.* The response time of a survey instrument may be defined as the time required for the instrument to attain 63% of its final reading in any radiation field. This time is determined by the product of the input capacity (in farads) of the detector and the shunting resistance (in ohms) across the detector, RC in Figure 9-1. The time constant is usually expressed in seconds. A survey instrument's time constant may have a strong influence on a radiation measurement. For example, if a measurement made with an ionization-type survey meter whose time constant is 3 seconds is made during a 0.2-second exposure of a diagnostic X-ray is 0.16 mR/h, then the true exposure rate is calculated with an adaptation of Eq. (9.9):

$$\dot{X}\,(\text{true}) = \frac{\dot{X}\,(\text{measured})}{1 - e^{-\frac{t}{RC}}} = \frac{0.16\ \text{mR/h}}{1 - e^{-\frac{0.2\ \text{s}}{3\ \text{s}}}} = 2.5\ \frac{\text{mR}}{\text{h}}.$$

A low value for the time constant means an instrument that responds to rapid changes in radiation level—such as would be experienced when passing the probe rapidly over a small area of contamination on a bench top or over a small crack in a radiation shield. A fast response time, however, may mean a decrease in sensitivity due to a smaller value of R. Furthermore, a fast response time may result in rapid fluctuations of the meter reading, thus making it difficult to obtain an average level. Most instruments offer a range of response times,

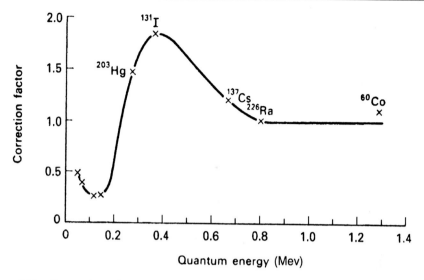

Figure 13-4. Energy dependence of a Geiger counter survey meter. The meter reading is multiplied by the correction factor appropriate to the quantum energy in order to obtain the true exposure rate. (Courtesy of Electronica Lombarda SPA.)

the appropriate one being selected by the surveyor, who turns the time constant selector switch to the desired value.

4. *Energy dependence.* Most radiation-measuring instruments have a limited span of energy over which the radiation dose is accurately measured. One of the figures of merit of a radiation dosimeter is the energy range over which the instrument is useful. This information must be known by the health physicist in order to choose a proper instrument for a particular application or to interpret the measurements properly. The energy dependence is usually specified by the manufacturer as "accurate to ±10% of the true value from 80 keV to 2 MeV" or by means of an energy-dependence curve (Fig. 13-4). The magnitude of the errors that can arise when the energy dependence factor is overlooked is shown in Table 13-2.

TABLE 13-2. Energy Dependence of Dose–rate Response of GM and Scintillation Counters—Meter Reading for a True Exposure Rate of 1 mR/h

ISOTOPE	GAMMA-RAY ENERGY (MeV)	GM COUNTER (mR/h)	SCINTILLATION COUNTER (mR/h)
^{60}Co	1.25	1.15	0.6
^{226}Ra	0.84	1.0	0.96
^{137}Cs	0.661	0.92	1.39
^{198}Au	0.411	0.82	2.65
^{203}Hg	0.279	1.29	7.5
^{141}Ce	0.145	2.4	14.1
^{241}Am	0.06	6.0	9.8

Surface Contamination

Surface contamination can be located by scanning with a sensitive detector, such as a thin-end window Geiger counter. Surface contamination is expressed in units of activity per unit area, Contamination limits usually are listed as disintegrations per minute per 100 cm² (Table 11-5).

EXAMPLE 13.5

A pancake-type Geiger-Müller (GM) counter, whose diameter is 4.37 cm, is used to scan a surface area that is believed to have become contaminated. The average of several measurements was 450 cpm. The detection efficiency of the counter is 4% and the counter's background is 50 cpm. Calculate the surface concentration, in dpm/100 cm².

Solution

The surface concentration, expressed as dpm/100 cm², is calculated:

$$C(\text{surface}) = \frac{\text{cpm(gross)} - \text{cpm(background)}}{\text{efficiency}} \times \frac{100\,\text{cm}^2}{\text{area of detector}} \qquad \textbf{(13.18)}$$

$$C = \frac{450\,\text{cpm} - 50\,\text{cpm}}{0.04\,\text{cpm/dpm}} \times \frac{100\,\text{cm}^2}{\dfrac{\pi}{4} \times (4.37\,\text{cm})^2} = 6.7 \times 10^4\,\frac{\text{dpm}}{100\,\text{cm}^2}.$$

After finding a contaminated spot or area, an appropriate dose-measuring instrument may be employed to measure the dose rate at a useful distance from the surface.

The main hazard from surface contamination is the transmission of the contamination from the surface into the body via inhalation or ingestion. To estimate this hazard, a *smear test* is performed to determine whether the surface contamination is fixed or whether it is loose and therefore transmissible. A smear test consists of wiping the suspected area with a piece of filter paper several centimeters in diameter and then measuring the activity in the paper. The area to be smeared varies according to the extent of the suspected contamination and the physical conditions under which the survey is made; a wipe area of 100 cm² is not uncommon. A smear survey is a systematic series of smears used to detect transmissible contamination. It is often done in a work area that is subject to contamination, where the background due to radiation sources is high enough to mask the activity due to contamination, or when detection with a survey meter is difficult, as is the case with ³H, ¹⁴C, or ³⁵S. It should be emphasized that a smear test is a qualitative or, at best, a semiquantitative determination whose chief purpose is to allow an estimate to be made of the degree to which surface contamination is fixed. If significant transmissible contamination is found and if, in the opinion of the health physicist, this contamination may be hazardous, then prompt decontamination procedures are instituted.

Decontamination can often be effected simply by wiping the surface with a damp cloth. If this is ineffective, then commercially available chemical solutions may be used. A simple method for removing tactilely transmissible surface contamination is to use masking tape. When the adhesive side of the tape is pressed to the contaminated surface, a good deal of the contaminant will adhere to the tape. Another method, which is more effective than the masking tape is the application of a polymer hydrogel that can seep into tiny crevices to engulf the contaminant. The hydrogel is applied with a roller and after it is dry, the hydrogel skin with the contaminant entrapped in it, is peeled off. Reasonably high decontamination efficiencies, depending on the nature of the surface and the contaminant, can be obtained. The agents that are used for decontamination, of course, become contaminated themselves, and are treated as low-level radioactive waste.

Leak Testing of Sealed Sources

Sealed gamma-ray, beta, bremsstrahlung, and neutron sources are used in a wide variety of applications in medicine, in research laboratories, in industry, and in antiterrorist activities such as examination of baggage and cargo containers. In all cases, the radioactive material is permanently enclosed either in a capsule or another suitable container. Before being shipped from the supplier, all such sources must pass an inspection for freedom from surface contamination and leakage. Either during transport from the supplier or in the course of time, however, the capsule may develop faults through which the radioactive source material may escape into the environment. Because of the potentially serious consequences of such an escape, a sealed source must be tested before being put into use and periodically thereafter for surface contamination and leakage. The testing cycle depends on the nature of the source and on the kind of use to which it is put. However, it is usually recommended that such tests be performed at least once every 6 months. The following techniques may be employed to perform these tests:

1. Wipe the source with either a piece of wet filter paper or a cotton swab. Repeat at least 7 days later. If less than 200 Bq (0.005 μCi) alpha or less than 2000 Bq (0.05 μCi) beta activity are wiped off each time, the source is considered free of leaks.
2. For high-activity sources such as those used in teletherapy, where wiping the source might be hazardous, accessible surfaces of the housing port or collimator should be wiped while the source is in the "off" position.
3. Immerse the source in ethanediol and reduce the pressure on the liquid to 100 mm Hg for a period of 30 seconds. A leak is indicated if a stream of fine bubbles issues from the source. This method is reliable only for such sources where enough gas would be trapped to produce a stream of fine bubbles.

AIR SAMPLING

Since no system of containment or control can be 100% effective all the time, it is inevitable that some radioactive material will be released to the atmosphere during normal operations involving unencapsulated radioactivity. Atmospheric radioactivity is a matter of concern because the inhalation pathway is a major avenue for the entry of contaminants into the body. We take in a larger mass of air than either food or water; the daily intakes by a reference person are only 1.9 kg of food and 2.2 kg of water, but 26 kg of air! Additionally, the area of interface in the lungs—between the body's internal milieu and the outside atmosphere—is 50–100 m^2. This large interface facilitates the transfer of noxious agents from the inhaled air into the body fluids. Therefore, if the quantity of radioactivity being handled is great enough to pose a significant inhalation hazard, in case of an accidental release of the radioactivity to the air, an air-sampling program is required to accurately assess the radioactivity content of the air.

Air-sampling programs are implemented in order to meet regulatory requirements, to verify the effectiveness of engineering and administrative methods for control of airborne radioactivity, and to supply data for public information purposes. Sampling strategies are determined by several different factors, including the reasons for sampling; the physical and radiological characteristics of the contaminant; environmental considerations (such as airflow patterns, dust, and radon); operational considerations, including whom, when, and where to sample; type of sample (area or personal); sample size; and so on. For example, general area sampling is useful for planning protective measures and detecting releases, but it is not suitable for determining workers' "actual exposure." To determine actual exposure, we must use breathing-zone samples or individual personal samplers (called *lapel samplers*) that are worn by the workers near their noses. These are among the many factors that must be considered in the design of an air-sampling program that will yield useful information.

Air-Sampling System

An air-sampling system includes three basic components: (1) a source of suction (a vacuum pump), for drawing the air to be sampled; (2) a collecting device, which separates the contaminant from the air; and (3) a metering device for measuring the quantity of air sampled. The concentration of airborne radioactivity is determined by dividing the quantity of collected activity by the volume of sampled air. It is essential that the air-sampling system—the pump, collector, and flowmeter—be properly calibrated. Proper calibration means that the three components of the system are calibrated together, as an integrated system.

Vacuum pumps are available in two basic designs, each with its own characteristics. Positive-displacement pumps—in which the air is pulled through a fixed volume by a rotating vane, a reciprocating piston, or a vibrating diaphragm—are characterized by high pumping rates against high resistance and a very slow decrease in flow rate as the resistance in the system increases. The second basic category includes centrifugal pumps, which are strongly influenced by the resistance in the system. Although centrifugal pumps can move large volumes of air against low resistance, their flow rate drops off rapidly with increasing resistance.

The choice of a collecting device depends on the nature of the contaminant to be collected. For airborne particles, filtration is the most commonly used collection method. Several different types of filter media are available: paper, glass fiber, and membrane (mixed cellulose ester is the most frequently used membrane filter).

Each of these has its own flow rate, filtering, and physical or chemical characteristics. Filters trap particles mainly by two mechanisms: (1) sieving, which captures particles that are larger than the pore size, and (2) impaction, which captures particles smaller than the pore size. In impaction, because of the inertia of the particles in the airstream, the particles tend to move in straight lines. As the air bends in its tortuous path through the filter's pores, the particles tend to continue in straight lines and thus strike the filter matrix, where they are captured. For this reason, the filtration efficiency of a filter increases as the flow rate through the filter increases. Filters made of glass fiber or paper trap particles within the matrix; membrane filters trap particles on the filter surface. This point is important when one is sampling for alpha or for low-energy beta particles because of the corrections for self-absorption that must be used. For this reason as well as for their very high retention efficiency for particles of respirable size, membrane filters are very widely used for the sampling of radioactive aerosols. Membrane filters may be made transparent with immersion oil, thus allowing direct microscopic observation of the particles for sizing or for particle concentration measurements. However, these filters retain a strong electrostatic charge. If the filter is placed into a windowless counter, this electrostatic charge would distort the electric field around the anode and thus would introduce a counting error. To prevent this, the membrane filter is treated with a mixture of dioxane and petroleum ether, which eliminates the static charges from the filter without interfering with the dust particles on it. The filtration efficiencies, at a sampling velocity of 0.61 m/s (2 ft/s), are shown in Table 13-3.

Airborne gases may be collected by a number of different techniques, including the following:

1. *Adsorption* is the process in which a monolayer of the gas binds to the surface of certain granular substances called *adsorbents*. Commonly used adsorbents include activated charcoal, silica gel (a hard, glassy form of SiO_2), activated alumina (a very porous form of $Al_2O_3 \cdot 3H_2O$), and molecular sieves (synthetic Na or Ca aluminosilicates of high porosity). The capacity of each adsorbent depends on its specific surface area (square meters per gram), the partial pressure of the gas, and the temperature. This binding capacity is represented by a curve called an *adsorption isotherm* (Fig. 13-5), in which the amount of gas adsorbed per gram of adsorbent is plotted against the equilibrium pressure at constant temperature. In use, the adsorbent is packed into a suitable container, and the air to be sampled is drawn through the adsorbent. If desired, the adsorbed gas can be driven off in the laboratory by the application of heat, or it may be chemically desorbed by passing an appropriate chemical absorber through the adsorbent bed.

TABLE 13-3. Collecting Efficiency of Certain Filters (Percent)

	<0.4	0.4–0.6	0.6–0.8	0.8–1.0	1–2	>2
Whatman 41	23	28	64	74	80	100
Whatman 4	23	32	38	79	84	100
MSA S	48	47	77	92	94	100
H-70	99.3	99.3				
Glass fiber	99.9	99.9				
Membrane	99.9	99.9				

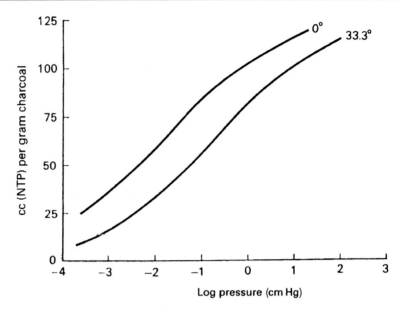

Figure 13-5. Adsorption isotherm of benzene by charcoal. (Reproduced with permission from McBain JW. *The Sorption of Gases and Vapours by Solids.* London, England: George Routledge & Sons; 1932.)

Adsorption is a widely used technique for sampling airborne radon and radioiodine. Radon is usually sampled with a passive collector. The air to be sampled diffuses through activated charcoal granules loosely packed in a canister that is open to the air, and the radon is adsorbed onto the carbon. After about 4–7 days of this exposure, the charcoal-containing canister is sealed shut and the gamma radiation from the radon and its daughters is counted with a scintillation counter. The counts are then compared to a calibration curve to determine the mean radon concentration during the sampling period.

In iodine sampling, the iodine-containing air is drawn through a cartridge containing activated carbon granules impregnated with triethylenediamine (TEDA). This is a chelating agent that binds the iodine to prevent desorption. Such charcoal cartridges also bind noble gases, such as ^{133}Xe. If noble gases are a possible contaminant when air is being sampled for iodine, we use a cartridge containing zeolite, impregnated with $AgNO_3$. This adsorbent captures elemental and organic iodine but is transparent to noble gases. In sampling for iodine vapors, it is customary to use a glass-fiber filter ahead of the iodine cartridge in order to remove particles that might otherwise be captured by the cartridge. The efficiency of the glass-fiber filters used for this purpose is 99.9% for 0.3-μm diameter dioctylphthalate (DOP) particles. We also use another charcoal cartridge behind the first iodine cartridge to capture any iodine that might break through the sampling cartridge. This breakthrough occurs if sampling continues after all the binding sites on the sampling cartridge are saturated with iodine or whatever other contaminant gas there might be in the atmosphere. The sampling train for iodine vapors thus consists of three sequential elements: a glass-fiber filter to remove particles, followed by the sampling cartridge (either activated charcoal or $AgNO_3$-impregnated zeolite), which is followed by another activated-charcoal

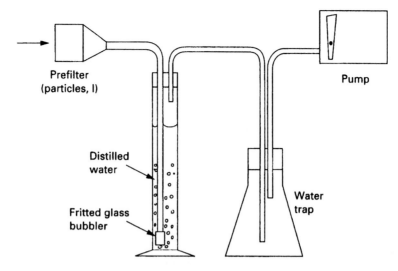

Figure 13-6. *Sampling tritiated water by absorbing it in ordinary water. An aliquot of the absorbing solution is counted in a liquid scintillation counter to determine the tritium concentration in the sampled air.*

cartridge to remove the iodine in the airstream in case of a breakthrough in the sampling cartridge.

2. *Absorption* is the process in which the air to be sampled is bubbled through a liquid with which the contaminant will interact. For example, tritiated water vapor will be absorbed in ordinary water, as shown in Figure 13-6. After bubbling a known volume of air through a known volume of collecting water, an aliquot of the water is counted in a liquid scintillation counter and the atmospheric concentration of the ^{3}H is calculated. Absorption also lends itself to the collection of $^{14}CO_2$. In this case, the air is bubbled through a solution of 0.5 N NaOH, and $Na_2^{14}CO_3$ precipitates. Counting the activity in the precipitate allows the calculation of the atmospheric concentration of the $^{14}CO_2$. For optimum operation, the gas must be brought into intimate contact with the absorbing solution, and it must remain in contact long enough for the desired reaction to take place. To accomplish this, the air is discharged into the absorbing solution through a fritted glass bubbler located deep into the absorbing solution. At a sampling rate of 1–5 L/min, the collection efficiency (for the gas appropriate to the absorbing solution) is close to 100%. In any particular application, the collection efficiency may easily be measured by connecting two collection setups in series, and measuring the activity in each one. If the two collectors are exactly the same, the collection efficiency, ε is given by

$$\varepsilon = 1 - \frac{A_2}{A_1}, \tag{13.19}$$

where A_1 and A_2 are the activities in the first and second solutions.

3. *Grab sample* is a process in which an evacuated container is opened to the atmosphere to be sampled, thus permitting the contaminated air to enter the container. The activity of this contaminated air may be determined by transferring

the gas to an ionization chamber and then measuring the ionization current due to the gaseous contaminant. Another method uses an evacuated container with a flat glass face that is coated on the inside surface with a scintillating medium, such as ZnS. Such a collector is called a Lucas cell. After it is coupled directly to a photomultiplier tube, the scintillations caused by the radioactive gas inside the Lucas cell are counted and the atmospheric concentration of the contaminant is determined from the count rate and the volume of air in the cell. This method is especially useful for alpha emitters, such as radon.

4. *Immersion monitoring* is a procedure in which a counter is immersed in a chamber through which the contaminated air flows. Except for tritium and ^{14}C and ^{35}S, all other gaseous contaminants have radiation characteristics that allow them to be measured with conventional beta–gamma detectors. This method is useful for continuous monitoring of airborne gas.

In health physics practice, the volume of air sampled is most often determined by measuring the sampling rate during the sampling time with a rotameter (Fig. 13-7). The rotameter, which is a variable area flowmeter, consists of a transparent glass or plastic vertical tube whose inside diameter is tapered—that is, is conical in shape—with the diameter increasing continuously from bottom to top. A ball whose diameter is slightly smaller than the bore at the bottom of the tube rests at the bottom of the tube when no air is flowing through the meter. Equation (8.15) tells us that the viscous force acting on a body that is immersed in a flowing fluid (air is a fluid in this context) is directly proportional to the relative velocity between the body and the flowing fluid. The viscous force exerted on the ball by the air that flows through the rotameter from the bottom to the top of the tube drags the ball to a height where the viscous force is exactly equal to the gravitational force acting on the ball. At this point, the ball remains stationary and appears to be "floating" in the airstream. If the

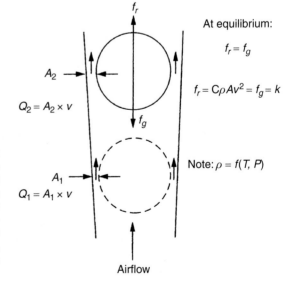

Figure 13-7. Operating principle of a rotameter. The velocity of the air flowing through the annular area A_2 is equal to the air velocity through the annular area A_1, thus resulting in equal viscous forces at both levels. When the ball is stationary anywhere in the rotameter tube, the upward viscous force acting on the ball is exactly equal to the downward gravitational force on the ball. Thus, the height of the "floating" ball is proportional to the volumetric airflow rate.

airflow is increased, the velocity of the air flowing through the annular space between the ball and the inside surface of the rotameter increases, thereby increasing the viscous force. This increased viscous force drags the ball upward, where the larger annular space leads to a decreased air velocity. At the height where the velocity of the increased volume of air through the annular space leads to a viscous force exactly equal to the gravitational force acting on the ball, the ball will come to rest. The new equilibrium position tells us what the new volumetric flow rate is.

The viscosity of the air depends on its density, which in turn depends on the temperature and pressure. If the rotameter is used at a temperature or pressure that differs significantly from the conditions under which it was calibrated, then the observed reading must be corrected to account for the different air density. The actual flow rate, Q_a, is related to the calibration reading of the rotameter, Q_0, by

$$Q_a = Q_0 \sqrt{\frac{\rho_0}{\rho_a}} = Q_0 \sqrt{\frac{p_0/T_0}{p_a/T_a}} = Q_0 \sqrt{\frac{p_0}{p_a} \times \frac{T_a}{T_0}}, \tag{13.20}$$

where the calibration and actual temperatures T_0 and T_a are in degrees absolute.

EXAMPLE 13.6

The rotameter on a pump was calibrated to read 2.0 L/min at an altitude of 575 ft (175 m), where the pressure was 29.31 in. Hg (745 mm Hg) and the temperature was 75°F (24°C). The pump was used in a uranium mine at an altitude of 7000 ft (2134 m), where the atmospheric pressure was 23.10 in. Hg (587 mm Hg) and the temperature 50°F (10°C).

(a) What was the actual flow rate if the rotameter reading was 2.0 L/min?

(b) What should the rotameter reading be for an actual flow rate of 2.0 L/min?

Solution

(a) If we substitute the respective values into Eq. (13.20), we find the actual flow rate to be

$$Q_a = 2.0 \times \sqrt{\frac{29.31}{23.10} \times \frac{460 + 50}{460 + 75}} = 2.2 \ \frac{L}{min}.$$

(b) Substituting into Eq. (13.20) and then solving for Q_0, we have

$$2 \ \frac{L}{min} = Q_0 \times \sqrt{\frac{29.31}{23.10} \times \frac{460 + 50}{460 + 75}}$$

$$Q_0 = 1.8 \ L/min.$$

Sampling Considerations

Certain problems exist when one is sampling for any kind of airborne contaminant (including nonradioactive contaminants), and there are problems that are unique to radioactivity sampling. These problems include what follows below.

Representative Sampling

The first problem is obtaining a sample of air *that is representative of the situation under investigation.* In most cases, we are interested in the radioactivity that a person might inhale. For this purpose, air samples are usually taken in the breathing zone—that is, at a height of about 6 ft above the ground. If the contaminant is a dust, then the collector should be oriented so that the collection orifice is vertical, so that it will collect respirable dust particles suspended in the air rather than nonrespirable particles that might fall down on the collector. There is a good deal of evidence showing that concentrations of airborne contamination vary significantly in time and location. Obtaining a "representative sample" of what a person might inhale is thus a fairly difficult task. To simplify this task, a worker may wear a personal air sampler whose collector is as near to his nose as practicable. Measurements made under actual working conditions with a personal air sampler and a fixed air sampler have shown that there is little correlation between the activity on the fixed air sampler and that of the personal air sampler.

Isokinetic Sampling

A special problem in obtaining a representative sample arises in sampling dusts that are moving at a high velocity, as in the case of an exhaust duct or chimney. Airborne particles are carried by an airstream, and they tend to follow the streamlines of flow. If the streamlines bend or curve, then the path of an airborne particle is determined by the ratio of the viscous forces (which tend to keep the particle in the streamlines) to the inertial force (which tends to cause the particle to cut across streamlines). Consider the case where a sampling device is oriented at right angles to the direction of flow in a duct—that is, the gas is blowing directly into the sampling device. If the gas is drawn through the sampler at a velocity less than that of the gas in the duct, then some of the gas must flow around the sampling device. Small particles will be carried by the air around the sampler, while large particles will, because of their inertia, tend to continue in a straight line and thus cut across the streamlines and enter into the sampler. This results in an excessive number of large particles in the collector, which leads to an overestimate of the mass or activity concentration in the gas. If the gas is drawn through the sampler at a higher velocity than that of the gas in the duct, then more of the smaller particles than the larger particles will be carried by the air into the collector, thus leading to a smaller deposition of mass or activity and consequently to an underestimation of the true concentration of particulate matter in the stream of gas. When the velocity of the gas through the sampler is equal to the velocity of gas in the duct, the streamlines of the gas are not disturbed by the sampling orifice and no sampling error due to the inertia of the suspended particles occurs. This condition is called *isokinetic sampling* and must be met if the dust sample is to be representative of the dusts in the airstream. The magnitude of the error due to *anisokinetic sampling* conditions increases as the mass of the particles increases and as the difference between the sampling velocity and the gas velocity increases.

Sample Size

The second problem is obtaining a sample *large enough to give a reasonably accurate estimate of the mean atmospheric concentration of the radioactivity*. This is relatively straightforward in the case of gaseous radioactivity. The sample size is determined by the sensitivity of the counting system and the concentration that we wish to measure. For the case of long-lived radionuclides (relative to the sampling time), these factors are related by

$$C = \frac{MDA}{V} = \frac{MDA}{S \times t}, \tag{13.21}$$

where

$$MDA = \text{minimum detectable activity, Bq or } \mu\text{Ci,}$$
$$V = \text{volume of air sampled, or sample size,}$$
$$S = \text{sampling rate, and}$$
$$t = \text{sampling time.}$$

EXAMPLE 13.7

Calculate the sampling time, at a rate of 4 L/min, to detect an ^{131}I concentration that is 10% of the derived air concentration (DAC) (DAC = 700 Bq/m^3) if the MDA of the counting system is 3.7 Bq ($10 \times 10^{-6} \mu$Ci).

Solution

Equation (13.21) is solved for t to give

$$t = \frac{MDA}{C \times S} = \frac{3.7 \text{ Bq}}{70 \text{ Bq/m}^3 \times 0.004 \text{ m}^3/\text{min}} = 13.2 \text{ minutes.}$$

In traditional industrial hygiene air sampling, the calculation for sampling time for airborne particles is the same as in the example above. However, the calculation for the sample size needed to determine the mean concentration of particulate radioactivity is more complex than that for gaseous activity. In the case of airborne radioactive particles, the particle concentration corresponding to the radiological DAC is very small; therefore, the probability of capturing an airborne particle is small. In the case of inorganic Pb, for example, the industrial hygiene permissible exposure limit (PEL) is 0.05 mg/m^3. The mass of a 1-μm aerodynamic equivalent Pb particle is 1.6×10^{-10} mg. The particle concentration corresponding to the PEL is

$$C(\text{PEL}) = \frac{0.05 \text{ mg/m}^3}{1.6 \times 10^{-10} \text{ mg/particle}} = 3.13 \times 10^8 \text{ particle/m}^3.$$

The DAC for ^{210}Pb is $1 \times 10^{-4}\,\mu\text{Ci/m}^3$ ($3.7\,\text{Bq/m}^3$), and the specific activity of ^{210}Pb is $79.2\,\text{Ci/g}$ ($2.93 \times 10^{12}\,\text{Bq/g}$). The activity of a 1-$\mu$m ^{210}Pb particle is

$$A = 1.6 \times 10^{-13}\,\frac{\text{g}}{\text{particle}} \times 79.2\,\frac{\text{Ci}}{\text{g}} = 1.27 \times 10^{-11}\,\frac{\text{Ci}}{\text{particle}}$$

$$= 1.27 \times 10^{-5}\,\frac{\mu\text{Ci}}{\text{particle}}.$$

The particle concentration corresponding to the radiological DAC is

$$C(\text{DAC}) = \frac{1 \times 10^{-4}\,\dfrac{\mu\text{Ci}}{\text{m}^3}}{1.27 \times 10^{-5}\,\dfrac{\mu\text{Ci}}{\text{particle}}} = 8\,\frac{\text{particles}}{\text{m}^3}.$$

The influence of this very small particle concentration on sample size may be illustrated by the following example.

EXAMPLE 13.8

Particles of ^{239}PuO$_2$ will be sampled with a membrane filter whose collection efficiency is given as 99%. What minimum sample size is needed to determine whether the Pu concentration exceeds 10% of the DAC (DAC $= 7 \times 10^{-12}\,\mu\text{Ci/mL}$)? The MDA for the counting system is $5 \times 10^{-7}\,\mu\text{Ci}$ ($0.0185\,\text{Bq}$).

Solution

The minimum sample size, if we did not have to consider the particle concentration is calculated from Eq. (13.21):

$$C = \frac{\text{MDA}}{V\,(\text{min}) \times \varepsilon},$$

$$V = \frac{5 \times 10^{-7}\,\mu\text{Ci}}{0.1 \times 7 \times 10^{-12}\,\mu\text{Ci/mL} \times 0.99} = 7.2 \times 10^5\,\text{mL} = 0.72\,\text{m}^3.$$

The PuO$_2$ particles, 1-μm AMAD (0.3 μm actual size), have a mean activity of $3.5 \times 10^{-7}\,\mu\text{Ci/particle}$. The DAC for class Y ^{239}Pu is $7 \times 10^{-12}\,\mu\text{Ci/mL}$ ($0.3\,\text{Bq/m}^3$). To meet the DAC means a particle concentration of

$$C(\text{DAC}) = \frac{7 \times 10^{-12}\,\mu\text{Ci/mL}}{3.5 \times 10^{-7}\,\mu\text{Ci/particle}} = 2 \times 10^{-5}\,\text{particle/mL} = 20\,\text{particle/m}^3.$$

For health physics purposes, we wish to detect 10% of the DAC (i.e., 2 particles/m^3) within $\pm20\%$ at the 95% confidence level (or confidence interval, CI). That is, we want to collect 2 ± 0.4 particles at the 95% confidence level.

$$95\%\,\text{CI} = 0.4 = \pm1.96\sigma_\text{C},$$

$$\sigma_\text{C} = \frac{0.4}{1.96} = 0.2$$

Poisson statistics apply here, because the probability of capturing any particular particle is very low. Therefore,

$$C \pm \sigma_C = \frac{N}{V} \pm \frac{\sqrt{N}}{N}. \tag{13.22}$$

Since

$$\frac{\sqrt{N}}{V} = \sqrt{\frac{N}{V} \times \frac{1}{V}} = \sqrt{\frac{C}{V}},$$

$$\sigma_C = 0.2 = \sqrt{\frac{C}{V}} = \sqrt{\frac{2}{V}}, \text{ and}$$

$$V = 50 \text{ m}^3.$$

Particle Sizing

We may adjust the DACs for aerosols whose sizes differ significantly from the 1-μm AMAD default size because the particle size determines the pulmonary deposition pattern and therefore the inhalation hazard from a given intake. The particle-size distribution of an aerosol can be determined with a cascade impactor, which separates airborne particles according to their aerodynamic size. The cascade impactor collects particles by impaction as a jet of high-velocity air strikes a surface perpendicular to its direction of travel and is thus abruptly deflected. Particulate matter, by virtue of its inertia, tends to continue in the original path and thus strikes the deflecting surface—which is also a collecting surface. The main advantage of the cascade impactor is that it separates particles according to their sizes (or their masses). How this is accomplished may be seen in Figure 13-8. The air is drawn through a series of openings of successively decreasing width, thus resulting in an increasing velocity through the successive stages. Because of their greater inertia, massive particles do not get past the first stage, while lighter particles can be carried by the airstream to the next stage. There the airstream passes through the opening at a higher velocity than through the first opening, thus imparting sufficient momentum to certain particles to cause them to impact on the second stage. In commercially available cascade impactors, this process is repeated four or more times, and then the air passes through a membrane filter that removes those particles small enough to have escaped impaction on the last stage. Each stage is thus uniquely associated with a certain *mass median aerodynamic diameter* (MMAD)—that is, the particle size that is collected with 50% efficiency by that stage. The various stages are glass slides coated with a very thin layer of adhesive material. The collected particles can either be examined microscopically or be determined either gravimetrically (for nonradioactive particles) or radiometrically.

To determine the size distribution of an aerosol with a calibrated cascade impactor, the dust is sampled and the total amount of collected material on each stage is determined. Table 13-4 shows a set of data for U_3O_8 dust (density = 8.3 g cm^{-3}) that were obtained in this manner.

Calibration curves (Fig. 13-9) for the four-stage cascade impactor, shown in Figure 13-8, show the collection efficiencies of the several stages for unit density particles

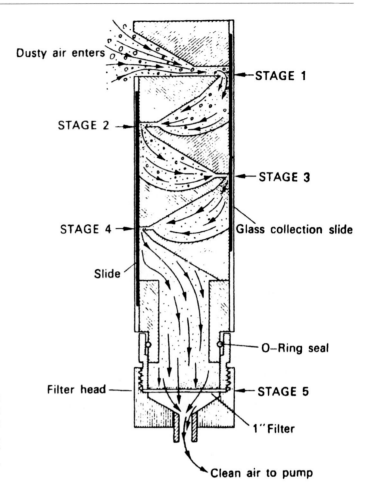

Figure 13-8. Cascade impactor. The dust particles are collected on two standard 1 in. × 3 in. glass microscope slides (stages 1, 2, 3, and 4) and on a membrane filter (stage 5). (Courtesy of Union Industrial Equipment Co.)

TABLE 13-4. Relationship Between Mass and Size Distribution in an Aerosol Sampled with a Cascade Impactor

STAGE	MMAD (μm)	PHYSICAL SIZE (μm)	% OF TOTAL MASS ON STAGE	CUMULATIVE PERCENT
1	12	4.26	11.2	94.4
2	3.9	1.35	12.4	71.0
3	1.5	0.52	49.6	40.0
4	0.43	0.16	12.2	9.1
5 (Filter)			3.0	3.0

Abbreviation: MMAD, mass median aerodynamic diameter.

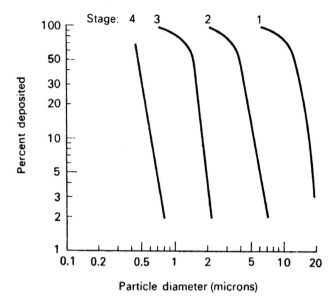

Figure 13-9. Particle-size distributions on the four stages of the cascade impactor shown in Figure 13-8 for unit density particles and a sampling rate of 17.5 L/min.

as a function of particle size. For particles whose density is not 1 g/cm^3, the physical equivalent size is calculated with Eq. (8.18). For example, Figure 13-9 shows that 1.5-μm particles of unit density are collected with 50% efficiency on stage 3. The actual physical size of this aerodynamically equivalent U$_3$O$_8$ particle whose density is 8.3 g/cm^3 is calculated by solving Eq. (8.1) for d_2 as follows:

$$\frac{d_1}{d_2} = \sqrt{\frac{\rho_2}{\rho_2}}$$

$$\frac{1.5\,\mu m}{d_2} = \sqrt{\frac{8.3\ \text{g/cm}^3}{1\ \text{g/cm}^3}}$$

$$d_2 = 0.52\,\mu m.$$

The MMADs for the four stages obtained from the calibration curves and corrected for density by Eq. (8.18) are plotted on log probability paper (Fig. 13-10) against the cumulative percentage up to the respective stage—that is, all the weight on the preceding stages plus one-half the weight on the stage in question. In plotting the data, greater emphasis is given to the weights on stages 2, 3, and 4, since the upper limit on stage 1 can be very large and the lower limit on stage 5 (the membrane filter) can be very small. From the curve of Figure 13-10, the count median diameter is found to be 0.7 μm and the geometric standard deviation σ_g is 3. The MMAD is calculated with Eq. (8.18), and is found to be 2.0 μm.

The particle size determined with the cascade impactor is the mass median diameter (MMD), that is, the diameter such that 50% of the mass (or volume) of the aerosol is in particles less than this diameter. The linear (or count) median diameter,

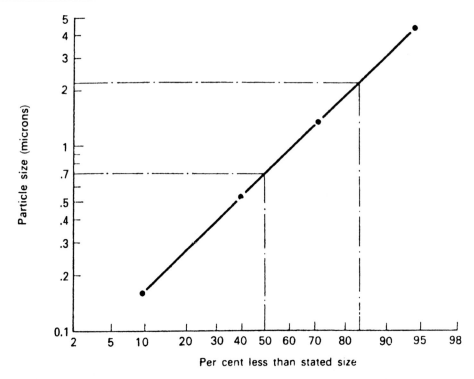

Figure 13-10. Data of Table 13-4 plotted on log-probability paper. The particle size corresponding to the 50% point is the geometric mean, 0.7 mm, and the ratio of the 84% size to the 50% size gives the geometric standard deviation as 3.

called CMD, is, the diameter below which 50% of the (or count) particles are smaller and 50% are larger, is related to the MMD by the equation

$$\log \text{ CMD} = \log \text{ MMD} - 6.9 \log^2 \sigma_g. \tag{13.23}$$

When we are interested in the surface of particles, as in the case of adsorption of gas on the particle or the plating of radon progeny on dust particles, then we use the surface median diameter, SMD, to characterize the aerosol. The SMD is that size below which we find less than 50% of the total surface area and above which we find 50% of the total surface area of the aerosol. The SMD is related to the MMD by

$$\log \text{ SMD} = \log \text{ MMD} - 1.51 \log^2 \sigma_g. \tag{13.24}$$

The standard deviation of the distribution of linear and surface diameters is exactly the same as that of the mass diameters. For the particles in Table 13-4, the CMD is calculated from Eq. (13.23) to be 0.02 μm, and we calculate the SMD using Eq. (13.24):

$$\log \text{ SMD} = \log \ 0.7 - 1.151 \ (\log \ 3)^2$$

$$\text{SMD} = 0.4 \ \mu\text{m}.$$

The geometric standard deviation is 3.

Since the size separation of particles in a cascade impactor depends on the velocity of the air in the jets, the sampling rate is very important. To avoid errors due to variations in the jet velocity, a critical orifice usually is used to keep the sampling rate constant.

Short-Lived Activity

Equation (13.21) implies that the sensitivity of our measurement of concentration can be increased without an end merely by increasing the sample size through increasing the sampling time. This is not exactly true, because there are practical limitations on the size of the sample. Within those limitations, we can, in most cases, adjust the sample size to be able to measure concentrations to at least 0.1 DAC. One important limitation on sample size is the half-life of the radionuclide being sampled. If the collected radionuclide decays significantly while it is being collected, then an equilibrium between the amount collected and the amount decaying will be reached. The equilibrium amount of collected activity will be determined by the difference between the collection rate and the decay rate.

If we sample for a radionuclide that decays significantly during sampling time, then the time rate of change of the collected activity is given by the activity-balance equation

$$\frac{dA}{dt} = \text{amount collected} - \text{amount decayed.} \tag{13.25}$$

If Q = sampling rate, C = atmospheric concentration, λ = transformation (decay) rate constant, and A = collected activity, then Eq. (13.25) becomes

$$\frac{dA}{dt} = Q\,\frac{m^3}{min} \times C\,\frac{Bq}{m^3} - \lambda\,min^{-1} \times A\,Bq. \tag{13.26a}$$

Equation (13.26a) can be written in traditional units as

$$\frac{dA}{dt} = Q\,\frac{mL}{min} \times C\,\frac{\mu Ci}{mL} - \lambda\,min^{-1} \times A\,Ci. \tag{13.26b}$$

If the sampling is done at a constant rate K, then Eqs. (13.26a) and (13.26b) become

$$\frac{dA}{dt} = K - \lambda A, \tag{13.27}$$

which can be written, when the variables are separated, as

$$\int_0^A \frac{dA}{K - \lambda A} = \int_0^t dt \tag{13.28}$$

and then integrated to give

$$A(t) = \frac{K}{\lambda}\left(1 - e^{-\lambda t}\right) = \frac{QC}{\lambda}\left(1 - e^{-\lambda t}\right). \tag{13.29}$$

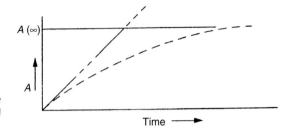

Figure 13-11. A plot of Eq. (13.29) shows the buildup of activity on the sampling medium and approach to the limiting value.

This equation is plotted in Figure 13-11. As time $\to \infty$, $e^{-\lambda t} \to 0$, and the collected activity approaches the limiting value

$$A(\infty) = \frac{QC}{\lambda}. \tag{13.30}$$

If the short-lived radionuclide decays while it is being counted, the instantaneous sample count rate will decrease from $\dot{N}_0$ to $\dot{N}$ during the time interval 0–t, according to the equation for radioactive decay:

$$\dot{N} = \dot{N}_0 e^{-\lambda t}.$$

The total number of counts during this time interval is given by

$$N = \int \dot{N}_0 e^{-\lambda t}\, dt = \frac{\dot{N}_0}{\lambda} \left(1 - e^{-\lambda t}\right) \tag{13.31}$$

and is represented graphically by the shaded area in Figure 13-12.

Equation (13.31) can be solved for the initial instantaneous count rate, which lets us determine the sample's activity at the start of the counting interval:

$$\dot{N}_0 = \frac{N \lambda}{1 - e^{-\lambda t}}. \tag{13.32}$$

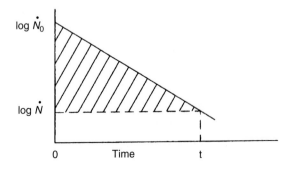

Figure 13-12. Decrease in instantaneous count rate while counting a short-lived radionuclide. The total number of counts during the counting interval is represented by the shaded area.

EXAMPLE 13.9

Argon-41, whose half-life is 1.83 hours, is sampled for 1 hour at a rate of 3 L/min. Counting of the sample started 0.5 hour after the end of the sampling period, and 5000 net counts were registered during a 30-minute counting period. If the counter efficiency was 10%, what was the ^{41}Ar concentration in the air?

Solution

The ^{41}Ar transformation rate constant is $0.693/T_{1/2} = 0.693/1.83\,\text{h} = 0.379\,\text{h}^{-1}$. The initial count rate, from Eq. (13.32), is

$$\dot{N}_0 = \frac{N\lambda}{1 - e^{-\lambda t}} = \frac{5000 \text{ counts} \times 0.379\,\text{h}^{-1}}{\left(1 - e^{-0.379 \text{ h} \times 0.5 \text{ h}^{-1}}\right) \times 60\,\dfrac{\text{min}}{\text{h}}} = 183 \text{ cpm}.$$

The activity of the sample at the beginning of the counting period, at 10% counting efficiency, was

$$\frac{183 \text{ cpm}}{0.1\,\dfrac{\text{cpm}}{\text{dpm}}} = 1830 \text{ dpm}.$$

Since 0.5 hour had elapsed between the end of the sampling period and the start of counting, the sample activity at the end of the sampling period is calculated from the radioactive decay equation:

$$1830 = A_0 e^{-0.379 \text{ h}^{-1} \times 0.5 \text{ h}}$$

$$A_0 = 2212 \text{ dpm}.$$

This activity, 2212 dpm, was the activity at the end of the sampling period $A(t)$ in Eq. (13.29). Solving Eq. (13.29) for C and substituting 2210 dpm for the activity at the end of the sampling period, we have

$$C = \frac{A(t) \times \lambda}{Q\left(1 - e^{-\lambda t}\right)}$$

$$= \frac{2212 \text{ dpm} \times 0.379\,\text{h}^{-1}}{3 \times 10^3\,\dfrac{\text{mL}}{\text{min}} \left(1 - e^{-0.379 \text{ h}^{-1} \times 1 \text{ h}}\right) \times 60\,\dfrac{\text{min}}{\text{h}} \times 2.2 \times 10^6\,\dfrac{\text{dpm}}{\mu\text{Ci}}}$$

$$C = 6.7 \times 10^{-9}\,\frac{\mu\text{Ci}}{\text{mL}}\left(248\frac{\text{Bq}}{\text{m}^3}\right).$$

Natural Airborne Radioactivity

Determination of a low-level airborne contaminant is complicated by the existence of naturally occurring radioactivity. This arises from the gaseous isotopes ^{222}Rn (radon) and ^{230}Rn (thoron), which seep out of the ground from the ubiquitous uranium and thorium series (the average concentration of uranium and thorium in the top 0.3 m of soil is 1 ton and 3 tons, respectively, per square mile) and from their transformation products. These transformation products attach themselves to airborne particles with which they come in contact, thus contaminating the dust particles with radioactivity. The limiting activity in the radon daughter chain is ^{214}Pb (RaB), a beta emitter whose half-life is 26.8 minutes. In the thoron daughter chain, the limiting activity is ^{212}Pb (ThB), a beta-emitting isotope with a half-life of 10.6 hours.

For routine monitoring of long-lived contaminants, allowance is made for these activities by (1) counting the air sample several hours after collection, thereby allowing the 26.8-minute activity to decay away, and (2) counting the air sample about two ThB half-lives later. From these two measurements, the activity of the long-lived contaminant can be calculated. The counting rate C_1 of the first measurement is due to the natural activity and the long-lived contaminant C_{LL}:

$$C_1 = C_{n_1} + C_{LL}; \tag{13.33}$$

when the second count is made, the natural activity has decayed to

$$C_{n_2} = C_{n_1} e^{-\lambda \Delta t}, \tag{13.34}$$

where λ, the decay constant of ThB, is 0.0655 h^{-1}, and Δt is the time interval in hours between the two counts. The second measurement, C_2, includes the following:

$$C_2 = C_{n_2} + C_{LL}, \tag{13.35}$$

$$C_2 = C_{n_1} e^{-\lambda \Delta t} + C_{LL}. \tag{13.36}$$

Solving Eqs. (13.35) and (13.36) simultaneously for the long-lived activity gives

$$C_{LL} = \frac{C_2 - C_1 e^{-\lambda \Delta t}}{1 - e^{-\lambda \Delta t}}. \tag{13.37}$$

EXAMPLE 13.10

In monitoring for airborne ^{90}Sr, a 10-m^3 air sample is taken with a membrane filter. The first measurement, taken 4 hours after sampling, gives a net counting rate of 100 cpm. The second count, 20 hours later, gives a net counting rate of 50 cpm. If the filter (after treatment to prevent electrostatic charge accumulation) was counted in a windowless 2π gas-flow counter, what was the mean concentration of ^{90}Sr in the air?

Solution

Substituting the respective values for C_1 and C_2 into Eq. (13.37) gives

$$C_{LL} = \frac{50 - 100 e^{-0.065 \text{ h}^{-1} \times 20 \text{ h}}}{1 - e^{-0.065 \text{ h}^{-1} \times 20 \text{ h}}} = 31.5 \text{ cpm}$$

for the long-lived (^{90}Sr) activity. Since the counter has an efficiency of 50% and the volume of air sampled was 10 m^3, the mean concentration of ^{90}Sr is calculated as follows:

$$C(^{90}\text{Sr}) = \frac{31.5 \text{ cpm}}{0.5 \dfrac{\text{cpm}}{\text{dpm}} \times 60 \dfrac{\text{dpm}}{\text{Bq}} \times 10 \text{ m}^3}$$

$$= 0.11 \frac{\text{Bq}}{\text{m}^3} \left(2.8 \times 10^{-12} \frac{\mu\text{Ci}}{\text{mL}} \right).$$

If the contaminant has such half-life that a significant amount will decay during the waiting period, then due allowance must be made for this fact. In this case, the activity in the sample at the times of the first and second counts is

$$C_1 = C_{n_1} + C_{C_1}, \tag{13.38}$$

$$C_2 = C_{n_2} + C_{C_2}, \tag{13.39}$$

where C_n is the naturally occurring activity and C_C is the activity of the contaminant. At the time of the second count the natural and contaminating activities will have decayed to

$$C_{n_2} = C_{n_1} e^{-\lambda_n \Delta t}, \tag{13.40}$$

$$C_{C_2} = C_{C_1} e^{-\lambda_C \Delta t}. \tag{13.41}$$

Solving these equations simultaneously gives

$$C_{C_1} = \frac{C_2 - C_1 e^{-\lambda_n \Delta t}}{e^{-\lambda_C \Delta t} - e^{-\lambda_n \Delta t}}. \tag{13.42}$$

Radon

Frequently used methods for environmental radon measurements include

- radon adsorption on activated charcoal,
- alpha-track detectors,
- electret ion chambers, and
- grab samples.

Activated Charcoal

To adsorb radon on charcoal, a canister of about 6–10 cm (diameter) × 2.5 cm (depth) is filled with activated charcoal. A diffusion barrier across the open top keeps the charcoal in the canister, but allows air to diffuse into the charcoal, and the radon penetrates into the charcoal pores by molecular diffusion. The charcoal-filled canister, thus, is a passive device that requires no power for its operation. The canister is tightly sealed after the diffusion barrier is put into place. Sampling is started by removing the seal after the canister is placed in the chosen location. The cover is removed to start the measurement. At the end of the measurement period, usually 2–7 days, it is resealed and sent to the laboratory for radiometric analysis by gamma-ray spectroscopy. The adsorbed radon activity is determined by placing the canister directly on a scintillation counter and counting the gammas from the adsorbed radon and its progeny. The charcoal adsorption system is calibrated by measuring the activity after exposing the canister to known concentrations of radon. Corrections for temperature and relative humidity must be made since these factors influence radon adsorption by the activated charcoal. The short half-life of radon requires that the exposed canister be measured as soon as possible after sampling is completed. The sensitivity of this method is about 0.5 pCi Rn/L (18.5 Bq/m^3), or about 2.5×10^{-3} working level (WL).

Alpha-Track Detectors

Long-term average Rn concentrations can be determined with alpha-track detectors. An alpha-track detector is a piece of plastic that suffers radiation damage when it is exposed to alpha radiation. In use, the detector is enclosed in a filter-covered container, and air diffuses through the filter into the container. Alpha particles from the airborne radon and its progeny strike the detector, and produce submicroscopic tracks in the plastic. At the end of the exposure period, the container is sealed and brought to the laboratory. There, the detector is removed from the container and the alpha tracks are "developed" by placing the detector into a caustic solution. This enlarges the submicroscopic tracks so that they are visible with a microscope. The track density is directly proportional to the total radon exposure. Because the alpha-track detector records the effects of radiation rather than to the radiation, and because the sensitivity and precision of the measurement depend on the total number of alpha tracks, long-term average radon concentrations can be measured simply by leaving the detector in place for a long period of time. The practical sensitivity of the system is about 0.2 pCi/L-month.

Electret Ion Chambers

An electret ion chamber (EIC) is an integrating monitor whose operating principle is similar to that of a capacitor-type pocket dosimeter. An electret is an electrostatically charged plastic (usually Teflon®) disc. In an EIC for measuring atmospheric radon, the electret is placed into a chamber that connects with the atmosphere through a filtered portal that is kept covered until the start of a measurement. During the measurement, usually a period of 3–7 days, the filtered portal is open and radon gas diffuses through the filter (whose function is to prevent airborne particles from entering into the ion chamber) into the chamber. The alphas from the radon and its progeny ionize the air in the chamber, and the ions neutralize charges on the electret's surface. The electret charge is measured before and after the exposure, and the rate of change of the charge (change divided by the time of exposure) is proportional to the average concentration of radon during the measurement period. Electrets are available for short-term exposures of 2–7 days, and for long-term exposures of 1–12 months. The sensitivity of this method is about 5 Bq/m^3 (0.14 pCi/L) for a 7-day measurement.

Grab Sample (Kusnetz Method)

If we wish to know the radon levels in an occupational setting, where higher radon levels may be expected, such as in a mine, in a gypsum factory, or in a phosphate ore processing plant, we can take a grab sample and analyze it for radon progeny. A

TABLE 13-5. Values of the Kusnetz Factor for Use in Equation (13.43)

TIME (MIN)	40	45	50	55	60	65	70	75	80	85	90
K	150	140	130	120	110	100	90	83	75	67	60

commonly used procedure for determining radon daughter concentration in units of WL is called the *Kusnetz* method. This method gives only the total concentration, and does not give the individual contributions of the several radon daughters to the total. The procedure consists of taking a 5-minute air sample at a volumetric sampling rate of 3–10 L/min, using a high-efficiency membrane filter to capture the radon progeny that had attached themselves to ambient dust particles. Then, after a delay of 40–90 minutes, the alpha activity on the filter is counted for 10 minutes. The counting data and the sample volume are used to calculate the radon daughter concentration in terms of WL:

$$\text{WL} = \frac{\text{Net alpha cpm}}{K \times V \times \varepsilon}, \tag{13.43}$$

where

$K =$ Kusnetz factor, which is a function of the delay time between end of sampling and start of counting; values for K are listed below in Table 13-5. The time in the table is the time from the end of sampling until the midpoint of the counting interval.
$V =$ volume of air sample.
$\varepsilon =$ counting efficiency.

EXAMPLE 13.11

A 5-minute air sample was taken at a rate of 5 L/min. Forty-five minutes after the end of sampling, the filter was placed into an alpha counter, and 10 minutes later, 600 alpha counts were recorded. A blank filter gave 4 counts during a 10-minute counting period. The counting efficiency was 49%. What was the radon daughter concentration?

Solution

Substituting the appropriate values into Eq. (13.43), we have

$$\text{WL} = \frac{\dfrac{600 \text{ counts}}{10 \text{ min}} - \dfrac{4 \text{ counts}}{10 \text{ min}}}{130 \times \dfrac{5L}{\text{min}} \times 5 \text{ min} \times 0.49} = 0.04 \text{ WL}.$$

CONTINUOUS ENVIRONMENTAL MONITORING

Continuous monitoring of the environment may be done to demonstrate compliance with regulations or to verify proper operation of equipment or procedures, or for immediate notification of a breakdown of control measures that could lead to a serious hazard. For example, if a threat to life could result from a source inadvertently left unshielded, then a continuous radiation monitor coupled to an alarm would be indicated. Continuous monitoring may also be required in a laboratory where low-level activities are measured and where precise knowledge of fluctuations in the background is therefore necessary. Another application of continuous monitoring is where the amount of radioactivity discharged into the environment must be known—as in the case of gaseous and particulate effluent from an incinerator used to burn radioactive waste, or a sewage line from a building in which much liquid radioactive waste is disposed of via the sink.

Continuous environmental monitors fall into three classes: those used to measure radiation levels (these are often called *area monitors*), those used to measure atmospheric radioactivity, and those used to measure liquid radioactivity.

Area monitoring systems usually consist of an appropriate detector, a ratemeter, a recorder, and, if necessary, an alarm that is actuated when a preset radiation level is exceeded. Liquids or gases may be monitored by letting them flow around or through a suitable detector. Basically, a liquid monitoring system is the same as the area monitoring system—except that the readout is calibrated to read in activity units, such as microcuries per cubic centimeter, rather than units of radiation dose. For airborne particles, air is sucked through a filter at a known rate. The filter is placed in close proximity to an appropriate detector that responds to the radioactive dust caught by the filter and is shielded against environmental radiation (Fig. 13-13). The pulses from the detector are measured by a ratemeter whose output may be recorded on a strip chart. Since radioactivity continues to accumulate on the filter as more air is sampled, the ratemeter reading continues to increase. The index of the degree of atmospheric contamination, therefore, is the rate of increase of the count rate rather than the value of the count rate. Monitors for airborne dust are therefore equipped with a derivative alarm that is actuated when the rate of increase of the counting rate exceeds a preset value.

COMBINED EXPOSURES

Very often, workers may be exposed to both radiation and harmful chemicals. According to United Nations Scientific Committee on the Effects of Atomic Radiation: "With the exception of radiation and smoking, there is little evidence from epidemiological data for a need to adjust for a strong antagonistic or synergistic combined effects. Although both synergistic and antagonistic effects occur at high exposures, there is no firm evidence for significant deviations from the additivity at controlled occupational or environmental exposures." The threshold doses for nonstochastic effects are much greater than the regulatory limits for either radiation or chemical exposure. Since such high exposures would be expected to occur only in the case of

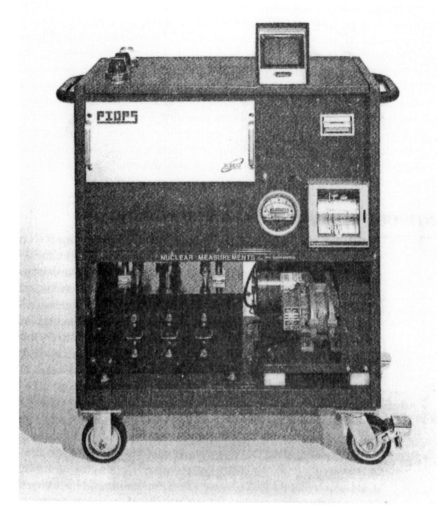

Figure 13-13. Continuous aerosol monitor for simultaneously measuring alpha, beta, and gamma activity at a sampling rate of 1 cfm (28.3 Lpm). The sensitivity at this sampling rate is $10^{-12}\mu$Ci/mL (0.037 Bq/m^3) of beta-gamma and of alpha activity. (Courtesy of Nuclear Measurements Corp.)

an accident, the recommended additivity of effects, although not explicitly stated, would apply to stochastic effects.

The regulatory limits for carcinogenic agents such as radiation or chemicals, such as formaldehyde, acetaldehyde, benzene, arsenic, and chromium are based on the linear, zero-threshold model, which postulates that there is no absolutely safe dose. Therefore, the limits are calculated to restrict the risk from exposure to these agents to a societally acceptable level (in return for the societal benefits to be reaped from the use of those agents). These regulatory limits are meant to be protective rather than predictive. Since both radiation and chemical carcinogens are regulated on a comparable basis, it is reasonable, for purpose of cancer prevention and ALARA planning, to limit combined exposure to the sum of the radiation and chemical exposure. If we make the very reasonable assumption that 1 PEL-hour of chemical exposure is equivalent in carcinogenic potential to 1 DAC-hour of radiation, which corresponds to a dose of 2.5 mrems (25 μSv), then we can add the mrem (or μSv) equivalent of the chemical exposure to the radiation dose to obtain the equivalent combined dose. For example, consider the case of worker in a radioisotope laboratory where the ambient radiation level is 0.3 mrem/h (3 μSv/h), and there is benzene in the air at a concentration of 6 ppm. The PEL for benzene listed by Occupational Safety and Health Administration (OSHA) in 29 CFR 1910.1000 is 30 ppm. For occupational safety purposes, the equivalent combined dose may be calculated as:

$$D \text{ (combined)} = \frac{6 \text{ ppm}}{30 \text{ ppm/PEL}} \times 4 \text{ h} \times 2.5 \frac{\text{mrems}}{\text{PEL-h}} + 0.3 \frac{\text{mrem}}{\text{h}} \times 4 \text{ h}$$

$$= 3.2 \text{ mrems}.$$

SOURCE CONTROL

The rise in worldwide terrorism led to a great deal of concern that some of the licensed widespread radioactive sources that are being used for peaceful purposes might be stolen or diverted to a terrorist group for use in a "dirty bomb," which refers to a high-explosive bomb that is packed with highly radioactive material. The dirty bomb actually is a radioactivity dispersal device. Detonation of the bomb results in the dispersal of the packed radioactivity, and thus creation of an area of high-level contamination that could lead to radiation casualties as well as to a terrorized public. Because of the international aspect of terrorism and the worldwide distribution of radioactive sources for peaceful uses, the International Atomic Energy Agency (IAEA) took the initiative in preventive action by formulating and adopting a *Code of Conduct in the Safety and Security of Radioactive Sources* in 2004. The Code offers guidance on actions to be taken by the member states to prevent the theft or diversion of legally licensed sources into the hands of unauthorized persons for malicious use to inflict harm on individuals, society, or on the environment.

The Code places all authorized sources into one of five categories, depending on the radionuclide, the quantity of radioactivity, its intended peaceful use (industrial radiography, radiation therapy, radiation sterilization, etc.), and the danger level posed by that source. A dangerous source is defined by the IAEA as "a source that could, if not under control, give rise to exposure sufficient to cause severe deterministic effects." The five categories as defind by the Code are the following:

• Category 1—This category consists of sources that are personally extremely dangerous. Being close to an unshielded category 1 source for a period of several minutes to an hour would probably lead to death.

If the activity were to be dispersed by an explosion, it could possibly (but unlikely) be life threatening to persons in the immediate vicinity. There would be little or no risk of immediate health effects to persons beyond a few hundred meters.

- Category 2—The sources falling in this category are personally very dangerous. Being close to the unshielded source for time periods of minutes to hours could cause permanent injury; and the exposure could be fatal for time periods of hours to days.

  Dispersed category 2 activity is very unlikely to be life threatening in the immediate vicinity of the bomb after the explosion. It would be virtually impossible for this source to contaminate a public water supply to a dangerous level.

- Category 3—The sources in this category are personally dangerous. Permanent injury may be caused following nearby exposure to the unshielded source for several hours; and could possibly (but unlikely) be fatal for a person who is close to the unshielded source for a period of days to weeks.

  The dispersed activity is extremely unlikely to permanently injure or kill a person in the immediate vicinity, and there exists little or no risk of immediate health effects beyond a few meters from the explosion.

- Category 4—The sources in this category are unlikely to be dangerous. The dispersed activity of a category 4 source would not permanently injure anyone.

- Category 5—The sources in this category are not dangerous. No one would be permanently injured either from the source or from the dispersed activity.

SUMMARY

Engineering and administrative measures are employed in order to provide a safe working environment for radiation workers. However, since there is no guarantee that protective measures will never break down, we keep the working environment and the workers under continuing surveillance to verify that all the protective systems are operating as designed. Should a breakdown occur, then the surveillance system should detect it in the early stages of the breakdown.

The workplace is monitored directly by two different methods: (1) by systematic and routine surveys that include measurement of external radiation, verification of the location and proper use of radiation sources, air sampling, and testing exposed surfaces for contamination, and (2) by fixed area monitors that continuously monitor external radiation fields and airborne radioactivity and have alarms that are preset to warn of high levels of radiation or airborne radioactivity. Individuals are monitored for external radiation with dosimeters, such as film badges, thermoluminescent dosimeters, and electronic dosimeters. For internally deposited radionuclides, workers are monitored by in vitro bioassay, in which the activity in excreta is measured, or by in vivo bioassay, in which the radiations originating in radionuclides inside the body are measured directly with appropriate counting instruments.

Monitoring data must be properly interpreted if it is to make a positive contribution to the overall radiation safety program.

To prevent authorized radioactive sources from falling into the hands of terrorists, the IAEA has formulated a code of practice that offers guidance on measures to be taken to secure the safety of radioactive sources.

PROBLEMS

13.1. A series of measurements with threshold detectors showed the following spectral distribution of neutrons:

ENERGY	PERCENT NEUTRONS
Thermal	40
1000 eV	20
0.01 MeV	10
0.1 MeV	10
1 MeV	10
10 MeV	10

When 500-mg ^{32}S was irradiated for 2 hours in this field and then counted in a 2π gas-flow counter 24 hours after the end of irradiation, the result was 500 cpm. What is the dose rate in this neutron field?

13.2. A sealed ^{90}Sr source is leak-tested. The wipe, counted in a 2π gas-flow counter, gave 155 counts in 5 minutes. The background was 130 counts in 5 minutes. At the 95% confidence level, is the source contaminated?

13.3. An air sample on a filter paper was counted in a 2π gas-flow counter and gave 800 counts in 5 minutes. A background count gave 260 counts in 10 minutes. What was the standard deviation of the net counting rate?

13.4. A radioisotope worker weighing 70 kg inadvertently drank water containing 3.7 MBq (100 μCi) ^{22}Na. Following this accidental exposure, his body burden was measured by whole-body counts made over a period of 2 months. The following retention function was fitted to the whole-body counting data:

$$Q(t) = 1.8 \exp(-0.082t) + 1.9 \exp(-0.052t) \text{ MBq.}$$

Calculate

(a) the cumulative activity, in Bq days.

(b) the initial dose rate, assuming the ^{22}Na to be uniformly distributed throughout the body (see Fig. 4-8 for ^{22}Na transformation scheme).

(c) the worker's dose commitment.

13.5. The maximum permissible skeletal burden of ^{90}Sr is 74 kBq (2 μCi). Calculate the number of transformations per minute per 24-hour urine sample that may be expected from one-fourth of this skeletal burden if 0.05% per day is eliminated in the urine.

13.6. Using the ICRP three-compartment lung model and the data for the reference man, calculate the ratio of concentration of soluble 1-μm AMAD uranium particulates in the air to uranium in the urine, Bq/m^3 air per Bq/L urine, for the case where a steady state has been attained through continuous inhalation of the uranium.

13.7. The body burden of ^{137}Cs at time t days following a single intake $Q(0)$ is given by

$$Q(t) = Q(0) \times (0.1\,e^{-0.693t} + 0.9\,e^{-0.011t}).$$

If the ratio of urinary to fecal excretion is $9:1$, calculate the activity per 24-hour urine sample 1 day and 10 days after ingestion of 50,000 Bq (1.35 μCi) ^{137}Cs.

13.8. A chemist accidentally inhaled a ^{14}C-tagged organic solvent that is readily absorbed from the lungs. The solvent is known to concentrate in the liver. That part of the solvent which is eliminated before deposition in the liver leaves in the urine; the detoxification products are eliminated from the liver into the GI tract and into the urinary tract; 25% is eliminated in the urine and 75% in the feces. Following the inhalation, 24-hour urine samples were collected over a 2-week period and the following data were obtained:

Days after inhalation	1	2	3	4	5	6	8	10	12	14
kBq/Sample	98	57	39	26	20	18	12	10	7.4	5.9

(a) How much activity was absorbed into the body?

(b) What was the total dose to the body during the 13 weeks after inhalation?

(c) What was the total dose to the liver during the 13 weeks after inhalation?

(d) What was the effective committed dose equivalent?

13.9. A health physicist samples waste water to ascertain that the water may be safely discharged into the environment. The water analysis is made by chemically separating the ^{90}Sr, allowing the ^{90}Y daughter to accumulate, then extracting and counting the ^{90}Y activity. The volume of the sample was 1 L, the ^{90}Y in growth time was 7 days, and the ^{90}Y activity was determined 15 hours after extraction in an internal gas-flow counter having an overall efficiency of 50%. The background counting rate, determined by a 60-minute count, was 35 cpm. The sample (including background) gave 2766 counts in 60 minutes. What was the ^{90}Sr concentration, at the 90% confidence level?

13.10. An air sample that was counted 4 h after collection gave 1450 counts in 10 minutes. The background was counted for 30 minutes, and gave a rate of 45 cpm. The sample was counted again 20 hours later, and gave 990 counts in 10 minutes;

a 60-minute background count gave 2940 counts. If the volume of the air sample was 1.0 m³ and the counting geometry was 50%, calculate the atmospheric concentration of the long-lived contaminant, in Bq/m^3 and mCi/cm^3, and the 95% confidence limits.

13.11. A film badge worn by a worker in a fast neutron field showed the following distribution of proton recoil tracks among 100 random microscopic fields of 2×10^{-4} cm² each:

NO. OF TRACKS PER FIELD	FREQUENCY
0	40
1	40
2	18
3	2

(a) If 2600 tracks/cm² correspond to 1 mSv (100 mrems), what was the fast-neutron dose?

(b) What is the 95% confidence limit of this measurement?

13.12. Using the three-compartment ICRP lung model and the physiologic data for the reference person, compute dose to the lungs and to the bone following a single acute exposure of 1 Bq-s (2.7×10^{-5} μCi-s) per m³ of a respirable aerosol, AMAD = 2 μm, of (a) strontium-90 titinate, (b) strontium-90 chloride.

13.13. The following size distribution was obtained on a sample of an aerosol:

PERCENT BY NUMBER	SIZE INTERVAL
10	0.5–1.0
15	1.0–1.5
15	1.5–2.0
10	2.0–2.5
10	2.5–3.0
10	3.0–3.5
10	3.5–4.5
10	4.5–6.0
5	6.0–8.0
5	8.0–10.0

(a) Plot the cumulative frequency distribution on linear graph paper, on linear probability paper, and on log probability paper by diameter (assume the particles to be spheres), surface area, and mass (assume the particles to have a density of 2.7 g/cm^3).

(b) Are the distributions normal or log-normal?

(c) Compute the geometric mean and standard deviations for each of the three types of distributions.

13.14. An instrument repairman suffered an accidental exposure to ^{131}I while working in a customer's laboratory. Two days later, his thyroid gland was found to contain 2×10^4 Bq (0.54 μCi) ^{131}I. Assuming he is a normal healthy man who weighs 70 kg, calculate

(a) the amount of ^{131}I activity originally deposited in the thyroid,

(b) the dose commitment to the thyroid as a result of the accident.

Note. The following thyroid retention function is given in ICRP 10:

$$R(t) = 0.7 \ \exp\left(-\frac{0.693}{0.35 \ \text{days}} t \ \text{days}\right) + 0.3 \ \exp\left(-\frac{0.693}{100 \ \text{days}} t \ \text{days}\right).$$

13.15. A 20-L breath sample was collected over 2 minutes. Analysis for ^{222}Rn showed the radon concentration to be 1×10^{-7} Bq/L. Estimate the body burden of ^{226}Ra from these data.

13.16. A laboratory worker accidentally ingested ^{210}Po by using a contaminated cup for his coffee. Twenty-four hour urine samples were taken over a 60-day period and analyzed. The following data were obtained:

Days After Ingestion	1	5	10	15	20	25	30	40	50	60
Bq per Sample	25	23	21	19	18	16	15	12	11	9

(a) Plot the data on semi-log paper and fit an equation to the elimination data.

(b) If 10% of ingested ^{210}Po is known to be eliminated in the urine, and 90% is eliminated in the feces, how much ^{210}Po was ingested?

(c) If 13% of the ^{210}Po was deposited in the kidneys, what was the committed dose equivalent to the kidneys from this accidental ingestion?

13.17. What is the dose commitment to the skeleton due to the ingestion of 100 Bq/d, for 1 year, of ^{90}Sr dissolved in drinking water?

13.18. An accidental release of ^{210}PoO$_2$ from a glove box leads to an atmospheric concentration of 1500 Bq/m^3 (4.05×10^{-8} μCi/cm^3). From a recording air monitor, whose alarm had failed, it was later learned that a worker had been exposed to the airborne ^{210}PoO$_2$ for 1 hour. Measurements made with a cascade impactor showed the activity-median aerodynamic particle size to be 0.5 μm. Using the data for the reference person, calculate

(a) the amount of activity deposited in the lung and

(b) the dose commitment to the lung from this accidental exposure.

13.19. A demineralizer 20 cm in diameter × 20 cm in height processes 200 L/min contaminated water and removes the following long-lived isotopes:

ISOTOPE	Bq/L	µCi/L
^{60}Co	1.48×10^4	0.4
^{137}Cs	1.11×10^5	3.0
^{144}Ce	1.85×10^6	50.0

The demineralizer operates for 180 days. Thirty days later,

(a) what is the activity of each of these isotopes in the demineralizer?

(b) if the demineralizer approximates a point source at 4 m, estimate the gamma-ray dose rate there.

(c) estimate the gamma-ray dose rate at the surface of the demineralizer.

13.20. In accidental releases to the air in a fuel reprocessing plant, the following mixture of isotopes is usually found. Using the DAC values for the air given in 10 CFR 20, calculate the atmospheric DAC for the total activity that must be applied during cleanup of the contamination.

ISOTOPE	% OF TOTAL ACTIVITY
^{89}Sr	7
^{90}Sr	1
^{91}Y	10
^{95}Zr	15
^{95}Nb	25
^{144}Ce	13
^{147}Pm	2

13.21. Tritiated water vapor was unknowingly released in a laboratory. An air sample was taken using a freeze-out technique (100% freeze out) when the leak was discovered. Further investigation revealed that the system had been leaking for 24 hours prior to the discovery. Five hundred liters of air were drawn through the cold trap, and the collected moisture was diluted to 50 mL. One milliliter of the dilution was counted for tritium betas in a liquid scintillation counter whose background was 12 cpm and whose counting efficiency was 30%. The 1-mL sample gave 3200 cpm.

(a) What was the tritium concentration in the air?

(b) A technician who had been working in the laboratory for 8 hours left for a vacation without leaving a urine sample. If the principal route of intake was inhalation and if all the inhaled tritium was taken up by the technician, estimate her dose commitment. (Use the biological data given for the reference person.)

(c) The technician submitted a urine sample 21 days later. What concentration of tritium would be expected in the urine?

13.22. A worker accidentally ingested an unknown amount of ^{60}Co activity. His body burden was measured by whole-body counting from day 1 until day 14 after the ingestion, with the following results:

Day	1	2	3	4	7	14
kBq	75.3	63.4	54.3	49.2	42.0	31.0

The whole-body intake retention fraction (IRF) for ingested ^{60}Co is given as

$$\text{IRF}(t) = 0.5e^{-1.386t} + 0.3e^{-0.1155t} + 0.1e^{-01155t} + 0.1e^{-8.663\times10^{-4}t}$$

(a) Estimate the amount of ingested activity.

(b) What was the committed dose from the ingested radiocobalt?

13.23. A rotameter is calibrated to read directly at a temperture of 25°C and a pressure of 760 mm Hg. It is used at an altitude of 5000 ft (1500 m), where the atmospheric pressure is 633 mm Hg and the temperature is 15°C. What was the actual flow rate when the rotameter reading was 2.5 L/min?

13.24. A rotameter that was calibrated for air at 25°C and 760 mm Hg was used to measure the flow rate of helium into a gas chromatograph in a laboratory where the temperature and pressure were the same as at calibration. The rotameter reading was 28.3 L/min (1 cfm). What was the actual flow rate of the helium?

13.25. The air in a laboratory with dimensions 10 m × 8 m × 5 m has airborne ^{239}Pu particles at a concentration of 0.1 DAC (DAC = 7×10^{-12} μCi/mL = 3×10^{-1} Bq/m^3). If all the airborne activity were to settle out, what would be the areal concentration of ^{239}Pu on the floor, in dpm/100 cm^2?

13.26. The continuous air monitor of a radiochemical manufacturing laboratory that synthesizes various ^{14}C-labeled compounds is set to alarm at 0.1 DAC. Long-term data show that the mix of ^{14}C in the air is 20% ^{14}CO, DAC = 7×10^{-4} μCi/mL; 70% ^{14}CO$_2$, DAC = 9×10^{-5} μCi/mL; and 10% labeled compounds, DAC = 1×10^{-6} μCi/mL. At what ^{14}C concentration should the alarm be set?

13.27. A high-volume air sampler, 10 cfm ± 1%, located at the site boundary, was activated by a process monitor that detected an accidental release of plutonium. A 1-hour air sample that was counted 4 hours after collection in an alpha counter that recorded 1200 counts during a 15-minute counting time. The alpha background after a 4-hour background count was 0.2 cpm. The sample was again counted 24 hours after the first measurement, and gave 3000 counts during a 1-hour-long counting time. Given the following information:

- filter collection efficiency = 95 ± 1%,
- self-absorption factor in filter = 0.5 ± 1%,
- filter diameter = 10 in. (25.4 cm),
- effective detector diameter = 4.5 in. (11.4 cm), and
- efficiency of counting system = 30 ± 2%,

calculate the Pu concentration and the 95% CI

(a) considering only the counting statistics.

(b) including all the statistical uncertainties.

13.28. The annual TEDEs of a radiation worker during the preceding 4 years were 35 mSv, 30 mSv, 25 mSv, and 10 mSv. According to the ICRP 60 recommendations, what is the maximum dose that he may receive during the fifth year?

13.29. A pancake GM counter, whose area is 15 cm^2, finds a contaminated surface whose diameter is about 50 cm, in a laboratory where ^{14}C is used. Several measurements are made over the contaminated area, and the average meter reading is 150 cpm. The counting efficiency for this type of measurement is 5%, and the background is 50 cpm. A wipe test over an area of 100 cm^2 gave 200 cpm above background in a counting system whose efficiency was 25%.

(a) Calculate the aerial concentration, in dpm/100 cm^2, of

(i) the total contamination.

(ii) the removable contamination.

(b) Calculate the total activity of the ^{14}C contamination in

(i) microcuries.

(ii) bequerels.

(c) Is the contamination within the 10 CFR 835 limits?

13.30. An amount of 18 μCi (666 kBq) of ^{137}Cs was found on the filter cartridges of a half-face respirator (protection factor, PF = 10) after a worker completed a job in a contaminated atmosphere. The inhalation ALI is 200 μCi. Calculate

(a) the estimated intake of ^{137}Cs.

(b) the committed effective dose equivalent (CEDE) from this exposure.

13.31. A laboratory worker was accidentally exposed to a single intake of highly soluble 1-μm ^{131}I particles. Measurements of the gammas from the thyroid showed the following activity in the thyroid at the respective times after exposure. The intake retention function (IRF) for the thyroid at each time is given in the table below. From these data

(a) estimate the intake activity.

(b) estimate the worker's committed effective dose from this exposure, using a dose conversion factor of 7.4×10^{-9} Sv/Bq.

	2 1/2 h	1 d	2 d	3 d	5 d	7 d	10 d
Bq	720	4941	5505	5268	4420	3692	2756
IRF	0.0213	0.133	0.149	0.142	0.120	0.0995	0.0751

13.32. An aerosol sample gave 5910 counts in 10 minutes, and a 30-minute count of a blank filter was 450 counts. The air sample size was $10 \pm 1/2$ ft^3, the aerosol collection efficiency was $95 \pm 2\%$, and the counting efficiency was $40 \pm 3\%$.

Calculate the activity concentration and the 95% confidence interval in the sampled air in (a) μCi/mL, and (b) Bq/m^3.

13.33. The DAC for ^{51}Cr is listed in 10 CFR 20 as 3×10^{-6} μCi/mL. An aerosol inhalation experiment uses CrO ($\sigma = 2.7$ g/cm^3) particles tagged with 0.01 atom percent ^{51}Cr. The laboratory worker's lapel monitor samples the air at a rate of 5 L/min.

   (a) Calculate the DAC in units of Bq/m^3.

   (b) What is the expected weight of an 8-hour air sample at 1 DAC?

   (c) The OSHA PEL for Cr is 1 mg/m^3. (For hexavalent Cr the PEL is 0.005 mg/m^3). What is the ^{51}Cr atmospheric concentration, in μCi/mL and Bq/m^3, that corresponds to OSHA's 1 mg/m^3 PEL for this case?

SUGGESTED READINGS

ATSDR. *Guidance Manual for the Assessment of Joint Toxic Action of Chemical Mixtures.* Agency for Toxic Substances and Disease Registry, U.S. Dept. of Health and Human Services, Public Health Service, Atlanta, GA, 2004.

AIHA. *Emergency Response Planning Guidelines & Workplace Environmental Exposure Levels.* American Industrial Hygiene Association, Fairfax, VA, 2006.

ACGIH. *Air Sampling Instruments for Evaluation of Atmospheric Contaminants,* 9th ed. American Conference of Governmental Industrial Hygienists, Cincinnati, OH, 2001.

ACGIH. *Threshold Limit Values and Biological Exposure Indices.* American Conference of Governmental Industrial Hygienists, Cincinnati, OH, 2007.

Bealieu, H. J., and Buchan, R. *Quantitative Industrial Hygiene.* Garland STPM Press, New York, 1981.

Blatz, H., ed. *Radiation Hygiene Handbook.* McGraw-Hill, New York, 1959.

Brodsky, A., ed. *Handbook of Radiation Measurements and Protection, Vol. II, Biological and Mathematical Information.* CRC Press, Boca Raton, FL, 1982.

Brodsky, A., ed. *Handbook of Radiation Measurements and Protection, Vol. I, Physical Science and Engineering Data.* CRC Press, West Palm Beach, FL, 1978.

Brodsky, A. Properly relating radiation protection requirements to relative radiotoxicity and risk, in Miller, K. L., ed. *Handbook of Management of Radiation Protection Programs,* 2nd ed. CRC Press, Boca Raton, FL, 1992.

Cadle, R. D. *Particle Size.* Reinhold, New York, 1965.

Clayton, G. D., and Clayton, F. E., eds. *Patty's Industrial Hygiene and Toxicology, Vol. I, General Principles,* 4th ed. John Wiley & Sons, New York, 1991.

Cohen, B. L., Cohen, E. S. Theory and practice of radon monitoring with charcoal adsorption. *Health Phys,* **45**:501–508, 1983.

Cooper, H. B. H., Jr., and Rossano, A. T., Jr. *Source Testing for Air Pollution Control.* McGraw-Hill, New York, 1971.

Cralley, L. J., and Cralley, L. V. *Patty's Industrial Hygiene and Toxicology, Vol. III, Theory and Rationale of Industrial Hygiene Practice.* Wiley Interscience, New York, 1979.

Currie, L. A. Limits for qualitative detection and quantitative determination: Application to radiochemistry. *Anal Chem,* **40**:586, 1968.

Dennis, R. G., ed. *Handbook on Aerosols.* TID-26608, National Technical Information Service, Springfield, VA, 1976.

DiNardi, S. R. *The Occupational Environment—Its Evaluation, Control, and Management,* 2nd ed. American Industrial Hygiene Association, Fairfax, VA, 2003.

Drinker, P., and Hatch T. F. *Industrial Dust.* McGraw-Hill, New York, 1954.

Eisenbud, M., and Gesell, T *Environmental Radioactivity,* 4th ed. Academic Press, New York, 1997.

Fleeger, A., and Lillquist, D. *Industrial Hygiene Reference & Study Guide,* 2nd ed. American Industrial Hygiene Association, Fairfax, VA, 2006.

George, A. C. Passive, integrated measurements of indoor radon using activated carbon. *Health Phys,* **46:**867–872, 1984.

Green, H. L., and Lane, W. R. *Particulate Clouds: Dusts, Smokes, and Mists.* D. Van Nostrand, Princeton, NJ, 1964.

Harbison, R.D., ed. *Hamilton & Hardy's Industrial Toxicology.* Mosby, St. Louis, MO, 1998.

Harper, F. T., Musolino, S. V., and Wente, W. B. Realistic radiological dispersal device hazard boundaries and ramifications for early consequence management decisions. *Health Phys,* **93:**1–16, 2007.

Harris, R. L., ed. *Patty's Industrial Hygiene and Toxicology, Vol. II, Recognition and Evaluation of Physical Agents, Biohazards, and Engineering Control,* 5th ed. John Wiley & Sons, New York, 2000.

Harris, R. L., Cralley, L. C., and Cralley, L. V., eds. *Patty's Industrial Hygiene and Toxicology, Vol. III, part A, Theory and rationale in industrial hygiene practice: The work environment,* 3rd ed. John Wiley & Sons, New York, 1994.

Hickman, D. P. In vivo measurements, in Raabe, O. G., ed. *Internal Radiation Dosimetry.* Medical Physics Publishing, Madison, WI, 1994.

International Atomic Energy Agency (IAEA), Vienna.

Procedures for the Systematic Appraisal of Operational Radiation Programs, TECDOC-430, 1987.

Radiodosimetry and Preventive Measures in the Event of a Nuclear Accident, TECDOC-893, 1998.

Code of Conduct on Safety and Security of Radioactive Sources, CODEOC, 2004.

Prevention of Inadvertent Movement and Illicit Trafficking of Radioactive Material, TECDOC-1311, 2002.

Detection of Radioactive Material at Borders, TECDOC-1312, 2002.

Characterization of Radioactive Sources, TECDOC-1344, 2003.

Safety Series No.

6. *Regulations for the Safe Transport of Radioactive Material,* 1985 ed., Supplement 1986, 1986.

9. *Basic Radiation Safety Standards for Protection Against Ionizing Radiation and the Safety of Radiation Sources,* 1995.

14. *Basic Requirements for Personnel Monitoring,* 1980.

18. *Environmental Monitoring in Emergency Situations,* 1966.

21. *Risk Evaluation for Protection of the Public in Radiation Accidents,* 1967.

32. *Planning for the Handling of Radiation Accidents,* 1969.

37. *Advisory Material for the IAEA Regulations for the Safe Transport of Radiaoactive Material,* 1985 ed., 3d ed. (as amended 1990) (1990).

45. *Principles for Establishing Limits for the Release of Radioactive Materials into the Environment,* 1978.

46. *Monitoring of Airborne and Liquid Radioactive Releases from Nuclear Facilities to the Environment,* 1978.

47. *Manual on Early Medical Treatment of Possible Radiation Injury,* 1978.

49. *Radiological Surveillance of Airborne Contaminants in the Working Environment,* 1979.

83. *Radiation Protection in Occupational Health,* 1987.

84. *Basic Principles for Occupational Radiation Monitoring,* 1987.

101. *Operational Radiation Protection: A Guide to Optimization,* 1990.

102. *Recommendations for the Safe Use and Regulation of Radiation Sources in Industry, Medicine, Research, and Teaching,* 1990.

103. *Provision of Operational Radiation Protection at Nuclear Power Plants,* 1990.

115. *International Basic Safety Standards for Protection against Ionizing Radiation and the Safety of Radiation Sources,* 1996.

120. *Radiation Protection and the Safety of Radiation Sources,* 1996.

RS-G-1.2. *Assessment of Occupational Exposure Due to Intakes of Radionuclides,* 1999.

RS-G-1.3. *Assessment of Occupational Exposure Due to External Sources of Radiation,* 1999.

RS-G-1.8. *Environmental and Source Monitoring for Purposes of Radiation Protection,* 2005.

RS-G-1.9. *Categorization of Radioactive Sources,* 2005.

International Commission on Radiological Protection (ICRP), Pergamon Press, Oxford, U.K.

ICRP Publication No.

7. *Principles of Environmental Monitoring Related to the Handling of Radioactive Materials,* 1965.

10. *Report of Committee IV on Evaluation of Radiation Dose to Body Tissues from Internal Contamination due to Occupational Exposure,* 1968.

10A. *The Assessment of Internal Contamination Resulting from Recurrent or Prolonged Uptakes,* 1971.

12. *General Principles of Monitoring for Radiation Protection of Workers,* 1969.

International Commission on Radiological Protection (ICRP). *Annals of the ICRP.* Pergamon Press, Oxford, U.K.

Report No.

24. *Radiation Protection in Uranium and Other Mines,* **1**(1), 1977.

28. *The Principles and General Procedures for Handling Emergency and Accidental Exposures of Workers,* **2**(1),1978).

29. *Radionuclide Release to the Environment: Assessment of Doses to Man,* **2**(2), 1979.

35. *General Principles of Monitoring for Radiation Protection of Workers,* **9**(4), 1983.

37. *Cost Benefit Analysis in the Optimization of Radiation Protection,* **10**(2,3), 1983.

43. *Principles of Radiation Monitoring for the Protection of the Public,* **15**(1), 1984.

47. *Radiation Protection of Workers in Mines,* **16**(1), 1986.

48. *The Metabolism of Plutonium and Related Elements,* **16**(2,3), 1987.

54. *Individual Monitoring for Intakes of Radionuclides by Workers: Design and Interpretation,* **20**(1), 1989.

60. *Recommendations of the International Commission on Radiological Protection,* **21**(1–3), 1991.

61. *Annual Limits on Intake of Radionuclides by Workers Based on the 1990 Recommendations,* **21**(4), 1991.

68. *Dose Coefficients for Intakes of Radionuclides by Workers,* **24**(4), 1994.

69. *Age-dependent Doses to Members of the Public from Intake of Radionuclides, Part 3, Ingestion Dose Coefficients,* **25**(1), 1995.

71. *Age-dependent Doses to Members of the Public from Intake of Radionuclides, Part 4, Inhalation Dose Coefficients,* **25**(3/4), 1996.

72. *Age-dependent Doses to Members of the Public from Intake of Radionuclides, Part 5, Compilation of Ingestion and Inhalation Dose Coefficients,* **26**(1), 1996.

88. *Doses to the Embryo and Fetus from Intakes of Radionuclides by the Mother,* **31**(1–3), 2001.

91. *A Framework for Assessing the Impact of Ionizing Radiation on Non-human Species,* **33**(3), 2003.

Kamath, P. R. *The Environmental Surveillance Laboratory.* WHO, Geneva, 1970.

Keith, L. H. *Principles of Environmental Sampling.* American Chemical Society, Washington, DC, 1987.

Kotrappa, P., Dempsey, J. C., Hickey J. R., and Stieff, L. K. An electret passive environmental Rn-222 monitor based on ionization measurements. *Health Phys,* **54**:47, 1988.

Kusnetz, H. Radon daughters in mine atmospheres—A field method for determining concentrations. *Am Ind Hyg Assoc J Quarterly,***17**:85, 1956.

Leidel, N. A., Busch, K. A., and Lynch, J. R. *Occupational Exposure Sampling Strategy Manual.* DHEW (NIOSH) Publication No. 77–173, National Institute for Occupational Safety and Health, Cincinnati, OH, 1977.

Lessard, E. T., et al. *Interpretation of Bioassay Measurements.* NUREG/CR-4884, BNL-NUREG-52063, U.S. Nuclear Regulatory Commission, Washington, DC, 1987.

Lodge, J. P., Jr., and Chan, T. L., ed. *Cascade Impactor Sampling and Data Analysis.* American Industrial Hygiene Association, Akron, OH, 1986.

Lovett, D. B. Track etch detectors for alpha exposure estimation. *Health Phys,* **16**:623, 1969.

Miller, K. L., ed. *Handbook of Management of Radiation Protection Programs,* 2nd ed. CRC Press, Boca Raton, FL, 1992.

Morgan, K. Z., and Turner J. E., eds. *Principles of Radiation Protection.* John Wiley, New York, 1967.

National Council on Radiation Protection and Measurements (NCRP). Bethesda, MD.

NCRP Report No.

38. *Protection against Neutron Radiation,* 1971.

39. *Basic Radiation Protection Criteria,* 1971.

48. *Radiation Protection for Medical and Allied Health Personnel,* 1976.

50. *Environmental Radiation Measurements,* 1976.

57. *Instrumentations and Monitoring Methods for Radiation Protection,* 1978.

58. *A Handbook of Radioactivity Measurements Procedures,* 1978.

59. *Operational Radiation Safety Program,* 1978.

62. *Tritium in the Environment,* 1979.

77. *Exposures from the Uranium Series with Emphasis on Radon and Its Daughters,* 1984.

78. *Evaluation of Occupational and Environmental Exposures to Radon and Radon Daughters in the United States,* 1984.

87. *Use of Bioassay Procedures for Assessment of Internal Radionuclide Deposition,* 1987.

96. *Comparative Carcinogenicity of Ionizing Radiation and Chemicals,* 1989.

97. *Measurement of Radon and Radon Daughters in Air,* 1988.

109. *Effects of Ionizing Radiation on Aquatic Organisms,* 1991.

114. *Maintaining Radiation Protection Records,* 1992.

116. *Limitation of Exposure to Ionizing Radiation,* 1993.

121. *Principles and Application of Collective Dose in Radiation Protection,* 1995.

122. *Use of Personal Monitors to Estimate Effective Dose Equivalent and Effective Dose to Workers for External Exposure to Low LET Radiation,* 1995.

127. *Operational Radiation Safety Program,* 1998.

138. *Management of Terrorist Events Involving Radioactive Material,* 2001.

Ness, S. A. *Air Monitoring for Toxic Substances, An Integrated Approach.* Van Nostrand Reinhold, New York, 1991.

Norwood, W. D. *Health Protection of Radiation Workers.* Charles Thomas, Springfield, IL, 1975.

Olishifishki, J. B., and Kerwin, M. A. Air-sampling instruments, in Plog, B, ed. *Fundamentals of Industrial Hygiene.* National Safety Council, Chicago, IL, 1988.

Ower, E., and Parkhurst, R. C. *The Measurement of Airflow,* 5th ed. Pergamon Press, Oxford, U.K., 1977.

Plog, B., and Quinlan, P., ed. *Fundamentals of Industrial Hygiene,* 5th ed. National Safety Council, Chicago, IL, 2002.

Poston, J.W., Sr. External dosimetry and personnel monitoring. *Health Phys,* **88:**289–296, 2005.

Raabe, O. G. Characterization of radioactive airborne particles, in Raabe, O. G., ed. *Internal Radiation Dosimetry.* Medical Physics Publishing, Madison, WI, 1994.

Saenger, E. L., ed. *Medical Aspects of Radiation Accidents.* U.S.A.E.C., Washington, DC, 1963.

Schleien, B. S., Slabeck, L. A., Jr, and Kent, B. K. *Handbook of Health Physics and Radiological Health.* Williams and Wilkins, Baltimore, MD, 1998.

Shapiro, J. *Radiation Protection,* 4th ed. Harvard University Press, Cambridge, MA, 2002.

Skrable, K. W., Chabot, G. E., French, C. S., and Labone, T. R. Estimation of intakes from repetitive bioassay measurements, in Raabe, O. G. ed. *Internal Radiation Dosimetry,* Medical Physics Publishing, Madison, WI, 1994.

Straub, C. P. *Public Health Implications of Radioactive Waste Releases.* WHO, Geneva, 1970.

Till, J. E., and Meyer, S. R., eds. *Radiological Assessment.* NUREG/CR-3332, U.S. Nuclear Regulatory Commission, Washington, DC, 1983.

U.S. Department of Energy (USDOE). *Radiological Control Manual.* DOE/EH-0256T, Washington, DC, 1992.

U.S. Environmental Protection Agency. *Integrated Risk Information System (IRIS).* National Center for Environmental Assessment, Washington, DC, 2002.

U.S. Nuclear Regulatory Commission. *Health Physics Surveys in Uranium Recovery Facilities.* Regulatory Guide 8.30, U.S. Nuclear Regulatory Commission, Washington, DC, May, 2002.

Wallace, R. B., and Doebbeling, B. N., eds. *Public Health & Preventive Medicine,* 14th ed. McGraw-Hill, New York, 1998.

Wight, G. D. *Fundamentals of Air Sampling.* Lewis Publishers, Boca Raton, FL, 1994.

Yang, R. S. H., ed. *Toxicology of Chemical Mixtures,* Academic Press, San Diego, CA, 1994.

Zenz, C. *Occupational Medicine,* 3rd ed. Mosby, St. Louis, MO, 1994.

14

NONIONIZING RADIATION SAFETY

Nonionizing radiation (NIR) generally means electromagnetic radiation whose quantum energy is less than 12 eV. However, although called "nonionizing" radiation, photons whose energy is as low as 3 eV may ionize certain molecules; an electron in a sodium atom, for example, requires only 2.3 eV of energy for its removal from the atom.

Safety practices to control the hazards from NIR received little attention before the end of World War II. At that time, we already had a good deal of experience with damage to the eyes from observing solar eclipses, from exposure to ultraviolet (UV) light among welders, and from exposure to infrared energy among glass blowers and steelworkers. We also had evidence of damage to the skin from exposure to UV and infrared radiation. However, it was the postwar boom in electronics and communications, based on the microwave portion of the electromagnetic spectrum, followed by the mushrooming use of lasers, that focused attention on the possible public health aspects of NIR, especially from these two sources of radiant energy. In 1968, the Radiation Control for Health and Safety Act (Public Law 90-602) was passed by the U.S. Congress for the purpose of regulating the hazards from consumer electronics products, and in 1970, the Occupational Safety and Health Act (PL 91-596) was passed to protect workers from hazards, including ionizing and nonionizing radiation hazards, associated with their occupations. These legislative acts, and acts in other countries, have led to the promulgation of safety regulations for microwaves, lasers, and UV radiation.

The International Commission on Radiological Protection (ICRP) limits its field of interest to ionizing radiation. NIR, therefore, received relatively little attention from the health physics community until the International Radiation Protection Association (IRPA) revised its constitution in 1977 to expand its area of activities to include NIR. The IRPA is a worldwide association of national radiation safety societies (such as the Health Physics Society in the United States). Until the Fourth International Congress in 1977, the IRPA dealt only with health and safety aspects of ionizing radiation. At that meeting, the IRPA decided to expand its interests to include the safe use of NIR. This expansion was immediately implemented by

TABLE 14-1. Radiometric Units

QUANTITY	SYMBOL	DESCRIPTION	UNITS
Radiant energy	U	Energy emitted from the source, per pulse	joule, J
Radiant power	P	Power emitted from the energy source	watt, W
Radiant intensity	I	Radiant power emitted per unit solid angle	W/sr
Radiance	L	Power emitted from the source per unit solid angle per unit area	$\dfrac{\text{W/sr}}{\text{cm}^2}$
Radiant emittance	W	Power emitted per unit area of the source	W/cm^2
Radiant exposure	H	Areal density of total radiant energy incident on a surface	J/cm^2
Irradiance[a]	E	Areal density of power incident on a surface	W/cm^2

[a]In the context of lasers, power per unit area is called *irradiance*. In the context of microwaves, power per unit area is called *power density*.

establishing the International Non-Ionizing Radiation Committee (INIRC), which was charged with (1) publishing NIR health criteria documents, (2) developing guidelines on the basis of these documents for occupational and public exposure limits, and (3) making recommendations on how to implement exposure limits for the safe use of NIR; INIRC evolved into the International Commission on Non-Ionizing Radiation Protection (ICNIRP). Although now a separate organization, ICNIRP maintains a close liaison and working relationship with IRPA. ICNIRP's charter specifies that its formal NIR safety recommendations be submitted to IRPA for comments before they are finalized. The recommendations of the ICNIRP are published in the radiation safety literature, such as the *Health Physics* journal and special reports published by the World Health Organization (WHO). In the United States, the National Council on Radiation Protection and Measurements (NCRP), the American Conference of Governmental Industrial Hygienists (ACGIH), and the American National Standards Institute (ANSI) make recommendations for the safe use of NIR.

UNITS

Illumination is measured in the *photometric* system of units. Photometric units relate to the response of the human eye to light. *Radiometric* units, on the other hand, are absolute physical units that are defined for the entire electromagnetic spectrum (Table 14-1). Safety standards and criteria for laser and microwave energy are specified in the radiometric system of units. Unlike ionizing radiation, where the quantum energy usually is expressed in electron volts, the energy of NIR usually is expressed either as wavelength or frequency. Of course, specifying either the quantum energy, the wavelength, or the frequency implicitly fixes the other two parameters, as shown in the example below:

EXAMPLE 14.1

Calculate the energy and frequency of a 400-nm UV photon.

Solution

The energy of a 400-nm UV photon is calculated with Eq. (2.77):

$$E = h\frac{c}{\lambda} = 6.6262 \times 10^{-34} \, \text{J} \cdot \text{s} \times \frac{3 \times 10^8 \, \frac{\text{m}}{\text{s}}}{400 \times 10^{-9} \, \text{m}} = 4.97 \times 10^{-19} \, \text{J}$$

$$= \frac{4.970 \times 10^{-19} \, \text{J}}{1.6 \times 10^{-19} \, \frac{\text{J}}{\text{eV}}} = 3.1 \, \text{eV},$$

and the frequency of this photon is calculated from Eqs. (2.76) and (2.77):

$$E = hf = h\frac{c}{\lambda},$$

$$f = \frac{c}{\lambda} = \frac{3 \times 10^8 \, \text{m/s}}{400 \times 10^{-9} \, \text{m}} = 7.5 \times 10^{14} \, \text{s}^{-1} = 750 \, \text{THz (terahertz)}.$$

UV LIGHT

UV radiation is defined by the WHO as light with wavelengths between 100 nm and 400 nm. The UV spectrum is divided into three regions: UVA, 320–400 nm; UVB, 280–320 nm; and UVC, 100–280 nm. Other common names for the different portions of the UV spectrum include *actinic UV*, UVA and UVB; *far UV*, UVC; and *near UV*, UVA. UVC is not transmitted through the atmosphere; it therefore is often referred to as *vacuum UV*.

Sources

The sun is the largest source of UV radiation; the sunlight that reaches the earth's surface consists mainly of UVA radiation, with a smaller component of UVB. All of the UVC is filtered by the ozone layer, and thus no UVC reaches the earth's surface. Man-made sources of UV radiation include:

- black light lamps
- carbon arcs
- dental polymerizing instruments
- fluorescence equipment
- germicidal lamps
- hydrogen lamps
- metal halide lamps
- mercury lamps
- plasma torches
- printing ink polymerization
- tanning equipment
- welding arcs

TABLE 14-2. Lethal Effectiveness of Colored Light against the Tubercle Bacillus

COLOR	KILLING TIME (min)
Clear	5–10
Blue	10–20
Red	20–30
Green	45

Biomedical Effects

Light, both visible and UV, has long been known to be biophysically active. Tanning and sunburn from exposure to sunlight are common experiences, and the use of UV lamps for bactericidal purposes is widespread. In an early-twentieth-century study on the lethal effects of filtered (by window glass of various colors) sunlight on the tubercle bacillus, the killing times shown in Table 14-2 were reported. For killing bacteria and bacterial spores, UV light in the wavelength range of 250–270 nm has been found to be the most effective. For *Escherichia coli*, for example, the most efficient wavelength is 265 nm; at this wavelength, the absorption of 14-MeV total energy is required to kill the bacterium.

Mechanisms of biological damage from light include both temperature effects due to absorbed energy and photochemical reactions. The chief mode of damage depends on the wavelength of the light and on the tissue being exposed. For control of hazards from UV and from lasers the critical organs are the eye and the skin.

Eye

The biomedical effects of UV radiation are strongly wavelength dependent. Generally, UV rays become increasingly penetrating into the eye as their wavelength increases. UVC, which is present in electric welding arcs, can damage the cornea and lead to photokeratitis, which is commonly called "welders flash." This is a painful inflammation of the cornea that may last for several days. UVB, which is also strongly present in electric arcs, is damaging to the lens as well as to the cornea, and is responsible for the formation of cataracts. It also stimulates the formation of a pterygium, which is a fleshy tissue that grows out of the corner of the eye and spreads over the cornea, thus blocking light from entering the eye. A pterygium is treated by surgical removal, and then by irradiation of the stump with betas from a ^{90}Sr–^{90}Y source. UVA is absorbed mainly in the lens, and it too is associated with cataract production. In addition to UV radiation, blue light, of wavelength around 440 nm, can produce scarring on the retina which, if severe, may lead to significant loss of vision.

Skin

All wavelengths of UV damage the collagen fibers in the skin, and thus accelerate the changes due to aging. In this regard, UVA plays a major role in the production of wrinkles. UVB is the UV component that is mainly responsible for the actinic (delayed photochemical) effects of UV radiation. It is responsible for tanning and erythema. UVB, together with UVA, are associated with the three types of skin cancers that are seen following long-term exposure. Basal-cell carcinoma has a very low degree of malignancy, and squamous-cell carcinoma has a higher degree of malignancy. Melanoma, the third skin cancer associated with exposure to UV radiation, is very highly malignant. Because of advances in diagnosis and treatment, the case mortality rate for melanoma has been reduced to about 50%.

Many persons can become photosensitive after taking certain medicines (including commonly used drugs such as tetracycline antibiotics, sulfa drugs, antihistamines, and nonsteroidal anti-inflammatory drugs) and after using certain common items, including cosmetics, deodorants, antibacterial soaps, and artificial sweeteners. A photosensitivity reaction occurs following a low-level exposure to UV radiation; the reaction usually is expressed as a rash or a severe sunburn when no sunburn is expected. There are two forms of photosensitivity: photoallergy and phototoxicity. In a photoallergic reaction, the initial UV radiation converts the agent into an antigen. Subsequent exposure to UV radiation triggers an antigen–antibody reaction. The photoallergic reaction usually occurs only on the exposed areas of the skin, although it may also spread beyond the exposed area.

Most cases of photosensitivity are of the phototoxic type. This involves an interaction between the agent molecule and a UV photon to produce an intradermal toxic substance. The signs and symptoms of a phototoxic reaction are similar to those of a photoallergic reaction. As with photoallergy, it occurs on the exposed areas of the skin.

Safety Standards and Guides

Although there are very few regulatory limits on exposure to UV radiation, numerous guidelines have been published, with all of them in general agreement. In the United States, the recommendations of the ACGIH are accepted as the basis for UV radiation safety practice. Rate of exposure to UV light is called the irradiance and is measured in watts per square meter (W/m^2) or in milliwatts per square centimeter (mW/cm^2); dose is called radiant exposure and is expressed in units of energy per unit area—joules per square meter (J/m^2) or millijoules per square centimeter (mJ/cm^2).

The fact that the potential for harmful effects is strongly dependent on the wavelength of the UV radiation leads to ranking the various wavelengths relative to 270 nm, which is the wavelength to which the biological systems are most sensitive. The recommended 8-hour radiant exposure threshold limit value (TLV), which is applicable to both the eye and the skin, is $30\,J/m^2$, or $3\,mJ/cm^2$ for 270-nm radiation. For other wavelengths, whose spectral effectiveness is less than that of 270-nm UV, the TLV is proportionately greater (Table 14-3). For heterochromatic UV radiation, the $3\,mJ/cm^2$ TLV applies to the *effective* spectral effective irradiance, which is defined by:

$$E_{\text{eff}} = \sum_{180}^{400} E_\lambda\, S(\lambda)\, \Delta\lambda, \tag{14.1}$$

where

E_{eff} = effective irradiance, in W/cm^2, relative to a monochromatic source at 270 nm,

E_λ = spectral irradiance, in $W/cm^2/nm$,

$S(\lambda)$ = relative spectral effectiveness, unitless, and

$\Delta\lambda$ = bandwidth, in nm.

TABLE 14-3.   Ultraviolet Radiation TLV® and Relative Spectral Effectiveness

WAVELENGTH, λ (nm)	TLV (mJ/cm²)	RELATIVE SPECTRAL EFFECTIVENESS, $S(\lambda)$
180	250	0.012
200	100	0.030
220	25	0.120
240	10	0.300
250	7.0	0.430
254	6.0	0.500
260	4.6	0.650
270	3.0	1.000
280	3.4	0.880
290	4.7	0.640
300	10	0.300
313	500	0.006
320	2.9×10^3	0.001
340	1.1×10^4	2.8×10^{-4}
360	2.3×10^4	1.3×10^{-4}
380	4.7×10^4	6.4×10^{-5}
400	1.0×10^5	3.0×10^{-5}

From ACGIH®, 2008 TLVs® and BEIs® Book. Copyright © 2008. Reprinted with permission.

In practice, the effective spectral irradiance is measured with a radiometer whose response to the different wavelengths is weighted by the relative spectral effectiveness factor, $S(\lambda)$. When the effective irradiance is known, the maximum exposure time to that irradiance can be calculated in order to remain within the recommended 3 mJ/cm² daily radiant exposure limit. The maximum exposure time is calculated as follows:

$$t \text{ (seconds)} = \frac{0.003\,\dfrac{\text{J}}{\text{cm}^2}}{E_{\text{eff}}\,\dfrac{\text{W}}{\text{cm}^2}}. \tag{14.2}$$

EXAMPLE 14.2

The measured effective irradiance at a distance of 10 cm from the center of a UV lamp is 2.4 mW/cm². Assuming the radiation to be isotropic, calculate

(a) the irradiance at a distance of 50 cm.

(b) the limiting exposure time at this irradiance?

Solution

(a) Using the inverse square law, we have

$$\frac{2.4 \dfrac{\text{mW}}{\text{cm}^2}}{E \dfrac{\text{mW}}{\text{cm}^2}} = \frac{(50 \text{ cm})^2}{(10 \text{ cm})^2}$$

$$E = 0.096 \text{ mW/cm}^2.$$

(b) With Eq. (14.2), we find

$$t = \frac{0.003 \dfrac{\text{J}}{\text{cm}^2}}{0.096 \times 10^{-3} \dfrac{\text{W}}{\text{cm}^2} \times 1 \dfrac{\text{J/s}}{\text{W}}} = 31.25 \text{ seconds.}$$

If a longer exposure time is required, then the laboratory worker must use a barrier cream or personal protective equipment, such as goggles and gloves that will absorb the UV radiation.

UV Protection

The basic principles for safe use of UV radiation are the same as for ionizing radiation: time, distance, and shielding. An additional safety consideration when working with intense UV sources is that short-wavelength UV can produce ozone (O_3) in measurable quantities. Ozone is a pulmonary irritant, and has an Occupational Safety and Health Administration (OSHA) permissible exposure limit (PEL) of 0.1 ppm.

Shielding, on a personal level, can be accomplished through the use of eyeglasses, goggles, or plastic face shields to protect the eyes and face. These items must, of course, be effective against the UV wavelengths in use. Ordinary glass blocks most UV light of wavelengths less than 330 nm, while transmitting most of the UV for longer wavelengths. Ordinary safety glasses and goggles use polycarbonate lenses, which absorb 100% of the UV. The UV-absorption properties of contact lenses, ordinary eyeglass lenses, sun glasses, and protective clothing can be determined by measuring the transmission of UV light with a radiometer.

Food and Drug Administration (FDA) regulations for sunscreen creams and lotions are published in 21 Code of Federal Regulations (CFR) 352. These blocking agents are designed only for UVB and UVA. The ability to block UVB is measured by the sun protection factor, SPF. The SPF is defined as the fraction of the incident UV that is transmitted by a thickness of 2 mg/cm^2. Thus, an SPF of 20 means that 1/20, or 5% of the incident radiation is transmitted, and 95% is absorbed. The percent of the incident UV that is absorbed is given by

$$\% \text{ absorbed} = \frac{\text{SPF} - 1}{\text{SPF}} \times 100. \tag{14.3}$$

EXAMPLE 14.3

Calculate the percentage of UVB absorbed by a sunscreen with an SPF $= 30$.

Solution

The percentage of UVB absorbed is calculated using Eq. (14.3):

$$\% \text{ absorbed} = \frac{30 - 1}{30} \times 100 = 96.7\%.$$

Thus we see that although an SPF of 30 is 50% greater than an SPF of 20, the difference between their absorptive capacities is very small.

LASERS

The word *laser* is an acronym for light amplification by stimulated emission of radiation. The laser is a device for producing a beam of monochromatic "light" in the UV, visible, or infrared regions of the electromagnetic spectrum, in which the waves are all in phase. That is, the light beam is said to be *coherent* in both space (since the waves are all in phase) and time (since the waves are all of the same frequency). As a result of this coherency, we have a beam that has relatively little divergence together with a high concentration of energy per unit area, both at the laser end and at the far end of the beam. This almost constant power density at both ends of the beam (which differs sharply from the inverse-square falloff of the intensity from a point source of incoherent light or of ionizing radiation, but see Problem 14.3) is a significant factor in the hazard potential of a laser.

All lasers include the three basic components (Fig. 14-1):

1. A high-Q optical cavity with one end completely mirrored and the other end partially mirrored—Q, as used here, has the same physical significance as the Q used to describe the quality of certain circuit configurations in electronics. Q is a figure of merit that gives the ratio of the energy stored in a particular device or circuit configuration to the energy dissipated per unit time interval:

$$Q = \frac{\text{energy stored}}{\text{energy dissipated/unit time interval}} = \frac{\text{energy stored}}{\text{dissipated power}}. \qquad \textbf{(14.4)}$$

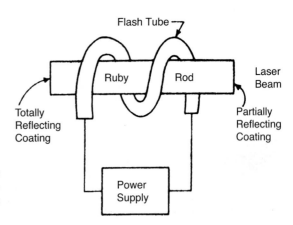

Figure 14-1. Components of a laser system, as illustrated by a schematic of a ruby laser with optical pumping, which is characteristic of solid-state lasers.

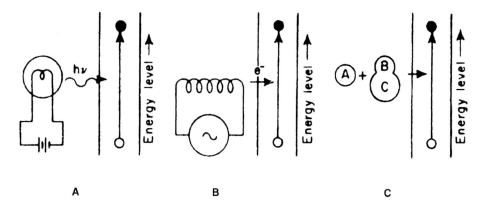

Figure 14-2. Energy-pumping systems for lasers. **A**. light (optical), **B**. electron collision (electrical), **C**. chemical.

2. Lasing medium—The lasing medium is a substance that can be excited to a metastable state through the addition of energy that is "pumped" into the lasing medium. The lasing medium may be either in solid, liquid, or gaseous form. Commonly used lasing media include ruby rods (a ruby consists of Al_2O_3 crystals in which about 0.5% of the Al has been replaced by Cr; the chromium atoms are the atoms that are excited to the metastable state and thus are responsible for the lasing action), neodynium in glass, gallium-arsenide, helium–neon, argon, and carbon dioxide.

3. Energy pump—The source of energy needed to excite the atoms of the lasing medium may be either an intense source of light that emits a wide range of photon energies and necessarily includes photons of exactly the right energy to excite the lasing atoms (Fig. 14-2) or, in the case of gas laser, a radiofrequency voltage generator of about 1000 V that accelerates ions, which in turn excites the lasing atoms by colliding with them. Semiconductor (or diode) lasers, such as gallium-arsenide, are pumped by passing an electric current of very high density, on the order of hundreds to thousands of amperes per square centimeter, across the P–N junction of the semiconductor.

Lasers are named according to the lasing medium. The various general categories of lasers are listed in Table 14-4.

TABLE 14-4. Laser Types and Typical Lasing Media

LASER TYPE	TYPICAL LASING MEDIUM	TYPICAL EXCITATION METHOD
Gas	He–Ne, CO_2	Electrical
Semiconductor	GaAlAs, GaN	Electrical
Solid State	YAG, Ti:sapphire	Optical
Dye	Rhodamine 6G	Optical
Metal Vapor	Copper	Electrical

Laser Operation

According to the Bohr atomic model (Chapter 3), photons of ordinary light are produced when excited electrons fall to a lower energy level. These electrons may be excited to the higher unstable energy levels through the addition of energy by one of several ways:

1. by absorbing energy from photons, as in the case of fluorescence,
2. by absorbing energy from charged particles, as in the case of luminescent paint or cathode-ray tube phosphors,
3. by heating, as in the case of an incandescent light bulb or a piece of metal or glass heated to a high temperature,
4. by collisions with other electrons, as in the case of a fluorescent lamp or a "neon" sign, or
5. by exothermic chemical reactions, as in the case of a flame.

The electronic transition, in the case of ordinary light, occurs randomly, and the photons, as a consequence, are unrelated to each other. In a laser, on the other hand, the electrons are excited by an energy "pump" into a relatively long-lived metastable state, where they remain until a passing photon of exactly the correct energy "stimulates" a transition to the lower energy level and all the excited atoms emit photons of the same energy at the same time. Einstein, in the development of the theory underlying the photoelectric effect (for which he was awarded the Nobel Prize in Physics in 1921), showed that a photon whose energy is exactly equal to that of an electron in an excited state can stimulate the excited electron to fall to the ground state and thus to emit a photon whose frequency corresponds to the excitation energy. Not only are the emitted and the stimulating photons of the same frequency, but they are also in phase.

Lasing Action

Under normal conditions, most of the atoms in any medium are in the ground state. Brownian motion leads to collisions among the atoms, in which sufficient energy to raise an atom to an excited level may be transferred. Thus, although most of the atoms are in the ground state, some atoms may be in one of the several possible excited states. The relationship between the number of atoms in any two energy levels is given by the Boltzmann equation,

$$N_2 = N_1 e^{\frac{(E_2 - E_1)}{kT}}, \tag{14.5}$$

where N_1 and N_2 are the numbers of atoms in energy levels E_1 and E_2, respectively; k is Boltzmann's constant, 1.38×10^{-23} J per degree K, and T is the absolute temperature, K.

In materials where the atoms can be excited to a metastable state, it is possible, by "pumping" large amounts of energy into them, to attain a population inversion, in which most of the atoms are in an excited state.

After a population inversion has been obtained, lasing action is initiated by a photon that is emitted from an excited atom whose electron spontaneously falls to the ground state. This photon then stimulates another excited atom to emit a photon by falling to a lower energy level. Most of these stimulated photons strike the walls of the

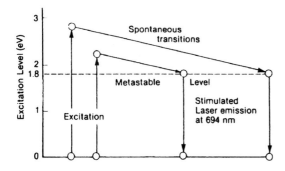

Figure 14-3. Energy-level diagram for a ruby laser. Electrons are excited to a high energy level by the pumping system. They then fall down spontaneously to the 1.8-eV metastable level, from which they are stimulated, and they all will cascade simultaneously to the ground state.

optical cavity and are lost. Those photons, however, which are released in a direction parallel to the long axis of the optical cavity continue to stimulate emission and to combine coherently with the emitted photons until they strike one of the mirrored ends of the optical cavity. Thus, as the photons progress within the optical cavity, the beam intensity continuously increases while the phase relationships remain constant, thereby maintaining the coherence of the beam. When the beam strikes the totally reflecting end, its direction is reversed, and it continues to stimulate emission of photons and to increase in intensity until it reaches the partially reflecting end. There, some of the beam escapes, and the remainder is reflected back to continue the process of stimulated photon emission. This lasing action continues as long as energy is supplied to the lasing medium in order to excite the atoms and thus to maintain a population inversion. The wavelength of this light depends on the difference between the energy level of the metastable state and of the lower energy level of the lasing medium. For a ruby laser, the wavelength is 694 nm; for a helium and neon (He–Ne) laser, the wavelength is 633 nm; and for a CO_2 laser, the emitted infrared energy has a wavelength of 10,600 nm. Figure 14-3 shows these energy levels for the ruby laser schematically; similar energy-level diagrams may be constructed for other lasing materials.

The laser is an extremely inefficient device. In most types of lasers, less than 0.1% of the energy pumped into the system is converted to useful coherent radiation.

Manner of Operation

Lasers operate in one of three different manners:

1. Continuous wave (CW),
2. Pulsed (long pulse or normal pulse), and
3. *Q*-switched (or *Q*-spoiled).

The optical cavity has one end that is completely reflecting and one end that is partially reflecting and partially transmitting. If the partially transmitting end allows a fraction of the light energy that strikes it to escape, and if energy can be pumped into the lasing medium at such a rate that the laser output can be maintained un-interruptedly, then we have a CW laser. Most CW lasers employ gas as the lasing medium, although solid-state lasers can also be made to operate in the CW mode. The first CW laser used a mixture of helium and neon (He–Ne), where the He atoms were excited by an applied radiofrequency high voltage. The excited He atoms, in turn, raised the Ne atoms to a metastable state by colliding with them. He–Ne CW lasers operate at power levels ranging from a fraction of a milliwatt to about 100 mW. At the high end of the CW power spectrum are CO_2 lasers, which operate at power levels up the kilowatts (kW) range. Pulsed lasers deliver their output in bursts of light whose duration range from femtoseconds (10^{-15} seconds) to 0.25 seconds. Lasers that emit pulses longer than 0.25 seconds are considered CW for safety purposes.

The ruby laser is an example of pulsed operating mode. A very intense flash of light, produced by discharging large capacitors across the flash lamp, pumps the lasing medium and creates a population inversion. The resultant stimulated radiation builds in intensity and emerges as a long pulse of coherent laser radiation. The energy content of a normal pulse from ruby lasers varies from a fraction of a joule to about 30 J, while the pulse repetition frequency (PRF) ranges from about 1/30 to 10 pulses per second.

A pulsed laser may also be operated in another manner, called *Q-switched* (or *Q-spoiled*). A *Q*-switch is an acousto-optical or electro-optical device within the optical cavity that is analogous to a shutter; it prevents laser emission until it is opened. In *Q*-switching, the *Q* of the optical cavity is suddenly increased from a low value, when lasing does not occur despite a large population inversion, to a high *Q*, when lasing can occur. The very large population inversion built up during the low-*Q* part of the operation suddenly falls to the ground state in a very short time, on the order of nanoseconds, to produce a very intense pulse. Because of the combination of high energy and narrow pulse width, very high powers, on the order of megawatts, are readily attainable with *Q*-switched lasers.

Transverse Electromagnetic Modes

The distribution of light energy across the laser beam is determined by diffraction effects within the optical cavity. It is described by the *mode pattern* of the transverse electromagnetic (TEM) waves, which is designated as TEM_{pq}, where p and q are integers. The TEM_{00} mode, which corresponds to a circular beam of laser light, has the least amount of diffraction and is the main mode of oscillation within the optical cavity. The light intensity across a TEM_{00} laser beam approximates a Gaussian distribution. Because of this variation in intensity across the beam and because the edge of the beam is not sharply defined as a result of diffraction effects at the edges of the mirrors, an arbitrary definition of the beam diameter is frequently used. One such value for describing the beam diameter when the laser is operating in the TEM_{00} mode is the $1/e$ power point. This is defined as the diameter of the circle that intercepts $1 - 1/e = 0.632$ of the energy in the laser beam and is used in all laser safety calculations. Laser manufacturers may also specify the beam diameter in terms of the $1 - 1/e^2$ diameter. To measure the beam diameter, we require a power meter whose aperture exceeds the circle that would enclose 100% of the laser beam and a coaxial iris diaphragm. A power measurement is first made with the iris wide open; the iris is then slowly closed until the power is down to 86.5% of the first reading. This gives the "$1/e^2$" diameter. The "$1/e$" diameter is determined by closing the iris until the power level is reduced to 63.2% of the wide-open measurement. Because the energy distribution across the cross section of the beam follows a Gaussian distribution from

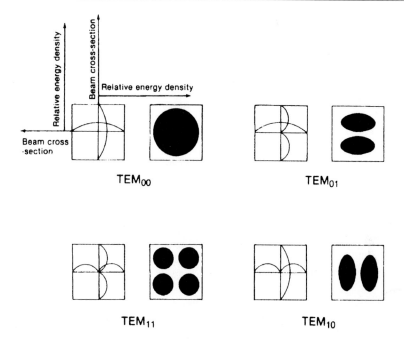

Figure 14-4. *Beam cross sections for four different TEM modes.*

the center outward, the two expressions of energy within a beam are not linear with energy. The $1/e$ diameter is related to the $1/e^2$ diameter by

$$D_{(1/e)} = \frac{D_{(1/e^2)}}{\sqrt{2}}. \tag{14.6}$$

Beam cross sections for several different TEM modes are shown in Figure 14-4.

Beam Divergence

Beam divergence is a measure of the spread of the beam after it leaves the laser. It is determined by measuring the beam diameter at two different distances from the laser, and then calculating the angle of divergence.

EXAMPLE 14.4

The $1/e^2$ diameters of a laser beam were found to be 2.82 mm at 0.5 m from the laser aperture and 5.30 mm at 4.5 m. What is the beam divergence?

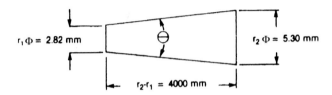

Solution

The length of an arc that subtends an angle Φ is given by

$l = r \times \Phi$, where Φ is the angle in radians.

The arc that subtends very small angles may be considered to be a straight line. The beam divergence is therefore calculated as

$$\text{diameter}_2 - \text{diameter}_1 = r_2\Phi - r_1\Phi = (r_2 - r_1)\Phi$$

$$\Phi = \frac{\text{diameter}_2 - \text{diameter}_1}{r_2 - r_1} = \frac{5.30\,\text{mm} - 2.82\,\text{mm}}{4500\,\text{mm} - 500\,\text{mm}} = 6.2 \times 10^{-4}\,\text{radian}$$

$$= 3.55 \times 10^{-2}\,\text{degree}.$$

Biological Effects

Mechanisms of damage from light include both heating effects due to absorbed energy and photochemical reactions. The chief mode of damage depends on the wavelength of the radiation and the rate at which the tissue is irradiated. The critical organs in the case of laser radiation are the eye and the skin.

Eye Damage

Laser irradiation of the eye may cause damage to the cornea, lens, or retina, depending on the wavelength of the light and the energy absorption characteristics of the ocular tissues. Figure 14-5 shows the percent transmission of light through the ocular media as a function of wavelength. The figure shows that most of the visible part of the electromagnetic spectrum is transmitted and that the transmission of the near UV and the near infrared drops very sharply. The visible light that is transmitted by the ocular media is strongly absorbed in the retina. Because of these transmission and absorption characteristics, we may infer that visible light is much less likely to damage the cornea, per unit of incident light energy, than to damage the retina. This expectation has been confirmed experimentally.

The threshold for minimum visible lesions (MVL) is the basis for setting laser safety standards. Maximum permissible exposure (MPE) limits to laser radiation are typically set at one-tenth the MVL. Evaluation of the MVL is performed 24 hours after exposure. The criterion for a retinal MVL is a minimum retinal lesion visible

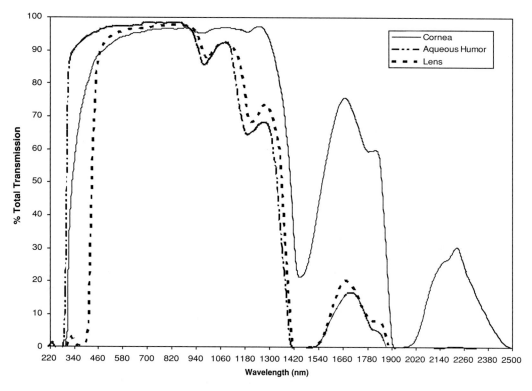

Figure 14-5. Transmission of light through human ocular media as a function of wavelength. (Based on data from Boettner EA, Dankovic D. *Ocular Absorption of Laser Radiation for Calculating Personnel Hazards.* USAF School of Aerospace Medicine; November 30, 1974. Final Report.)

through an ophthalmoscope. Retinal injuries at the MVL or greater exposures can lead to permanent blind spots. The magnitude of the damage and the latent period before a visible lesion is seen are functions of the irradiated area, exposure rate, and total exposure. The basic factor in retinal damage is the rate at which heat energy can be removed from the irradiated tissue and the consequent temperature change. A temperature increase of only several degrees greater than that experienced during fevers is believed to be capable of producing permanent retinal damage. Threshold values for retinal damage from visible light are listed in Table 14-5.

TABLE 14-5. Retinal Damage Thresholds

LASER TYPE	WAVELENGTH	PULSE	LEVEL
Continuous wave	White light	—	6 W/cm^2
Normal pulse	694 nm	200 ms	0.85 J/cm^2
Q-switched pulse	694 nm	30 ns	0.07 J/cm^2

Reproduced with permission from Sliney DH, Palmisano WA. The evaluation of laser hazards. *AIHA J.* 1968;29(5):425–431. With permission of Taylor & Francis. (http: // www. informaworld.com)

TABLE 14-6. *Skin Damage Thresholds*

LASER	λ(nm)	EXPOSURE TIME	AREA (cm²)	MRD (J/cm²)
Ruby, normal pulse	694	0.2 ms	2.4–3.4 X 10⁻³	14–20
Argon	500	6 s	95 × 10⁻³	13–17
CO_2	1060	4–6 s	1	4–6
Ruby, Q-switched	694	10–12 ns	0.33–1.0	0.5–1.5

Reproduced with permission from Goldman L. The skin. *Arch Environ Health*. March 1969;12:434–436. Copyright © 1969 Heldref Publications.

Skin Damage

Acute exposure of the skin to sufficiently high amounts of energy from lasers may lead to burns that do not differ from ordinary thermal or solar burns. The overexposed skin undergoes nonspecific coagulation necrosis whose extent depends on the degree of overexposure. The incident radiant energy is converted to heat, which is not rapidly dissipated because of the poor thermal conductivity of the tissue. The resulting local temperature rise leads to denaturation of the tissue proteins. If enough energy is absorbed, the water in the tissue may be vaporized, and the tissue itself may be heated to incandesence and carbonized. The response of the skin to laser light depends mainly on the wavelength and pulse duration of the laser. Skin pigmentation too plays a role on skin damage thresholds; generally, the response to laser light increases as the pigmentation increases. Table 14-6 lists the minimal reactive doses (MRD) to the flexor surface forearm of a Caucasian adult from laser light under several different conditions of exposure.

Scars may develop when severe lesions from acute overexposure heal. Chronic low-level exposure to visible laser light generally does not lead to injury. It should be pointed out, however, that UV light can lead to skin cancer. Experimental evidence suggests that in the absence of photosensitizing substances, UV in the wavelength range of 290–320 nm is carcinogenic. Epidemiological studies show that exposure to sunlight, which includes this band of wavelengths, is associated with an increased incidence of skin cancer, including melanoma, a highly malignant form of skin cancer. These studies show the incidence of all types of skin cancer to double about every 8° to 10° latitude as the equator is approached.

Protection Guides and Standards

In contrast to ionizing radiation, where our protection standards are based mainly on the conservative assumption of a zero threshold for harmful stochastic effects, all the harmful effects from overexposure of the eye and skin to laser radiation have well-documented thresholds. Based on these thresholds, ICNIRP and national organizations, such as the ACGIH and the ANSI have recommended maximum exposure limits for laser radiation. MPEs to the skin are listed in Table 14-7.

In setting safety standards for the eyes, the focusing action of the crystalline lens must be considered. The total amount of light energy entering the eye is determined by the area of the pupillary opening. The transmitted light energy that reaches the retina is absorbed by the pigmented epithelium, where most of it is converted into heat. Because of the focusing action of the lens, the image of the limiting aperture

TABLE 14-7. Maximum Permissible Exposure (MPE) for Skin to a Laser Beam[a]

λ (nm)	EXPOSURE TIME (s)	MPE[a]
400–1400	10^{-9}–10^{-7}	$2C_A \times 10^{-2}$ J/cm^2
400–1400	10^{-7}–10	$1.1C_A t^{0.25}$ J/cm^2
400–1400	10–3 × 10^4	$0.2C_A$ W/cm^2
1400–1500	10^{-9}–10^{-3}	0.1 J/cm^2
1400–1500	10^{-3}–10	$0.56\ t^{0.25}$ J/cm^2
1400–10^6	10–3 × 10^4	0.1 W/cm^2
1500–1800	10^{-9}–10	1.0 J/cm^2
1800–2600	10^{-9}–10^{-3}	0.1 J/cm^2
1800–2600	10^{-3}–10	$0.56\ t^{0.25}$ J/cm^2
2600–10^6	10^{-9}–10^{-7}	1×10^{-2} J/cm^2
2600–10^6	10^{-7}–10	$0.56\ t^{0.25}$ J/cm^2

[a]$C_A = 1.0$ for $\lambda = 400$–700 nm; $C_A = 10^{2(\lambda-700)}$ for $\lambda = 700$–1050 nm; $C_A = 5.0$ for $\lambda = 1050$–1400 nm.

Reproduced with permission from Laser Institute of America from *The Safe Use of Lasers* (ANSI Z136.1–2000).

(the pupillary opening) formed on the retina is very much smaller than the pupillary opening. For light of wavelength λ cm, and an eye whose pupillary diameter is d_p and whose lens has a focal length f cm, the diameter of the image on the retina, d_r, is given by

$$d_r = \frac{2.44\lambda f}{d_p}. \tag{14.7}$$

Since radiant exposure (H) or irradiance (E) is related to the illuminated area by

$$H\,(\text{or } E) = \frac{\text{energy}}{\text{area}}, \tag{14.8}$$

the ratio of H or E of the cornea to that of the retina varies inversely with the square of the ratio of the pupillary diameter to the diameter of the image on the retina:

$$H\,(\text{retina}) = H\,(\text{cornea}) \times \left(\frac{d_p}{d_r}\right)^2. \tag{14.9}$$

 # EXAMPLE 14.5

A Q-switched ruby laser, $\lambda = 694.3$ nm, emits 15 J/pulse. If a pulse of this radiation, in a beam 1.6 cm in diameter, were accidentally to fall on an eye whose iris was opened to 7-mm diameter, and the focal length of the lens is 1.7 cm, calculate the radiant exposure at

(a) the cornea and

(b) the retina.

Solution

(a) The radiant exposure at the cornea is given by

$$H = \frac{\text{energy}}{\text{area}} = \frac{15\,\text{J}}{\frac{\pi}{4}(1.6\,\text{cm})^2} = 7.46\,\frac{\text{J}}{\text{cm}^2}.$$

(b) If the focal length of the lens is 1.7 cm, the diameter of the image on the retina is found from Eq. (14.7) to be

$$d_r = \frac{2.44 \times 694.3 \times 10^{-7}\,\text{cm} \times 1.7\,\text{cm}}{0.7\,\text{cm}} = 4.11 \times 10^{-4}\,\text{cm},$$

and the radiant exposure at the retina is, from Eq. (14.9),

$$H(\text{retina}) = H(\text{cornea}) \times \left(\frac{d_p}{d_r}\right)^2 = 7.46\,\frac{\text{J}}{\text{cm}^2} \times \left(\frac{0.7\,\text{cm}}{4.11 \times 10^{-4}\,\text{cm}}\right)^2$$

$$= 2.16 \times 10^7\,\frac{\text{J}}{\text{cm}^2}.$$

The maximum exposure of the retina must allow for this enormous concentration of light energy due to the focusing action of the lens. On the basis of retinal damage thresholds and concentration of the light on the retina by the eye's optical system, the exposure limits listed in Tables 14-8, 14-9, and 14-10 have been recommended by the several organizations. It should be noted that the recommendations of the scientific and technical committees of the several professional organizations are substantially equivalent. Portions of the ANSI exposure limits for direct intrabeam exposure and for exposure to diffuse reflected light are listed in Tables 14-7 and 14-8. Table 14-8 lists some of the frequency- and time-dependent limits for exposure of the eye. Table 14-9 lists the ocular exposure limits for direct viewing and the skin exposure limits for some common types of CW lasers. Because the size

TABLE 14-8. Maximum Permissible Exposure (MPE) for Direct Ocular Exposure, Intrabeam Viewing a Laser Beam[a]

λ (μm)	EXPOSURE TIME (s)	MPE
0.400–0.700	10^{-13}–10^{-11}	1.5×10^{-8} J/cm^2
0.400–0.700	10^{-11}–10^{-9}	$2.7\,t^{0.75}$ J/m^2
0.400–0.700	10^{-9}–18×10^{-6}	5.0×10^{-7} J/cm^2
0.400–0.700	18×10^{-6}–10	$1.8\,t^{0.75} \times 10^{-3}$ J/cm^2
0.500–0.700	10–3×10^4	1×10^{-3} W/cm^2
0.700–1.050	18×10^{-6}–10	$1.8\,C_A\,t^{0.75} \times 10^{-3}$ J/cm^2
1.050–1.400	50×10^{-6}–10	$9.0\,C_C\,t^{0.75} \times 10^{-3}$ J/cm^2
2.600–10^3	10–3×10^4	0.1 W/cm^2

[a]$C_A = 10^{2(\lambda-0.700)}$ for $\lambda = 0.700$–1.050, $C_C = 1.0$ for $\lambda = 1.050$–1.150, $C_C = 10^{18(\lambda-1.150)}$ for $\lambda = 1.150$–1.200; $C_C = 8$ for $\lambda = 1.200$–1.400.

Reproduced with permission from Laser Institute of America from *The Safe Use of Lasers* (ANSI Z136.1–2000).

TABLE 14-9. Maximum Permissible Exposures (MPE) for the Skin and for Direct Intrabeam Viewing for Selected Lasers

LASER TYPE	WAVELENGTH (nm)	EXPOSURE TIME (s)	EYE MPE	SKIN MPE
Argon	275	$10–3 \times 10^4$	3×10^{-3} J/cm^2	3×10^{-3} J/cm^2
He–Cd	325	10–1000	1 J/cm^2	1 J/cm^2
Argon	351	10–1000	1 J/cm^2	1 J/cm^2
He–Cd	441.6	0.25	2.5×10^{-3} W/cm^2	0.2 W/cm^2
Argon	488	10–58	1×10^{-3} W/cm^2	0.2 W/cm^2
	488	58–100	5.8×10^{-2} J/cm^2	0.2 W/cm^2
	488	>100	5.8×10^{-4} W/cm^2	0.2 W/cm^2
	514.5	$10–3 \times 10^4$	1×10^{-3} W/cm^2	0.2 W/cm^2
He–Ne	632	0.25	2.5×10^{-3} W/cm^2	—
	632	$10–3 \times 10^4$	1×10^{-3} W/cm^2	0.2 W/cm^2
Krypton	647	0.25	2.5×10^{-3} W/cm^2	—
	647	$10–3 \times 10^4$	1×10^{-3} W/cm^2	0.2 W/cm^2
InGaAlP	670	0.25	2.5×10^{-3} W/cm^2	
GaAs	905	$10–3 \times 10^4$	2.6×10^{-3} W/cm^2	0.5 W/cm^2
Neodynium:YAG	1064	$10–3 \times 10^4$	5×10^{-3} W/cm^2	1 W/cm^2
InGaAsP	1310	$10–3 \times 10^4$	4×10^{-2} W/cm^2	—
InGaAsP	1550	$10–3 \times 10^4$	0.1 W/cm^2	—
CO$_2$	10600	$10–3 \times 10^4$	0.1 W/cm^2	0.1 W/cm^2

Reproduced with permission from Laser Institute of America from *The Safe Use of Lasers* (ANSI Z136.1–2000).

of the image on the retina varies inversely with the pupil diameter, the degree of concentration of light on the retina increases as the diameter of the pupil increases. For this reason, to be conservative, the MPE values listed in Table 14-8 for visible light are based on a pupil diameter of 7 mm, which is considered to be the maximum opening of the iris diaphragm of the eye. For other wavelengths, where retinal damage is not the limiting harmful effect, the incident laser energy is averaged over a 1-mm-diameter circle. Tables 14-7, 14-8, and 14-9 are shown here for purposes of illustration only. For practical application in any real situation, the complete tables in the latest edition of the respective organizations recommendations should be consulted.

Regulatory Requirements

In the United States, laser safety standards coordinated in the Federal Laser Product Performance Standard (FLPPS) and regulations are promulgated by two agencies: the Department of Health and Human Services through the Center for Radiological Health and Devices (CRHD) and the Department of Labor (DOL) through the OSHA. The CRHD regulates manufacturers only, not users, through requirements for performance specifications. Several different organizations, such as ANSI, International Electrochemical Commission (IEC) and the U.S regulatory agencies classify lasers according to the level of potential hazard. The U.S. laser safety classifications are unified in the FLPPS. Except for minor differences, all the laser classification are essentially equivalent. All lasers are classified into one of four different classes, depending on the level of risk from the laser. Class I is the least hazardous and class IV

TABLE 14-10. Summary of Laser Classes According to their Hazard Potential

Class I:	Laser cannot cause injury either because it is too low powered or because of engineered safety controls.
Class II:	May be viewed for less than 0.25 second. The aversion response, which leads to a blink in <0.25 second, is sufficient to prevent injury to the eye. Maximum power level = 1 mW.
Class IIIA:	Can injure the eye in intrabeam viewing for <0.25 second, or viewing A specular reflection for <0.25 second. Maximum power = 5 mW.
Class IIIB:	Same as IIIA, except that maximum power = 500 mW, maximum radiant exposure = 10 J/cm^2 per pulse.
Class IV:	Hazardous to the eyes and the skin during intrabeam and diffuse exposure. Potential fire hazard. Power level >500 mW.

The classes are from the FLPPS. Other classes are defined by ANSI and IEC which do not differ substantially from the FLPPS classification. ANSI has added three additional sub-classes, 1M, 2M, and 3R. 1M lasers can produce eye injury only when viewed with optical instruments, such as binoculars. Class 2M lasers with expanding beams are unsafe for viewing >0.25 second with an optical aid. Class 3R is essentially the same as Class IIIA.

Sources: OSHA Technical Manual and reproduced with permission from Laser Institute of America from *The Safe Use of Lasers* (ANSI Z136.1–2000).

is the most hazardous. Table 14-10 lists the potentially hazardous capabilities of the lasers in each of the four classes.

According to the laser's class, certain engineering and labeling requirements are specified in the regulations. The engineering requirements include the following:

1. A protective housing, which prevents the exposure to laser radiation not necessary for the performance of the intended function of the laser (leakage radiation).
2. Safety interlocks, designed to prevent human access to laser radiation upon removal or displacement of the protective housing.
3. A remote-control connector to allow additional interlocks and remote on–off controls.
4. Lockout and Tagout, key control to prevent unauthorized use of the laser. The key must be removable and the laser must be inoperable unless the key control is turned on by the key.
5. Beam stops to properly and safely terminate the beam.
6. Activation warning system that notifies personnel in and adjacent to the area in which the laser is active.
7. A beam attenuator that is independent of other means of stopping the beam.

The labeling requirements include information to be prominently displayed on the appropriate signs, warning of a laser hazard, and information about the laser and its output radiation, which must be prominently affixed to the laser. The engineered features and labeling requirements for each laser class are listed in the FDA regulations in 21 CFR 1040, and in the ANSI and IEC standards; they are summarized in Table 14-11. The OSHA regulates the use of lasers in industry and specifies user qualifications, posting and labeling requirements, MPE levels, and suitable laser safety goggles. According to OSHA regulations (29 CFR, 1926.54), employees shall

TABLE 14-11. Summary of Laser-Engineered Safety Features and Labeling Requirements

	CLASS			
	I	**II**	**III**	**IV**
Safety feature				
Protective housing	X	X	X	X
Safety interlock	X	X	X	X
Remote connector			X	X
Key control			X	X
Emission indicator		X	X	X
Beam attenuator		X	X	X
Label				
Certification and Manufacturer	X	X	X	X
Class designation and warning logotype		X	X	X
Aperture label		X	X	X
Radiation output				
Noninterlocked protective housing		X	X	X

Source: 21CFR 1040.10.

not be exposed to light intensities above 1 mW/cm^2 for direct staring, 1 mW/cm^2 for incidental observing, and 2 W/cm^2 for diffuse reflected light.

Direct Viewing

Intrabeam exposures to laser energy (Fig. 14-6) are specified in units of *radiant exposure*, H, J/cm^2, or in units of *irradiance*, E, W/cm^2. Irradiance is related to radiant exposure by

$$H = E \times t, \tag{14.10}$$

where t is the exposure time in seconds. The corresponding quantities at the laser aperture are called *emergent radiant exposures*, H_0, and *emergent irradiance*, E_0, respectively, and are specified by the energy output J in joules per pulse per unit area of the laser aperture or the laser power output, P, per unit area of laser aperture (E_0).

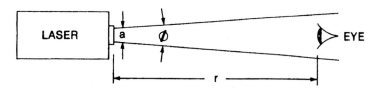

Figure 14-6. Intrabeam viewing of the primary or direct beam. (Reprinted with permission from ACGIH® *A Guide for Control of Laser Hazards*. 4th ed. Cincinnati, OH: American Conference of Governmental Industrial Hygienists; 1990. Copyright © 1990.)

EXAMPLE 14.6

What is the MPE value for direct ocular exposure for 5 seconds to the 442-nm light from a He–Cd laser operating at a power level of 20-mW CW?

Solution

Table 14-8 lists the MPE for this exposure condition as

$$\text{MPE } (H) = 1.8t^{0.75} \times 10^{-3} \, \frac{\text{J}}{\text{cm}^2}.$$

For $t = 5$ seconds, we have

$$\text{MPE } (H) = 1.8 \, (5)^{0.75} \times 10^{-3} = 6.02 \times 10^{-3} \, \frac{\text{J}}{\text{cm}^2} = 6.02 \, \frac{\text{mJ}}{\text{cm}^2}.$$

Since

$$H \, \frac{\text{mJ}}{\text{cm}^2} = E \, \frac{\text{mW}}{\text{cm}^2} \times t \text{ seconds},$$

$$\text{MPE } (E) = \frac{6.02 \, \dfrac{\text{mJ}}{\text{cm}^2}}{5 \text{ seconds}} = 1.2 \, \frac{\text{mW}}{\text{cm}^2}.$$

Thermal injury from pulsed radiation delivered in narrow, repetitive pulses is more severe than that from the same average amount of energy delivered at a uniform rate. Therefore, for scanning CW lasers and for repetitively pulsed lasers, the MPE per pulse is reduced. In the context of laser safety a repetitively pulsed laser is one that generates a continous train of pulses lasting less than 0.25 s with a pulse repetition frequency (PRF) ≥ 1 Hz. For repetitively pulsed lasers, the MPE is calculated according to three different criteria, and the lowest MPE is the one that is applied. The three rules, according to ANSI Z136.1-2007, are the following:

1. *Single pulse limit—Assuming exposure to only one pulse from a multiple pulse laser, the MPE that is applied is for that pulse only.*
2. *Average power limit—The MPE is based on the sum of all the energy deposited in the irradiated tissue, divided by the number of pulses during the exposure period, to give the average energy per pulse.*
3. *Repetitive pulse limit—To prevent pulse-cumulative thermal injury from exposure to n pulses from a repetitively pulsed laser, the MPE for single pulse in the train is reduced by the multiple pulse correction factor C_p:*

$$C_{\text{p}} = n^{-0.25}, \tag{14.11}$$

where n = number of pulses during viewing time.

EXAMPLE 14.7

A ruby laser, $\lambda = 694.3$ nm, is pulsed at a rate of 2 min^{-1}, and each pulse is 10 microseconds wide. What is the MPE for

(a) direct ocular exposure and

(b) skin exposure?

Solution

(a) Since for safety analysis this is not considered a repetitively pulsed laser, we find (Table 14-8) that the maximum permissible radiant exposure for a pulse width (or exposure time) of 10 microseconds is

$$H(\text{MPE}) = 5 \times 10^{-7} \frac{\text{J}}{\text{cm}^2}.$$

In terms of irradiance, this corresponds to

$$E(\text{MPE}) = \frac{H}{t} = \frac{5 \times 10^{-7} \frac{\text{J}}{\text{cm}^2}}{10 \times 10^{-6} \text{ s}} = 0.05 \frac{\text{W}}{\text{cm}^2} = 50 \frac{\text{mW}}{\text{cm}^2}$$

during each pulse.

(b) From Table 14-7, the MPE for skin exposure to 10 microseconds of 0.6943-mm light is found to be

$$H(\text{MPE}) = 1.1 \times C_{\text{A}} \times t^{0.25} \frac{\text{J}}{\text{cm}^2} = 1.1 \times 1 \times \left(10 \times 10^{-6}\right)^{0.25}$$

$$= 0.062 \frac{\text{J}}{\text{cm}^2}.$$

EXAMPLE 14.8

An argon laser, $\lambda = 0.5145 \ \mu$m, produces pulses 10 nanoseconds wide at a PRF of 1 MHz. What is the MPE level for direct intrabeam viewing for a total exposure time of 0.5 second?

Solution

According to rule 1, the MPE for a single 10-nanosecond pulse of 0.5145-μm light is found in Table 14-8 to be

$$H(\text{MPE})_{\text{rule 1}} = 5 \times 10^{-7} \ \text{J/cm}^2.$$

According to rule 2, the maximum total energy deposited during the 0.5-second viewing time is given in Table 14-8:

$$H(\text{MPE}) = 1.8 \; t^{0.75} \times 10^{-3} \; \text{J/cm}^2 = 1.8 \, (0.5)^{0.75} \times 10^{-3} = 1.1 \times 10^{-3} \; \text{J/cm}^2$$

is the MPE for the entire pulse train. Since the PRF is 1 MHz, the total number of pulses entering the eye during 0.5 second is

$$n = 0.5 \, \text{s} \times 1 \times 10^6 \, \frac{\text{pulses}}{\text{s}} = 5 \times 10^5 \, \text{pulses}.$$

The limiting radiant exposure per pulse, therefore, is

$$H\,(\text{MPE})_{\text{rule 2}} = \frac{1.1 \times 10^{-3} \, \dfrac{\text{J}}{\text{cm}^2}}{5 \times 10^5 \, \text{pulses}} = 2.2 \times 10^{-9} \, \frac{\text{J/cm}^2}{\text{pulse}}.$$

The irradiance (E) limit that corresponds to a given $H(\text{MPE})$ for a repetitively pulsed beam for an exposure time t seconds is given by

$$E\,(\text{MPE})_{\text{group}} = \text{PRF} \times t \times H(\text{MPE}) \, \frac{\text{J/cm}^2}{\text{pulse}}, \tag{14.12}$$

where PRF is the pulse repetition frequency. When we substitute the appropriate values into Eq. (14.12), we obtain

$$E\,(\text{MPE}) = 5 \times 10^5 \frac{\text{pulses}}{\text{s}} \times 0.5 \, \text{second} \times 2.2 \times 10^{-9} \, \frac{\text{J/cm}^2}{\text{pulse}}$$

$$= 5.5 \times 10^{-4} \, \frac{\text{W}}{\text{cm}^2} = 0.55 \, \frac{\text{mW}}{\text{cm}^2}.$$

According to rule 3, the MPE per pulse must be reduced by the factor $C_{\text{p}} = n^{-0.25}$. Since the number of pulses n during the exposure period $= 5 \times 10^5$, the reduced MPE per pulse is calculated from

$$H\,(\text{MPE})_{\text{rule 3}} = n^{-0.25} \times \text{MPE}_{\text{single pulse}}$$

$$= \left(5 \times 10^5\right)^{-0.25} \times 5 \times 10^{-7} \, \frac{\text{J}}{\text{cm}^2} = 1.9 \times 10^{-8} \, \frac{\text{J/cm}^2}{\text{pulse}},$$

and the corresponding irradiance, from Eq. (14.11) is:

$$E\,(\text{MPE})_{\text{rule 3}} = 5 \times 10^5 \, \frac{\text{pulses}}{\text{s}} \times 0.5 \, \text{second} \times 1.9 \times 10^{-8} \, \frac{\text{J/cm}^2}{\text{pulse}}$$

$$= 4.75 \times 10^{-3} \, \frac{\text{W}}{\text{cm}^2} = 4.75 \, \frac{\text{mW}}{\text{cm}^2}.$$

The lowest calculated MPE, 2.2×10^{-9} J/cm^2 per pulse, corresponding to 0.55 mW/cm^2, is the MPE that applies to this case.

The MPE calculated according to rule 2 will generally give the governing MPE for PRF > 55 kHz for radiation in the wavelength range of 0.4–1.05 μm, and PRF > 22 kHz for radiation in the wavelength range of 1.05–1.4 μm. These two frequencies are called *critical* frequencies in the context of retinal hazards from lasers.

EXAMPLE 14.9

A small He–Ne laser, of the type often used in the classrooms, has the following characteristics:

Wavelength = 632.8 nm,
Power output = 0.5-mW CW radiation,
Aperture diameter = 2 mm,
Beam divergence = 0.2 milliradians.

Calculate

(a) the emergent irradiance;

(b) the irradiance at a distance of 1 m;

(c) the irradiance at a distance of 10 m;

(d) the hazardous intrabeam viewing distance—that is, the distance at which the irradiance (from Table 14-9) exceeds 2.5 mW/cm^2.

Solution

(a) The emergent irradiance is

$$E_0 = \frac{\text{power output}}{\text{aperture area}} \tag{14.13}$$

$$= \frac{0.5\,\text{mW}}{\dfrac{\pi}{4}\,(0.2\,\text{cm})^2} = 15.9\,\text{mW/cm}^2.$$

(b) Irradiance at a distance from the aperture will be less than the emergent irradiance because of beam divergence. Absorption of the laser light by air is negligible unless the path is very long. For visible laser light, the attenuation coefficient varies from about 10^{-2} m^{-1} in thick fog to about 10^{-5} m^{-1} in clean air.

From Figure 14-7, we see that the irradiance at a distance r cm is given by

$$E = \frac{Pe^{-\mu r}}{A_L} = \frac{Pe^{-\mu r}}{\pi \left(\dfrac{1}{2} D_L\right)^2} = \frac{Pe^{-\mu r}}{\pi \left(\dfrac{1}{2}\,(a + r\phi)\right)^2}, \tag{14.14}$$

where

E = irradiance, mW/cm^2,
P = power output of the laser, mW,

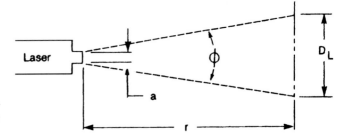

Figure 14-7. Geometry for evaluating irradiance at a distance r from the laser aperture.

A_L = area of laser beam at distance r cm, cm^2,
a = laser aperture, cm,
D_L = diameter, cm, of laser beam at distance r cm,
ϕ = beam divergence, radians, and
μ = attenuation coefficient of air, cm^{-1}.

At a distance of 1 m, $e^{-\mu r} \approx 1$, the irradiance from this laser, whose emergent beam irradiance E_0 is 15.9 mW/cm^2, is

$$E = \frac{0.5 \text{ mW}}{\pi \left[\frac{1}{2}(0.2 \text{ cm} + 100 \text{ cm} \times 0.0002 \text{ radian}) \right]^2} = 13.15 \frac{\text{mW}}{\text{cm}^2}.$$

(c) At a distance of 10 m (1000 cm), the irradiance decreases to

$$E = \frac{0.5 \text{ mW}}{\pi \left[\frac{1}{2}(0.2 \text{ cm} + 1000 \text{ cm} \times 0.0002 \text{ radian}) \right]^2} = 3.98 \frac{\text{mW}}{\text{cm}^2}.$$

It is important to note that the light intensity from a laser does not follow the inverse square law when distances are measured from the laser aperature.

(d) The hazardous intrabeam viewing distance may be calculated by neglecting air attenuation, rearranging Eq.(14.14) to solve for r, and substituting MPE = 2.5 mW/cm^2 for E to give the equation for calculating the *nominal ocular hazard distance*, NOHD. The NOHD is the distance beyond which exposure is less than the MPE, and no ocular hazard exists. The area within the NOHD is also called the *nominal hazard zone*, NHZ. The NOHD can be calculated by solving Eq.(14.14) for r after substituting E (MPE). If we neglect the beam attenuation by the atmosphere, we obtain

$$r_{\text{NOHD}} = \frac{1}{\phi \text{ radians}} \sqrt{\frac{P \text{ mW}}{\frac{\pi}{4} \times E \text{ (MPE)} \frac{\text{mW}}{\text{cm}^2}} - (a \text{ cm})^2}. \tag{14.15}$$

When we substitute the respective values into Eq. (14.15), we have

$$r_{\text{NOHD}} = \frac{1}{2 \times 10^{-4} \text{ radians}} \sqrt{\frac{0.5 \text{ mW}}{\frac{\pi}{4} \times 2.5 \frac{\text{mW}}{\text{cm}^2}} - (0.2 \text{ cm})^2} = 2317 \text{ cm}.$$

TABLE 14-12. Reflecting Materials

TYPE	MATERIAL	REFLECTION COEFFICIENT
Specular	Mirrored glass	0.8–0.9
	Aluminum foil	0.84–0.87
	Rhodium	0.7–0.9
	Aluminum, polished	0.6–0.7
	Chromium	0.60–0.65
	Stainless steel	0.55–0.65
	Black structural glass	0.04–0.05
Mixed	Aluminum, oxidized	0.70–0.85
	Aluminum, brushed	0.54–0.58
	Aluminum paint	0.6–0.7
	Stainless steel, satin	0.51–0.56
Diffuse	White plaster	0.90–0.92
	White paint, flat	0.75–0.90
	Limestone	0.35–0.65
	Sandstone	0.30–0.42

For higher-power lasers, the "safe" viewing distance can become very great. If the power of the laser in this example is increased to 100 mW, then the "safe" viewing distance is found to be 3.57×10^4 cm, or 357 meters!

Reflections

When a laser beam falls on a surface, some fraction of the incident light, depending on the nature of the surface and on the wavelength of the light, will be reflected. If the reflecting surface is polished and mirrorlike and the angle of incidence of the beam is equal to the angle of reflection, we have specular reflection. On the other hand, if the reflecting surface is rough or dull and the illuminated surface appears equally bright at all viewing angles, the surface is matte, and we have diffuse reflection. We have mixed reflections if some of the incident light is diffusely reflected and some undergoes specular reflection. The reflection coefficient of a surface gives the fraction of the incident light reflected by that surface. Reflection coefficients for some materials are listed in Table 14-12.

An *extended source* is a source whose wavelength is in the retinal hazard range, 400–1400 nm, and whose dimensions are large relative to the viewing distance. In this case, the source can be resolved into a geometrical image on the retina (which cannot be done with a point source). Typically, direct viewing of laser diodes are extended sources; and diffuse reflections may be extended sources. For purposes of laser hazard control, we have an extended source when the source subtends a viewing angle $>1.5 \times 10^{-3}$ radians. As long as the eye views a reflection of an extended source, the intensity of the light energy on the retina is independent of the viewing distance, since the light intensity variation with distance is exactly compensated by the change in the subtended viewing angle (Fig. 14-8). The relationship among the size of the reflection, D_L; the viewing distance, r_1; and the angle subtended by the eye, α, is given by

$$\alpha = \frac{D_L \times \cos\theta_V}{r_1}. \tag{14.16}$$

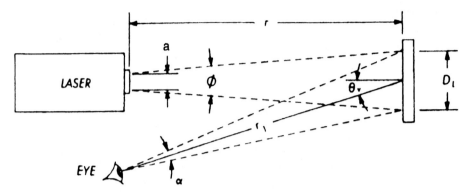

Figure 14-8. Extended source viewing of a diffuse reflection. (Reprinted with permission from ACGIH® *A Guide for Control of Laser Hazards*. 4th ed. Cincinnati, OH: American Conference of Governmental Industrial Hygienists; 1990. Copyright © 1990.)

EXAMPLE 14.10

A doubled Nd:YAG laser (532 nm) is used in a laser light show and illuminates a 3-cm-diameter circle. How close must a viewer be to consider this an extended source?

Solution

If into Eq.(14.16) we substitute the limiting angle, 1.5×10^{-3} radian, $\cos \theta_V = 1$ (which is the maximum possible value) and $D_L = 3$ cm, we have

$$(r_1)_{max} = \frac{3 \text{ cm} \times 1}{1.5 \times 10^{-3} \text{ radians}} = 2000 \text{ cm} = 20 \text{ m}.$$

At distances less than 20 m, this reflection is treated as an extended source for purpose of hazard evaluation. At greater distances, it is considered a point source.

EXAMPLE 14.11

A CW He–Ne laser, $\lambda = 0.633$ μm, having a power output (P) of 1 mW, a 3-mm aperture diameter, a, and a beam divergence, ϕ, of 1 milliradians is used in a darkened laboratory. The beam illuminates a white painted matte wall, whose reflection coefficient, ρ, is 0.8, at a distance of 10 m. May the reflected spot be viewed for 60 seconds from a point that is 30° off the beam's central axis ($\theta_V = 30°$) and at a distance of 1 m ($r_L = 1$ m) from the wall without eye protection?

Solution

Since the energy distribution within a laser beam follows a Gaussian distribution, the beam diameter does not change linearly with distance. Instead, the beam diameter as a function of distance, r, from the aperture is given by

$$D_{\rm L} = \sqrt{a^2 + (r \times \phi)^2} \qquad\qquad (14.17)$$

$$D_{\rm L} = \sqrt{(0.3\ {\rm cm})^2 + (1000\ {\rm cm} \times 1 \times 10^{-3}\ {\rm radian})^2} = 1\ {\rm cm}$$

To determine whether the reflection is treated as a point source or an extended source, we calculate the viewing angle subtended by the reflection, and compare it to the 1.5×10^{-3}-radian maximum angle subtended by a "point" source. The viewing angle subtended by the 1-cm-diameter reflection, when viewed at a distance of 100 cm is calculated with Eq. (14.16)

$$\alpha = \frac{D_{\rm L} \times \cos \theta_{\rm V}}{r_1} = \frac{1\ {\rm cm} \times \cos 30°}{100\ {\rm cm}} = 8.7 \times 10^{-3}\ {\rm radian}.$$

Since the viewing angle exceeds 1.5×10^{-3} radian, we have an extended source. The brightness of the reflection is given by

$$E = \frac{\rho \times P \times \cos \theta_{\rm V}}{\pi \times r_{\rm L}^2}. \qquad\qquad (14.18)$$

When we substitute the respective values into Eq. (14.18), we have

$$E = \frac{\rho \times P \times \cos \theta_{\rm V}}{\pi \times r_{\rm L}^2} = \frac{0.8 \times 1 \times 10^{-3}\ {\rm W} \times \cos 30°}{\pi (100\ {\rm cm})^2} = 2.2 \times 10^{-8} \frac{\rm W}{\rm cm^2}.$$

From Table 14-13, we find that the maximum permissible irradiance, $E_{\rm MPE}$ for 632.8-nm light, for an exposure time of 60 seconds, is calculated as follows:

$$E_{\rm MPE} = 1.8 \times C_{\rm E} \times T_2^{-0.25} \times 10^{-3}\ {\rm W/cm^2}$$

$$T_2 = 10 \times 10^{(\alpha - 1.5)/98.5} = 10 \times 10^{\left(\frac{8.7 - 1.5}{98.5}\right)} = 11.8$$

$$C_{\rm E} = \frac{\alpha}{1.5} = \frac{8.7}{1.5} = 5.8,$$

therefore,

$$E_{\rm MPE} = 1.8 \times 5.8 \times (11.8)^{-0.25} \times 10^{-3}\ {\rm W/cm^2} = 5.6 \times 10^{-3}\ {\rm W/cm^2}.$$

Since the reflected exposure is less than the MPE, no eye protection is required to view the reflection from the specified location.

TABLE 14-13. Maximum Permissible Exposure (MPE) for Extended Source Ocular Exposure to a Laser Beam for Exposure Durations >0.7 second

λ (μm)	EXPOSURE TIME (s)	MPE
Photochemical		
For $\alpha \leq 11$ milliradian, the MPE is expressed as irradiance and radiant exposure		
0.400–0.600	0.7–100	$C_B \times 10^{-2}$ J/cm^2
0.400–0.600	100–3 $\times$ 10^4	$C_B \times 10^{-4}$ W/cm^2
For $\alpha > 11$ mrad, the MPE is expressed as radiance and integrated radiance		
0.400–0.600	0.7–1 $\times$ 10^4	100C_B J/cm^2/sr
0.400–0.600	1 $\times$ 10^4–3 $\times$ 10^4	$C_B \times 10^{-2}$ W/cm^2/sr
Thermal		
0.400–0.700	0.7–T_2	$1.8C_E \times t^{0.75} \times 10^{-3}$ J/cm^2
0.400–0.700	T_2–3 $\times$ 10^4	$1.8C_E \times T_2^{-0.25} \times 10^{-3}$ W/cm^2

$C_B = 1$ for $\lambda = 0.400$ to 0.450 μm and for $\lambda = 0.450$ to 0.600 μm, $C_B = 10^{20(\lambda - 0.450)}$. $C_E = 1$ for $\alpha < 1.5$ mrad, $\alpha/1.5$ mrad for 1.5 mrad $< \alpha < 100$ mrad, and $\alpha^2/150$ for $\alpha > 100$ mrad.

$T_2 = 10 \times 10^{(\alpha - 1.5)/98.5}$ for $\lambda = 0.400$ to 1.400 μm. Wavelengths must be expressed in μm and the angle α in milliradians for calculations.

For exposures >0.7 second and for $\lambda = 0.400$ to 0.600 μm, MPEs are based on retinal hazards that include both thermal and photochemical effects. Normally, both effects have to be calculated, and the more conservative value is used.

Reproduced with permission from the Laser Institute of America from *The Safe Use of Lasers* (ANSI Z136.1–2000).

Protective Eyewear

The eye can be protected against laser radiation by means of protective goggles that attenuate the intensity of the laser light while transmitting enough ambient light for safe visibility. The attenuation of light by a protective goggle is given by its *optical density*, OD, which is defined by

$$OD = \log \frac{E \text{ (or } H)}{\text{MPE}}, \tag{14.19}$$

where MPE is the maximum allowable exposure on the cornea, E is the irradiance, and H is the radiant exposure. The determination of the minimum required density is illustrated in the following example:

EXAMPLE 14.12

A 10-W CO$_2$ laser (10.6 μm, CW) is used for polymer welding. The aperture is 3.5 mm and the divergence, ϕ, is 4 milliradians. An aversion response time of 10 seconds is assumed for this "invisible" laser. What is the OD of laser safety eyewear for the "worst-case" exposure?

Solution

The irradiance at the aperture of the laser is given by Eq. (14.13):

$$E = \frac{P}{\text{area}} = \frac{10 \text{ W}}{\frac{\pi}{4} (0.35 \text{ cm})^2} = 103.9 \frac{\text{W}}{\text{cm}^2}.$$

The MPE for the eye is found in Table 11-8 to be 0.1 W/cm². The required OD is calculated with Eq. (14.19):

$$\text{OD} = \log \frac{E}{\text{MPE}} = \log \left(\frac{103.9 \text{ W/cm}^2}{0.1 \text{ W/cm}^2} \right) = 3.$$

EXAMPLE 14.13

A He–Ne laser has a power output of 15 mW CW. The $1/e^2$ beam diameter at the aperture is 1.7 mm, and the beam divergence is 1.0 milliradian. What is the minimum OD of goggles in order to comply with the MPE recommended in the ANSI standard for intrabeam exposure to the 632.8-nm (0.6328-μm) radiation from this laser at a distance of 1 m from the aperture?

Solution

Since laser safety calculations are made on the basis of the $1/e$ diameter, the $1/e^2$ diameter must be converted into the $1/e$ diameter. The relationship between the $1/e$ diameter and the $1/e^2$ diameter is given by Eq. (14.6) as

$$D_{(1/e)} = \frac{D_{(1/e^2)}}{\sqrt{2}}.$$

From the above relation, the aperture diameter used to evaluate laser safety is given by

$$a = \frac{0.17 \text{ cm}}{\sqrt{2}} = 0.12 \text{ cm aperture diameter.}$$

Neglecting the attenuation of the beam by 100 cm of air, we find the irradiance at 100 cm from the laser aperture, with Eq. (14.14), to be

$$E = \frac{P}{\frac{\pi}{4} \left[a^2 + r^2 \phi^2 \right]} = \frac{1.5 \times 10^{-3} \text{ W}}{\frac{\pi}{4} \left[(0.12 \text{ cm})^2 + (100 \text{ cm})^2 (1 \times 10^{-3} \text{ radian})^2 \right]}$$

$$E = 7.8 \times 10^{-2} \frac{\text{W}}{\text{cm}^2}.$$

In Table 14-9, we find that the MPE for the eye for 0.25-second viewing time (the aversion response time) of a He–Ne beam is 2.5×10^{-3} W/cm². The minimum required OD is, from Eq. (14.19):

$$OD = \log \frac{E}{MPE} = \log \frac{7.8 \times 10^{-2} \dfrac{W}{cm^2}}{2.5 \times 10^{-3} \dfrac{W}{cm^2}} = 1.5.$$

EXAMPLE 14.14

A ruby laser, $\lambda = 694$ nm, is pulsed at a rate of 2 pulses per minute. Each pulse is 20 nanoseconds wide and contains 10 J of energy. The 1/e diameter of the exit beam is 18 mm, and the beam divergence is 7 milliradians. What is the minimum OD required to comply with the recommendations in ANSI Z136.1, assuming a worst-case exposure?

Solution

The radiant exposure per pulse is

$$H = \frac{10\,J}{\dfrac{\pi}{4}(1.8\text{ cm})^2} = 3.93 \frac{J}{cm^2}.$$

From Table 14-8, we find that the MPE value for a pulse 2×10^{-8} second wide is

$$H\,(MPE) = 5.0 \times 10^{-7}\,J/cm^2,$$

and since the time between pulses is more than 0.25 second, they are considered singly. The minimum required OD, therefore, is:

$$OD = \log \frac{H}{MPE} = \log\left(\frac{3.93\ J/cm^2}{5 \times 10^{-7}\ J/cm^2}\right) = 6.9 \text{ at } 694 \text{ nm.}$$

The optimum eyewear provides maximum attenuation of the laser light while transmitting the maximum amount of ambient light. When specifying laser safety eyewear, therefore, the *luminous transmission* must be considered along with the OD. The optimum goggle is the one that provides maximum attenuation of the laser light while transmitting the maximum amount of ambient light. Luminous transmission is given as the percent transmission of light from a standard source whose spectral distribution is equivalent to that of a blackbody at 6500 Å. This source

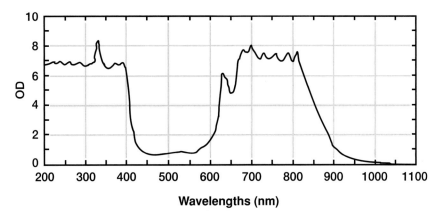

Figure 14-9. Optical density variation with wavelength from one of the commercially available goggles for protection against laser light. The luminous transmission of this glass for a standard C source is 12%. (Courtesy of ThorLabs, Inc., Newton, NJ.)

is known as the Commission International d'Electricité (CIE) standard source C and is approximately equivalent to average daylight. Figure 14-9 shows the light-absorbing properties of one of the commercially available goggles. The curve shows that although these goggles provide an OD of 8 for the 694-nm wavelength light from a ruby laser, they are almost useless for protection against the 455–515-nm wavelengths from He–Ne lasers.

When choosing laser safety eyewear for protection against laser light, the resistance of the lenses to damage from the laser beam must be considered. The absorption of laser energy by the lenses of the protective eyewear leads to an increase in temperature of the lens. The lens must be capable of absorbing the amount of energy under the expected operating conditions without suffering changes in light transmission, without softening or shattering, and without suffering other surface damage that might impair its usefulness or create a hazard to the user. It must be understood that no single lens material is useful for all wavelengths and all radiant exposures. In choosing protective eyewear, therefore, careful consideration must be given to the laser operating parameters, the MPE levels, the conditions of use, and the response of the protective eyewear to the insult from the laser beam under the most severe conditions of use. Pulse duration is another special consideration for short-pulse protective eyewear, since nonlinear effects can occur and defeat the protective characteristics of the protective eyewear. The protective eyewear that is finally chosen must meet the safety criteria in each of these categories.

 EXAMPLE 14.15

A Nd:YAG pulsed laser is used for cutting stainless steel sheet metal; it has the following specifications:

$\lambda = 1064$ nm,
PRF $= 300$ Hz,
Pulse width $= 0.1$ millisecond $= 0.1 \times 10^{-3}$ second,
$Q = 30$ J/pulse,
$a = 7$ mm $= 0.7$ cm, and
$\phi = 6$ milliradians $= 6 \times 10^{-3}$ radian.

(a) What is the radiant exposure, J/cm² per pulse, at the laser's aperture?

(b) Calculate the MPE for this laser for an exposure time $T = 10$ seconds, which is the aversion response time for nonvisible light. Use all three rules for pulsed lasers.

(c) What OD is required for laser safety goggles for this laser if exposure may be at the aperture?

(d) What is the diffuse reflection eye-hazard distance for this laser?

(e) What is the eye-hazard distance for direct intra-beam viewing?

Solution

(a) The radiant energy at the aperture is given by Eq. (14.8):

$$H = \frac{\text{Energy}}{\text{Area}} = \frac{30\dfrac{\text{J}}{\text{pulse}}}{\pi \left(\dfrac{0.7\text{cm}}{2}\right)^2} = 78\dfrac{\text{J}}{\text{cm}^2}\dfrac{}{\text{pulse}}.$$

(b) *MPE according to rule 1 (exposure to only 1 pulse)*—Using the values given in Table 14-8, the MPE for 1.064 μm, 0.1-millisecond exposure is

$$\text{MPE} = 9.0\; C_C t^{0.75} \times 10^{-3} \text{ J/cm}^2,$$

where

$$C_C = 1$$
$$t = 0.1 \times 10^{-3} \text{ seconds}$$

$$\text{MPE}_{\text{rule 1}} = 9.0 \times 1.0 \times (0.1 \times 10^{-3})^{0.75} \times 10^{-3} = 9 \times 10^{-6} \text{ J/cm}^2.$$

MPE according to rule 2 (average power limit)—Here we calculate the MPE based on the viewing time divided by the number of pulses during the viewing time. Using the MPE expression from Table 14-8, and using $t = 10$ seconds, we have the total quantity of energy that enters the eye during the 10-second exposure.

$$H = 9.0 \times 1.0 \times (10)^{0.75} \times 10^{-3} = 5.1 \times 10^{-2} \text{ J/cm}^2.$$

During the 10-second exposure time the total number of pulses that enter the eye is

$$n = 300 \frac{\text{pulses}}{\text{s}} \times 10 \text{ seconds} = 3000 \text{ pulses.}$$

The average radiant exposure per pulse, therefore, is the MPE for radiant exposure per pulse.

$$\text{MPE}_{\text{rule 2}} = \frac{5.1 \times 10^{-2} \frac{\text{J}}{\text{cm}^2}}{3 \times 10^3 \text{ pulses}} = 1.7 \times 10^{-5} \frac{\text{J/cm}^2}{\text{pulse}}.$$

MPE according to rule 3—Here we calculate the MPE by multiplying the single pulse MPE by a dose-reduction factor, C_p. From Eq. (14.11), we calculate C_p:

$$C_p = n^{-0.25} = (3 \times 10^3)^{-0.25} = 0.135.$$

Then, the MPE according to rule 3 is calculated as

$$\text{MPE}_{\text{rule 3}} = \text{MPE}_{\text{rule 1}} \times C_p = 9 \times 10^{-6} \text{ J/cm}^2 \times 0.135 = 1.2 \times 10^{-6} \text{ J/cm}^2.$$

The MPE according to rule 3, 1.2×10^{-6} J/cm^2, is the smallest MPE, and therefore, is the one be applied in this case.

(c) The OD required for eye protection is calculated with Eq. (14.19):

$$\text{OD} = \log \frac{H}{\text{MPE}} = \log \left(\frac{78 \frac{\text{J}}{\text{cm}^2}}{1.2 \times 10^{-6} \frac{\text{J}}{\text{cm}^2}} \right) = 7.8.$$

(d) The diffuse reflection eye-hazard distance for the MPE of 1.2×10^{-6} J $\cdot$ cm^{-2} is calculated with the aid of Eq. (14.18), and using the MPE(H) instead of the MPE(E), and the energy in a pulse, Q, rather than the power P in the equation.

$$E = \frac{\rho \times P \times \cos \theta_V}{\pi \times r_L^2}.$$

If we solve Eq. (14.18) for r_L, which in this case is the *nominal ocular hazard distance*, r_{NOHD}, we have, for CW lasers:

$$r_{\text{NOHD}} = \sqrt{\frac{\rho \times P \times \cos \theta_V}{\pi \times \text{MPE}(E)}}, \tag{14.20a}$$

or, for pulsed lasers that emit Q J/pulse:

$$r_{\text{NOHD}} = \sqrt{\frac{\rho \times Q \times \cos \theta_V}{\pi \times \text{MPE}(H)}}.$$ (14.20b)

The worst viewing scenario is 100% reflection, $\rho = 1$, and very close to a viewing angle, θ_V, of $0°$. Since we are dealing here with a pulsed laser, we use Eq. (14.20b).

$$r_{\text{NOHD}} = \sqrt{\frac{1 \times 30\,\text{J} \times \cos 0°}{\pi \times 1.2 \times 10^{-6}\,\dfrac{\text{J}}{\text{cm}^2}}} = 2.82 \times 10^3 \text{ cm}.$$

(e) To calculate the NOHD for intrabeam viewing of a pulsed laser we modify Eq. (14.15) by substituting the pulse energy, J, for the power, P, and the $\text{MPE}(H)$ for the $\text{MPE}(E)$:

$$r_{\text{NOHD}} = \frac{1}{\phi \text{ radians}} \sqrt{\frac{Q\,\text{J}}{\dfrac{\pi}{4} \times \text{MPE}(H)\dfrac{\text{J}}{\text{cm}^2}} - (a \text{ cm})^2}.$$ (14.21)

When we substitute the respective numbers into Eq. (14.21), we have

$$r_{\text{NOHD}} = \frac{1}{6 \times 10^{-3} \text{ rad}} \sqrt{\frac{30\,\text{J}}{\dfrac{\pi}{4} \times 1.2 \times 10^{-6}\,\dfrac{\text{J}}{\text{cm}^2}} - (0.7 \text{ cm})^2}$$

$$= 9.4 \times 10^5 \text{ cm} = 9.4 \text{ km}.$$

Safety Measurements

Evaluation of the safety aspects of a laser includes measurement of power or energy and beam divergence. Two general types of power and energy instruments are used: one based on the photoelectric effect, which is very fast and is suitable for Q-switched measurements; and one based on a thermal effect, which is very stable and wavelength-independent but is slower and less sensitive than photoelectric devices.

Power and Energy

Photoelectric Devices. These instruments employ either photomultipliers or photodiodes as the detection elements. In either case, the output signal is directly proportional to the irradiance, and the meter is usually calibrated to give average power levels for CW or high PRFs; connectors are provided to display pulses on an oscilloscope and thus to determine the energy per pulse, pulse width, pulse frequency,

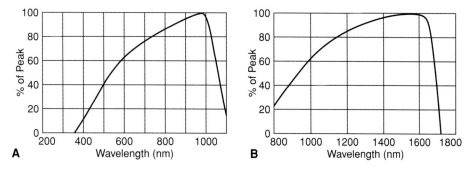

Figure 14-10. Calibration curve for a photoelectric detector. **A.** Silicon diode **B.** In GaAs detector. (Courtesy of Coherent, Inc, Santa Clara, CA.)

and peak power. Like most quantum electronic devices, photoelectric detectors are highly energy-dependent and each instrument must be calibrated. A typical calibration curve, as supplied by the manufacturer, is shown in Figure 14-10.

EXAMPLE 14.16

The output from a 60-Hz pulsed ruby laser, $\lambda = 694.3$ nm, is measured with a photodiode-type meter. With the aid of an oscilloscope, we find rectangular pulses as shown below:

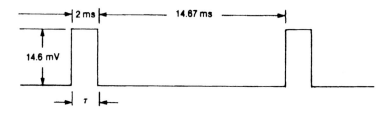

The meter reading, which is proportional to the average power, is 35 μA. Calculate the

(a) duty cycle (fraction of time that lasing actions occurs),

(b) average power, P, μW,

(c) peak power, P_0, μW, and

(d) energy per pulse, J.

Solution

(a) The duty cycle is calculated as follows:

$$\text{duty cycle} = \frac{\text{on time}}{\text{on time} + \text{off time}} = \frac{2}{2 + 14.67} = 0.12.$$

(b) The meter was calibrated at 920 nm (0.92 μm), where its calibration curve shows the relative response to be 0.98. At 694.3 nm, the relative response is 0.9; the calibration chart informs us that the meter's average current output is 0.48 μA/μW. The average power represented by a meter reading of 35 μA is

$$P = \frac{\dfrac{0.98}{0.9} \times 35\,\mu\text{A}}{0.48\dfrac{\mu\text{A}}{\mu\text{W}}} = 79.4\,\mu\text{W}.$$

(c) Peak power P_0 may be calculated by any of the following methods:

$$P_0 = \frac{\text{average power}}{\text{duty cycle}} = \frac{79.4\,\mu\text{W}}{0.12} = 662\,\mu\text{W}; \tag{14.22}$$

$$P_0 = \frac{\text{average power}}{\text{pulse frequency} \times \text{pulse width}} = \frac{P}{n \times \tau} \tag{14.23}$$

$$= \frac{79.4\,\mu\text{W}}{60\text{ s}^{-1} \times 2 \times 10^{-3}\text{ s}} = 662\,\mu\text{W};$$

$$P_0 = \frac{\text{pulse height}}{\text{calibration factor}}$$

$$= \frac{\dfrac{0.98}{0.9} \times 14.6\text{ mV}}{24\dfrac{\text{mV}}{\text{mW}}} = 0.662\text{ mW} = 662\,\mu\text{W}. \tag{14.24}$$

(d) Energy per pulse, U, is given by

$$Q_0 = P_0\text{ W} \times 1\,\frac{\text{J/s}}{\text{W}} \times \tau \text{ seconds}$$

$$= P_0\text{ W} \times \tau \text{ seconds} \times 1\,\frac{\text{J/s}}{\text{W}} \tag{14.25}$$

$$= 662 \times 10^{-6}\text{ W} \times 2 \times 10^{-3}\text{ seconds} \times 1\frac{\text{J/s}}{\text{W}} = 1.32 \times 10^{-6}\,\frac{\text{J}}{\text{pulse}}.$$

Thermal Devices. Light energy can also be measured by transforming it into heat energy and then measuring the heat. Thermocouples and bolometers are the commonly used transducers for this purpose. A *thermocouple* consists of two wires of different metals joined together at the ends. If the two junctions are at different temperatures, a current, whose magnitude depends on the temperature difference, flows through the circuit. This current can be measured and its magnitude related to the intensity of the light incident on the detector. In practice, in order to increase the sensitivity of the instrument, a number of thermocouples are joined together to form a thermopile. Bismuth–silver, copper–constantan, and manganim–constantan are the metals used in thermopiles. The surfaces that receive the light energy are coated either with lampblack, gold black, or parson's black, all of which have very high absorbances ($\geq 95\%$) for the wavelengths associated with most lasers.

A *ballistic thermopile* is a frequently used transducing element for measuring the energy in a laser pulse. This device employs two absorbers, one of the absorbers absorbs energy from the laser light to which it is exposed and thus experiences a temperature rise, while the other is a reference absorber that is exposed only to the ambient light. The temperature difference between them generates a voltage difference that is quantitatively related to the energy in the pulse of laser light. The ballistic thermopile is useful for measuring pulses in the range of about 1 mJ to 100 J.

A *bolometer* is a resistive element whose electrical resistance is a function of temperature. One special form of such a circuit element is the *thermistor*, which is a semiconductor with a high negative-temperature coefficient of resistivity. The resistive element, enclosed in a light-receiving case that is treated with lampblack to maximize energy absorption, forms one of the arms of a bridge that is balanced in the absence of the laser light. The incident light raises the temperature of the bolometer, thus changing its resistance and unbalancing the bridge. The degree of unbalance is quantitatively related to the incident light energy.

Pyroelectric detectors are sensitive detectors that depend on the pyroelectric properties of certain polar crystals, such as tourmaline and gallium nitride (GaN). Pyroelectric materials generate an electrical potential difference when positive and negative charges move to opposite ends of the crystal as a result of a temperature change. Laser light incident on the surface of the detector increases the temperature of the surface, thereby creating a current flow within the crystal and a voltage change across the crystal. The change in voltage is proportional to the illumination from the laser. The response of a pyroelectric detector is energy dependent, and depends on the type of crystal.

Detectors based on thermal effects are generally less sensitive than quantum devices. However, they are wavelength-independent, very stable, and easy to calibrate; they retain their calibration for long periods of time.

RADIOFREQUENCY RADIATION AND MICROWAVES

Radiofrequency (RF) radiation is defined arbitrarily as electromagnetic radiation in the frequency range of 3 kHz to 300 MHz, while the arbitrary definition of microwaves includes electromagnetic radiation whose frequencies range from 300 MHz to 3000 GHz. Frequency band designations are listed in Table 14-14; industrial, scientific, and medical applications of RF radiation and microwaves have been assigned

TABLE 14-14. Microwave and Radio-frequency Band Designations

FREQUENCY (MHz)	BAND	DESCRIPTION
0–0.00003	SELF	Sub-extremely-low frequency
0.00003–0.0003	ELF	Extremely low frequency
0.0003–0.003	VF	Voice frequency
0.003–0.03	VLF	Very low frequency
0.03–0.3	LF	Low frequency
0.3–3	MF	Medium frequency
3–30	HF	High frequency
30–300	VHF	Very high frequency
300–3,000	UHF	Ultrahigh frequency
3,000–30,000	SHF	Superhigh frequency
30,000–300,000	EHF	Extremely high frequency
300,000–3,000,000	SEHF	Supra-extremely-high frequency

Reproduced with permission from *A Practical Guide to the Determination of Human Exposure to Radiofrequency Fields.* Bethesda, MD: National Council on Radiation Protection & Measurement; 1993. NCRP Report 119.

the frequency bands listed in Table 14-15, and radar frequency bands are listed in Table 14-16.

Although RF and microwaves are non-ionizing radiations, many devices, such as klystrons, that generate these radiations also generate X-rays. Survey meters that are used to check for the presence of X-rays from microwave generators are specially designed for use in the presence of RF or microwave radiation. Such specially designed survey meters must be used, otherwise erroneous X-ray readings will be obtained that may lead to unsafe conditions.

Sources

NIR devices are widely encountered in our daily lives, including radio and television transmitters; communication systems, such as mobile telephones, GPS, and radar, both civilian and military; home appliances and convenience gadgets, such as garage-door openers, remote auto-door openers and engine starters, and microwave ovens; industrial heat sealers; and medical diathermy and imaging machines. Generally, the power densities to which the members of the public are exposed in the sea of electromagnetic energy radiating from these sources are on the order of microwatts per square centimeter, which is very low relative to their potential for harm.

TABLE 14-15. Industrial, Scientific, and Medical (ISM) Frequency Bands

FREQUENCY (MHz)	λ
13.56	22.12 m
27.12	11.06 m
40.68	7.37 m
915	32.8 cm
2,450	12.2 cm
5,800	5.2 cm
22,125	1.4 cm

TABLE 14-16. *Radar Bands*

FREQUENCY (GHz)	BAND
1–2	L
2–4	S
4–8	C
8–12	X
12–18	Ku
18–27	K
27–40	Ka
40–75	V
75–110	W
110–300	mm
300–3000	μm

Communications

The short wavelengths in the microwave frequency bands, on the order of millimeters to centimeters, contrast sharply with the very much longer wavelengths, on the order of tens to hundreds of meters, in the RF portion of the electromagnetic spectrum. This wavelength difference is the basis for the widespread application of microwaves in communications and in radar. The short wavelengths allow electromagnetic energy to be transmitted through the air or through free space in sharply focused, intense beams similar to a beam of light. Furthermore, these focused, high-frequency beams can carry more information than can be transmitted by the more conventional RF waves. This increased information-carrying capacity of microwaves is due to the bandwidths associated with microwaves. Information is transmitted in a band of frequencies. For example, speech requires a bandwidth of about 3000 Hz, music is transmitted in a bandwidth of about 20,000 Hz, and television requires a bandwidth of about 4 MHz. In the case of microwaves, a 200-MHz bandwidth centered on 2000 MHz carrier frequency—that is, a 10% bandwidth—has more frequency bands available for transmission of speech and music than all the AM and FM frequencies combined.

In radar applications, a short, intense, highly focused pulse of microwave radiation is emitted from an antenna. If this emitted radiation pulse strikes an object, some of the incident energy is reflected back to the radar antenna, which is connected to a receiver as well as a transmitter, and is detected as an incoming signal by the receiver. The distance between the object and the radar is determined from the time between the emitted pulse and the arrival of the reflected signal. The direction of the object is determined from the direction in which the antenna was pointed. From these two measurements, the location of the object, in polar coordinates, can be determined at any moment. If the object is moving, it can be tracked by continuous measurements; its speed and direction can thus be determined.

Antennas

The focusing of energy into relatively narrow, intense beams is possible because the size of microwave antennas greatly exceeds the wavelength of the emitted radiation. A microwave antenna usually consists of a microwave-feeding device, such as a dipole or a horn connected to the microwave generator, and a parabolic reflector, as shown in Figure 14-11.

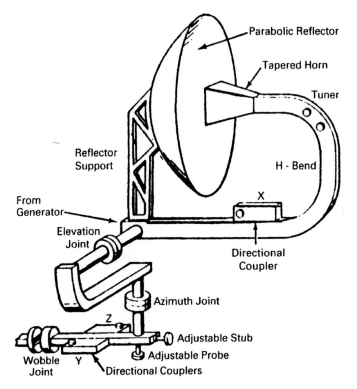

Figure 14-11. Microwave antenna showing the feeder (tapered horn) and the parabolic reflector.

In a dipole, electromagnetic energy is radiated from solid conductors that are coupled to a transmitter. The horn is an opening in a waveguide from which electromagnetic radiation emerges in the direction in which the aperture is facing. The microwave feed is mounted at the focus of the parabolic reflector and emits radiation into the reflector. The radiation is then reflected in a (theoretically) parallel beam. However, the beam does spread, with the amount of spread being inversely proportional to the size of the reflector. The measure of beam spread is called the *beamwidth*. The beamwidth is defined by the width of the beam at the half-power points and is measured in degrees. The ability of an antenna to concentrate the radiated electromagnetic energy into a beam is described by a figure of merit called the *antenna gain*. The gain of an antenna is defined as the ratio of the intensity of the radiated signal in the far-field beam to the intensity at the same point if the same amount of transmitter power were radiated by an isotropic antenna.

$$\text{Antenna gain} = G = \frac{\text{power from antenna}}{\text{power from isotropic radiator}} = \frac{P}{P_0}. \tag{14.26}$$

The gain of an antenna is related to its area and to the wavelength of the radiation. For a parabolic antenna, this relationship is given by

$$G = \frac{4\pi A}{\lambda^2}, \tag{14.27}$$

where A is the area of the antenna aperture and λ is the wavelength of the radiation.

All microwave antennas can be used either for transmission or reception of microwave energy, depending on whether the dipole or horn is connected to a transmitter or to a receiver. In either case, the gain of the antenna is the same in both applications. Antenna gain is usually expressed in decibels (dB) relative to a reference power density, rather than as a power density ratio, as in Eq. (14.26). Gain in decibels is given by

$$G = 10 \log \frac{P_2}{P_1} \text{ dB,} \qquad\qquad (14.28)$$

where P_1 is a reference power density and P_2 is the power density of interest. Gain does not increase the power of a transmitter, it simply concentrates the energy into a beam of higher energy density than in the case of 4π (isotropic) radiation. As a rough rule of thumb, a 6-dB increase in gain will double the range of the microwave device. Generally, the antenna gain increases as the size of the dish increases relative to the wavelength of the radiation increases. Thus, when the diameter of the dish is equal to the wavelength, the antenna gain is 2.55 dB, when the dish diameter is eight times greater than the wavelength, the antenna gain is 8.5 dB.

 EXAMPLE 14.17

A "standard gain horn" designed for use in the 1.7- to 2.6-GHz frequency range has a gain of 16.5 dB with reference to an isotropic radiator. To what power ratio does this gain correspond?

Solution

Substituting the value for the gain into Eq. (14.28) gives

$$16.5 = 10 \log \frac{P_2}{P_1}$$

$$\frac{P_2}{P_1} = \log^{-1} \frac{16.5}{10} = 44.7.$$

 EXAMPLE 14.18

A 16 in. (0.41 m) diameter parabolic dish antenna for a WiFi application operates at a frequency of 2.5 GHz. What is the antenna gain in dB?

Solution

The antenna gain is calculated with Eq. (14.27). The area of the aperture is

$$A = \frac{\pi}{4} (0.41 \text{ m})^2 = 0.13 \text{ m}^2, \text{ and the wavelength is}$$

$$\lambda = \frac{c}{f} = \frac{3 \times 10^8 \dfrac{\text{m}}{\text{s}}}{2.5 \times 10^9 \text{ s}^{-1}} = 0.12 \text{ m}.$$

Therefore,

$$G = \frac{4\pi A}{\lambda^2} = \frac{4\pi \times 0.13 \text{ m}^2}{(0.12 \text{ m})^2} = 113.5,$$

$$G_{\text{dB}} = 10 \times \log G = 10 \times \log 113.5 = 20.5.$$

The quantitative nature of the radiation fields changes with increasing distance from the antenna (Fig. 14-12). Close to the antenna is a region, called the *near field,* where not all the energy in the electromagnetic field around the antenna is radiated. Part of the energy, called the *reactive* energy, is stored in the field and is recovered and reemitted during successive oscillations, in a manner analogous to the stored electrical and magnetic energy that is interchanged between the capacitor and inductor in a low-frequency resonant circuit. In the near field, the electric and magnetic fields are not perpendicular to each other. Their exact orientation varies from point to

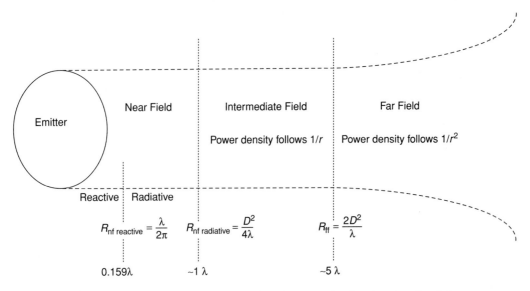

Figure 14-12. Radiation zones. Distances from antenna for approximating the several radiation zones as a function of antenna size and radiation wavelength.

point because the radiator is not an ideal "point source," but is a geometric object with actual dimensions. This leads to differences in path length of the radiation due to different points of origin on the antenna, which in turn lead to differences in phase and destructive and constructive interference of the electromagnetic waves. The end results of the interference are alternating points of maxima and minima in radiation intensity. Thus, the simple relationship among power density, electric field strength, and magnetic field strength illustrated in Example 2.17 and Eq. (2.74) does not apply to near-field conditions. At a distance less than $\lambda/2\pi$, the reactive energy exceeds the radiated energy, and that potion of the near field is called the *reactive near field*; the reactive energy is equal to the radiated energy at this distance. At distances from the antenna aperture greater than $\lambda/2\pi$, the proportion of reactive energy decreases rapidly until the end of the near field, at a distance R_{nf} from the antenna

$$R_{nf\,radiative} = \frac{D^2}{4\lambda}, \tag{14.29}$$

where D is the maximum linear dimension of the parabolic reflecting dish.

Beyond the end of the near field and the start of the far field is a transition region called the *intermediate field* (also called the *Fresnel* region), where the simple relationship of Eq. (2.74) still does not exist. In this region, electric and magnetic field strengths decrease linearly with distance from the aperture; that is, they follow a $1/r$ relationship.

In the far field (also called the *Fraunhofer region*), the electric and magnetic fields are perpendicular to each other, thus making possible meaningful measurements of power density. The electric and magnetic field strengths decrease linearly with increasing distance from the antenna, and the power density follows the inverse square law, that is, it falls off as the square of the distance from the antenna (in the context of microwave radiation safety, the microwave energy flux is called the *power density*; it is represented by S and is expressed as power per unit area, i.e., as W/m^2 or as mW/cm^2).

$$\frac{S_1}{S_2} = \frac{R_2^2}{R_1^2}. \tag{14.30}$$

The distance to the start of the far-field region from the radiator depends on the size of the antenna and on the wavelength of the radiation. Although there is no sharp boundary marking the beginning of the far-field region, *for measurement and hazard-estimation purposes*, its distance from a parabolic antenna whose greatest linear dimension is D may be approximated by

$$R_{ff} = \frac{2D^2}{\lambda}. \tag{14.31}$$

A rule of thumb says that the far-field distance starts at about 10 times the diameter of the reflecting dish.

EXAMPLE 14.19

At about what distance from a 2-m-diameter antenna that is transmitting a beam of 3000-MHz (10 cm) microwaves can we expect to find far-field conditions?

Solution

From Eq. (14.31), the estimated distance is

$$R_{ff} = \frac{2D^2}{\lambda} = \frac{2\,(2\text{ m})^2}{0.1\text{ m}} = 80\text{ m}.$$

Until this distance, the beam undergoes very little divergence; at this distance, the beam starts to spread and to become conical in shape.

The average power density at a uniformly illuminated antenna aperture is simply

$$S_0 = \frac{P}{A}, \tag{14.32}$$

where

S_0 = average power density,
P = microwave power output, and
A = area of aperture.

In the near field, the maximum is four times greater than the average power density. The maximum power density in the near field, therefore, is

$$S_{nf} = \frac{4P}{A} = 4S_0. \tag{14.33}$$

For purposes of safety assessment, the power density throughout the near field is considered to be $4S_0$. In the intermediate field, the power density decreases linearly with distance. The power density within the intermediate field at a distance R from the antenna may therefore be estimated from

$$S_{if} = S_{nf}\frac{R_{nf}}{R} = 4S_0\frac{R_{nf}}{R}. \tag{14.34}$$

In the far field, for distances R from the antenna greater than $2\,D^2/\lambda$, the power density at a distance R from an antenna whose aperture area is A and whose gain is G, without reflection from the ground, is

$$S_{ff} = G \times \frac{P}{4\pi R^2} = \frac{AP}{\lambda^2 R^2}. \tag{14.35}$$

Ground reflection of the radiation increases the power density by a factor of 4, or 6 dB ($10 \times \log 4 = 6$).

EXAMPLE 14.20

To estimate the hazard from a dipole antenna that radiates 1000 W of 3000-MHz microwaves from a circular parabolic reflector 0.75 m in diameter, calculate

(a) the mean power density at the aperture,

(b) the maximum power density in the near field,

(c) the distance to the far field,

(d) the power density at a distance of 250 m, and

(e) the distance at which the power density will be 10 mW/cm² (100 W/m²).

Solution

(a) $S_0 = \dfrac{P}{A} = \dfrac{1000 \text{ W}}{\dfrac{\pi}{4}(0.75 \text{ m})^2} = 2263\ \dfrac{\text{W}}{\text{m}^2} = 226.3\ \dfrac{\text{mW}}{\text{cm}^2}.$

(b) $S_{nf} = 4 S_0 = 4 \times 226.3\ \dfrac{\text{mW}}{\text{cm}^2} = 905\ \dfrac{\text{mW}}{\text{cm}^2}.$

(c) $R_{ff} = \dfrac{2D^2}{\lambda}$, where

$$\lambda = \frac{c}{f} = \frac{3 \times 10^8\ \frac{\text{m}}{\text{s}}}{3000 \times 10^6 \text{s}^{-1}} = 0.1 \text{ m}.$$

Therefore,

$$R_{ff} = \frac{2(0.75 \text{ m})^2}{0.1 \text{ m}} = 11.25 \text{ m}.$$

(d) $S_{ff} = \dfrac{AP}{\lambda^2 R^2} = \dfrac{\left[\dfrac{\pi}{4}(0.75 \text{ m})^2\right] \times 1000 \text{ W}}{(0.1 \text{ m})^2 \times (250 \text{ m})^2} = 0.71\ \dfrac{\text{W}}{\text{m}^2} = 0.071\ \dfrac{\text{mW}}{\text{cm}^2}.$

(e) If we solve Eq. (14.35) for R, and substitute the appropriate values, we have

$$R = \sqrt{\frac{AP}{\lambda S_{ff}}} = \sqrt{\frac{\left[\dfrac{\pi}{4}(0.75 \text{ m})^2 \times 1000 \text{ W}\right]}{(0.1 \text{ m})^2 \times 100\dfrac{\text{W}}{\text{m}^2}}} = 21 \text{ m}.$$

Power level is sometimes expressed in terms of dBm or dBw. The reference power for dBm is 1 mW, and for dBw the reference power is 1 W. A power output of 1 mW, expressed as dBm, would be

$$dBm = 10 \log \frac{P}{1 \text{ mW}}$$

$$= 10 \log \frac{1 \text{ mW}}{1 \text{ mW}} = 0. \tag{14.36}$$

EXAMPLE 14.21

An internet wireless access point that is IEEE 802.11g compliant has an output power level of 15 dBm. What is the power output of this unit?

Solution

According to Eq. (14.36),

$$15 \text{ dBm} = 10 \log \frac{P}{1 \text{ mW}}$$

$$P = 31.6 \text{ mW}.$$

Thermal Effects

In its interaction with matter, microwave energy may either be reflected, as in the case of metals; transmitted with little energy loss to the transmitting medium, as in the case of glass; or absorbed by the irradiated matter and thus raise the temperature of the absorber. This heating is attributed to two effects: the main mechanism is believed to be joule heating due to ionic currents induced by the electric fields that are set up within the absorbing medium by the radiation. The second mechanism is due to the interaction between polar molecules in the absorber and the applied high-frequency electric field. The alternating electric field causes these polar molecules to oscillate back and forth in an attempt to maintain the proper alignment in the electric field. These oscillations are resisted by other intermolecular forces, and the work done by the alternating electric field in overcoming these resistive forces is converted into heat.

The 27-MHz band is widely used in industry in *dielectric heating*, that is, for heating materials that are not electrically conducting, such as in the case of wood being dried or glued, plastics being heat-sealed, textiles undergoing heat treatment, etc. The 915- and 2450-MHz bands are used for *microwave heating* in industry and in the home. Heating in both these modes is very rapid. In dielectric heating, the object to be heated is placed between two electrodes across which a high-frequency voltage, on the order of 100,000 V/m, is applied. Effectively, we have an electrical capacitor, in which the material to be heated is the dielectric. Most dielectric materials—such as ceramics, wood, paper, plastics, etc.—absorb energy when placed in an alternating electric field, because these "nonconductors" exhibit some degree of conductivity as polar molecules rotate under the influence of the alternating electric field. The *loss tangent*, or the degree of lossiness of a dielectric material, is a measure of energy absorption by this mechanism. (Lossiness should not be confused with leakage of charge through an insulater, as in the case of the pocket dosimeter shown in Fig. 6-2.) The degree of lossiness for any given material, as shown in Eq. (2.63), is a function of the frequency of the alternating electric field. Generally, the efficiency of dielectric heating is 50–60%. An application of industrial dielectric heating is given in the following example:

 EXAMPLE 14.22

A total of 500 kg of resin-bonded sand cores are to be baked in a dielectric-core oven every hour. The sand mix contains 3% water, and resin that cures at 107°C. If the specific heat of the resin-sand mixture is 1250 J/kg/°C (0.3 Btu/lb/°F), the ambient temperature is 18°C, and the overall efficiency is 50%. Calculate

(a) the power required to heat the water in the mixture from 18°C to 100°C (specific heat of water = 4178 J/kg/°C).

(b) the power required to vaporize the water (latent heat of vaporization of water = 2.25×10^6 J/kg).

(c) the power required to heat the sand–resin mixture from 18°C to 107°C.

(d) the total power required.

Solution

(a) The required power to heat the water in the mixture from 18°C to 100°C is

$$P = 0.03 \times 500 \, \frac{\text{kg}}{\text{h}} \, (100°C - 18°C) \times 4178 \, \frac{\text{J/kg}}{°C}$$

$$\times \frac{1 \text{ hour}}{3600 \text{ seconds}} = 1428 \, \frac{\text{J}}{\text{s}}.$$

(b) The required power to vaporize the water is

$$P = 0.03 \times 500 \, \frac{\text{kg}}{\text{h}} \times 2.25 \times 10^6 \, \frac{\text{J}}{\text{kg}} \times \frac{1 \text{ hour}}{3600 \text{ seconds}}$$

$$= 9375 \, \frac{\text{J}}{\text{s}}.$$

(c) The required power to heat the sand–resin mixture from 18°C to 107°C is

$$P = 0.97 \times 500 \,\frac{\text{kg}}{\text{h}} \times (107°\text{C} - 18°\text{C}) \times 1250 \,\frac{\text{J/kg}}{°\text{C}}$$

$$\times \frac{1 \text{ hour}}{3600 \text{ seconds}} = 14{,}988 \,\frac{\text{J}}{\text{s}}.$$

(d) Total power dissipated in the cores is

$$1428 + 9375 + 14{,}988 = 25{,}791 \,\frac{\text{J}}{\text{s}},$$

and, at 50% efficiency, the required power is

$$P = \frac{25{,}791 \text{ J/s}}{0.5} \times \frac{1 \text{ W}}{\text{J/s}} \times \frac{1 \text{ kW}}{1000 \text{ W}} = 51.6 \text{ kW}.$$

Microwave cooking is widely used because of the speed with which food can be heated in this way. In a conventional oven, the oven's interior, including the walls and the air, must be heated. Heat then is transferred from the hot air to the surface of the food, and it then flows by conduction into the material being cooked. The overall process is relatively inefficient and slow. In microwave cooking, on the other hand, the oven and its interior environment are not heated. All the microwave energy is absorbed by the food. Furthermore, because of the penetration of the microwaves to a depth of 1–2 cm below the surface of the food, direct deep heating of the food occurs. The volume of food that must be heated by conduction from the outer layers is thus greatly diminished. This combination of efficient energy utilization and deep heating leads to rapid cooking, as shown in Example 14.23. The deep-heating effect of microwave irradiation is the basis of medical microwave diathermy, in which beneficial amounts of heat can be applied to inflamed or injured joints and tissues inside the body without overheating the skin.

 EXAMPLE 14.23

How long will it take to heat 0.45 kg of fresh peas in 0.05-L water to a temperature of 75°C from a room temperature of 18°C in a microwave oven whose microwave power output is 700 W if the specific heat of the pea-and-water mixture is 3760 J/kg/°C?

Solution

The required amount of heat energy is

$$Q = 0.5 \text{ kg} \times 3760 \,\frac{\text{J/kg}}{°\text{C}} \times (75°\text{C} - 18°\text{C}) = 1.1 \times 10^5 \text{ J}.$$

Since there is 1 J/s in a watt,

$$1.1 \times 10^5 \, \text{J} = 700 \, \text{W} \times 1\frac{\text{J/s}}{\text{W}} \times t \text{ seconds}$$

$$t = 157 \text{ seconds} = 2.6 \text{ minutes.}$$

A microwave oven consists of a microwave generator—usually a magnetron whose maximum power output is 600–1200 W, a waveguide for conducting the microwaves from the generator to the oven cavity, the oven cavity, and a metallic rotating "stirrer" that produces a relatively uniform radiation field inside the oven by preventing the establishment of standing waves within the oven cavity. Additionally, for safety reasons, all microwave ovens have doors that are interlocked with the microwave generators, and which stop the generation of microwaves if the door should be opened while the oven is operating. If the door is not properly closed, the interlocks prevent the activation of the microwave generator. If the oven door were not properly closed, then microwave radiation would leak through the gap between the oven cavity and the door, thus creating a possible health hazard. Verification of the proper operation of the door interlock is thus an important part of the safety evaluation of a microwave oven.

Penetration Depth

As microwaves pass through a medium, they lose energy to the medium through joule heating from ionic currents induced by the electric field and through the vibration of polar molecules, such as those in water, under the influence of the changing electric field. This resulting continuous decrease in the intensity of the electromagnetic field is related exponentially to the depth of penetration into the absorbing medium by

$$E_2 = E_1 e^{-2\alpha t}, \tag{14.37}$$

where

E_1 = incident power density,
t = absorber thickness,
E_2 = power density at depth t, and
α = absorption coefficient.

The absorption coefficient α is dependent on the frequency of the radiation and on the conductivity, permittivity, and permeability of the absorber:

$$\alpha = \omega \sqrt{\frac{\mu\epsilon}{2}} \left\{ \left[1 + \left(\frac{\sigma}{\omega\epsilon} \right)^2 \right]^{\frac{1}{2}} - 1 \right\}^{\frac{1}{2}}, \tag{14.38}$$

where

ω = angular frequency = $2\pi f$,

σ = conductivity, (ohm-meter)$^{-1}$,

ϵ = permittivity = relative dielectric constant $\times \epsilon_0$, and

μ = permeability. Since the permeability of biological substances is very close to that of free space, we may use $\mu = \mu_0 = 4\pi \times 10^{-7}$ N/A.

 EXAMPLE 14.24

Calculate

(a) the absorption coefficient of muscle tissue for 2450-MHz radiation, given that $\sigma = 2.21$ per ohm-meter and the relative dielectric coefficient is 47.

(b) by what depth will 95% of the radiation be absorbed?

Solution

Substituting the appropriate values into Eq. (14.38) gives

$$\alpha = 2\pi \times 2.45$$

$$\times 10^9 \text{ s}^{-1} \sqrt{\frac{\left(4\pi \times 10^{-7}\dfrac{\text{N}}{\text{A}}\right) \times 47 \times 8.85 \times 10^{-12} \dfrac{\text{C}^2}{\text{N} \cdot \text{m}^2}}{2}}$$

$$\times \left\{ \left[1 + \left(\frac{2.21 \left(\dfrac{1}{\text{ohm} \cdot \text{m}} \right)}{2\pi \times 2.45 \times 10^9 \text{ s}^{-1} \times 47 \times 8.85 \times 10^{-12} \dfrac{\text{C}^2}{\text{N} \cdot \text{m}^2}} \right)^2 \right]^{\frac{1}{2}} - 1 \right\}^{\frac{1}{2}}$$

$$= 59.87 \text{ m}^{-1} = 0.6 \text{ cm}^{-1}.$$

(b) At the depth that will include 95% of the absorbed energy, the power density will be 5% of the initial power density. Therefore, from Eq. (14.37), we have

$$\frac{E_2}{E_1} = 0.05 = e^{-2\times 0.6 \text{ cm}^{-1}\times t \text{ cm}}$$

$$\ln 0.05 = -2 \times 0.6 \times t$$

$$t = 2.5 \text{ cm}.$$

The effectiveness of an absorber for radiation of any given wavelength is measured by the *penetration depth* in the absorber. At an absorber thickness $t = 1/\alpha$, the power density is reduced by absorption to

$$\frac{E_2}{E_1} = e^{-2} = 0.135$$

of its original value. Since the power density is reduced to 13.5%, this means that 86.5% of the energy is absorbed in a thickness equal to $1/\alpha$. This thickness is called the penetration depth, δ, and its exact value depends on the frequency of the radiation and on the electrical and magnetic properties (μ, σ, and ϵ) of the absorber. In the case of the 2450-MHz radiation of Example 14.24, the penetration depth in muscle tissue is

$$\delta = \frac{1}{\alpha} \qquad\qquad (14.39)$$

$$\delta = \frac{1}{0.6 \text{ cm}^{-1}} = 1.67 \text{ cm.}$$

The rate of heat generation in any absorber, such as biological tissue, is inversely proportional to the square of the penetration depth. Thus, a tissue with a relatively small penetration depth because of high water content, such as muscle, will heat much faster under microwave radiation than will a tissue such as fat, whose penetration depth is relatively large because of its very low water content. At 2450 MHz, for example, the penetration depths in muscle and fat are 1.7 and 11.2 cm, respectively. The rate of heating in the muscle, therefore, from a given power density, will be about $(11.2/1.7)^2 = 43.4$ times greater than in the fat. Table 14-17 lists the dielectric parameters and penetration depth for muscle tissue for several frequencies and Table 14-18 lists these parameters for several other frequencies for muscle and for fat. Note that the penetration depth decreases with increasing frequency, and that at a frequency of 100,000 MHz (100 GHz), only a very thin layer of tissue, 0.03 cm, absorbs 86.5% of the incident energy.

TABLE 14-17. Penetration Depth and Dielectric Parameters for Muscle Tissue *vs.* Frequency

FREQUENCY (MHz)	RELATIVE DIELECTRIC CONSTANT ϵ_T	CONDUCTIVITY, σ (S/m)	PENETRATION DEPTH, δ (cm)
0.1	1850	0.56	213
1.0	411	0.59	70
10	131	0.68	13.2
100	79	0.81	7.7
1000	60	1.33	3.4
10000	42	13.3	0.27
100000	8	60	0.03

Reproduced with permission from Adair ER, Peterson RC. Biological effects of radiofrequency/microwave radiation. *IEEE Trans Microw Theory Tech.* 2002; 50(3):953–962.

TABLE 14-18. Electrical Properties of Human Muscle and Fat

FREQUENCY (MHz)	MUSCLE					FAT				
	Wavelength in air (cm)	Dielectric constant ϵ_m	Conductivity σ_m (mho/m)	Depth of penetration (cm)	Wavelength in tissue (cm)	Dielectric constant ϵ_f	Conductivity σ_f (millimho/m)	Depth of penetration (cm)	Wavelength in tissue (cm)
27.12	1006	113	0.612	14.3	68.1	20	10.9–43.2	159	241
40.68	738	97.3	0.693	11.2	51.3	14.6	12.6–52.8	118	187
100	300	71.7	0.889	6.66	27	7.45	19.1–75.9	60.4	106
433	69.3	53	1.43	3.57	8.76	5.6	37.9–118	26.2	28.8
750	40	52	1.54	3.18	5.34	5.6	49.8–138	23	16.8
915	32.8	51	1.60	3.04	4.46	5.6	55.8–147	17.7	13.7
1500	20	49	1.77	2.42	2.81	5.6	70.8–171	13.9	3.41
2450	12.2	47	2.21	1.70	1.76	5.5	96.4–213	11.2	5.21

Adapted with permission from Guy AW, Lehmann JF, Stoneridge JB. Therapeutic applications of electromagnetic power. *Proc IEEE.* 1974; 62(1):55–75. Copyright © 1974 IEEE.

Biological Effects

It should be understood that we must distinguish between biological effects and harmful or detrimental biological effects. Thus, the biological effect of hot and humid weather is perspiration, and the effect of dim light or bright light is to open or reduce the opening of the iris diaphragm. Clearly, these are not harmful biological effects. A biological effect becomes harmful when the body's homeostatic mechanisms become overwhelmed (usually by too large a dose) and cannot deal with the insult that led to the biological effect.

The biological effects of RF radiation are frequency dependent, and can be grouped into three categories according to frequency:

Electrostimulatory effects (3 kHz–5 MHz)—At high enough levels, an electric field can generate painful nerve impulses.

Thermal effects (100 kHz–3 GHz)—Temperature rise, either whole body or localized, when the body absorbs energy faster than its thermoregulatory system.

Skin heating effects (3–300 GHz)—At frequencies greater than 3 GHz, the energy is absorbed mainly in the skin, and the microwave radiation behaves in a fashion similar to that of infrared radiation. An increase in skin temperature to about 45°C will cause sufficient pain for the person to leave the exposure area. This effect is associated mainly with exposure to an open waveguide from a high powered source.

Organs and tissues are made of a structural matrix that is bathed in biological fluids. The structural matrix is built of fixed molecules that often are electrically polarized, while the biological fluids contain ions of dissolved electrolytes and macromolecules. Under the influence of the electric fields from high-frequency electromagnetic radiation, these polar molecules and ions are subjected to electric forces whose magnitude is proportional to the product of the electric field intensity and the charge on the ion or on the polar molecule, Eq. (2.36),

$$f = \varepsilon q.$$

Because of the electrical properties of tissue, a person in an external electric field greatly perturbs that field, and the electric field in the tissues of the person in that field is about 5–7 orders of magnitude smaller than the external electric field in which he is immersed. On the other hand, the magnetic permeability of tissue is not very much different from that of air, and the magnetic field inside a person is about the same as that in which the person is immersed. These induced forces lead to current flow in the case of the dissolved ions and consequently to joule heating of the biological material. The rapidly alternating electrical forces on the immobile structural molecules may cause them to vibrate or rotate, which, in turn, leads to heat production. Additionally, the electric-field-induced forces may change the spatial distribution of polar molecules from a random orientation to an orientation aligned with the electric field. In all cases of microwave irradiation of living material (single cells to complex organisms), both of these induced-force effects occur simultaneously. When biological effects are due mainly to heating, we say that we have *thermal effects*; when a biological effect cannot be attributed to heating, we say that we have a *nonthermal effect*. Thermal effects are associated with exposures greater than 10 mW per cm, while nonthermal effects generally are associated with exposures less than 10 mW per cm.

Animal studies show that microwave radiation, in frequencies ranging from 200–24,000 MHz, is lethal if the product of exposure intensity and time is sufficiently great to increase the body temperature beyond the body's homeostatic capabilities ($\geq 5°C$) for a sustained period. For example, rats exposed to 3000-MHz radiation at a power density of 300 mW cm^{-2} suffered a temperature increase of 8–10°C and died after 15 minutes of exposure; at a power density of 100 mW cm^{-2}, rats died after 25 minutes of exposure, when their body temperature had risen by 6–7°C.

The temperature rise in any absorbing medium is related to the absorbed power density P_a, by

$$P_a = \frac{\rho \frac{\text{kg}}{\text{m}^3} \times c \frac{\text{J/kg}}{°C} \times \Delta T °C}{t \text{ seconds}} \frac{\text{W}}{\text{m}^3}, \tag{14.40}$$

where

ρ = density of the absorbing medium,
c = specific heat of the absorbing medium,
ΔT = temperature increase, and
t = exposure time.

If the absorbing medium is a living tissue, the temperature increase will differ from that predicted by Eq. (14.40) because of heat loss due to evaporative cooling, and convective and conductive heat loss or gain. The net amount of heat stored in the body is given by the heat balance equation

$$S = M \pm R \pm C - E, \tag{14.41}$$

where

M = metabolic heat rate,
R = radiative heat gain or loss,
C = conductive and convective heat gain or loss,
E = heat loss due to evaporative cooling, and
S = rate of heat storage.

While resting, a person generates metabolic heat at a rate of about 75 W; while engaged in moderate work or exercise, the metabolic heat output increases to about 300 W. This metabolic heat is dissipated in the environment when the temperature and humidity do not exceed the comfort range. If the temperature and humidity are too high to dissipate the metabolic heat, the person's body temperature increases. The additional heat load due to absorption of microwave energy must be dissipated in exactly the same manner as any other heat load. An unacceptable heat stress results when the combination of heat load and environmental conditions lead to an increased body temperature of 1°C or more. The "comfort range" is measured by the *temperature–humidity index* (THI), which is defined by

$$\text{THI} = 0.72(T_d + T_w) + 40.6, \tag{14.42}$$

where

T_d = dry bulb temperature, °C and
T_w = wet bulb temperature, °C.

In terms of percent relative humidity, RH, Eq. (14.42) may be approximated by

$$\text{THI} = 1.44\,T_d + 0.1\,\text{RH} + 30.6. \tag{14.43}$$

Values of THI from 65 to 80 are usually considered comfortable. As the THI value increases above 80, the heat stress on a person becomes increasingly difficult, and additional heat loads may lead to overheating.

Now let us consider the thermal stress from absorption of microwave radiation. If we assume the projected area of a person to be 0.9 m^2, an incident radiation beam whose power density is 10 mW/cm^2 will deliver energy to a person at a rate of

$$0.9\,\text{m}^2 \times 10\,\frac{\text{mW}}{\text{cm}^2} \times 10^4\frac{\text{cm}^2}{\text{m}^2} \times 10^{-3}\frac{\text{W}}{\text{mW}} = 90\,\text{W}$$

if all the incident energy is absorbed. This additional heat load is about the same as that which a person generates in the course of his normal activities and usually can be dissipated without undue thermal strain if the THI does not exceed about 70. As the THI increases above 80, a radiation exposure at 10 mW/cm^2 could lead to unacceptable thermal stress. Thus, we see that the biological thermal stress from whole-body exposure at power densities on the order of 1–10 mW/cm^2 depends strongly on the THI.

Most of the documented harmful biological effects in humans from microwaves are attributed to hyperthermia. These include damage mainly to the eyes and to the testicles. Both these tissues are relatively ischemic and thus are unable to efficiently dissipate energy that is absorbed at a rate greater than 10–15 mW/cm^2. The lens of the eye is avascular and encapsulated, and thus is particularly vulnerable to heat buildup and temperature rise from high radiation intensities. Figure 14-13 shows the relationship between energy absorption in the lens of the eye and the consequent temperature rise. Microwave radiation through heating, and possibly through a nonthermal mechanism, initiates a chain of events that may ultimately lead to cataracts. The site of the initially observed lesions from microwave radiation is not in the lens substance but rather on the posterior surface of the lens capsule. The pathogenesis of cataracts from ionizing radiation is similar to that of microwave-induced cataracts. "Senile" cataracts (those due to aging), on the other hand, originate in the anterior surface of the lens.

Although the time–intensity relationship for cataractogenesis is not precisely known, one of the principal factors in microwave cataractogenesis is the increased temperature of the lens. Time–intensity exposure conditions that lead to an intraocular temperature of 45°C or higher are believed to be cataractogenic. When translated to practical conditions, a high risk of developing a cataract is associated with exposures on the order of a hundred or more milliwatts per square centimeter.

Testicular function is strongly influenced by temperature. Normally the temperature of the testicles, which are outside the core of the body, is about 2°C less than the core temperature of 37°C. Increase of the testicular temperature even to 37°C

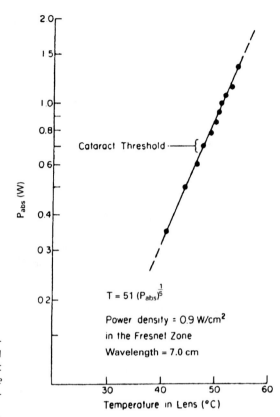

Figure 14-13. A log–log plot of power absorption versus temperature rise in the lens. (Reproduced from Hirsch FG. *Microwave cataracts: A case report reevaluated.* In: *Electronic Product Radiation and the Health Physicist.* Rockville, MD: Bureau of Radiological Health; 1970. BRH/DEP 70–26.)

depresses spermatogenesis. This effect is reversible and spermatogenesis again proceeds normally when the temperature of the testes is lowered. Animal experiments have shown the threshold for minimal reversible testicular damage, consisting of depressed spermatogenesis and degeneration of the epithelial lining of the seminiferous tubules, to be greater than 10 mW/cm^2.

Workers and members of the public seem to be concerned mainly with four possible effects of microwave radiation:

- Cancer—The transformation of normal cells to cancer cells involves changes to the DNA. Such changes can be induced by ionizing radiation and by certain chemicals (carcinogens). There is no evidence that low microwave levels, at frequencies up to 300 GHz directly changes the cellular DNA and initiates a carcinogenic transformation.
- Birth defects—Increased body temperature of pregnant female animals have been found to be teratogenic. Increasing the body temperature by 2.5°C or more, regardless of the method of attaining the hyperthermia, leads to significant birth defects. In studies on several rodent species, raising the core temperature to 43°C by exposure at a dose rate of 11 W/kg led to developmental abnormalities and

to fetal death. Exposure at 6–7 W/kg resulted in fetal growth retardation and to post-natal behavioral changes. Exposure at 4 W/kg produced no direct effect.

- Genetic (heritable) defects—Generally, temperature increases of $\leq 1°C$ have been found not to be mutagenic and do not lead to somatic mutations or to hereditary effects.
- Behavioral effects—Although the biological mechanisms for nonthermal behavioral effects are not clearly understood, many such effects have been observed in the laboratory. The main impetus for experimental study of nonthermal effects was the persistent reports from the East European countries of behavioral and physiological effects on workers who had prolonged histories of exposure to low-level (<10 mW/cm^2) microwave exposure. Because of the lack of dosimetric quantification of the radiation fields and also because all the symptoms described in these reports are normally associated with a population that is simply growing older, it is difficult to evaluate the public health significance of these reports. However, animal studies have shown nervous-system effects from hyperthermia. The investigators found that "the maximum heat dose without obvious complications after localized hyperthermia in regions of the central nervous system (CNS) lies in the range of 40–60 minutes at 42–42.5°C or 10–30 minutes at 43°C."

Epidemiologic studies in human populations have failed to demonstrate a clear relationship between RF or microwave radiation and either cancer or birth defects. A review of the published studies on nonthermal effects shows the experimental findings to be contradictory and inconclusive. These facts, together with the absence of biological mechanisms that can satisfactorily explain the reported results, have led the U.S. National Research Council to conclude that "the connections among the various experimental findings and the theoretical constructs do not yet lead to a comprehensive conceptual structure for the reported phenomena sufficient to enable an evaluation of the significance of the theories." The National Institute of Environmental Health concluded that "The NIEHS does not believe that either cancers or noncancer health outcomes provide sufficient evidence of a risk to currently warrant a concern."

Laboratory studies with animals at high doses (relative to recognized safety standards and exposure limits) confirm teratogenic effects and developmental abnormalities following in utero exposure, changes in electroencephalograms, alterations in the blood–brain barrier, alteration of cell membrane permeability, hematologic effects, central nervous system effects, and behavioral changes. Until dosimetry problems are solved and uncertainties in the dose–response relationships for repeated and continuous low-level exposure are eliminated, a prudent degree of conservatism continues to be exercised in the control of hazards from RF and microwave radiation and the exposure limits that form the basis for these controls.

Microwave Measurements

In electromagnetic fields, we may measure the electric field intensity or the magnetic field. When the relationship between the electric and magnetic field intensities is known, as in the case of the far field, the power density can be calculated from measured values of ε or H, as illustrated in Example 2.17. In any case, the electromagnetic field is probed by an antenna that interacts with the electromagnetic field. In the case of a dipole antenna, for example, a voltage is induced across the antenna. This voltage is proportional to the electric field intensity:

$$V = l\frac{\varepsilon_0}{\sqrt{2}} \qquad\qquad (14.44)$$

where l, the constant of proportionality, is the effective length of the antenna and ε_0 is the maximum electric field strength. Thus, the electrical response of any given dipole probe is quantitatively related to the intensity of the electric field. By using a calibrated probe, therefore, we can measure the electric field strength in units of V/m or V^2/m^2. The magnetic field strength is measured in units of A/m with a probe that has orthogonal loops in which currents interact with the magnetic field, or by the Hall effect, in which charges are separated when a conductor is oriented perpendicular to the magnetic field. The separated charges lead to a potential difference across the conductor, which is determined by the strength of the magnetic field. For far-field conditions, the power density can be readily calculated from electric field strength using Eq. (2.72). Radiation survey meters are usually calibrated to read the far-field power density corresponding to the measured electric field intensity. In the near field, both electric field and magnetic field strengths must be measured.

The devices most often used in microwave probes to convert the microwave energy into electric current or voltage are crystal diodes and bolometers. The crystal diode is a nonlinear device that rectifies the received signal and has an output voltage that is proportional to the antenna power input (typically, the sensitivity is on the order of 5 mV/mW). Since microwave power density is proportional to the square of the electric field strength, the crystal detector is called a "square-law" detector. This square-law response is seen only for small power inputs; when the input power exceeds about 10 mW, the square-law response starts to change into a linear response; at input powers in excess of 100 mW, the departure from the square-law response is significant and may lead to serious measurement errors.

The bolometer often used in microwave measurements is the thermistor. Since the resistance of a thermistor decreases with increasing temperature and the temperature increase is proportional to the intensity of the microwave radiation, the radiation field strength may be determined by measuring changes in thermistor resistance. Thermistors are characterized by long time constants, on the order of 0.1–1 second, and therefore are useful for measuring average power. A *barretter* is a resistive element whose electrical resistance increases with temperature. Barretters are characterized by short time constants, on the order of 250–500 μ seconds, and thus are suitable for measuring peak power. Thermistors and barretters can be used over a power range of 1 μW to several milliwatts.

A dipole probe with a thermocouple is another temperature-sensitive device. Absorption of microwave energy heats one junction of the thermocouple to establish a temperature difference between the heated junction and the cold junction. This temperature difference generates a voltage whose magnitude depends on the temperature difference, which in turn is proportional to the microwave power density. The meter is calibrated to read in units of power per unit area.

A power meter may be a bridge, one arm of which is the transducing element. The bridge is balanced in the absence of microwave radiation, and the voltage drop across the transducer due to the absorption of microwave energy unbalances the bridge, with the degree of imbalance being proportional to the absorbed microwave power. Because the response of the detector follows the square law only for a low power, it is common to use an attenuator between the receiving antenna and the detector. The degree of attenuation is given in decibels. For example, a 20-dB attenuator will attenuate the input to measure the power density received by the antenna. In this case, the power density is related to the measured power by the relationship

$$S = \alpha \frac{4\pi\, P}{\lambda^2 G_a},$$ **(14.45)**

where

$S =$ power density,
$P =$ absorbed power,
$G_a =$ antenna gain, absolute power gain, not decibels,
$\alpha =$ actual attenuation factor, not decibels,
$\lambda =$ wavelength.

EXAMPLE 14.25

A 200-ohm thermistor whose sensitivity is 25 ohms/mW is used with an antenna whose gain is 16 dB at 10,000 MHz and a 30-dB attenuator to measure the power density in a 10,000-MHz field. From the resistance change, the absorbed power is found to be 0.4 mW. What is the power density in the microwave field?

Solution

Antenna gain, G_a: 16 dB $= 10 \log G_a$

$$G_a = \log^{-1} \frac{16}{10} = 40.$$

Wavelength, λ: $f \times \lambda = 3 \times 10^{10} \, \frac{\text{cm}}{\text{s}}$

$$\lambda = \frac{3 \times 10^{10}\, \frac{\text{cm}}{\text{s}}}{1 \times 10^{10}\, \text{s}^{-1}} = 3\,\text{cm}.$$

Attenuation factor, α: 30 dB $= 10 \log \alpha$

$$\alpha = \log^{-1} \frac{30}{10} = 1000.$$

Power density, S: $S = \alpha \dfrac{4\pi P}{\lambda^2 G_a} = 1000 \times \dfrac{4\pi \times 0.4\ \text{mW}}{(3\,\text{cm})^2 \times 40} = 14\ \dfrac{\text{mW}}{\text{cm}^2}.$

RF detector probes can burn out if they absorb too much power. There therefore is an upper limit on the power density that can be measured with any particular probe.

Several factors must be considered when choosing or using a microwave-radiation monitoring instrument. First, introduction of the detector probe causes some distortion of the field, and the power density that is measured while the probe is in the field is not necessarily the power density at that point in the absence of the probe. This source of error can be minimized by using a small probe. A second factor is polarization. If we have a dipole-receiving antenna and if the dipole is oriented perpendicularly to the plane of polarization of the electric field, then no voltage will be induced in the dipole and no microwave energy will be detected. On the other hand, aligning the dipole parallel to the plane of polarization results in an induced voltage, and thus to detection of the microwave field. One method of accounting for polarization is to use a probe that contains three mutually perpendicular dipoles. The sum of the induced voltage in each of the three dipoles will be the same regardless of their orientation. Third, microwave detectors are frequency-dependent, and the frequency response of the probe must be matched to the frequency of the field being measured. Finally, detector probes will burn out if they absorb too much power. There is an upper limit, therefore, on the power density that can be measured with any particular probe. Most survey meters read the average power level rather than the power in an individual pulse. Damage to probes, therefore, occurs more frequently from pulsed sources rather than from CW sources.

EXAMPLE 14.26

Measurements are to be made in a 2.45-GHz field that is pulsed at a rate of 1600 Hz, with a pulse width of 0.25 μ seconds. If the probe's damage level is 1.75×10^5 mW/cm^2 and full-scale reading on the instrument is 100 mW/cm^2, will the instrument reach full-scale reading before the probe burns out?

Solution

According to Eq. (14.23)

$$P_0 = \frac{\text{average power}}{\text{pulse frequency} \times \text{pulse width}} = \frac{P}{n \times \tau},$$

the average power, P, corresponding to a peak power, $P_0 = 1.75 \times 10^5$ mW/cm^2 is

$$P = P_0 \times n \times \tau = 1.75 \times 10^5 \, \frac{\text{mW}}{\text{cm}^2} \times 1.6 \times 10^3 \, \frac{\text{pulses}}{\text{s}} \times 0.25 \times 10^{-6} \, \frac{\text{s}}{\text{pulse}}$$

$$= 70 \, \frac{\text{mW}}{\text{cm}^2}.$$

Thus, the probe will be burned out if the meter reads ≥ 70 mW/cm^2.

Dosimetry

Dosimetry of ionizing radiation is based on energy absorption from the radiation field by means of collisions between the particles of radiation and the atoms in the absorbing media. This basic mechanism is relatively simple and well understood; therefore, the distribution of absorbed energy can be calculated and measured. The quantity of ionizing radiation dose then is simply given by the concentration of absorbed energy, and we are confident that this quantity is a reasonable predictor of the biological effect of the radiation exposure. For NIR too, the basic dosimetric quantity is absorbed energy per unit mass, but the rate of energy absorption is biologically significant. The basic NIR dosimetric quantity, therefore, is the *specific absorption rate* (SAR). The SAR is a measure of the time rate of energy absorption per unit mass and is specified in units of joules per kilogram per second, or watts per kilogram.

$$\text{SAR} = \frac{\Delta\left(\dfrac{E \text{ J}}{t \text{ seconds}}\right)}{\Delta m \text{ kg}} = \frac{\text{W}}{\text{kg}}. \tag{14.46}$$

In terms of electrical parameters, the SAR can be calculated by

$$\text{SAR} = \frac{\sigma E^2}{\rho}, \tag{14.47}$$

where

σ = conductivity of the tissue, Ω/m,
E = rms electric field strength *in the tissue*, V/m, and
P = density of the tissue, kg/m^3.

The SAR can be measured by

$$\text{SAR} = \frac{c\Delta T}{\Delta t}, \tag{14.48}$$

where

ΔT = change in temperature. °C,
Δt = duration of exposure, seconds, and
c = specific heat of the irradiated tissue, J/kg/°C.

When RF waves and microwaves interact with living systems, the transferred energy causes charged particles, such as ions in solution, to move along the lines of the electric field and polar molecules to rotate under the influence of the electric and magnetic fields. The motion of the charged particles and the polar molecules, in turn, produce new electric and magnetic fields. The electric and magnetic fields within the body are therefore very different from the external electromagnetic fields. Thus, the SAR depends in a very complex manner on the electrical and magnetic properties of the various tissues, on the orientation of the electromagnetic field relative to the person, and on whether or not the person is grounded. Irradiation of people and animals leads to complex, frequency-specific, nonuniform energy absorption patterns that are difficult to calculate theoretically and to measure experimentally. Equation (14.38) shows the absorption coefficient for microwaves to depend on

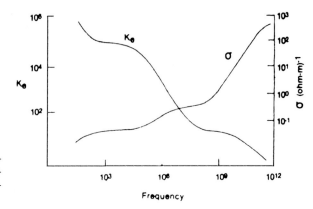

Figure 14-14. Curves showing the dependence of conductivity and dielectric coefficient of muscle tissue on frequency of the irradiating electromagnetic field.

frequency, the dielectric properties of the absorber, the magnetic properties of the absorbing medium, and the electrical conductivity of the absorbing medium. Figure 14-14 and Table 14-18 show the frequency dependence of electrical conductivity and dielectric coefficient for muscle and for fat. These electrical properties are strongly dependent on the amount of water in the absorber, and thus energy absorption by different organs and tissues in living systems is strongly dependent on the degree of hydration of organs or tissues. For example, skin, muscle, and internal organs all have large water contents and, therefore, high absorption coefficients; fat, bone, and yellow bone marrow have small water contents and therefore have low absorption coefficients.

The situation is further complicated by reflections at interfaces between different types of tissue, such as the interface between skin and fat, fat and muscle, and muscle and bone. This effect is implicit in the influence of physical size and geometry on energy absorption, as illustrated in Figure 14-15, which shows the relative cross section of spheres as a function of their radii and wavelength of the radiation. Figure 14.16 shows the dependence of SAR on frequency and orientation of the electromagnetic field for an adult person. The complexities and unknowns in relating the internal fields to the specific absorption rate make it virtually impossible to design an instrument analogous to the tissue equivalent chamber for ionizing radiation for measuring SAR. It is therefore not practical to set safety limits in terms of the SAR. Instead, radiation safety standards are specified in terms of radiation exposure, such as environmental power density, which is expressed in milliwatts per square centimeter (or watts per square meter), or electric field strength in units of volts per meter, or magnetic field strength in units of amperes per meter. Power density is applicable to far-field conditions, while electric and magnetic field intensities are appropriate for near-field conditions.

Safety Guides and Standards

Recommendations for the protection of workers and members of the public from the harmful effects of RF and microwave radiation have been made by numerous international and professional organizations, and regulatory agencies in many countries have promulgated legally enforceable standards and exposure limits. On the international level, the WHO, the International Labor Organization (ILO), and the

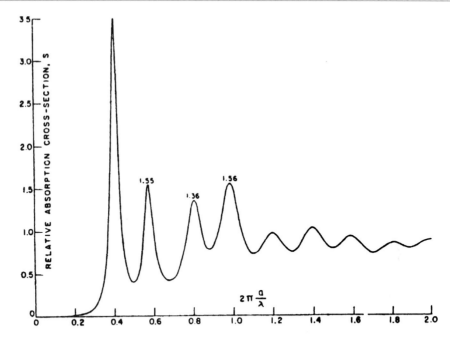

Figure 14-15. Curve showing the dependence of energy absorption cross section (for 28.8-GHz radiation) of a sphere of muscle-equivalent material on the ratio of size to wavelength. $f = 2880$ MHz; $a =$ radius of the sphere; and $\lambda =$ wavelength. (Reproduced from Sher LD. Interaction of microwave and RF energy on biological material. In: *Electronic Product Radiation and the Health Physicist.* Rockville, MD: Bureau of Radiological Health; 1970. BRH/DEP 70–26.)

ICNIRP have published recommended exposure limits. Professional organizations such as the American Industrial Hygiene Association (AIHA), the Institute of Electrical and Electronic Engineers (IEEE) through the ANSI, and the NCRP in the United States, the Deutsche Institute für Normeln (DIN) in Germany, and the Standards Association of Australia have also recommended exposure limits for RF and microwave radiation.

It should be noted that all the recommendations are designed to protect individuals. They do not protect medical devices such as cardiac pacemakers, nor electro-explosive devices unless explicitly stated. It is also important to emphasize that the safety standards are not designed to protect health physics surveying instruments, installed radiation monitoring instruments, and other electronic measuring devices that have safety functions. These instruments may be sensitive to RF radiation. If they should be irradiated by RF radiation, they would fail to respond properly to ionizing radiation. Health physics instruments and all safety related instruments that may be exposed to RF radiation must be designed to be immune to the RF radiation.

Regulations for the protection of workers in the United States have been promulgated by OSHA. A maximum exposure level of 10 mW/cm^2 incident electromagnetic power density for frequencies of 10 MHz to 100 GHz inclusive, averaged over any 6-minute period, has been set by OSHA. The U.S. Public Health Service Bureau of Devices and Radiological Health is charged with the responsibility of protecting the public from harmful radiation effects from consumer products. For the case of radiation from microwave ovens, the bureau set a limit of 1 mW/cm^2 leakage

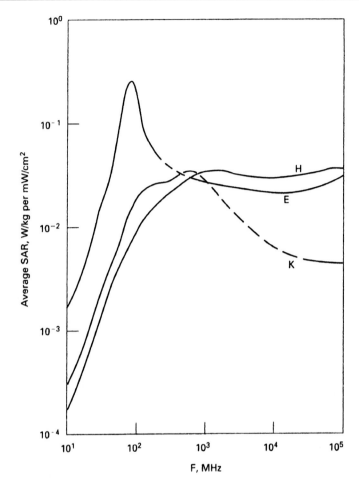

Figure 14-16. Calculated whole-body average SAR as a function of frequency for models of an average person in three radiation fields at the same power density of 1 mW/cm^2, but three different orientations. In curve E, the electric field is parallel to the long dimension of the person; in curve H it is perpendicular to the long dimension; and in curve K, the electric field is between the other two orientations. For humans, an absorption resonance occurs at a frequency of about 70 MHz. Generally, an absorption resonance occurs at a frequency whose wavelength is approximately twice the longest dimension of the absorber. (Reproduced with permission from *A Practical Guide to the Determination of Human Exposure to Radiofrequency Fields*. Bethesda, MD: National Council on Radiation Protection & Measurement; 1993. NCRP Report 119.)

radiation at a distance of 5 cm from the oven when the oven leaves the factory. Furthermore, the oven must be so designed and built that the maximum leakage that may be expected during its lifetime will not exceed 5 mW/cm^2 at 5 cm. The Federal Communications Commission (FCC) is responsible for setting RF radiation safety standards for exposure from broadcasting.

The OSHA maximum occupational exposure level of 10 mW/cm^2 in the United States was set on the basis of thermal effects only. It was believed to be the maximum sustained heat load that the homeostatic thermoregulatory system of a healthy adult worker can accommodate. The available information on the NIR bioeffects, nonthermal as well as thermal, shows that the SAR threshold for harmful bioeffects is

TABLE 14-19. Occupational Exposure Reference Levels for Radiofrequency Electromagnetic Fields

| FREQUENCY | UNPERTURBED RMS FIELD STRENGTH | | Power density (W/m²) |
	Electric field (V/m)[a,b]	Magnetic field (A/m)[a,b]	
<1 Hz	—	1.63×10^5	—
1–8 Hz	20,000	$1.63 \times 10^5/f^2$	—
8–25 Hz	20,000	$2 \times 10^4/f$	—
0.025–0.82 kHz	500/f	20/f	—
0.82–65 kHz	610	24.4	—
0.065–1 MHz	610	1.6/f	—
1–10 MHz	610/f	1.6/f	—
10–400 MHz	61	0.16	10
400–2000 MHz	$3f^{0.5}$	$0.008^{0.5}$	f/40
2–300 GHz[c]	137	0.36	50

[a] f as indicated in the frequency column

[b] For f between 100 kHz and 10 GHz, measurements averaged over any 6 minute period

[c] For f > 10 GHz, average over $68/f^{1.05}$ minute period, f in GHz

Reproduced with permission from ICNIRP. Guidelines for limiting exposure to time-varying electric, magnetic, and electromagnetic fields (up to 300 GHz). *Health Phys.* 1998; 74(4):494–522.

much higher than 0.4 W/kg. Exposure of a person at an SAR of 0.4 W/kg represents an increase of about 35% in metabolic rate. An SAR ten times greater, 4 W/kg, would increase the core temperature by about 1°C, an increase that can be accommodated by healthy adult workers. Accordingly, the limits for occupational exposure recommended by the professional and international organizations are based on an upper SAR limit of 0.4 W/kg. It is believed that adherence to the frequency-dependent derived exposure limits, which are given in terms of electric or magnetic field strength or power density, will ensure that the SAR under all conditions of exposure will not exceed 0.4 W/kg. Figure 14-16 shows the calculated SAR, W/kg per mW/cm² exposure, as a function of frequency.

The guidelines of the ICNIRP for occupational exposure are given in Table 14-19. The ANSI/IEEE recommendations are listed in Table 14-20, and the ACGIH recommended limits for occupational exposure are listed in Table 14-21. Because of the

TABLE 14-20. MPEs for Exposure to Radiofrequency Radiation in a Controlled Environment

FREQUENCY (MHz)	ELECTRIC FIELD E (RMS V/m)	MAGNETIC FIELD H (RMS A/m)	POWER DENSITY S (RMS W/m²)	AVERAGING TIME (minutes)
0.1–1.0	1842	$16.3/f_M$		6
1.0–30	$1842/f_M$	$16.3/f_M$		6
30–100	61.4	$16.3/f_M$		6
100–300	61.4	0.163	10	6
300–3000	—	—	$f_M/30$	6
3000–30 000	—	—	100	$19.63/f_G^{1.079}$
30 000–300 000	—	—	100	$2.524/f_G^{0.476}$

NOTE: f_M = frequency in MHz, f_G = frequency in GHz.

Pulsed RF fields between 100 kHz and 300 GHz have two safety criteria in addition to the MPEs listed in Table 14.19.

Abstracted with permission from ANSI/IEEE C95.1-2005. *IEEE Standards for Safety Levels with Respect to Human Exposure to Radiofrequency Electromagnetic Fields.* New York, NY: IEEE; 2006:Table 8.

TABLE 14-21. Radio Frequency/Microwave Threshold Limit Values

	PART A—ELECTROMAGNETIC FIELDS[a] F = FREQUENCY IN MHz			
FREQUENCY	Power density, S (mW/cm²)	Electric field strength (V/m)	Magnetic field strength (A/m)	Averaging time E^2, H^2, or S (minutes)
30 kHz–100 kHz		614	163	6
100 kHz–3 MHz		614	16.3/f	6
3 MHz–30 MHz		1842/f	16.3/f	6
30 MHz–100 MHz		61.4	16.3/f	6
100 MHz–300 MHz	1	61.4	0.163	6
300 MHz–3 GHz	f/300			6
3 GHz–15 GHz	10			6
15 GHz–300 GHz	10			$616,000/f^{1.2}$

	PART B—INDUCED AND CONTACT RADIO-FREQUENCY CURRENTS[b] MAXIMUM CURRENT (mA)			
FREQUENCY	Through both feet	Through each foot	Contact	Averaging time
30 kHz–100 kHz	2000f	1000f	1000f	1 second
100 kHz–100 MHz	200	100	100	6 minutes

[a]The exposure values in terms of electric and magnetic field strengths are the values obtained by spatially averaging values over an area equivalent to the vertical cross section of the human body (projected area).

[b]It should be noted that the current limits given above may not adequately protect against static reactions and burns caused by transient discharges when contacting an energized object.

nonmagnetic nature of tissue, there is little interaction of static magnetic fields with tissue. Exposure in static magnetic fields as high as 2 T (2×10^4 G or 1.59×10^6 A/m) have been found to produce no harmful biomedical effects. However, alternating magnetic fields induce electrical currents in biological materials. Currents resulting from pulsed magnetic fields on the order of 1 mT (10 G or 796 A/m) peak field strength can affect cellular physiology, including increase in the rate of repair of bone fractures in humans. For this reason, frequency-dependent limits on magnetic field strength are included in the safety standards. To meet the safety standards, the following criteria must be satisfied:

Criterion 1—The peak electric field strength may not exceed 100 kV per meter.
Criterion 2—The aerial energy density, J/m², during any 0.1-second time interval, may not exceed 1/5 of the total aerial energy density during the frequency-dependent averaging time specified in Table 14-19.

$$\sum_{0}^{0.1\,s} \left(S_{\text{peak}} \times \tau \right) \leq \frac{1}{5} \left(\text{MPE}_{\text{avg}} \times t_{\text{avg}} \right). \tag{14.49}$$

The detectors in RF microwave survey meters are built to respond to either electric or magnetic field intensity or to power density. In the far field, the power density is related to the electric and magnetic fields by

$$S = \frac{\varepsilon^2}{377} = 377 H^2, \tag{14.50}$$

where

S = power density, W/m^2,
ε = electric field strength, V/m, and
H = magnetic field strength, A/m.

The relationship in Eq. (14.50) is valid for the far field only. In the near field, the phase relationship between the electric and magnetic fields is variable and ordinarily is not known. Even though NIR survey meters may read in power density, they usually measure only the electric or magnetic field, and their measurements are converted to an "equivalent" plane-wave power density by Eq. (14.50) for readout. In making near-field measurements, we must, therefore, measure both the electric field and the magnetic field.

EXAMPLE 14.27

A radar has the following characteristics

- Frequency, $f = 2.45$ GHz,
- Pulse width, $T = 25$ milliseconds,
- PRF = 0.002 (1 pulse every 500 seconds), and
- Peak power density, $S = 100,000$ W/m^2.

Does this radar meet the IEEE safety standards for exposure in a controlled environment?

Solution

To meet the safety standard, the radar must satisfy two criteria:

(1) the peak electric field limit of 100 kV/m and

(2) the energy density limit.

Criterion 1—The electric field intensity is calculated with Eq. (14.50)

$$S = \frac{\varepsilon^2}{377}$$

$$\varepsilon = \sqrt{377 \times S_P} = \sqrt{377 \times 100,000} = 6140 \ \frac{\text{V}}{\text{m}}.$$

Since this is less than 100 kV/m, safety criterion 1 is satisfied.
Criterion 2—The energy density criterion requires the energy density to be

$$\sum_0^{0.1\,\text{s}} \left(S_{\text{peak}} \times \tau \right) \le \frac{1}{5} \left(\text{MPE}_{\text{avg}} \ \text{W/m}^2 \times t_{\text{avg}} \ \text{seconds} \right).$$

The $\text{MPE}_{t\,\text{avg.}}$, according to Table 14-20 is

$$\text{MPE}_{t\,\text{avg}} = \frac{f_{\text{MHz}}}{30} = \frac{2450}{30} = 81.7 \; \frac{\text{W}}{\text{m}^2},$$

and the averaging time, according to Table 14-20 is 6 minutes, or 360 seconds. Therefore, the aerial density in the controlled area must be less than

$$\frac{1}{5}\left(81.7 \; \frac{\text{W}}{\text{m}^2} \times 360 \text{ seconds}\right) = 5880 \; \frac{\text{J}}{\text{m}^2}.$$

In this case, where we have one pulse every 500 seconds, so all the energy of the pulse is included in the 0.1-second time interval. The resulting aerial energy density is

$$\text{Energy density} = 100,000 \; \frac{\text{W}}{\text{m}^2} \times 25 \times 10^{-3} \text{ second} = 2500 \; \frac{\text{J}}{\text{m}^2},$$

which is less than the permissible exposure limit of 5880 J/m^2 calculated above. Since both safety criteria are met, the radar is therefore safe for operation within the controlled area.

Multiple Sources

Since the SAR is frequency-dependent, we cannot simply add the field measurements if a worker is exposed to radiation from two or more sources of different frequencies. To determine compliance with the exposure limits, we measure the field strength, F_i, at each of the different frequencies and determine the fraction of the permissible exposure, L_i, represented by each different frequency. To comply with the exposure limit, the sum of these fractions may not exceed unity.

$$\frac{F_1}{L_1} + \frac{F_2}{L_2} + \cdots + \frac{F_n}{L_n} \leq 1. \tag{14.51}$$

 EXAMPLE 14.28

Measurements of electric and magnetic field strengths were made in a workplace where induction heaters and dielectric heaters were being used at the same time and the data listed below were obtained. Is the total exposure within the ICNIRP guidelines for occupational exposure?

SOURCE	f (MHz)	MEASURED		ICNIRP LIMIT	
		ε (V/m)	H(A/m)	ε (V/m)	H(A/m)
IH_1	0.90	20	1.1	614	1.8
IH_2	3600	26	0.3	137	0.36
DH_1	31	18.2	0.1	61	0.16
DH_2	7.5	9.8	0.05	81.9	0.21

Induction heating is the result of magnetically induced electric currents in a conducting material. The material to be heated is placed inside a high-frequency induction coil. The high-frequency alternating magnetic fields generated in the coil induce an electric current in the conducting material, which results in joule heating of the conductor as the current surges back and forth under the influence of the high-frequency magnetic field. Dielectric heating is used for nonconducting materials, such as plastics. Many dielectric materials absorb energy when placed in a high-voltage alternating electric field. Although called "nonconductors," they show some degree of conductivity due mainly to rotation of polar molecules in the alternating electric field (*dielectric loss*) and to a lesser degree movement of free ions (*conduction loss*). Because they do absorb energy from an alternating electromagnetic field, such nonconductors are called *lossy dielectrics*. The degree of "lossiness" is a function of the frequency of the applied electric field. The energy absorbed from the electric field heats the nonconducting material.

Solution

To determine whether the exposure is within the ICNIRP guidelines, we must see whether the conditions of Eq. (14.51) are met for both the electric and magnetic fields. For the electric field, we have

$$\sum_i \frac{E_i}{L_i} = \frac{20}{614} + \frac{26}{137} + \frac{18.2}{61} + \frac{9.8}{81.3} = 0.64$$

and for the magnetic field, substituting the appropriate values into Eq. (14.51), we obtain

$$\sum_i \frac{H_i}{L_i} = \frac{1.1}{1.8} + \frac{0.3}{0.36} + \frac{0.1}{0.16} + \frac{0.05}{0.21} = 2.31.$$

The sum of the fractional exposures to the electric field is less than 1; therefore, the electric field intensity is within the ICNIRP guideline. For the magnetic field, however, the sum of the fractional exposures is greater than 1; therefore, the guideline limit is exceeded.

PRINCIPLES OF RADIATION SAFETY

The principles of radiation protection for NIR are the same as those for ionizing radiation—namely, time, distance, and shielding. Most of the recommended exposure limits are 6-minute time-weighted averages, and some are based on frequency. Thus, in the case of a 6-minute averaging period, a worker may be exposed at twice the guideline level for a 3-minute period during any 6-minute interval. Generally, the maximum exposure time during any t_{avg} interval when the field intensity exceeds the guideline limit is given by

$$t_{max} = \frac{t_{avg.} \times F}{L},$$ (14.52)

where

t_{avg} = frequency-dependent averaging time,
F = measured field intensity, either electric or magnetic, or power density, and
L = limiting exposure.

Shielding against magnetic fields is easily accomplished through the use of ferromagnetic materials, such as iron or alloys of high permeability (Table 14.22). Attenuation of electric field intensity is accomplished through the use of solid metal shields. The exact degree of attenuation is determined by the electrical properties of the shielding material, the shield thickness, and the frequency of the radiation. The relationship among these factors is given by

$$A = 3.34 \times t \times \sqrt{\mu \times \sigma \times f},$$ (14.53)

TABLE 14-22. Electric Conductivity and Magnetic Permeability of Selected Radio-Frequency Shielding Materials

METAL	RELATIVE CONDUCTIVITY	RELATIVE PERMEABILITY
Silver	1.05	1
Copper, annealed	1.00	1
Copper, hard-drawn	0.97	1
Gold	0.70	1
Aluminum	0.61	1
Magnesium	0.38	1
Zinc	0.29	1
Brass	0.26	1
Cadmium	0.23	1
Nickel	0.20	1
Phosphor-bronze	0.18	1
Iron	0.17	1000
Tin	0.15	1
Steel, SAE 1045	0.10	1000
Beryllium	0.10	1
Lead	0.08	1
Hypernick	0.06	80,000
Monel	0.04	1
Mu metal	0.03	80,000
Permalloy	0.03	80,000
Steel, stainless	0.02	1000

where

A = attenuation, dB,
t = shield thickness, inches,
μ = relative (to copper) permeability,
σ = relative (to copper) conductivity, and
f = frequency, Hz.

 ## EXAMPLE 14.29

Calculate the reduction in electric field intensity by a shield of copper foil 1-mil (0.001-inch) thick at a frequency of 27 MHz.

Solution

Substituting the appropriate values from Table 14-22 into Eq. (14.53), we have

$$A = 3.34 \times 0.001 \times \sqrt{1 \times 1 \times 27 \times 10^6} = 17.4\,\text{dB}.$$

The attenuation in decibels, if the incident radiation level is I_0 and the transmitted intensity is I, is given by

$$A, \text{db} = 10 \log \frac{I_0}{I}. \tag{14.54}$$

$$\frac{I_0}{I} = \log^{-1}\frac{A}{10} = \log^{-1}\frac{17.4}{10} = 55.$$

The transmitted electric field intensity is thus seen to be only 1/55 of the incident intensity.

For shielding against microwave radiation, it is convenient to use wire mesh. The reduction factor by which a wire-mesh shield reduces the electric field intensity is given by

$$\frac{I_0}{I} = \frac{1}{4}\left\{\frac{\lambda}{a} \times \frac{1}{\ln\left[\frac{0.83e^{\frac{2\pi r}{a}}}{\left(\frac{2\pi r}{e^a - 1}\right)}\right]}\right\}^2, \tag{14.55}$$

where

λ = wavelength,
a = center-to-center distance between wires,
r = radius of wire,
I_0 = incident radiation intensity, and
I = transmitted radiation intensity.

EXAMPLE 14.30

Window screen, 16 in. × 16 in. mesh, 10-mil wire, is used to shield against 2450-MHz radiation.

(a) By what factor will the incident radiation be reduced?

(b) What is the reduction expressed in dB?

Solution

(a) If we substitute the following numerical values into Eq. (14.55),

$$\lambda = \frac{c}{f} = \frac{3 \times 10^{10} \dfrac{\text{cm}}{\text{s}}}{2.45 \times 10^9 \text{ s}^{-1}} = 12.24 \text{ cm}$$

$$a = \frac{1}{16} \text{ inch} = 0.0625 \text{ in.}$$

$$r = \frac{0.010 \text{ in.}}{2} = 0.005 \text{ in.}$$

$$\frac{r}{a} = \frac{0.005 \text{ in.}}{0.0625 \text{ in.}} = 0.080$$

$$\frac{\lambda}{a} = \frac{12.24 \text{ cm}}{0.0625 \text{ in} \times 2.54 \dfrac{\text{cm}}{\text{in.}}} = 77.102,$$

we find that $\dfrac{I_0}{I} = 1385.$

(b) The reduction expressed in dB is given by

$$\text{dB} = 10 \log \frac{I_0}{I} = 10 \log 1385 = 31.4 \text{ dB}.$$

SUMMARY

Nonionizing radiation, as the name implies, does not possess the ability to ionize atoms by knocking out electrons or to break apart molecules, although the shorter wavelengths of visible light and UV light are sufficiently energetic to ionize some molecules. The nonionizing electromagnetic radiations discussed in this chapter fall into three separate categories: UV light, laser radiation, and RF and microwave radiation. UV light includes wavelengths from 100 nm to 400 nm. The biological hazard is mainly to the eyes, with the production of cataracts; and to the skin, with the production of erythema and skin cancer. The use of protective clothing and sunblocking creams is effective in preventing skin damage. Sunglasses that absorb UV light are effective in preventing eye injury.

Laser radiation includes radiation in the UV, visible, and infrared portions of the electromagnetic spectrum; its wavelengths span the range from about 100 nm to about 1 mm. Microwave wavelengths range from about 1 mm to the order of meters, and RF wavelengths range from meters to kilometers. The biological hazards from laser radiation are mainly to the eye and skin. Maximum exposure levels depend on the characteristics of the source (wavelength, pulsed or CW, duty cycle) and exposure time. Exposure limits are specified as radiant exposure, J/cm^2, or irradiance, W/cm^2. Lasers are classified according to their power output and thus to their potential hazard.

The absorption of energy from RF and microwave radiation can lead to systemic effects due to temperature rise (thermal effects) and due to realignment of molecules and electric fields within the body. Dosimetry is based on the rate per unit mass of energy absorption from the external field. The quantity of dose is called the specific absorption rate (SAR) and is measured in units of watts per kilogram. Because of the extreme difficulty of measuring the SAR in a biologically meaningful way, environmental safety standards are specified in terms of maximum values for the electric and magnetic fields and for the power density. Radiation monitoring instruments are designed to measure these quantities. These derived exposure limits, which are frequency-dependent, are set at levels to ensure that the average whole-body dose does not exceed 0.4 W/kg. Radiation safety measures include minimizing exposure time, maximizing distance from the source, and interposing shielding when necessary.

PROBLEMS

14.1. The lethal absorbed dose of 265-nm UV light for *E. coli* bacteria is 14 MeV. How many photons of this UV radiation does the lethal absorbed dose represent?

14.2. An yttrium–aluminum-garnet (YAG) laser emits near-infrared radiation 1060 nm in wavelength at a power level of 10-W CW. The exit aperture is 3 mm in diameter, and the beam divergence is 5 milliradians. Calculate

(a) the $1/e^2$ diameter at the aperture,

(b) the $1/e^2$ diameter at a distance of 10 m, and

(c) the irradiance at a distance of 10 m.

14.3. A 0.1-J ruby laser has an aperture of 7 mm and a beam divergence of 1 milliradian.

(a) What is the radiant exposure at distances of 5 and 10 m from the aperture?

(b) How far behind the laser aperture is the virtual focal point from where the laser light seems to originate?

(c) Is the inverse square law applicable if distances are measured from the virtual focal point of the laser beam?

14.4. The output of a CW pumped Nd:YAG laser is Q-switched at a pulse repetition frequency of 10 kHz. If each pulse is 50 nanoseconds wide and if the mean power output is 10 W, calculate

  (a) the duty cycle,

  (b) the peak power per pulse, and

  (c) the energy per pulse.

14.5. What is the recommended MPE value, in mW/cm^2, for direct ocular exposure for 1 second to a beam from a He–Ne laser operating at a power level of 5-mW CW?

14.6. What is the protection standard (i.e., the maximum permissible irradiance for a direct intrabeam exposure) to a 0.8-millisecond-wide pulse from a 694.3-nm ruby laser?

14.7. A pulsed ruby laser, $\lambda = 694.3$ nm, is operated in a laboratory at a level of 5×10^{-4} J/pulse, 100-μ second pulse width, and a PRF of 60 pulses/s. The beam exit aperture is 1 mm in diameter, and the beam divergence is 0.1 milliradian. What optical density is required for protective goggles for

  (a) incidental exposure for as long as 2 seconds and

  (b) continuous exposure?

14.8. A He–Ne laser, $\lambda = 632.8$ mm, is operated at a power level of 3-W CW. The laser aperture diameter is 0.9 mm, and the beam divergence is 0.9 milliradian. If the possibility exists for momentary accidental intrabeam ocular exposure not exceeding 0.25 second, calculate the minimum required optical density of protective goggles for

  (a) exposure at the laser,

  (b) exposure at a distance of 100 m, and

  (c) continuous intrabeam viewing for up to 100 seconds at a distance of 100 m?

14.9. A scanning He–Ne laser that scans at a rate of 10 s^{-1} emits 5 mW through an aperture of 0.7 cm. If the beam divergence is 5 milliradian, then, for an intrabeam-viewing distance of 200 cm, calculate

  (a) the time during each scan that the pupil of the eye can be exposed,

  (b) the radiant exposure per scan,

  (c) the average irradiance at the cornea, and

  (d) the hazard class that should be assigned to this laser?

14.10. A microwave beam is pulsed 100 times per second, the pulse width is 1 μ second, and the peak power is 1 MW.

  (a) What is the duty cycle?

  (b) What is the average power?

14.11. A radar operates at an average power level of 20 W; its pulse width is 1 μ second, and the PRF is 1000 s^{-1}. Calculate

  (a) the duty cycle and

  (b) the peak power.

14.12. Calculate the gain of a 30-cm-diameter parabolic antenna used to transmit at a frequency of 3000 MHz. Express the answer

   (a) as the power ratio and

   (b) in decibels.

14.13. A far-field measurement shows the power density in a 1000-MHz radiation field to be 4 mW/cm^2. Calculate

   (a) the electric field strength, in V/m, and the square of the electric field strength,

   (b) the magnetic field strength, in A/m, and the square of the magnetic field strength, and

   (c) the energy density, in pJ/cm^3.

14.14. How many decibels attenuation of power density are required to reduce a 1 W/cm^2 field to 1 mW/cm^2?

14.15. What is the maximum magnetic intensity in a plane electromagnetic wave whose maximum electric intensity is 100 V/m?

14.16. A dipole antenna with a 50-cm parabolic dish radiates 100 W of power at a frequency of 2400 MHz. Calculate the

   (a) mean power density at the aperture,

   (b) maximum power density in the near field,

   (c) distance to the far field,

   (d) power density at 1 m, and

   (e) distance at which the power density is down to 1 mW/cm^2.

14.17. A rectangular horn antenna, 17 cm × 24 cm and operating at a frequency of 2400 MHz, has an effective area of 200 cm^2. If the radiated power is 100 W, calculate the

   (a) mean power density at the aperture,

   (b) maximum power density in the near field,

   (c) distance to the start of the far field,

   (d) power density in the far field, at a distance of 5 m, and

   (e) distance at which the power density is down to 1 mW/cm^2.

14.18. A radar installation, using a parabolic dish antenna 1.2 m in diameter, has a peak power output of 2 MW of 10-GHz radiation. If the PRF is 200 s^{-1} and the pulse width is 5 μ seconds, calculate the

   (a) duty cycle,

   (b) average power output,

   (c) antenna gain, in decibels, and

   (d) downrange distance to an average power density of 1 mW/cm^2.

14.19. A radar that rotates at 3 rpm operates at a frequency of 10 GHz and peak power of 2 MW. The PRF is 400 s^{-1}, the pulse width is 3 μ seconds, the beam width is 4.5°, and the parabolic dish is 0.5 m in diameter. Calculate the

(a) duty cycle,

(b) average power,

(c) power density at a distance of 50 m, and

(d) energy density per 6-minute exposure at a distance of 50 meters. Is this calculated exposure within the OSHA limit?

14.20. Show by dimensional analysis that the unit for α in Eq. (14.38) is per meter.

14.21. Calculate the wavelength of 100-MHz microwaves in muscle and in fat.

14.22. Calculate the penetration depth of 100-MHz radiation in fat and in muscle.

14.23. How many decibels attenuation will reduce a field of 800 mW/cm^2 to the power density of 1 mW/cm^2 recommended by ICNIRP for occupational exposure to 300-GHz radiation?

14.24. **(a)** How far from a 10-GHz radar transmitter would the far field be expected to begin if the antenna diameter is 0.6 m?

(b) A power meter, whose calibration at 10 GHz gives –10 dB as the power level that corresponds to 1 mW/cm^2, is used to measure the power density at the distance calculated in part (a). The meter reading is +3.5 dB. What is the power density at this point?

(c) At what distance from the antenna will the power density be down to –7 dB?

14.25. A microwave survey meter that reads in decibels is calibrated to read – 8 dB in a field whose power density is 0.01 mW/cm^2. It is then used in a radiation survey and gives a reading of +2.5 dB at a certain point in a microwave field. What is the power density at the point?

14.26. A power meter reads 5 mW in a 10-GHz microwave field. If the standard gain horn has a gain of 16 dB at this frequency and if a 30-dB attenuator was used, what is the power density in the microwave field?

14.27. A radar whose beamwidth is 12° rotates at 3 rpm. What is the exposure time for a person who remains in the scanning field for 0.1 hours?

14.28. A radar has the following characteristics:

$f = 10$ GHz	Beamwidth = 2.5°
Peak power = 2 MW	Rotational frequency = 4 rpm
PRF = 200 pulses/s	Dish diameter = 1.22 m
Pulse width = 5 μ seconds	

(a) What is the duty cycle?

(b) What is the average power?

(c) What is the power density at 100 m?

(d) A person spends 1 hour at this distance. According to OSHA standards, is his exposure within acceptable limits?

14.29. A worker is simultaneously exposed to four different radiation sources. Measurements of the electric and magnetic fields produced by each source alone are listed below. Does this work area meet the ACGIH safety requirements listed in Table 14-21?

SOURCE	FREQUENCY (MHz)	E (V/m)	H (A/m)
1	7.5	140	0.2
2	30	24	0.07
3	950	13	0.18
4	2450	54	0.20

14.30. An experimental setup employing a 2450-MHz magnetron produces a leakage radiation field of 100 mW/cm². It is proposed to use a chicken-wire screen, 4 in. × 4 in. whose wire diameter = 0.025 in., as a shield. What will the power density be outside the proposed shield?

14.31. A laser pointer used in a classroom emits 633-nm radiation (red) at a power of 5 mW; the 1/e diameter of the beam at the aperture is 7 mm. Assume that the normal aversion response time applies.

   (a) Calculate the irradiance of the beam at the aperture.

   (b) Calculate the MPE (E) for this exposure condition.

   (c) Does this laser meet the MPE limit?

14.32. Photons whose λ = 270 nm are effective in damaging DNA molecules. What is the energy of an individual 270-nm photon, in joules, ergs, and electron volts?

14.33. The sterilization dose for *Streptococcus lactis* is 88 J/m². If a "germicidal" UV lamp, λ = 254 nm, is specified, and will be located at a distance of 0.1 m from the bacteria, what power light is needed, assuming an isotropic point source?

14.34. A white fluorescent lamp is used in an office. At a point where a worker will be located, the UVA, λ_{eff} = 380 nm, is 23 mW/m²; and the UVC, λ_{eff} = 254 is 5 μW/m². What is the MPE, J/cm² for an 8-hour exposure? Is the MPE exceeded?

14.35. A compact fluorescent lamp that is used in an office has a UVA, λ_{eff} = 390 nm, output of 50,000 mW/m² and UVC, λ_{eff} = 254 nm, 5 μW/m² at a point occupied by a worker. Is her UV dose within the AIHA guideline for an 8-hour exposure?

14.36. A nitrogen laser whose aperture is 1 mm in diameter, produces 10 mJ pulses 20 × 10⁻⁹ second wide. The beam diameter at a distance of 100 m is 10 cm. What is the

   (a) MPE for intrabeam viewing, J/cm²,

   (b) beam divergence, and

   (c) nominal ocular hazard distance (NOHD)?

14.37. A 532-nm doubled Nd:YAG laser is pulsed at 25 Hz with an energy of 7.5 mJ per 6-nanosecond-wide pulse. The data plate on the laser says that that the aperture is 3 mm in diameter, and the beam divergence is 0.1 milliradian. What is the

   (a) MPE for intrabeam viewing,

   (b) NOHD?

14.38. A supermarket uses a door-opening device that operates at 10.5 GHz. If the power output is 10 mW and the antenna gain is 6 dB, what is the distance to the MPE?

14.39. A point-to-point microwave relay tower has two CW emitters: one operates at a power level of 5 W and a frequency of 4 GHz, the other at 12.5 W and 6 GHz. The antenna gain is 24 dB. Calculate the

   (a) MPE and

   (b) distance to the MPE.

14.40. A Bluetooth device operates at 2.45 GHz and a PRF of 1600. Assuming a point source of emission, and an omni-directional antenna whose gain is 3 dB, what is the maximum allowable energy per pulse if the antenna is expected to be 1 cm from the operator of this device?

SUGGESTED READINGS

ACGIH. *A Guide for Control of Laser Hazards*, 4th ed. American Conference of Governmental Industrial Hygienists, Cincinnati, OH, 1990.

ACGIH. *2007 Threshold Limit Values & Biological Exposure Indices*. American Conference of Governmental Industrial Hygienists, Cincinnati, OH, 2007.

AIHA Nonionizing Radiation Committee. *Radio-Frequency and Microwave Radiation*, 3rd ed. American Industrial Hygiene Association, Fairfax, VA, 2004.

American National Standards Institute (ANSI). New York.

   ANSI Z-136-1-2000. *The Safe Use of Lasers*, 2000.

   ANSI/IEEE C95.1-2005. *Standard for Safety Levels with Respect to Human Exposure to Radiofrequency Electromagnetic Fields, 3 kHz to 300 GHz*, 2006.

   ANSI/IEEE C95.3-2002. *IEEE Recommended Practice for Measurement and Computations of Radiofrequency Electromagnetic Fields with Respect to Human Exposure*, 2002.

Bahr, A., Boltz, T., and Hennes, C. Numerical dosimetry and ELF: Accuracy of the method, variability of models and parameters, and the implication for quantifying guidelines. *Health Phys*, **92:**521–530, 2007.

Baranski, S., and Czerski, P. *Biological Effects of Microwaves*. Dowden, Hutchinson, and Ross, Stroudsburg, PA, 1976.

Barat, K. *Laser Safety Management*. CRC, Boca Raton, FL, 2006.

Carlson, F. P. *Introduction to Applied Optics for Engineers*. Academic Press. New York, 1971.

Department of the Air Force. *Laser Health Hazards Control*. AFM 161-8. Department of the Air Force, Washington, DC, 1969.

Duchêne, A. S., Lakey, J. R. A., and Repacholi, M. H., eds. *IRPA Guidelines on Protection Against Non-ionizing Radiation*. Pergamon Press, New York, 1991.

Durney, C. H., Johnson, C. C., Barber, P. W., et al. *Radiofrequency Radiation Dosimetry Handbook*, 2nd ed. SAM-TR-78-22. School of Aerospace Medicine, Brooks Air Force Base, TX, 1978.

Gandhi, O. P. ed. *Biological Effects and Medical Applications of Electromagnetic Energy*, Prentice-Hall, Englewood Cliffs, NJ, 1991.

Geeraets, W. J., and Berry, E. R. Ocular spectral characteristics as related to hazards from lasers and other light sources. *Am J Ophthalmol*. **66:**15, 1968.

Goldman, L., Rockwell, R. J. Jr., and Hornby, P. Laser laboratory design and personnel protection from high energy lasers, in N. C. Steere, ed. *Handbook of Laboratory Safety*, 2nd ed. Chemical Rubber Publishing Company, Cleveland, OH, 1971.

Gordon, Z. V. Occupational health aspects of radiofrequency electromagnetic radiation, in *Ergonomics and Physical Environmental Factors*. Occupational Safety and Health Series, No. 21. International Labor Office, Geneva, 1970.

Grandolfo, M., and Vecchia, P. Physical aspects of radiofrequency electromagnetic field interactions, in Repacholi, M. H., ed. *Non-Ionizing Radiations*. IRPA-INIRC, Australian Radiation Laboratory, Yallambie, Australia, 1988.

Halliday, D., Resnick, R., and Walker, J. *Fundamentals of Physics*, 7th ed. Wiley, New York, 2004.

Hazzard, D. G., ed. *Symposium on Biological Effects and Measurement of Radiofrequency/Microwaves.* HEW Publication (FDA) 77-8026. Bureau of Radiological Health, Rockville, MD, 1977.

Henderson, R., and Schulmeister, K. *Laser Safety,* 2nd ed. Taylor and Francis, London, 2008.

Heinrich, H. Assessment of non-sinusoidal pulsed, or intermittent exposure to low frequency electric and magnetic fields. *Health Phys,* **92:**541–546, 2007.

Hitchcock, R. T., Moss, C. E., Murray, W. E., Patterson, R. M., and Rockwell, R.J. Non-ionizing radiation, in *The Occupational Environment: Its Evaluation and Control.* American Industrial Hygiene Association, Fairfax, VA, 2003.

Hitz, C. B., Ewing, J. J., Hecht, J., eds. *Introduction to Laser Technology.* Wiley-IEEE Press, New York, 2001.

ICNIRP. Guidelines for limiting exposure to time varying electric, magnetic, and electromagnetic fields (up to 300 GHz). *Health Phys,* **74:**494–532, 1998.

ICNIRP. Guidelines on limits of exposure to ultraviolet radiation of wavelengths between 180 nm and 400 nm. *Health Phys,* **87:**171–186, 2004.

ICNIRP. ICNIRP statement on far infrared radiation exposure. *Health Phys,* **91:**630–645, 2006.

ICNIRP. International workshop on EMF dosimetry and biophysical aspects relevant to setting exposure guidelines. *Health Phys,* **92**(6), 2007.

IRPA/INIRC. Protection of the patient undergoing a magnetic resonance examination. *Health Phys,* **61:**923–928, 1991.

International Labor Office (ILO), Geneva.

Occupational Safety and Health Series No.

53. *Occupational Hazards from Non-Ionising Electromagnetic Radiation,* 1985.

57. *Protection of Workers against Radiofrequency and Microwave Radiation: A Technical Review,* 1986.

69. *Protection of Workers from Power Frequency Electric and Magnetic fields: A Practical Guide,* 1994.

70. *Visual Display Units: Radiation Protection Guidance,* 1994.

71. *Protection of Workers from RF Heaters and Sealers,* 1998.

Johnson, C. C., Durney, C. H., Barber, P. W., et al. *Radiofrequency Radiation Dosimetry Handbook.* SAM TR-76-35. USAF School of Aerospace Medicine, Brooks Air Force Base, TX, 1976.

Jokela, K. Assessment of complex EMF exposure situations including inhomogeneous field distribution. *Health Phys,* **9:**531–540, 2007.

Largent, E. J., and Olishifski, J. B. Non-ionizing radiation, in J. B. Olishifsky, ed. *Fundamentals of Industrial Hygiene.* National Safety Council, Chicago, IL, 1979.

Laufer, G. *Introduction to Optics and Lasers in Engineering,* Cambridge University Press, Cambridge, U.K., 1996.

Lin, J. C. Dosimetric comparison between different quantities for limiting exposure in the RF Band: Rationale and implications for Guidelines. *Health Phys,* **92:**547–553, 2007.

Marshal, W., Sliney, D., ed. *LIA Laser Safety Guide,* 10th ed. Laser Institute of America, Cincinnati, OH, 2000.

Martens, L. Different basic dosimetric quantities for the characterization of exposure to low frequency electric and magnetic fields and the implication for practical exposure conditions and guidelines. *Health Phys,* **92:**515–520, 2007.

Lengyel, B. A. *Introduction to Laser Physics.* Wiley, New York, 1966.

Magid, L. M. *Electromagnetic Fields, Energy and Waves.* Wiley, New York, 1972.

Marshall, W. J. Laser reflections from relatively flat specular surfaces. *Health Phys,* **56:**753–757, 1989.

Mooradian, A., Jaeger, T., and Stokseth, P., eds. *Tunable Lasers and Applications.* Springer-Verlag, New York, 1976.

National Council on Radiation Protection and Measurements (NCRP), Bethesda, MD.

Report No.

67. *Radiofrequency Electromagnetic Fields—Properties, Quantities and Units, Biophysical Interaction, and Measurements,* 1981.

86. *Biological Effects and Exposure Criteria for Radiofrequency Electromagnetic Fields,* 1986.

119. *A Practical Guide to the Determination of Human Exposure to Radiofrequency Fields,* 1993.

National Research Council. *Non-thermal Effects of Non-ionizing Radiation.* National Academy Press, Washington, DC, 1986.

Peterson, R. C., Radiofrequency/Microwave protection guides. *Health Phys,* **61:**59–67, 1991.

Polk, C., and Postow, E., eds. *Handbook of Biological Effects of Electromagnetic Fields.* CRC Press, Boca Raton, FL, 1986.

Rayner, S., and Rickert, L. W. Perception of risk: The social context of public concern over non-ionizing radiation, in Repacholi, M. H., ed. *Non-Ionizing Radiations*. IRPA-INIRC, Australian Radiation Laboratory, Yallambie, Australia, 1988.

Repacholi, M. H. ed. *Non-Ionizing Radiations: Physical Characteristics, Biological Effects, and Health Hazard Assessment*. IRPA-INIRC. Australian Radiation Laboratory, Yallambie, Australia, 1988.

Sliney, D. H. Measurement of optical radiation, in Repacholi, M. H., ed. *Non-Ionizing Radiations*. IRPA-INIRC. Australian Radiation Laboratory, Yallambie, Australia, 1988.

Stuchly, M. A. Biological effects of radiofrequency fields, in Repacholi, M. H., ed. *Non-Ionizing Radiations*. IRPA-INIRC. Australian Radiation Laboratory, Yallambie, Australia, 1988.

Stuchly, M. A., and Stuchly, S. S. Experimental radio and microwave dosimetry, in Polk, C., and Postow, E., eds. *Handbook of Biological Effects of Electromagnetic Fields*. CRC Press, Boca Raton, FL, 1986.

World Health Organization Protection (WHO). *Environmental Health Criteria (EHC)*, World Health Organization, Geneva, Switzerland.

No. 16. *Radiofrequency and Microwaves*, 1981.

No. 23, *Lasers and Optical Radiation*, 1982.

No. 35, *Extremely Low Frequency (ELF) Fields, 1992*.

No. 69, *Magnetic Fields, 1987*.

No. 137, *Electromagnetic Fields*, 1992.

No. 160, Ultraviolet Radiation, *2nd ed., 1994*.

APPENDIX A

Values of Some Useful Constants

VALUE	SYMBOL	QUANTITY	SI	cgs
Electron charge	e	$1.6\,E-19$ C	$4.8\,E-10$ SC	
Electron mass	m_0	$9.1085\,E-31$ kg	$9.1085\,E-28$ g	0.000548 amu
				0.000548 amu
Proton mass	m_p	$1.6726\,E-27$ kg	$1.6726\,E-24$ g	1.007276 amu
				1.007276 amu
Neutron mass	m_n	$1.67492\,E-27$ kg	$1.67492\,E-24$ g	1.008665 amu
				1.008665 amu
Atomic mass unit	amu	$1.6604\,E-27$ kg	$1.6604\,E-24$ g	931 MeV 931 MeV
Speed of light	c	$2.997928\,E8$ m/s	$2.997928\,E8$ m/s	
Avogadro's number	N	$6.0247\,E23$ mole^{-1}	$6.0247\,E23$ mole^{-1}	
Planck's constant	h	$6.6262\,E-34$ Js	$6.6262\,E-27$ ergs	
Gas constant	R	8.3144 J mole$^{-1}\,^\circ K^{-1}$	$8.3144\,E7$ ergs mole$^{-1}\,^\circ K^{-1}$	0.082 L atm. mole$^{-1}\,^\circ K^{-1}$
Boltzmann's constant	k	$1.38062\,E-23$ J $^\circ K^{-1}$	$1.38062\,E-16$ erg $^\circ K^{-1}$	
Acceleration of gravity	g	9.807 m s^{-2}	980.665 cm s^{-2}	
Gravitational constant	r	$6.673\,E-11$ Nm^2 kg^{-2}	$6.673\,E-8$ dyne cm^2 g^{-2}	

APPENDIX B

Table of the Elements

NAME	SYMBOL	ATOMIC NO.	ATOMIC WEIGHT
Actinium	Ac	89	227
Aluminum	Al	13	26.98
Americium	Am	95	(243)
Antimony	Sb	51	121.76
Argon	A	18	39.944
Arsenic	As	33	74.92
Astatine	At	85	(210)
Barium	Ba	56	137.36
Berkelium	Bk	97	(249)
Beryllium	Be	4	9.013
Bismuth	Bi	83	208.99
Boron	B	5	10.82
Bromine	Br	35	79.916
Cadmium	Cd	48	112.41
Calcium	Ca	20	40.08
Californium	Cf	98	(251)
Carbon	C	6	12.011
Cerium	Ce	58	140.13
Cesium	Cs	55	132.91
Chlorine	Cl	17	35.457
Chromium	Cr	24	52.01
Cobalt	Co	27	58.94
Columbium,	see Niobium		
Copper	Cu	29	63.54
Curium	Cm	96	(247)
Dysprosium	Dy	66	162.51
Einsteinium	E	99	(254)
Erbium	Er	68	167.27
Europium	Eu	63	152.0
Fermium	Fm	100	(253)
Fluorine	F	9	19.00
Francium	Fr	87	(223)
Gadolinium	Gd	64	157.26
Gallium	Ga	31	69.72
Germanium	Ge	32	72.60
Gold	Au	79	197.0

(*Continued*)

Table of the Elements (*Continued*)

NAME	SYMBOL	ATOMIC NO.	ATOMIC WEIGHT
Hafnium	Hf	72	178.50
Hahnium	Ha	105	(262)
Helium	He	2	4.003
Holmium	Ho	67	164.94
Hydrogen	H	1	1.0080
Indium	In	49	114.82
Iodine	I	53	126.91
Iridium	Ir	77	192.2
Iron	Fe	26	55.85
Kurchatovium	Ku	104	(261)
Krypton	Kr	36	83.80
Lanthanum	La	57	138.92
Lawrencium	Lw	103	(260)
Lead	Pb	82	207.21
Lithium	Li	3	6.940
Lutetium	Lu	71	174.99
Magnesium	Mg	12	24.32
Manganese	Mn	25	54.94
Mendelevium	Mv	101	(256)
Mercury	Hg	80	200.61
Molybdenum	Mo	42	95.95
Neodymium	Nd	60	144.27
Neon	Ne	10	20.183
Neptunium	Np	93	(237)
Nickel	Ni	28	58.71
Niobium (columbium)	Nb	41	92.91
Nitrogen	N	7	14.008
Nobelium	No	102	(254)
Osmium	Os	76	190.2
Oxygen	O	8	16.000
Palladium	Pd	46	106.4
Phosphorus	P	15	30.975
Platinum	Pt	78	195.09
Plutonium	Pu	94	(242)
Polonium	Po	84	210
Potassium	K	19	39.100
Praseodymium	Pr	59	140.92
Promethium	Pm	61	(147)
Protactinium	Pa	91	231
Radium	Ra	88	226
Radon	Rn	86	222
Rhenium	Re	75	186.22
Rhodium	Rh	45	102.91
Rubidium	Rb	37	85.48
Ruthenium	Ru	44	101.1
Selenium	Se	34	78.96
Samarium	Sm	62	150.35
Scandium	Sc	21	44.96
Silicon	Si	14	28.09
Silver	Ag	47	107.873
Sodium	Na	11	22.991
Strontium	Sr	38	87.63
Sulfur	S	16	32.066

(*Continued*)

Table of the Elements (*Continued*)

NAME	SYMBOL	ATOMIC NO.	ATOMIC WEIGHT
Tantalum	Ta	73	180.95
Technetium	Tc	43	(99)
Tellurium	Te	52	127.61
Terbium	Tb	65	158.93
Thallium	Tl	81	204.39
Thorium	Th	90	232
Thulium	Tm	69	168.94
Tin	Sn	50	118.70
Titanium	Ti	22	47.90
Tungsten (wolfram)	W	74	183.86
Uranium	U	92	238.07
Vanadium	V	23	50.95
Xenon	Xe	54	131.30
Ytterbium	Yb	70	173.04
Yttrium	Y	39	88.91
Zinc	Zn	30	65.38
Zirconium	Zr	40	91.22

APPENDIX C

The Reference Person Overall Specifications

PARAMETER	MALE	FEMALE
Weight, kg	70	58
Height, cm	170	120
Surface area, m^2	1.8	1.6
Specific gravity	1.07	1.04
Total body water, per kg	0.62	0.52
Intracellular water, per kg	0.34	0.32
Total blood volume, L	5.2	3.9
Total blood weight, kg	5.5	4.1

Weight of Selected Organs of the Adult Human Body

ORGAN	MALE, GRAMS	FEMALE, GRAMS
Total Body	70,000	58,000
Muscle, skeletal	28,000	17,000
Fat	13,500	16,000
Skeleton		
Without bone marrow	7,000	4,200
Red marrow	1,500	1,300
Yellow marrow	1,500	1,300
Blood	5,500	4,100
Skin and sub-cutaneous tissue	2,600	1,790
Liver	1,800	1,400
Brain	1,400	1,200
Gastrointestinal tract	1,200	1,100
Contents of the GI tract		
Stomach	250	ng[a]
Small intestine	400	ng
Upper large intestine	220	ng
Lower large intestine	135	ng
Lungs, including blood	1,000	800
Lymphoid tissue	700	580
Breast	26	380
Kidneys (2)	310	275
Heart, without blood in chambers	330	240
Spleen	180	150
Pancreas	100	85
Salivary glands (6)	85	70
Uterus, non-pregnant		80
Teeth	46	41
Urinary bladder	45	45
Testes (2)	35	
Spinal cord	30	28
Thymus	20	20
Thyroid gland	20	17
Prostate gland	16	
Eyes (2)	15	15
Adrenal glands (2)	14	14
Ovaries (2)		11

[a]ng 5 not given.

Source: ICRP 23. Reproduced with permission from International Commission on Radiological Protection (ICRP). *Report of the Task Group on Reference Man.* Oxford, England: Pergamon Press; 1965. ICRP Report 23. Copyright © 1965 International Commission on Radiological Protection.

Chemical Composition

ELEMENT	PROPORTION, %	APPROXIMATE WEIGHT, G
Oxygen	61.0	43,000
Carbon	23.0	16,000
Hydrogen	10.0	7,000
Nitrogen	2.6	1,800
Calcium	1.4	1,000
Phosphorus	1.1	780
Sulfur	0.2	140
Potassium	0.2	140
Sodium	0.14	100
Chlorine	0.12	95
Magnesium	0.027	19
Iron	0.006	4.2
Zinc	0.0033	2.3
Copper	0.0001	0.072
Iodine	0.00002	0.013
Manganese	0.00002	0.012

Applied Physiology

Data for adults for normal activity in a temperate zone

1. *Water balance[a]*

DAILY WATER INTAKE, ML	MEN	WOMEN
Water of oxidation	350	250
In food	700	450
As fluids	1,950	1,400
Total	3,000	2,100

DAILY WATER OUTPUT, ML	MEN	WOMEN
Sweat	650	420
Insensible	850	600
In feces	100	90
Urine	1,400	1,000
Total	3,000	2,100

2. *Respiratory data[a]*

	ADULT MEN	ADULT WOMEN
Total lung capacity (TLC), L	5.6	4.4
Functional residual capacity (FRC), L	2.2	1.8
Vital capacity (VC), L	4.3	3.3
Anatomical dead space (ADS), L	0.16	0.13
Minute volume (MV), L/m		
Resting	7.5	6.0
Light activity	20.0	19.0
Total inhaled volume, L		
8 h at work	9,600	9,100
8 h light activity	9,600	9,100
8 h resting	3,600	2,900
Daily total, L	2.3E4	2.1E4
% breathed at work	42	43
Gas exchange area, m^2	75	66

TLC: Amount of gas in the lungs at the end of a maximal inhalation.

FRC: Volume of gas in the lungs at the end of a resting exhalation.

VC: Maximal volume of air that can be expelled from the lungs after a maximal inhalation.

ADS: Volume of the respiratory tract where no gas exchange occurs. It includes the "ducts" that carry the inhaled air to the deep respiratory tract, where gas exchange occurs.

MV: Amount of air inhaled in one minute.

Duration of Exposure

1. *Occupational exposure*

The following figures have been adopted in calculations pertaining to occupational exposure:
   8 hours per day
   40 hours per week
   50 weeks per year
   50 years continuous work period

2. *Nonoccupational exposure*
A nominal lifetime of 70 years has been adopted

Source: Data from ICRP 30.

Blood Counts, Normal Values for Adults

BLOOD COMPONENTS	MEN	FEMALE
Red blood count ($3\,10^6$/mL)	5.4 ± 0.8	4.8 ± 0.6
Hemoglobin (g/100 mL)	16.0 ± 2.0	14.0 ± 2.0
Hematocrit (volume %)	47.0 ± 7.0	42.0 ± 5.0
White blood counts (leukocytes)		
Total leukocytes:	4,300–10,800/mL percent	
Segmented neutrophils	34–75	
Band neutrophils	0–8	
Lymphocytes	12–50	
Monocytes	3–15	
Eosinophils	0–5	
Basophils	0–3	

Reproduced with permission from Berkow R et al. *The Merck Manual of Diagnosis and Therapy.*
15th ed. Rahway, NJ: Merck Sharp & Dohme Research Laboratories: 1987:101–105. Copyright
© 1987 by Merck & Co., Inc., Rahway, NJ.

APPENDIX D

Source in Bladder Contents

	ENERGY IN MeV					
	0.01	**0.015**	**0.020**	**0.030**	**0.050**	**0.10**
Bladder wall	8.49E–04	1.40E–03	1.43E–03	9.83E–04	4.49E–04	2.56E–04
Stomach wall	2.83E–18*	4.25E–18[†]	1.20E–11[†]	3.28E–08[†]	4.53E–07	1.05E–06
Small intestine plus contents	1.52E–10*	2.28E–10[†]	1.76E–07	5.11E–06	1.24E–05	1.22E–05
Upper large intestine wall	1.71E–10*	2.57E–10[†]	1.02E–07[†]	3.04E–06	8.59E–06	8.31E–06
Lower large intestine wall	3.42E–07*	5.12E–07	7.80E–06	3.51E–05	4.16E–05	3.01E–05
Kidneys	1.52E–19*	2.28E–19[†]	3.95E–12[†]	2.46E–08[†]	4.05E–07	9.98E–07
Liver	2.61E–19*	3.91E–19[†]	2.37E–12[†]	2.05E–08	2.72E–07	5.55E–07
Lungs	4.25E–29*	6.39E–29[†]	5.55E–17[†]	7.65E–11[†]	1.31E–08	8.89E–08
"Other tissues" (suggested for muscle)	2.00E–07^	2.02E–06^	5.42E–06^	9.69E–06^	9.26E–06^	6.86E–06^
Ovaries	6.23E–09*	9.35E–09[†]	1.62E–06[†]	2.78E–05	3.58E–05	2.82E–05
Pancreas	3.63E–22*	5.45E–22[†]	2.11E–13[†]	6.51E–09[†]	2.92E–07	7.24E–07
Skeleton (suggested for total endosteal cells)	2.56E–11*	3.84E–11%	1.60E–08	1.16E–06	4.30E–06	4.06E–06
Red marrow	2.84E–08*	4.25E–08*	5.67E–08	3.88E–06	1.23E–05	1.00E–05
Skin	2.66E–08*	3.99E–08	3.75E–07	1.70E–06	2.26E–06	2.12E–06
Spleen	2.63E–22*	3.94E–22[†]	1.52E–13[†]	4.78E–09[†]	1.96E–07	3.87E–06
Testes	1.79E–09*	2.69E–09[†]	1.39E–06	1.54E–05	2.75E–05	1.88E–05
Thymus	5.91E–37*	8.87E–37[†]	1.32E–20[†]	2.05E–12[†]	2.06E–09[†]	2.67E–08[†]
Thyroid	6.20E–25*	9.31E–25[†]	1.24E–24[†]	2.86E–14[†]	1.55E–10[†]	4.05E–09[†]
Uterus	3.88E–06*	5.83E–06	4.28E–05	1.09E–04	1.02E–04	6.21E–05
Total body	1.43E–05	1.43E–05	1.42E–05	1.31E–05	1.00E–05	7.28E–06
Bladder wall	2.47E–04	2.56E–04	2.22E–04	2.07E–04	1.97E–04	1.57E–04
Stomach wall	1.02E–06	1.10E–06	1.86E–06	1.30E–06	1.83E–06	1.53E–06
Small intestine plus contents	1.03E–05	8.97E–06	8.84E–06	8.17E–06	8.42E–06	6.65E–06
Upper large intestine wall	8.37E–06	8.18E–06	6.19E–06	6.15E–06	5.80E–06	5.29E–06
Lower large intestine wall	2.51E–05	2.44E–05	2.09E–05	2.16E–05	2.02E–05	1.36E–05
Kidneys	1.00E–06	1.33E–06	1.17E–06	1.69E–06	1.26E–06	1.37E–06
Liver	7.70E–07	9.76E–07	1.02E–06	9.60E–07	1.19E–06	1.04E–06
Lungs	9.33E–08	1.65E–07	2.83E–07	3.07E–07	3.31E–07	4.61E–07
"Other tissues" (suggested for muscle)	6.28E–06^	6.13E–06^	5.71E–06^	5.42E–06^	5.11E–06^	4.27E–06^
Ovaries	2.72E–05	2.17E–05	1.35E–05	2.31E–05	1.66E–05	1.48E–05
Pancreas	1.10E–06	8.92E–07	1.00E–06	8.00E–07	1.40E–06	8.26E–07
Skeleton (suggested for total endosteal cells)	2.70E–06	2.03E–06	1.78E–06	1.72E–06	1.71E–06	1.55E–06

(Continued)

Source in Bladder Contents (*Continued*)

	ENERGY IN MeV					
	0.01	0.015	0.020	0.030	0.050	0.10
Red marrow	6.10E–06	4.33E–06	3.72E–06	3.47E–06	3.36E–06	3.07E–06
Skin	2.01E–06	2.24E–06	2.35E–06	2.22E–06	2.12E–06	1.89E–06
Spleen	5.29E–07	7.80E–07	8.59E–07	6.34E–07	1.12E–06	4.63E–07
Testes	1.59E–05	1.75E–05	1.57E–05	1.28E–05	1.40E–05	1.21E–05
Thymus	6.22E–08†	1.10E–07†	1.54E–07†	1.78E–07†	1.94E–07†	2.10E–07†
Thyroid	1.33E–08†	3.27E–08†	5.68E–08†	7.33E–08†	8.55E–08†	1.05E–07†
Uterus	5.51E–05	5.11E–05	4.68E–05	3.98E–05	4.04E–05	3.30E–05
Total body	6.58E–06	6.44E–06	5.98E–06	5.63E–06	5.35E–06	4.44E–06

* Extrapolation from higher energy
† Build up factor method
% Calculated by difference

APPENDIX E

Total Mass Attenuation Coefficients, μ/ρ, cm²/g

	0.1 MeV	0.15 MeV	0.2 MeV	0.3 MeV	0.4 MeV
H	0.295	0.265	0.243	0.212	0.189
	0.173	0.160	0.140	0.126	0.113
	0.103	0.0876	0.0691	0.0572	0.0502
	0.0446	0.0371	0.0321		
Be	0.132	0.119	0.109	0.0945	0.0847
	0.0773	0.0715	0.0628	0.0565	0.0504
	0.0459	0.0394	0.0313	0.0266	0.0234
	0.0211	0.0180	0.0161		
C	0.149	0.134	0.122	0.106	0.0953
	0.0870	0.0805	0.0707	0.0636	0.0568
	0.0518	0.0444	0.0356	0.0304	0.0270
	0.0245	0.0213	0.0194		
N	0.150	0.134	0.123	0.106	0.0955
	0.0869	0.0805	0.0707	0.0636	0.0568
	0.0517	0.0445	0.0357	0.0306	0.0273
	0.0249	0.0218	0.0200		
O	0.151	0.134	0.123	0.107	0.0953
	0.0870	0.0806	0.0708	0.0636	0.0568
	0.0518	0.0445	0.0359	0.0309	0.0276
	0.0254	0.0224	0.0206		
Na	0.151	0.130	0.118	0.102	0.0912
	0.0833	0.0770	0.0676	0.0608	0.0546
	0.0496	0.0427	0.0348	0.0303	0.0274
	0.0254	0.0229	0.0215		
Mg	0.160	0.135	0.122	0.106	0.0944
	0.0860	0.0795	0.0699	0.0627	0.0560
	0.0512	0.0442	0.0360	0.0315	0.0286
	0.0266	0.0242	0.0228		
Al	0.161	0.134	0.120	0.103	0.0922
	0.0840	0.0777	0.0683	0.0614	0.0548
	0.0500	0.0432	0.0353	0.0310	0.0282
	0.0264	0.0241	0.0229		
Si	0.172	0.139	0.125	0.107	0.0954
	0.0869	0.0802	0.0706	0.0635	0.0567
	0.0517	0.0447	0.0367	0.0323	0.0296
	0.0277	0.0254	0.0243		
P	0.174	0.137	0.122	0.104	0.0928
	0.0846	0.0780	0.0685	0.0617	0.0551
	0.0502	0.0436	0.0358	0.0316	0.0290
	0.0273	0.0252	0.0242		

(*Continued*)

Total Mass Attenuation Coefficients, μ/ρ, cm^2/g (Continued)

	0.1 MeV	0.15 MeV	0.2 MeV	0.3 MeV	0.4 MeV
S	0.188	0.144	0.127	0.108	0.0958
	0.0874	0.0806	0.0707	0.0635	0.0568
	0.0519	0.0448	0.0371	0.0328	0.0302
	0.0284	0.0266	0.0255		
Ar	0.188	0.135	0.117	0.0977	0.0867
	0.0790	0.0730	0.0638	0.0573	0.0512
	0.0468	0.0407	0.0338	0.0301	0.0279
	0.0266	0.0248	0.0241		
K	0.215	0.149	0.127	0.106	0.0938
	0.0852	0.0786	0.0689	0.0618	0.0552
	0.0505	0.0438	0.0365	0.0327	0.0305
	0.0289	0.0274	0.0267		
Ca	0.238	0.158	0.132	0.109	0.0965
	0.0876	0.0809	0.0708	0.0634	0.0566
	0.0518	0.0451	0.0376	0.0338	0.0316
	0.0302	0.0285	0.0280		
Fe	0.344	0.183	0.138	0.106	0.0919
	0.0828	0.0762	0.0664	0.0595	0.0531
	0.0485	0.0424	0.0361	0.0330	0.0313
	0.0304	0.0295	0.0294		
Cu	0.427	0.206	0.147	0.108	0.0916
	0.0820	0.0751	0.0654	0.0585	0.0521
	0.0476	0.0418	0.0357	0.0330	0.0316
	0.0309	0.0303	0.0305		
Mo	1.03	0.389	0.225	0.130	0.0998
	0.0851	0.0761	0.0648	0.0575	0.0510
	0.0467	0.0414	0.0365	0.0349	0.0344
	0.0344	0.0349	0.0359		
Sn	1.58	0.563	0.303	0.153	0.109
	0.0886	0.0776	0.0647	0.0568	0.0501
	0.0459	0.0408	0.0367	0.0355	0.0355
	0.0358	0.0368	0.0383		
I	1.83	0.648	0.339	0.165	0.114
	0.0913	0.0792	0.0653	0.0571	0.0502
	0.0460	0.0409	0.0370	0.0360	0.0361
	0.0365	0.0377	0.0394		
W	4.21	1.44	0.708	0.293	0.174
	0.125	0.101	0.0763	0.0640	0.0544
	0.0492	0.0437	0.0405	0.0402	0.0409
	0.0418	0.0438	0.0465		
Pt	4.75	1.64	0.795	0.324	0.191
	0.135	0.107	0.0800	0.0659	0.0554
	0.0501	0.0445	0.0414	0.0411	0.0418
	0.0427	0.0448	0.0477		
Tl	5.16	1.80	0.866	0.346	0.204
	0.143	0.112	0.0824	0.0675	0.0563
	0.0508	0.0452	0.0420	0.0416	0.0423
	0.0433	0.0454	0.0484		
Pb	5.29	1.84	0.896	0.356	0.208
	0.145	0.114	0.0836	0.0684	0.0569
	0.0512	0.0457	0.0421	0.0420	0.0426
	0.0436	0.0459	0.0489		

Total Mass Attenuation Coefficients, μ/ρ, cm^2/g (*Continued*)

	0.1 MeV	0.15 MeV	0.2 MeV	0.3 MeV	0.4 MeV
U	1.06	2.42	1.17	0.452	0.259
	0.176	0.136	0.0952	0.0757	0.0615
	0.0548	0.0484	0.0445	0.0440	0.0446
	0.0455	0.0479	0.0511		
Air	0.151	0.134	0.123	0.106	0.0953
	0.0868	0.0804	0.0706	0.0655	0.0567
	0.0517	0.0445	0.0357	0.0307	0.0274
	0.0250	0.0220	0.0202		
NaI	1.57	0.568	0.305	0.155	0.111
	0.0901	0.0789	0.0657	0.0577	0.0508
	0.0465	0.0412	0.0367	0.0351	0.0347
	0.0347	0.0354	0.0366		
H_2O	0.167	0.149	0.136	0.118	0.106
	0.0966	0.0896	0.0786	0.0706	0.0630
	0.0575	0.0493	0.0396	0.0339	0.0301
	0.0275	0.0240	0.0219		
Concrete*	0.169	0.139	0.124	0.107	0.0954
	0.0870	0.0804	0.0706	0.0635	0.0567
	0.0517	0.0445	0.0363	0.0317	0.0287
	0.0268	0.0243	0.0229		
Tissue[†]	0.163	0.144	0.132	0.115	0.100
	0.0936	0.0867	0.0761	0.0683	0.0600
	0.0556	0.0478	0.0384	0.0329	0.0292
	0.0267	0.0233	0.0212		

Reproduced from Etherington H. *Nuclear Engineering Handbook*. New York, NY: McGraw-Hill; 1958.

Mass Energy Absorption Coefficients, μ_a/ρ, cm^2/g

	0.1 MeV	0.15 MeV	0.2 MeV	0.3 MeV	0.4 MeV
H	0.0411	0.0487	0.0531	0.0575	0.0589
	0.0591	0.0590	0.0575	0.0557	0.0533
	0.0509	0.0467	0.0401	0.0354	0.0318
	0.0291	0.0252	0.0255		
Be	0.0183	0.0217	0.0237	0.0256	0.0263
	0.0264	0.0263	0.0256	0.0248	0.0237
	0.0227	0.0210	0.0183	0.0164	0.0151
	0.0141	0.0127	0.0118		
C	0.0215	0.0246	0.0267	0.0288	0.0296
	0.0297	0.0296	0.0289	0.0280	0.0268
	0.0256	0.0237	0.0209	0.0190	0.0177
	0.0166	0.0153	0.0145		
N	0.0224	0.0249	0.0267	0.0288	0.0296
	0.0297	0.0296	0.0289	0.0280	0.0268
	0.0256	0.0238	0.0211	0.0193	0.0180
	0.0171	0.0158	0.0151		
O	0.0233	0.0252	0.0271	0.0289	0.0296
	0.0297	0.0296	0.0289	0.0280	0.0268
	0.0257	0.0238	0.0212	0.0195	0.0183
	0.0175	0.0163	0.0157		
Na	0.0289	0.0258	0.0266	0.0279	0.0283
	0.0284	0.0284	0.0276	0.0268	0.0257
	0.0246	0.0229	0.0207	0.0194	0.0185
	0.0179	0.0171	0.0168		
Mg	0.0335	0.0276	0.0278	0.0290	0.0294
	0.0293	0.0292	0.0285	0.0276	0.0265
	0.0254	0.0237	0.0215	0.0203	0.0194
	0.0188	0.0182	0.0180		
Al	0.0373	0.0283	0.0275	0.0283	0.0287
	0.0286	0.0286	0.0278	0.0270	0.0259
	0.0248	0.0232	0.0212	0.0200	0.0192
	0.0188	0.0183	0.0182		
Si	0.0435	0.0300	0.0286	0.0291	0.0293
	0.0290	0.0290	0.0282	0.0274	0.0263
	0.0252	0.0236	0.0217	0.0206	0.0198
	0.0194	0.0190	0.0189		
P	0.0501	0.0315	0.0292	0.0289	0.0290
	0.0290	0.0287	0.0280	0.0271	0.0260
	0.0250	0.0234	0.0216	0.0206	0.0200
	0.0197	0.0194	0.0195		

(*Continued*)

Mass Energy Absorption Coefficients, μ_a/ρ, cm^2/g (*Continued*)

	0.1 MeV	0.15 MeV	0.2 MeV	0.3 MeV	0.4 MeV
S	0.0601	0.0351	0.0310	0.0301	0.0301
	0.0300	0.0298	0.0288	0.0279	0.0268
	0.0258	0.0242	0.0224	0.0215	0.0209
	0.0206	0.0206	0.0206		
Ar	0.0729	0.0368	0.0302	0.0278	0.0274
	0.0272	0.0270	0.0260	0.0252	0.0242
	0.0233	0.0220	0.0206	0.0199	0.0195
	0.0195	0.0194	0.0197		
K	0.0909	0.0433	0.0340	0.0304	0.0298
	0.0295	0.0291	0.0282	0.0272	0.0261
	0.0251	0.0237	0.0222	0.0217	0.0214
	0.0212	0.0215	0.0219		
Ca	0.111	0.0489	0.0367	0.0318	0.0309
	0.0304	0.0300	0.0290	0.0279	0.0268
	0.0258	0.0244	0.0230	0.0225	0.0222
	0.0223	0.0225	0.0231		
Fe	0.225	0.0810	0.0489	0.0340	0.0307
	0.0294	0.0287	0.0274	0.0261	0.0250
	0.0242	0.0231	0.0224	0.0224	0.0227
	0.0231	0.0239	0.0250		
Cu	0.310	0.107	0.0594	0.0368	0.0316
	0.0296	0.0286	0.0271	0.0260	0.0247
	0.0237	0.0229	0.0223	0.0227	0.0231
	0.0237	0.0248	0.0261		
Mo	0.922	0.294	0.141	0.0617	0.0422
	0.0348	0.0315	0.0281	0.0263	0.0248
	0.0239	0.0233	0.0237	0.0250	0.0262
	0.0274	0.0296	0.0316		
Sn	1.469	0.471	0.222	0.0873	0.0534
	0.0403	0.0346	0.0294	0.0268	0.0248
	0.0239	0.0233	0.0243	0.0259	0.0276
	0.0291	0.0316	0.0339		
I	1.726	0.557	0.260	0.100	0.0589
	0.0433	0.0366	0.0303	0.0274	0.0252
	0.0241	0.0236	0.0247	0.0265	0.0283
	0.0299	0.0327	0.0353		
W	4.112	1.356	0.631	0.230	0.121
	0.0786	0.0599	0.0426	0.0353	0.0302
	0.0281	0.0271	0.0287	0.0311	0.0335
	0.0355	0.0390	0.0426		
Pt	4.645	1.556	0.719	0.262	0.138
	0.0892	0.0666	0.0465	0.0375	0.0315
	0.0293	0.0280	0.0296	0.0320	0.0343
	0.0365	0.0400	0.0438		
Tl	5.057	1.717	0.791	0.285	0.152
	0.0972	0.0718	0.0491	0.0393	0.0326
	0.0301	0.0288	0.0304	0.0326	0.0349
	0.0354	0.0406	0.0446		
Pb	5.193	1.753	0.821	0.294	0.156
	0.0994	0.0738	0.0505	0.0402	0.0332
	0.0306	0.0293	0.0305	0.0330	0.0352
	0.0373	0.0412	0.0450		

(Continued)

Mass Energy Absorption Coefficients, μ_a/ρ, cm^2/g (*Continued*)

	0.1 MeV	0.15 MeV	0.2 MeV	0.3 MeV	0.4 MeV
U	0.963	2.337	1.096	0.392	0.208
	0.132	0.0968	0.0628	0.0482	0.0383
	0.0346	0.0324	0.0332	0.0352	0.0374
	0.0394	0.0443	0.0474		
Air	0.0233	0.0251	0.0268	0.0288	0.0296
	0.0297	0.0296	0.0289	0.0280	0.0268
	0.0256	0.0238	0.0211	0.0194	0.0181
	0.0172	0.0160	0.0153		
NaI	1.466	0.476	0.224	0.0889	0.0542
	0.0410	0.0354	0.0299	0.0273	0.0253
	0.0242	0.0235	0.0241	0.0254	0.0268
	0.0281	0.0303	0.0325		
H$_2$O	0.0253	0.0278	0.0300	0.0321	0.0328
	0.0330	0.0329	0.0321	0.0311	0.0298
	0.0285	0.0264	0.0233	0.0213	0.0198
	0.0188	0.0173	0.0165		
Concrete*	0.0416	0.0300	0.0289	0.0294	0.0297
	0.0296	0.0295	0.0287	0.0278	0.0272
	0.0256	0.0239	0.0216	0.0203	0.0194
	0.0188	0.0180	0.0177		
Tissue[†]	0.0271	0.0282	0.0293	0.0312	0.0317
	0.0320	0.0319	0.0311	0.0300	0.0288
	0.0276	0.0256	0.0220	0.0206	0.0192
	0.0182	0.0168	0.0160		

Reproduced from Etherington H. *Nuclear Engineering Handbook*. New York, NY: McGraw-Hill; 1958.

ANSWERS TO PROBLEMS

2.1   0.53 m/s to the left

2.2   a. 6.25×10^5 m/s^2
     b. 3.125×10^4 N
     c. 25 (kg m)/s
     d. 25(kg m)/s

2.3 6.02×10^{24} kg

2.4   17.4 km/h @ 9.5° to auto's direction

2.5   0.0017 radian

2.6 2×10^{-4} C

2.7 9.8×10^{-8} C

2.8   1.44 V

2.9   a. 0.73×10^7 m/s
       1.03×10^7 m/s
     b. 1.16×10^{-6} N

2.10 electron: v/c = 0.941
      m/m$_0$ = 2.96
      proton: v/c = 0.046
      m/m$_0$ = 1.001

2.11 2.77×10^{-13} m

2.12 1.4×10^{-8} m

2.13 3.73 eV

2.14 5.4×10^{-10} m

2.15 a. 816 V
     b. 0.83 MeV
     c. 1.24 MeV

2.16 1.92×10^{-5} m/s

2.17 a. 1.88×10^7 m/s
     b. 1.07×10^{-9} s

2.18 a. 1.9×10^7 m/s
     b. 1.65×10^{-9} s

2.19 1.04×10^{-18} J

2.20 1500 W

2.21 1×10^{-4} C
     2×10^{-4} C

2.22 a. 45.55 V
     b. 4×10^6 m/s

2.23 1.42×10^{-10}

2.24 a. 0.8 kg
     b. 2.7×10^9 kg

2.25 a. 3.83×10^{26} W
     b. 4.3×10^6 tonnes/s

2.26 10.5 MeV

2.27 a. 0.39 Å
     b. 6.614×10^{-24} m
     c. 2.86×10^{-14} m

2.28 a. 1.05×10^3 J/Btu
     b. 4186 J/(kg° C)

2.29 a. 0.73 A/m
     b. 194.5 V/m
     c. 10 mW/cm^2

2.30 a. 1.33×10^{-6} mW/cm^2
     b. 2.65×10^{-4} A/m

2.31 a. 1.59×10^{-7} mW/cm^2
     b. 3.5×10^{-2} V/m
     c. 9.1×10^{-5} A/m

2.32 714 V/m, 1.89 A/m

2.33 1.61×10^5 m^3

2.34 a. 6.8×10^7 m/s
     b. 2.65%

2.35 a. 8.375×10^{-16} J
     b. 8.375×10^{-9} erg
     c. 5234 eV

2.36 a. 3.077 m/s
     b. 4.9×10^{-12} N

2.37 a1. 2.1×10^6 m/s
     a2. 2.999×10^8 m/s
     b. 50

3.1 4.3×10^{-14} m

3.2 3.29×10^{22} atoms

3.3   a. 2.49×10^{-11} cm
    b. 2.8×10^3 eV

3.4   54.4 eV

3.5   1.1 mA

3.6   0.0075

3.7 1.1×10^5 per cm

3.8 1.46×10^{-15} g(cm/s)
    0.4 MeV

3.9   193 nm

3.10 a. 5.7×10^{11} J
     b. 0.48 MeV

3.11 Be: 2.3×10^{14} g/cm^3
     Pb: 2.3×10^{14} g/cm^3

3.12 K: 2e, L: 8e, M: 3e

3.13 13.6 eV

3.14 0.42 eV

3.15 a. 2.93×10^6 m/s
     b. 50.7 nm

3.16 3.19×10^{16} photons/s

3.17 7.587 MeV

3.18 102.3 nm, 12.11 eV
     2.93×10^{15} s^{-1}, 97 nm
     12.78 eV, 3.085×10^{15} s^{-1}

3.19 V$_H$ = 2.2×10^6 m/s
     V$_{He}$ = 4.5×10^6 m/s

3.20 2.6 eV

3.21 15.99937 amu

3.22 35.45273 amu

3.23 Na: 9.27×10^{19}
     Cl: 9.27×10^{19}
     H: 6.69×10^{22}
     O: 3.34×10^{22}

3.24 2×10^4 phot/cm^2/s

3.25 4.14 MeV

3.26 6.69×10^{22}

3.27 8.198×10^{-14} J
  0.512 MeV
  0.042 Å

3.28 1.47×10^{-6} g

3.29 1.545 Å

3.30 2952 Å

3.31 a. $f_e = 57.6$ N
  b. $f_g = 1.84 \times 10^{-34}$

3.32 4.34 eV

4.1 0.156 MeV

4.2 1.3 MBq, 35.1 μCi

4.3

	^{198}Au, %	^{131}I, %
t(0)	65	35
t(3)	52	48
t(8)	32	68
t(16)	11	89

  $A(t) = 37e^{-0.26t} + 20e^{-0.086t}$

4.4 b. 14.3 d
  c. 0.049 d^{-1}
  d. $A(t) = 5500e^{-0.049t}$
  e. ^{32}P

4.5 289.3 mCi, 10.7 GBq

4.6 4×10^4

4.7 1.2 μg

4.8 299 years

4.9 a. 55 d
  b. 5 d
  c. 160 d
  d. 1200 d

4.10 36%

4.11 3.25×10^{15}

4.12 9.96×10^5

4.13 a. 598 d
  b. 86.6 d

4.14 39 tonnes

4.15 4.2 g

4.16 U-4: 0.029 Ci/ton
  U-5: 0.00132 Ci/ton
  U-8: 0.029 Ci/ton

4.17 U-4: 0.34 μCi
  U-5: 0.016 μCi
  U-8: 0.34 μCi

4.18 1.3°C

4.19 23 μCi/tonne

4.20 6.28

4.21 104 hours

4.22 $A(t) = 100e^{-0.087t} + 10e^{-0.115t}$

4.23 $\sim$ 7 h

4.24 2.6 μg

4.25 0.27 g U-8
  0.26 g U-5
  0.58 g Th-232

4.26 70 y, 1.1×10^{14} Bq

4.27 26 min.

4.28 0.12 Bq

4.29 5.2×10^{16} Bq/m^3

4.30

	^{35}S	^{14}C
a.	7.8×10^{-9} W/MBq	7.9×10^{-9} W/MBq
b.	1.3×10^4 W/kg	1.3 W/kg

4.31 a. 1.8×10^{-7} W/MBq
  b. 972 W/kg

4.32 5.2×10^9 J

4.33 a. 4.5×10^8 W/kg
  b. 4.5×10^8 W/kg

4.34 6.4×10^{-5} mL

4.35 23.3 atm.

4.36 a. 9.47×10^{11} Bq
  b. 5.7×10^{-3} MeV/t

4.37 a. 136.5 h
  b. 0.035 μg

4.38 a. 3×10^4 Ci
  b. Yes

4.39 1.15×10^9 Bq

4.40 7.1×10^{16} Bq/year

4.41 U-8/U-5 = 34.6

4.42 a. U-4: 3.5×10^6 Bq
  U-5: 7.56×10^4 Bq
  U-8: 631 Bq
  b. 3.58×10^{16} Bq

4.43 a. 73 mCi
  b. 73 mCi
  c. 0.92 mg
  d1. 0
  d2. 4.6×10^3 Ci/g
  d3. $15.8 \times \mu$g

4.44 a. 6.93 m
  b. 10 m

4.45 b. 128.7 mrems/y

4.46 a1. 7μ Ci/g
  a2. 2.6×10^5 Bq/g
  b. 2.9×10^{-8} Ci

4.47 a. 1.58×10^5 Ci/g
  b. 2.5×10^{-17} g
  c. 1.3×10^{-9} mole
  d. 0.041 mole
  e. 2.75×10^{-18}%

4.48 7.35×10^8 y

4.49 a. 5.42 MBq
  b. 2.63×10^{15} atoms
  c. 4.36×10^{-9} mole
  d. 0.107 μL

4.50 7.2 dpm

4.51 1.24 μg

4.52 5.65 mL

5.1 4.08×10^{23}

5.2 Si: 2.65×10^{22}
  O: 5.3×10^{22}

5.3 Al: 3.9×10^{23} elec/cm^2
  Fe: 3.8×10^{23} elec/cm^2

5.4 ^{32}P

5.5 E = 1.17 MeV
  ^{210}Bi

5.6 0.083 cm

5.7 a. 1.09 MeV
  b. 1.30 MeV

5.8 a. 0.077 MeV
  b. 0.023 MeV

5.9 a. 0.22 MeV
  b. 0.22 MeV

5.10 0.48 MeV

5.11 0.61 MeV

5.12 a. 0.047 MeV
  b. 0.617 MeV
  c. 1.12 MeV

5.13 a. 0.63 per cm
  0.056 cm^2 /g
  19.2 barns
  b. 1.25 MeV

5.14 a. beta and gamma
  b. $\sim$1 MeV
  c. 0.4 MeV
  d. ^{198}Au
  e. $900e^{-24t} + 100e^{-0.25t}$

5.15 41.3

5.16 1:0.8:1.2

5.17 a. 6.25×10^9 phot/cm^2 /s
  b. 1.12×10^3 ergs/g/s
  0.112 J/kg/s

5.18 a. HVL

  0.1MeV $\left\{ \begin{array}{l} \text{Al 1.59 cm} \\ \text{Cu 0.18 cm} \end{array} \right\}$

  0.8 MeV $\left\{ \begin{array}{l} \text{Al 3.75 cm} \\ \text{Cu 1.12 cm} \end{array} \right\}$

TVL

$0.1 \text{ MeV} \begin{cases} \text{Al } 5.3 \text{ cm} \\ \text{Cu } 0.6 \text{ cm} \end{cases}$

$0.8 \text{ MeV} \begin{cases} \text{Al } 12.4 \text{ cm} \\ \text{Cu } 3.7 \text{ cm} \end{cases}$

1 TVL = 3.3 HVL

5.19 14.3 cm

5.20 a. 1.24 cm
0.063

5.21 a. 0.4
b. 0.285
c. 0.044
d. 0.042

5.22 2.8 MeV

5.23 0.37 mW/cm^2

5.24 100,000 V

5.25 3,300 ion pairs

5.26 1.2×10^5 n/s/MBq
4.4×10^3 n/s/μCi

5.27 4.4×10^5 cm/s
1159 K, 886°C

5.28 6.4×10^8 n/cm^2 /s

5.29 0.0059 cm

5.30 2.6×10^6 n/s

5.31 58.1 days

5.32 4.4×10^{-7} μCi

5.33 1.39×10^{-11}

5.34 1.0089 amu

5.35 a. 0.0091:1
b. 96:1

5.36 0.0175 cm

5.37 a. 4.82×10^{-4} cm
b. 21 m

5.38 44 collisions
117 collisions

5.39 6.5 MBq
175 μCi

5.40 a. 0.249 per cm
b. 1.96×10^{10} n/s

5.41 4.1×10^{-5} mol Li/L

5.42 4.2 cm

5.43 a. 0.031 cm
b. 0.79 cm
c. 1.1 cm

5.44 a. 88.7%
b. 44%
c. 7.25%

5.46 5,134 J/s
1,465 cal/s

5.47 0.022 per cm

5.48 2.62×10^{-5} μg/g

5.49 a. 0.21 MeV
b. 1.12 MeV

5.50 a. 0.144 MeV
b. 0.177 MeV

6.1 148 V
0.33 μC/kg per h

6.2 1.3 mR/h

6.3 0.083

6.4 0.0012°C

6.5 a. 0.03 mGy/h
b. 3.5 mGy/h

6.6 0.95 mGy/h

6.7 a. 1.04×10^{10}
b.

	mR/h	C/kg/h
incident	5.9×10^6	1.52
emergent	1.9×10^3	4.9×10^{-4}

incident : 5.7×10^4 mGy/h
emergent : 18 mGy/h

6.8 a. 6.6×10^5
b. 1.06×10^{-4} W/m^2
1.06×10^{-5} mW/cm^2

6.9 1.14 rads to body
461 rads to kidney

6.10 3.6 h

6.11 108 MBq

6.12 3.6 mrads/y

6.13 0.17 mGy/y

6.14 284 mGy/s

6.15 8.9 mGy

6.16 a. 0.77 Gy
b. 3.9×10^{-7} C

6.17 1.24×10^4 Gy
2.6×10^{18} ion pairs/g

6.18 3 mGy
4.6 mGy

6.19 a. $A = 1.8e^{-0.63t} + 2.2e^{-0.11t}$
b. 0.19 mGy,
0.26 mGy
c. 0.32 mGy

6.20 5.75×10^5 Gy/s

6.21 a. 4.2×10^{-6} W/kg
b. 1.1×10^{-6} W/kg

6.22 12.7 mGy/h, 0.14 mGy/h

6.23 0.1 mGy gamma
0.17 mGy neutrons

6.24 a. 0.046 mGy/h
b. 0.31 mGy

6.25 ^{197}Hg: 180 mrads
^{203}Hg: 389 mrads

6.26 a. 4.16 h
b. 5.84 mrads
58.4 μGy

6.27 a. 0.7 rad
b. 2.5 rads
c. 0.1 rad

6.28 22 Gy

6.29 0.0024°C/h

6.30 a. $A(t) = 555e^{-0.064t}$
b. 3.4×10^{-7} Gy

6.31 a. 3 h
b. 6 h
c. 4.33 h
d. 2.15 mrads

6.32 a. 7.5 days
b. 9.24% per day

6.33 6.5×10^9 phot/cm^2 /s

6.34 a. Liver: 0.022 Gy
Kidneys: 0.127 Gy
Rest of body: 0.0041 Gy
b. 0.438 Sv

9.1 a. 0.02
b. 0.38

9.2 a. 2.37, 1.32 cpm
b. 2.71 cpm
c. 30.0±4.5 cpm
30.0±7.0 cpm

9.3 75.0±6.9 cpm

9.4 a. 60.6±2.8 cpm
b. 4.65%

9.5 a. Yes
b. No

9.6 Yes

9.7 Impossible

9.8 a. 17.0±3.7 cpm
b. 11%

9.9 85 min.

9.10 a. 50±20 cpm
b. 50±8 cpm

9.11 a. 0.271
b. 0.09
c. 0.135

9.12 No

9.13 a. 0.056
b. 0.68
c. 0.16

9.14 a. 12 cpm
  b. 4.6 cpm
  c. 3.3 cpm
9.15 1.6 Bq
9.16 0.3, 0.23 cpm
9.17 Yes
9.18 13.1 mR/h
9.19 57 keV
9.20 305 mR/h
  $7.9 \times 10^3 \ \mu C/kg/h$
9.21 0.275 MeV
9.22 7.8×10^{-13} A
9.23 122 mR/h
9.24 a. 1×10^{10} ohms
  b. 2.5 s
  c. 11.5 s
9.25 40 V
9.26 a. 2×10^6 ohms
  b. 0.64 V
9.27 12.5%
9.28 2×10^{-5} V
9.29 3.95 cps
  per $n/cm^2/s$
9.30 5×10^{-5} A
9.31 892 y
9.32 6.4×10^{-16}
  A per n/cm^2 /s
  1.4×10^{-15}
  A per n/cm^2 /s
9.33 26.7 m
9.34 2000 n/cm^2 /s
9.35 132 cps
9.36 1%
9.37 0.0955 Gy
  9.55 rads
9.38 Not satisfactory
9.39 500±107
9.40 90±8%
9.41 3.84×10^4
9.42 10 min.
9.43 16.7 mR
9.44 600±70 cpm
9.45 a. 1.74 s
  b. 92 mR/h
10.1 a. 44 cm
  b. 0.08 m/cm^2 /s
  c. 0.014 mGy/h
    1.4 mrads/h
10.2 $^1/_4$ inch

10.3 N wall: 1/8 inch Pb
  W wall: 1 inch Pb
10.4 74 cm
10.5 0.32
10.6 a. 3.19 cm^2 /g
    33.2 cm^{-1}
  b. 0.097 cm
10.7 6 mm
10.8 71 cm = 28 in.
10.9 0.79 g/cm^2
10.10 1.6×10^3 MBq
10.11 4h 17 min.
10.12 5.7 cm
10.13 7 mR/h
10.14 1.4 mSv/h
10.15 24 μSv/h
10.16 13.5 cm
10.17 269 cm
10.18 3%
10.19 0.76 μCi/cm^3
10.20 a. ^{125}I: 9.45 mrem· m^2/h
    ^{198}Au: 24.8 mrem· m^2/h
    ^{24}Na: 99.4 mrem· m^2/h
  b. 12.9 cm Pb
10.21 1.1 cm polyethylene
  plus 5 cm Pb
10.22 .8 HVL
  9.4 cm
10.23 a. 1 TVL = 2,22 mm
  b. 1 HVL = 2/3 mm
  c. 1 TVL = 3.3 HVL
10.24 2.31 mm
10.25 0.16 mrem/h
10.26 1 h 25 min
10.27 264 mR/s
10.28 a.

$$2.7 \times 10^{-7} \times \frac{mrem/y}{\mu Ci/cm^2} = \frac{mSv/y}{Bq/m^2}$$

$$0.6 \times \frac{mrem/h}{dpm/100 \, cm^2} = \frac{Sv/h}{Bq/m^2}$$

b. $1.58 \times 10^{-8} \dfrac{Sv/y}{Bq/m^2}$

11.1 13 wk: 35 mGy
  1 y: 40 mGy
11.2 a. 6.4×10^3 rads
  b. 2.34 rads
11.3 52.5 rads
  0.02 rad

11.4 a. No
  b. 2.6×10^5 Bq
  c. 42.6 d
  d. 21.9 mSv
  e. 38.8 mSv
  f. 38.8 mSv
11.5 Yes
11.6 a. No
  b. 0.12 ppm, 50 ppm
11.7 a. 1.36, 2.71
  b. 1.00002
  c. 1.2 μCi/millimole
11.8 a. 1.8×10^7 Bq/s
  b. 3.1×10^3 m
11.9 a. thyroid: 1.4×10^{-10} Gy
  b. 3.6×10^{-11} Gy
  c. body: 2.5×10^{-13} Gy
  d. body: 5.3×10^{-14} Gy
11.10 58 μCi/week
11.11 7.1×10^5 Bq/m^3 @ 800 m
11.12 a. 8.26×10^{16} Bq
  b. 3.8×10^4 y
11.13 3.2×10^{-7} Sv
11.14 14.4 m^3/min.
11.15 a.

Nuclide	pCi/s	Bq/s
U	650	24.1
^{232}Th	1950	72.2
^{228}Ra	650	24.1
^{226}Ra	650	24.1

b.

Nuclide	pCi/m^3	Bq/m^3
U	4×10^{-5}	1.5×10^{-6}
^{232}Th	1.2×10^{-4}	4.5×10^{-6}
^{228}Ra	4×10^{-5}	1.5×10^{-6}
^{226}Ra	4×10^{-5}	1.5×10^{-6}

c. 2×10^{-8} Sv
  24.4%
  6.24×10^{-6} μCi/mL
  2.3×10^5 Bq/m^3
11.18 a. 0.13 DAC· h
  b. 0.33 mrem
    33 μSv
11.19 797 days
11.20 587 μCi
12.1 ^{24}Na: 92 Bq/L
  ^{36}Cl: 3.2×10^{-5} Bq/L
  ^{35}S: 0.47 Bq/L
  ^{38}Cl: 431 Bq/L

12.2

Nuclide	Bq/L	pCi/mL
^{24}Na	1200	32
^{36}Cl	3.2×10^{-3}	8.6×10^{-5}
^{35}S	46	1.2
^{38}Cl :	233	6.3

12.3   1 μGy/h

12.4   a. 75.4 Ci @ 1 h
        14.2 Ci @ 8 h
        0.46 Ci @ 7 d
        0.08 Ci @ 30 d

12.5   1000 Ci

12.6   <u>Dose rate, rads/h</u>

Δt	surface	@25 ft.
1 m	466	0.31
1 h	3.4	2.3×10^{-3}
1 d	0.076	5×10^{-5}
7 d	0.007	4.8×10^{-6}

12.7   3.72 Ci

12.8   a. 151.4 g/L
        b. 20.64 g/L

12.9   1.94 n/fission

12.10 a. 35.5 mGy
        b. 264 mGy

12.11 a. 1023 neutrons
        b. 279 generations

12.12 710 min. later

12.13 25 mGy gamma
        22.5 mGy neutrons

12.14 a. <u>element   barns</u>

O	2.8×10^{-4}
Si	0.171
Ca	0.430
Al	0.230
Na	0.525
Fe	2.56
K	2.1
H	0.332

        b. 0.011 cm^{-1}

12.15

Δt d	Bq $\times 10^{18}$	MCi
8	1.37	37.01
30	2.54	68.54
60	2.72	73.64
180	2.74	74.05

12.16 2.9×10^4 Ci
        1.1×10^{15} Bq

13.1   7.6 Sv/h

13.2   No

13.3   5.9 cpm

13.4   a. 58.5 MB·q
        27.4 μGy/h

13.5   555 tpm

13.6   1 Bq/m^3 per 3.6 Bq/L

13.7   2700 Bq @ 1 d
        450 Bq @ 10 d

13.8   a. 1.3 MBq
        b. 2.87 μGy
        c. 3.35 mGy
        d. 0.17 mSv

13.9   0.52±0.09 Bq/L

13.10 1.05±0.23 Bq/m^3
        (28.4±6.1) $\times 10^{-12}$ μCi/mL

13.11 1.58±0.34 mSv

13.12

H, Sv	
Lungs	Bone
a. 3.6×10^{-12}	8×10^{-11}
b. 6×10^{-14}	1.5×10^{-10}

13.13 b. log-normal
        c. CMD = 2.5 μm $\times /\div 2$
        SMD = 8.2 μm $\times /\div 2$
        MMD = 10.6 μm $\times /\div 2$

13.14 a. 6.5×10^4 Bq
        b. 0.4 Gy

13.15 2000 Bq

13.16 a. U(t) = $25.4e^{-0.017t}$
        b. 2.06×10^4 Bq
        c. 38 mGy

13.17 68 mSv

13.18 a. 787.5 Bq
        31 mSv

13.19 a. 19.9 Ci ^{60}Co
        155 Ci ^{137}Cs
        1950 Ci ^{144}Ce
        b. 9 rads/h
        c. 8100 rads/h

13.20 3×10^{-8} μCi/mL

13.21 a. 1.77×10^4 Bq/m^3
        b. 2.6 μGy
        c. 894 Bq/L

13.22 a. 130 kBq
        b. 2.9 mSv

13.23 2.7 L/m

13.24 76.2 L/m

13.25 0.078 dpm/100 cm^2

13.26 9×10^{-7} μCi/mL

13.27 a. (3.9±0.32) $\times$
        10^{-11} μCi/mL
        b. (3.9±0.6) $\times$
        10^{-11} μCi/mL

13.28 No exposure

13.29 a1. 1.33×10^4
        dpm/100 cm^2
        a2. 800 dpm
        b1. 0.12 μCi
        b2. 4.37×10^3

13.30 a. 2 μCi
        b. 50 mrems

13.31 a. 3.65×10^4 Bq
        b. 0.27 mSv

13.32 a. (2.42±0.37) $\times 10^{-8}$
        μCi/mL
        b. 914±140 Bq/m^3

13.33 a. 1.1×10^5 Bq/m^3
        b. 1 μg CrO

14.1 3×10^6

14.2   a. 2.79 mm
        b. 5 cm
        c. 509 mW/cm^2

14.3   a. 0.172 J/cm^2
        0.085 J/cm^2
        b. 7 m
        c. No

14.4   a. 5×10^{-4}
        b. 2×10^4 W
        c. 0.001 J

14.5   1.8 mW/cm^2

14.6   10.7 mW/cm^2

14.7   a. 5.1
        b. 8.3

14.8   a. 5.3
        b. 1.3
        c. 1.9

14.9   a. 6.1×10^{-3} s
        b. 6.5×10^{-5} J/cm^2
        c. 2.6×10^{-4} W/cm^2
        d. Class III

14.10 a. 10^{-4}
        b. 100 W

14.11 a. 1×10^{-3}
        b. 20,000 W

14.12 a. 88.8
        b. 19.5 dB

14.13 a. 122.8 V/m
        b. 0.325 A/m
        c. 0.133 pJ/cm^3

14.14 30 dB

14.15 0.27 A/m

14.16 a. 51 mW/cm^2
     b. 204
     c. 4 m
     d. 102 mW/cm^2
     e. 11.2 m

14.17 a. 500 mW/cm^2
     b. 2000 mW/cm^2
     c. 138 cm
     d. 0.5 mW/cm^2
     e. 358 cm

14.18 a. 1×10^{-3}
     b. 2000 W
     c. 42 dB
     d. 320 m

14.19 a. 1.2×10^{-3}
     b. 1.2×10^3 mW/cm^2
     c. 21 mW/cm^2
     d. Yes

14.20 Derivation

14.21 27 cm, 106 cm

14.22 fat: 60 cm
     muscle: 6.7 cm

14.23 29 dB

14.24 a. 24 m
     b. 22.4 mW/cm^2
     b. 80 m

14.25 0.11 mW/cm^2

14.26 175 mW/cm^2

14.27 12 s

14.28 a. 1×10^{-3}
     b. 2000 W
     c. 26 mW/cm^2
     c. Yes

14.29 No

14.30 1.4 mW/cm^2

14.31 a. 13 mW/cm^2
     b. 2.5 mW/cm^2
     c. No

14.32 4.6 eV

14.33 0.2 W

14.34 380 nm: 4.7×10^4 mJ/cm^2
     260 nm: 4.6 mJ/cm^2

14.35 No

14.36 a. 6.65×10^{-3} J/cm^2
     b. 1×10^{-3} radian
     c. 13.4 m

14.37 a. 3.2×10^{-7} J/cm^2
     b. 17.3 km

14.38 1.8 cm

14.39 a. 100 W/m^2
     b. 1.9 m

14.40 1963 W/pulse
     3.9×10^{-4} J/pulse

INDEX

Page numbers followed by "t" denote tables; those followed by "f" denote figures.